Nature's
MEDICINES

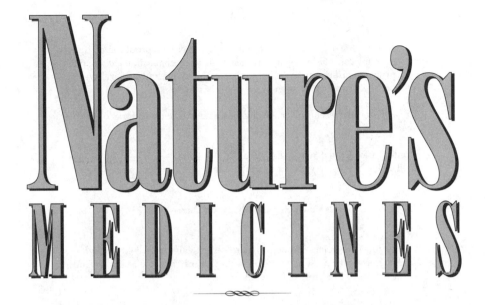

Nature's MEDICINES

From Asthma to Weight Gain,
From Colds to High Cholesterol—
The Most Powerful All-Natural Cures

By Gale Maleskey
and the Editors of
PREVENTION
Health Books

Medical Reviewer: Alan R. Gaby, M.D., past president
of the American Holistic Medical Association and professor of nutrition
at Bastyr University in Bothell, Washington

RODALE

Library of Congress Cataloging-in-Publication Data

Maleskey, Gale.
   Nature's medicines : from asthma to weight gain, from colds to high cholesterol—the most powerful all-natural cures / by Gale Maleskey and the editors of Prevention Health Books
       p.   cm.
   Includes index.
   ISBN-13 978–1–57954–028–9 hardcover
   ISBN-10 1–57954–028–7 hardcover
   1. Naturopathy.   I. Prevention Health Books.   II. Title.
RZ440.M34 1999
615.5'35—dc21   99–15694

Distributed to the trade by Holtzbrinck Publishers

14 16 18 20 19 17 15 13   hardcover

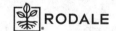 **RODALE**

WE **INSPIRE** AND **ENABLE** PEOPLE TO IMPROVE
THEIR LIVES AND THE WORLD AROUND THEM

FOR PRODUCTS & INFORMATION
WWW.RODALESTORE.COM
WWW.PREVENTION.COM

(800) 848-4735

About *Prevention* Health Books

The editors of *Prevention* Health Books are dedicated to providing you with authoritative, trustworthy, and innovative advice for a healthy, active lifestyle. In all of our books, our goal is to keep you thoroughly informed about the latest breakthroughs in natural healing, medical research, alternative health, herbs, nutrition, fitness, and weight loss. We cut through the confusion of today's conflicting health reports to deliver clear, concise, and definitive health information that you can trust. And we explain in practical terms what each new breakthrough means to you, so you can take immediate, practical steps to improve your health and well-being.

Every recommendation in *Prevention* Health Books is based upon interviews with highly qualified health authorities, including medical doctors and practitioners of alternative medicine. In addition, we consult with the *Prevention* Health Books Board of Advisors to ensure that all of the health information is safe, practical, and up-to-date. *Prevention* Health Books are thoroughly factchecked for accuracy, and we make every effort to verify recommendations, dosages, and cautions.

The advice in this book will help keep you well-informed about your personal choices in health care—to help you lead a happier, healthier, and longer life.

Notice

This book is intended as a reference volume only, not as a medical manual. The information given here is designed to help you make informed decisions about your health. It is not intended as a substitute for any treatment that may have been prescribed by your doctor. If you suspect that you have a medical problem, or if you are pregnant or nursing, we urge you to seek competent medical care.

The supplements in this book should not be given to children. Pregnant women should consult their doctors and use caution when taking supplements, as some may affect their health, cause miscarriage, or affect the health of the unborn child. If you are taking prescription medications or being treated for a chronic health condition, it is advisable to consult your doctor before taking supplements.

Nature's Medicines Staff

Senior Managing Editor: Edward Claflin

Writers: Gale Maleskey, with Julie Evans, Diane Gardiner Kozak, Nanci Kulig, Joely Johnson, James McCommons, Judith Springer Riddle

Art Director: Darlene Schneck

Interior and Cover Designer: Richard Kershner

Book Project Researcher: Christine Dreisbach

Editorial Researchers: Adrien Drozdowski, Jan Eickmeier, Carol J. Gilmore, Grete Haentjens, Jennifer L. Kaas, Mary Kittel, Terry Sutton Kravitz, Mary S. Mesaros, Deborah Pedron, Kathryn Piff, Paula Rasich, Staci Ann Sander, Teresa A. Yeykal, Nancy Zelko

Senior Copy Editor: Jane Sherman

Layout Designer: Pat Mast

Associate Studio Manager: Thomas P. Aczel

Manufacturing Coordinators: Brenda Miller, Jodi Schaffer, Patrick Smith

Rodale Healthy Living Books

VICE PRESIDENT AND PUBLISHER: Brian Carnahan

VICE PRESIDENT AND EDITORIAL DIRECTOR: Debora T. Yost

EDITORIAL DIRECTOR: Michael Ward

VICE PRESIDENT AND MARKETING DIRECTOR: Karen Arbegast

PRODUCT MARKETING MANAGER: Denyse Corelli

BOOK MANUFACTURING DIRECTOR: Helen Clogston

MANUFACTURING MANAGERS: Eileen F. Bauder, Mark Krahforst

RESEARCH MANAGER: Ann Gossy Yermish

COPY MANAGER: Lisa D. Andruscavage

PRODUCTION MANAGER: Robert V. Anderson Jr.

OFFICE MANAGER: Jacqueline Dornblaser

OFFICE STAFF: Julie Kehs, Suzanne Lynch, Mary Lou Stephen

Susan Olson, Ph.D. Clinical psychologist, transition therapist, and weight-management consultant in Seattle

Mary Lake Polan, M.D., Ph.D. Professor and chairman of the department of gynecology and obstetrics at Stanford University School of Medicine

David P. Rose, M.D., Ph.D., D.Sc. Chief of the division of nutrition and endocrinology at Naylor Dana Institute, part of the American Health Foundation, in Valhalla, New York, and an expert on nutrition and cancer for the National Cancer Institute and the American Cancer Society

Maria A. Fiatarone Singh, M.D. Scientist I in the nutrition, exercise physiology, and sarcopenia laboratory at the Jean Mayer USDA Human Nutrition Research Center on Aging at Tufts University in Boston, associate professor at Tufts University School of Nutrition Science and Policy in Medford, Massachusetts, and professor of exercise and sports science and medicine at the School of Health Sciences at the University of Sydney in Australia

Yvonne S. Thornton, M.D. Associate clinical professor of obstetrics and gynecology at Columbia University College of Physicians and Surgeons in New York City and director of the perinatal diagnostic testing center at Morristown Memorial Hospital in New Jersey

Lila Amdurska Wallis, M.D., M.A.C.P. Clinical professor of medicine at Weill Medical College of Cornell University in New York City, past president of the American Medical Women's Association, founding president of the National Council on Women's Health, director of continuing medical education programs for physicians, and Master and Laureate of the American College of Physicians

Andrew T. Weil, M.D. Director of the program in integrative medicine and clinical professor of internal medicine at the University of Arizona College of Medicine in Tucson

E. Douglas Whitehead, M.D. Associate clinical professor of urology at Albert Einstein College of Medicine in the Bronx, associate attending physician in urology at Beth Israel Medical Center, and co-founder and director of the Association for Male Sexual Dysfunction, both in New York City

Richard J. Wood, Ph.D. Laboratory chief of the mineral bioavailability laboratory at the Jean Mayer USDA Human Nutrition Research Center on Aging at Tufts University in Boston and associate professor at the Tufts University School of Nutrition Science and Policy in Medford, Massachusetts

Susan Zelitch Yanovski, M.D. Director of the obesity and eating disorders program in the division of digestive diseases and nutrition at the National Institute of Diabetes and Digestive and Kidney Diseases in Bethesda, Maryland

foreword

During my medical school training, I was dismayed to learn from my professors that "doctors don't cure disease; we merely help patients live with their illnesses."

It wasn't long before I found out how right they were. As I continued my studies, I discovered that most of the drugs we prescribed relieved symptoms but did not address the cause of the problem. Moreover, adverse side effects resulting from our therapies were far too common.

In the 20 years since I graduated from medical school, things have not gotten much better, just more expensive.

Modern medicine presents us with a paradox. On the one hand, new drugs and technological advances have enabled us to achieve better results than ever before in cases of severe infections, trauma, and surgical emergencies. In contrast to these exciting developments in acute-care medicine, the conventional treatment of most chronic diseases leaves a lot to be desired.

As I came to recognize these limitations, I began to investigate various alternatives, including the use of dietary modifications, nutritional supplements, and herbs. It soon became clear that the natural approach was safer, less expensive, and often more effective than the methods that were being taught in medical schools. Patients who had failed to respond to the best that modern medicine had to offer frequently had dramatic results with these "alternative" treatments.

I also discovered that many effective natural therapies had already been scientifically documented in medical journals, although most of these reports were not widely known in the conventional medical community.

During the past several years, there has been renewed interest in natural medicine and, at the same time, an explosion of research documenting the effectiveness of the alternative approach. Unfortunately, the average doctor still has little knowledge or understanding of how to use natural medicines, and even practitioners who emphasize nutrition and herbal therapies do not always agree about what works and what does not.

When it comes to using alternative medicine and unconventional therapy, many decisions are yours to make. Of course, you want to make informed choices, particularly when those choices affect your own health and that of your family. You need up-to-date and reliable sources of information. This book is such a resource, with comprehensive information about more than 95 vitamins, minerals, herbs, and other natural supplements that are in common use.

In this book, Gale Maleskey and the editors of *Prevention* Health Books—along with a team of 15 researchers—have done an admirable job of reviewing important research and interviewing innovative practitioners in order to provide you with an extensive and reliable overview of natural therapies.

The first part of the book provides detailed descriptions of the scores of supplements that are available to you today. The benefits of each of these remedies is discussed, and appropriate precautions are provided concerning possible interactions and side effects. The second part reviews more than 75 common medical conditions and describes exactly how natural therapies may be helpful.

As new research is published and as the conventional medical community becomes more open to the potential of natural medicine, many of the remedies described here will become standard practice in the new millennium. Others may fall by the wayside if additional studies fail to confirm the initial impressions of forward-looking researchers, practitioners, and medical professionals.

In this book, you'll discover which remedies are scientifically documented and which require additional study. Much of the information presented here is supported by solid scientific research that has been published in medical journals. In addition, you'll find recommendations that are based primarily on the clinical experience, opinions, or theories of the doctors and health practitioners who were interviewed for the book. It's a responsible overview of an exciting, promising, and still-controversial field of health care.

Alan R. Gaby, M.D.
Professor of nutrition
Bastyr University, Bothell, Washington

contents

3: *Fighting Disease with Supplements*

introduction

health rewards from mother nature

Sometimes, the keys to good health come in very small packages.

Many of those packages are sitting, right now, on the shelves of your nearest drugstore, supermarket, or health food store. That's where you'll find supplements that scientists, nutritionists, and doctors have distilled from nature's storehouse of healing remedies.

Some of these supplements—truly, nature's medicines—are derived from fruits and vegetables. Others come from minerals—yes, the same minerals that make up stone and soil. Still others are highly concentrated versions of many herbs that have been used for centuries in healing teas, tinctures, and tonics.

Alongside the nutritional and herbal supplements, however, you'll also find substances so unusual that they almost seem bizarre—from bee pollen and brewer's yeast to shark cartilage and fish oil. Even some living, beneficial organisms have their place among nature's medicines.

Faced with so many choices, how do you know which of these natural supplements are right for you?

That's where this book comes in.

In *Nature's Medicines,* you'll find out exactly how and when to take these supplements to improve and maintain your health. You'll discover how they can protect you from disease, keep your immune system powered up, and help you maintain sturdy, strong bones. Some will free you from aches and pains; others can help relieve heartburn or indigestion. Nature's medicines can even help your blood carry all of the necessary nutrients to your greedy cells.

The benefits don't stop there. In these pages, you'll discover how to keep your skin healthy and flexible and free of itching, rashes, and infections. You'll learn how to restore worn-out tissue, fight cancer, and help your liver, kidneys, and bladder do the cleanup chores that they're supposed to do. You'll find out which supplements can help keep your heart trust-worthy, your arteries clean, and your lungs clear.

In this book, you have a complete, authoritative guide to the most ef-fective supplements that are currently available. You'll find specific, sound advice from many experts, including medical doctors, researchers, and a wide range of naturopaths, herbalists, and other practitioners of alternative medicine.

Look in part 1 to learn how nature's medicines were first discovered and how to choose among the many vitamins, minerals, herbs, and other supplements that are available today. Then turn to part 2 for an A-to-Z guide to the healing power of the world's most effective natural medicines. In part 3, you can look up your specific health concerns: There you'll find out which of the powerful healing supplements can help protect you or speed your recovery from disease.

There are many ways to use this wealth of information. Want the most up-to-date and reliable evidence about leading supplements? You'll find that in parts 1 and 2. Want to know which remedies are most highly recom-mended by leading experts for specific health concerns? Turn to part 3 for authoritative answers, plus advice on appropriate dosages.

On every page, you'll learn how nature's medicines go hand in hand with other health measures such as a nutritious diet and stress-relieving, im-munity-boosting exercise. By combining these strategies, you can provide the best all-around health care for yourself and your family.

At the same time, however, it's important to know which of nature's medicines might not be appropriate. Before taking any supplement, you should note the cautions that are described in the "Supplement Snapshots" in part 2. If you are pregnant, nursing, or have a chronic illness, be sure to consult a medical doctor or other qualified health-care practitioner before using any of the supplements described in this book. If you are taking pre-scription medication or treatments, always talk to your doctor about pos-sible interactions or side effects before taking supplements. Also, do not give these supplements to children.

1

what you
need to know
about
supplements

vitamins and minerals

essential ingredients for a healthy body

Hippocrates got it right in one sentence: "Let food be thy medicine."

It took an additional 2,000 years of observation, plus a century of modern scientific research to find out why food has the healing powers that Hippocrates ascribed to it—and the details are still being worked out.

Take vitamins, for instance. Ancient Greek and Egyptian physicians prescribed "liver juice" for night blindness. They had no way of knowing that their prescription contained a remarkable amount of vitamin A. It wasn't until 1930, in fact, that Swiss researchers determined the chemical structure of vitamin A and its precursor, beta-carotene. We now know that people who don't get enough vitamin A can experience night blindness, an early symptom of deficiency.

The discovery of vitamin C followed a parallel route. By 1601, some astute observers had noted that consuming citrus fruits prevented scurvy, a disease that wiped out countless crews of sailors who lived on salted meat and dried biscuits while at sea. It took two more centuries before British navy ships were required to carry rations of lime or lemon juice, and even then, the advocates of this practice had no idea why these tart fruits should help prevent the dreaded sailors' disease. It wasn't until more than 100 years later that vitamin C was finally isolated.

As vitamin C revealed the power of vitamins, iron was the telltale clue to the potential of minerals. "Metals of heaven"—iron-rich meteorites—were used therapeutically by the ancient civilizations of the eastern Mediterranean. The oldest surviving manuscript, the *Ebers Papyrus*, details two iron-rich remedies. In 1932, iron deficiency was officially recognized as the cause of chlorosis, a type of anemia found in teenage girls, and we were also well into the twentieth century before scientists proved that iron is a component of hemoglobin, a protein in red blood cells. Now, it's universally recognized that we all need iron to help rebuild blood.

What Makes a Mighty Multi?

Scan the supplement shelves of your local pharmacy, and you're likely to see a multitude of multivitamin/mineral supplements. Obviously, each contains a wide variety of vitamins and minerals, and if you carefully compare labels, you'll find that some brands have a little more of this, while others have a little more of that. Beyond shaking the bottles, checking the prices, and comparing labels, how should you look for a multi?

No matter what the state of your health, it's smart to take a supplement that contains 100 percent of the Daily Value (DV) for most essential vitamins and minerals. The trouble is, none of the multis contains 100 percent of what you need. If you eat a healthful diet, you'll get many of the vitamins and minerals that you'll find in a multi, but many diets come up short on the following nutrients, experts say. You can get them by taking a multi along with a few individual supplements. Here are the suggested amounts.

Daily Multivitamin/Mineral Supplement

- Vitamin A/beta-carotene: 5,000 international units (mixed carotenoids)
- Vitamin B_6: 2 milligrams
- Vitamin D: 400 international units
- Folic acid: 400 micrograms

Small Stuff, Big Action

The scientific definition of a vitamin is "an organic compound, not a lipid or amino acid, required in very small amounts for essential functions in the body." Anything that's organic—from mulch and tree trunks to toenails and earlobes—contains the element carbon, the same element that's found in every vitamin. Lipids (fats) and amino acids are also organic, but they are not vitamins.

The customary means of getting vitamins into our bodies is to eat plants or animals that make or store these compounds. Plants use sunlight, air, water, and nutrients from the soil to synthesize folate in their leaves. Some plants and animals make their own vitamin C. Vitamins can also be synthesized from organic compounds in a laboratory. Thus, when you buy a vitamin supplement, you might be getting compounds that have been put

- Chromium: 200 micrograms
- Copper: 2 milligrams
- Magnesium: 100 milligrams
- Selenium: At least 100 micrograms
- Zinc: 15 milligrams

As for iron, unless you have iron-deficiency anemia, look for a supplement that doesn't include it. You probably don't need extra iron, and studies have linked high iron levels with increased risk of heart attack and atherosclerosis (hardening of the arteries). Some premenopausal women, however, may need extra iron to compensate for menstrual blood loss.

Additional Supplements

You won't find the optimal dose of the following nutrients in most multi, so buy these supplements separately.

- Vitamin C: 250-milligram tablets. The optimal dose is 500 milligrams a day, but you'll absorb more if you take two doses spaced 12 hours apart.
- Vitamin E: 100 to 400 international units (mixed tocopherols) once a day.
- Calcium: 500 to 1,000 milligrams once a day.

together by plants and animals, or you might be getting identical, look-alike compounds that have been assembled in a laboratory.

Minerals are inorganic, but these, too, are available from organic sources. Plants absorb minerals from the ground, and animals get them from the plants they eat, so the root source of all minerals is the Earth.

By definition, anything officially labeled a "vitamin" is in some way absolutely necessary to human health. "If a substance found in food has a defined biochemical function in the human body, it is considered essential," says Forrest Nielsen, Ph.D., director of the U.S. Department of Agriculture (USDA) Human Nutrition Research Center in Grand Forks, North Dakota. It may take many years of research, however, before scientists know whether a component is essential, he adds.

Essential nutrients may be parts of hormones. The trace mineral iodine,

Where Phytos Finish in the Nutrient Race

When it comes to stocking your body with nutrients, the essentials are just that—essential. They include protein, carbohydrates, fats, vitamins, minerals, and water.

Then there are the phytonutrients. *Phyto* means "plant," so phytonutrients are simply nutrients derived from plants. Phytonutrients may promote good health, but unlike vitamins, they have not been found to be essential, says Cyndi Thomson, R.D., Ph.D., clinical nutrition research specialist at the University of Arizona Cancer Prevention Center in Tucson.

Then where does that leave our green vegetables? Weren't we all told to eat our peas and broccoli or we'd wither and fade away?

Despite what you were told, or even what you told your kids, "you will not die if you do not eat broccoli—but you may not be as healthy, either," Dr. Thomson says. In fact, there's only one class of phytonutrients, the carotenoids, that has been shown to have vitamin activity. The beta-carotene that you get from carrots and some other fruits and vegetables is changed by your body into different compounds, one of which is much-needed vitamin A.

So, even though you can survive without vegetables, you do need them. While it's true that some phytonutrients are available as nutritional supplements, no matter how "complete" the supplements are, they're bound to leave out many of the phytos that are found in fruits and vegetables. Not only that, but the mixture of these nutrients that you get naturally from carrots, blueberries, broccoli, and other plant foods provides some benefits that generally can't be duplicated by a laboratory-produced pill.

You're better off supplementing your diet with a wide range of fresh fruits and vegetables. Especially good sources of the phytonutrients that will help you thrive are berries, garlic, dark leafy greens, deep yellow and orange fruits and vegetables, grape juice, tomatoes, and, yes, broccoli.

for instance, is needed to manufacture thyroxine, the thyroid gland's major hormone. Nutrients may also be needed to break down food for energy, as many of the B vitamins are.

Nutrients can also break down wastes that are subsequently eliminated from the body. The trace mineral manganese serves this role, converting the toxic ammonia that we form in our bodies into urea, which is excreted in urine.

Some nutrients appear to be essential even though their biochemical functions have yet to be defined, Dr. Nielsen says. Chromium, nickel, and boron are examples. Arsenic, a substance that we label as poison, is one of the possibly essential nutrients under investigation, since we don't know why our bodies need it.

It's likely that more nutrients will make the "essential" list as research continues. "There are a lot of gray areas left to explore," says Gerald Combs Jr., Ph.D., professor of nutrition at Cornell University in Ithaca, New York. He cites omega-3 fatty acids and the amino acid carnitine as two examples. "Now we realize that omega-3 fatty acids are required for neurological development and eye development in infants," says Dr. Combs. "Some experts also think that carnitine may be required for infants under some circumstances."

As we develop better technology, we can scrutinize the additional properties of vitamins and minerals even more closely, Dr. Combs adds. "We can measure things we couldn't even conceive of earlier." Within the last four decades, for example, the ability to measure zinc has improved tremendously. "Twenty-five years ago, we thought there were five or six zinc-containing enzymes because that's all we could measure," Dr. Combs observes. "Now we know there are two or three hundred, simply because we can detect tinier and tinier amounts."

Getting Your DVs

Although each of us has somewhat different needs for vitamins and minerals, we all need a certain basic supply of nutrients. Based on research, experts have drawn up a set of nutrition guidelines that are universally used as a standard of measurement by the federal government. The nutrition information that you'll find on any packaged food—and on most bottles of vitamins and minerals—is based on those guidelines.

Wherever you see the abbreviation DV, it stands for Daily Value. The DV column on a label lists the percentages of the DV for vitamins or minerals in a serving of a food or in a single dose of a supplement, based on an intake of 2,000 calories a day. The DV for vitamin C, for instance, is 60 milligrams, so a supplement containing 60 milligrams has 100 percent of the

DV. The label of a supplement containing 30 milligrams of vitamin C would indicate that it has 50 percent of the DV.

Since each of us has different needs, your vitamin C requirement might be higher than the DV if you're older, if your immune system needs some boosting, or if you're recovering from an infection. Smokers, for instance, have an enhanced risk of many kinds of diseases, so the recommended dose for them is 100 milligrams, more than 160 percent of the DV that applies to most nonsmokers.

Age differences, sex differences, and stage of life can also affect your nutrient needs, meaning that your actual daily requirements for vitamins and minerals may vary from the DV for many reasons. For both men and women, vitamin and mineral requirements are likely to change somewhat with age, and very active or athletic people are likely to need more than those who are less active. All of these factors have an impact on individual nutrient requirements.

Some of these differences are readily apparent. Consider the needs of infants. Per pound of body weight, nutrient needs are highest when an infant is growing rapidly, as it does during the first year of life, says Kathryn Kolasa, Ph.D., professor of nutrition education at East Carolina University School of Medicine in Greenville, North Carolina. Nutrient needs are also high during teenage growth spurts, usually from ages 12 to 20 for boys and 10 to 18 for girls.

A Little Something Extra

To help us get our DVs of vitamins and minerals as well as meet other basic nutritional requirements, nutrients are routinely added to foods that many of us eat nearly every day. When this is done, the foods are called fortified or enriched. This program, regulated by the federal government, has been highly successful in helping to eliminate severe nutritional deficiencies.

In the United States, iodine has been added to salt since 1930. Before then, in areas where people had little or no iodine in their food supplies, it was fairly common to see the medical condition called goiter. An enlargement of the thyroid gland, goiter is a direct result of iodine deficiency, says Paul Lachance, Ph.D., professor and executive director of the Nutraceutical Institute at Rutgers University in New Brunswick, New Jersey.

Slightly less than ½ teaspoon of iodized salt a day provides enough iodine to prevent goiter. Non-iodized salt, such as kosher salt, is still available, but manufacturers are required by law to offer the iodized version as well. People are so used to buying iodized salt that goiter problems have been virtually eliminated.

Vitamin D is another cause célèbre of the government's nutrition program. Since the 1940s, vitamin D has routinely been added to milk to help prevent childhood rickets, a disease that causes bones to become deformed or soften. This fortification program helped make childhood rickets virtually unknown in the United States, Dr. Lachance says.

In a quart of fortified milk, you're supposed to get 400 international units (IU) of vitamin D, which is the DV. Not all milk contains this amount, and fat-free milk seems to be skimpiest, according to a study from researchers at Boston University. Sadly, vitamin D deficiencies are still prevalent in middle-aged and older adults, leading to problems that result in the softening of the skeleton (osteomalacia) or loss of bone (osteoporosis). Still, the vast majority of young Americans are getting enough vitamin D from milk and other sources to ensure that they aren't at risk for childhood rickets.

Vitamin A is also added to milk, particularly reduced-fat, low-fat, and fat-free milk. In the 1940s, when this vitamin was found to improve immune response and correct some vision problems in children and women, the government began requiring that it be added. Whole milk naturally contains some vitamin A—about one-third of the DV in a quart—but extra vitamin A is sometimes added. Most powdered milk contains vitamin A, along with vitamin D.

Since 1942, white flour, cornmeal, and polished (white) rice have been enriched with three B-complex vitamins—thiamin, riboflavin, and niacin—and with iron. In 1998, folic acid was added to the list of required fortifications. Whole wheat flour is not enriched because it naturally contains these and other nutrients.

Even with this fortification program, we can't take all of these nutrients for granted, Dr. Lachance says. While fortification has made serious deficiencies much less likely to develop, iron deficiency is still the most common in the United States, he says. It's also possible that you're not getting enough vitamin A or D if you don't drink much milk. In fact, people consuming adequate vitamin D through milk can still be vitamin D deficient during the winter months.

Deficiency Detection

When someone is deficient in an essential nutrient, some symptoms are sure to crop up after a while. Health problems ensue. Fatigue, muscle weakness, irritability, reduced resistance to infection, poor healing, and slowed growth, are common to many vitamin and mineral deficiencies.

Despite these well-known signs, the detective work isn't easy. Anemia, for example, is a condition that's characterized by many of the symptoms of overall nutrient deficiencies—particularly fatigue and muscle weakness. It occurs when there's a reduction in the number of red blood cells, but there are many possible causes of that reduction. In some people, anemia is caused by iron deficiency. Others may display symptoms of other kinds of anemia because they're short on vitamins A, B_6, B_{12}, C, and E, folate, riboflavin, or copper. Sometimes looking at red blood cells (or bone marrow cells, where red blood cells originate) under a microscope gives a clue to what type of anemia it is.

In other cases, initial symptoms are more distinct or tend to show up first in a certain area of the body. If a wound takes longer than usual to stop bleeding, for instance, that slow clotting time might indicate a vitamin K deficiency, or someone may develop poor night vision, a tip-off for vitamin A deficiency. These days, a suspected vitamin or mineral deficiency can usually be confirmed with tests that measure blood levels of the nutrient or that test a particular enzyme or cell function associated with the nutrient, Dr. Nielsen says.

There are some nutrients that we can take for granted, however. We get lots of them every day in our diets. These include sodium, phosphorus, sulfur, and chloride.

Adequate versus Optimal

Over the years, as researchers have explored the effects of different amounts of vitamins and minerals, a new approach has emerged. In the past, they tried to determine the minimum necessary amounts of nutrients that were needed to prevent deficiencies and thereby prevent the health problems caused by deficiencies. Today, scientists are paying greater attention to the amounts of nutrients needed for *optimal* nutrition.

"We're asking different questions than we used to," Dr. Combs says. "For the last hundred years, since the first vitamin, thiamin, was discovered, the questions have been 'Do you need this vitamin? Will it keep you alive?

Will it prevent a deficiency disease, such as scurvy or beriberi?' Now that those diseases are pretty much gone from our society, we are looking at other health problems related to diet."

Among the leading problems related to nutrition, Dr. Combs points out, are cancer, heart disease, and certain kinds of diabetes. "Thus, we are asking different questions to determine whether there may be benefits at higher levels," he says.

Vitamin E, for example, is currently being studied for its apparent ability to help prevent heart disease. "In population studies, groups taking vitamin E supplements clearly had a lower risk of heart disease," Dr. Combs says. "However, these people possibly had other healthier behaviors than those who didn't take supplements, so it still needs to be determined if this big reduction in heart disease can indeed be directly attributed to vitamin E." Research continues to find out how much prevention vitamin E does offer to those who are at risk for heart attack.

Supplement-Making Made Simple

How are vitamin and mineral supplements made, tested, packaged, and sold? How do you know if you're getting what the label says?

Vitamins, whether synthetic or "natural," are processed in huge, modern plants. There are only about six large companies worldwide that produce most vitamins so that hundreds of companies can purchase them as ingredients for vitamin pills.

Each vitamin is produced by a unique series of steps. Vitamin C, for instance, can be made from natural-source dextrose, a type of sugar. The process involves nine steps. Technically complex, those steps mimic the way animals manufacture the vitamin in their bodies.

Vitamin B_{12}, another vitamin in high demand, requires the use of a particular kind of bacteria that can break down sugar into alcohol. It's no coincidence that the French, who are famous wine producers, are also the world's leading producers of vitamin B_{12}.

Making vitamin E, on the other hand, is a much different process. This vitamin is oil-soluble, which means that it's dissolved and carried in a medium of vegetable oil. The natural-source vitamin E must be isolated from soybean oil, while the synthetic form is synthesized by a chemical process.

Once isolated, each vitamin can be run through a series of chemical analyses to make sure that it is pure and has the right chemical structure.

Sustenance from Sunbeams— And Other Sources

Most of our nutrients come from food, but there are notable exceptions.

Given enough exposure to the sun's ultraviolet rays, our bodies convert one kind of fat in the skin to vitamin D. Sunlight has traditionally been considered health-reviving for that reason.

Getting adequate vitamin D helps prevent crippling bone deformities like rickets, which began to appear more than 200 years ago as northern European countries became industrialized. With more people living in cities and more cities darkened by the overhang of smoke from industrial production, sunlight was fighting a losing battle with manmade interferences.

A Polish doctor named Sniadecki first made the connection between the need for sunlight and the bone diseases that appeared like a slow-moving epidemic in these industrialized areas. He advised parents to take their rickets-ridden children into the country, or at least carry them into the sunlight as often as possible. He had no idea what healing power was in the rays, but whatever it was, he surmised, these children needed it.

There are also instances in which lifestyle does the doctoring. In countries such as India, people who are strict vegetarians suffer from shortages of vitamin B_{12} in their diets. Some of the lack is made up from an unusual source—bacteria in food. Unappetizing as it seems, certain bacteria synthe-

Manufacturers of any vitamin made in the United States or imported for use do these appraisals voluntarily.

All vitamins sold in the United States must meet the quality standards set by the U.S. Pharmacopeia (USP), a scientific, standard-setting organization for the drug industry. Even if the vitamins are made in China, for example, they have to meet USP standards to be sold here, says Frank Girardi, director of market services at Roche Vitamins in Parsippany, New Jersey.

Minerals are a different story. Unlike most vitamins, minerals are obtained from natural sources. Often, that means mining. Sent to manufacturing laboratories, the minerals go through a purification process. Finally, they're usually combined with some other ingredient to make them stable, nontoxic, and more absorbable.

Sabinsa, for example, a company in Piscataway, New Jersey, makes a product called selenomethionine. At the heart of that supplement is the minsize vitamin B_{12}. Our bodies need only a tiny amount of this vitamin, and bacteria make enough to compensate.

Some forms of yeast, which is actually a living fungus, also synthesize B_{12}. Since this is especially true of brewer's yeast, a strict vegetarian who drinks beer may have a ready source of this vitamin, says Gerald Combs Jr., Ph.D., professor of nutrition at Cornell University in Ithaca, New York. (Of course, the average beer contains only 0.06 microgram of B_{12}, so even if vegetarians have an occasional cold one, they must take supplements to get the Daily Value of 6 micrograms.)

Extra minerals can also be obtained in some unusual ways. Take iron, for instance. The iron in cast-iron pots or skillets is actually transferred to food when we cook with those utensils. Although the transfer might seem insignificant, it can increase the iron content of foods by two to six times.

The skins of fruits and vegetables, especially root vegetables like carrots and potatoes, are also good mineral "supplements" because trace minerals are concentrated in the pores of the skins. True, you need to wash these foods before eating them to remove unwanted bacteria and pesticides, but you'll still get some minerals once you start munching.

eral selenium. Sabinsa buys selenium from producers around the world and purifies it. Then the manufacturer uses a chemical process to bond the pure selenium with methionine, an amino acid. The purpose of this process is to make selenium more available to the body.

Many companies worldwide prepare minerals for use in multivitamin/mineral supplements. Most handle only one or two types of minerals, though, so a supplement manufacturer that offers many kinds of minerals may purchase them from a wide range of suppliers.

Mineral product manufacturers also use the USP standards of testing. Since the companies that do the formulations are buying batches of vitamins and minerals from hundreds of different suppliers around the world, testing is important. An incoming batch that was previously tested is tested again upon arrival at the manufacturer to make sure that it meets certain specifications.

Keep or Toss?

Vitamins can be an investment—and the best way to protect that investment is to store supplements in a cool, dry place.

But what's considered a cool, dry place?

The bathroom's out because the steamy shower jacks up the humidity, and the cupboard above the stove is out because it gets hot up there. You have a lot of other choices, though.

"Keep them in a spot that's not exposed to direct sunlight, excess humidity, or heat," says V. Srini Srinivasan, Ph.D., senior scientist with the U.S. Pharmacopeia, a private standard-setting organization for the drug industry. For most people, a kitchen cupboard fits that bill, as long as it's well away from the stove.

To find out how long a supplement is likely to remain effective, check the expiration date on the bottle before you buy it. The label might carry a code such as 010108, which simply means that the expiration date is January 1, 2008. An expiration date may be two to four years from the date of manufacture, depending on the nutrient.

Experts say it's best not to buy or use expired supplements because of reduced potency. As long as a product is properly stored, though, it's guaranteed to meet the potency listed on the label up to the expiration date. After that, the product begins to degrade, and its potency slowly drops.

You'll lengthen the life of your supplements if you store them in the refrigerator or freezer. If you do, though, don't leave the cap off after you take them, since moisture will condense inside the bottle. Recap the bottle quickly and return it to the refrigerator or freezer.

Some additional tips: Always keep bottles tightly closed, and don't leave supplements inside a hot car. It's also important to keep them out of the reach of children: Even though they're not as poisonous as many household products, an overdose can be dangerous or even fatal. Discard any product that begins to look or smell strange. It might have become contaminated by mold, bacteria, or other harmful organisms.

The first step is to "culture" the batch to see if any unwanted bacteria or yeast starts to grow. After that, individual ingredients are weighed out, mixed together, sampled and tested again, and put into tablets or capsules. Finally, they are bottled and placed on store shelves.

Natural versus Synthetic

Looking at this vast and profitable manufacturing process, you may begin to wonder whether the selected, purified nutrients that end up in supplements are really very natural at all.

Of course, food is the most obvious natural source of vitamins, and the Earth is the most natural source of minerals, but the vitamins and minerals in supplements are several times removed from their original sources. While some manufacturers isolate vitamin E from soybean oil and derive vitamin C from acerola berries, supplemental vitamins aren't often made that way these days.

Although some people think "natural" means "better," there's a practical reason for synthetic vitamins: The laboratory process is much more efficient and less expensive than isolating these nutrients from foods. Also keep in mind that even vitamins labeled "natural" undergo several steps in processing before they arrive in the final product form.

In some cases, the chemical structure of so-called synthetic vitamins is slightly different from what's found in nature, but manufacturers can change concentrations or quantities to compensate for the differences. Natural vitamin E, for example, is better retained by the body than the synthetic form, but manufacturers can make up for this by adding more synthetic vitamin E to capsules. Thus, although natural E may offer some added protection, the synthetic product is processed to ultimately have the same strength.

In other cases, the synthetic form of a vitamin may be better than the natural form. Some research indicates that synthetic folic acid—in the form of supplements or in fortified foods such as cereals—is often better absorbed than the natural folate found in many leafy green vegetables. Biotin and niacin show similar characteristics: In both cases, the synthetic vitamins are absorbed better than the natural forms in many foods.

With minerals, the question of natural versus synthetic never comes up. Since minerals are elements, they can only be purified—not created—in the lab. If they aren't mined from the ground, they're separated from other natural sources. Calcium, for instance, is derived from limestone, oyster shells, eggshells, or naturally occurring beds of calcium carbonate.

What is synthetic in the case of minerals is the combination that makes them less toxic and easier for our bodies to absorb. Chromium picolinate, for instance, is a patented form of chromium that's been combined with picolinic acid. In this form, the metal chromium is easier to absorb, Dr. Nielsen says.

Do Dinosaurs Have What You Need?

If you have youngsters, it's possible that you have some vitamins around that are grape-flavored and resemble prehistoric cartoon characters. Dinosaur-shaped vitamins are fine for the kids, but will they do you any good?

It's perfectly okay to take one or two each day, says Cathy Kapica, R.D., Ph.D., assistant professor of nutrition and clinical dietetics at Finch University of Health Sciences/The Chicago Medical School in North Chicago. In fact, "if you have trouble swallowing, chewable vitamins are a reasonable way to supplement," she says. Liquid vitamins are also available, she notes.

Most chewables will not provide adequate nutrition for an adult. You'll want to read labels to compare what you get in a children's vitamin to what you'd get in an adult multivitamin. This will vary by brand. If you're looking for high amounts of antioxidant nutrients, for instance, you won't find them in dinosaur-shaped, multicolored chewables. Even if you have a dinosaur as a supplement appetizer now and then, you're better off with adult-size supplements for adult-size doses, Dr. Kapica advises. Some brands even have chewables for grown-ups.

Meeting Special Needs

In the "Supplement Snapshots" in part 2 of this book, you'll find the DV listed for each of the vitamins and minerals discussed. Keep in mind, though, that as we've mentioned, your specific needs may exceed the DV, depending on your sex, age, and various health factors.

Pregnant women need twice as much iron as nonpregnant women, and their requirements for vitamin D and folic acid are more than double. Expectant mothers also need much more vitamin C and E and all of the B vitamins. Among minerals, extra calcium is critical for pregnant women, and more zinc and magnesium are also required.

If a woman nurses her baby, requirements for some nutrients during the first six months of nursing soar even higher than the levels required during pregnancy, Dr. Kolasa says. This is true for vitamins A, C, and E and most of the B vitamins, along with magnesium, zinc, and selenium. "That's why women are advised to continue taking their prenatal vitamins until they wean their babies," she says.

Women also have an increased need for iron during their childbearing years because they normally lose iron every month during menstruation. If you're a woman whose menstrual flow is heavy and you often feel tired, you should probably see your doctor about an iron supplement, says Dr. Kolasa.

The iron requirements for men are generally less than those for women because men normally have larger iron stores. Men don't lose much iron unless they have chronic internal bleeding, such as from a bleeding ulcer. Since high iron stores have been associated with an increased risk for conditions such as heart disease and cancer, men are usually advised not to take supplemental iron unless they have been tested for deficiency and advised by a doctor, Dr. Kolasa says.

The need for some nutrients, such as the B vitamins, which are used to help metabolize food, are based on calorie intake. These nutrient requirements are higher for men, who usually eat more calories each day, than for women. The differences are slight, however.

Calcium is often singled out as a nutrient that's needed more by women in menopause than by premenopausal women, but men also need it, Dr. Kolasa points out. "Men get osteoporosis, too," she says.

Upping Your Supplements as You Age

Research by the Food and Drug Administration shows that we need a higher maintenance dose of certain nutrients as we age, says Robert Russell, M.D., associate director of the Jean Mayer USDA Human Nutrition Research Center on Aging at Tufts University in Boston.

"It's simple," Dr. Russell says. "Older people are eating less food. They are less active." Since we have more sedentary lifestyles when we're older, we're likely to eat less—and that means that we probably don't get enough nutrients.

Contrary to popular belief, Dr. Russell says, most older people can absorb most nutrients just as well as younger people. In fact, their absorption of vitamin A appears to go up, which means that they have to be careful not to overdo it with this potentially toxic nutrient.

There are exceptions. Absorption of one form of vitamin B_{12} can be a

Safety with Supplements

Like prescription and over-the-counter drugs, any kind of supplement needs to be taken responsibly, says Mark Stengler, N.D., a naturopathic doctor and author of *The Natural Physician: Your Health Guide for Common Ailments*. Before you start taking any supplements that are new to you, heed the following suggestions from Dr. Stengler.

• To avoid or minimize any side effects, start with a lower dosage than the one stated on the label, then gradually increase the dosage until you reach recommended levels.

• Consult a knowledgeable physician or health practitioner before using any new supplements. Certain vitamins, herbs, and emerging dietary supplements can be toxic in higher doses.

• If you are pregnant or nursing, avoid all supplements unless they have been prescribed or approved by your doctor. Also, check with your physician before using supplements if you are taking prescription medication. People who are taking anticoagulant (blood-thinning) medications, for example, should not take high doses of vitamin E, sweet clover, or a number of other supplements that thin the blood.

problem for up to one-third of older people. They don't need larger amounts of it, but they need to take it in the form that their bodies can use, says Dr. Russell. That form can be found in fortified food products or in supplements, which is why a lot of senior multi formulas have it.

Older people also have trouble with vitamin D. "Their skin doesn't manufacture it as well as it did when they were younger, so they need to get more from foods or supplements," Dr. Russell says. He recommends 400 IU of vitamin D a day for people ages 50 to 70 and 600 IU for people who are over 70.

Riboflavin, too, can be a problem for older people, Dr. Russell notes. Since many seniors have smaller appetites, they often get less riboflavin than they should in their diets. To adjust the balance, you'd have to consume several servings of dairy products each day, he says. He recommends at least 1.3 milligrams of riboflavin a day for men age 50-plus and at least 1.1 milligrams for women.

Vitamin B_6 requirements also seem to be higher among seniors. About

one-third of older people show signs of deficiency, Dr. Russell says. He recommends that men 50 and older get 1.7 milligrams and women take 1.5
milligrams.

Older people might also benefit from getting more than the DV of thiamin, especially if they drink alcohol, Dr. Russell says. In one study, when
women who got an average of less than 1 milligram a day of thiamin were
given supplements of 10 milligrams a day, they reported sleeping better
and having better appetites. They also reported that they felt more
cheerful.

Studies also indicate that it might be helpful for older people to get
more of the antioxidant nutrients—vitamins C and E and selenium. In research done at Tufts University, a study showed that healthy elderly people
who got 800 IU of vitamin E a day had improved immune function. It's important to check with a doctor before taking amounts of vitamin E over 400
IU, however.

As for minerals, the DVs are usually adequate for older people. In fact,
the DVs for some minerals, such as chromium and magnesium, may even
be set too high, Dr. Russell says. If many older people don't get the recommended amounts, it's possibly because they aren't eating the foods that
supply these needed nutrients.

How Do You Know When Enough Is Enough?

If you take in more supplements than your body can handle, what was
beneficial at a lower dose becomes potentially toxic, says Henry Lukaski,
Ph.D., research leader for mineral nutrient functions at the USDA research
center in North Dakota.

In the "Supplement Snapshots" in part 2, you'll find information about
cautions and side effects to help ensure that you take safe and reasonable
doses. This advice comes from doctors and researchers, based on studies
and observations.

When scientists talk about the *toxicity* of a vitamin or mineral, they are
referring to the concentration at which it becomes harmful—the point at
which it begins to act more like a poison than a medicine.

Each vitamin and mineral with known toxicity has its own unique
symptoms. If you get way too much of the trace mineral selenium, for instance (as once happened to people who took an improperly made dietary
supplement), you might lose your hair and fingernails and develop a gar-

Memory Joggers:
How to Remember to Take 'Em

One man put the bottle in his shoe. "He could remember to take his pills in the evening, but he could never remember in the morning," says Joyce Cramer, a medical researcher in psychiatry at West Haven–Yale Veterans Affairs Medical Center in Connecticut and an authority on drug-taking behavior. He had one pair of sneakers that he wore every day, "so he put his pill bottle in there."

Sound silly? "It worked for him," Cramer says. "And if it works for you, do it. It's just like car keys. Some people put them in their pocket, some hang them by the door—whatever it takes to remember to take them when you leave the house."

If you've been forgetting to take your daily supplements and you want some easy memory joggers, you might want to try one or both of the following tactics.

• Use a daily chore as a cue. Using a habit as a reminder can go a long way, but if it's going to work, you have to get it established. The cue needs to be something that you do at a regular time every day, like drinking a morning cup of juice. If you always take a vitamin after drinking your juice, your mind will cue you, "Oops, I forgot something" if you neglect to do it.

• If you take a number of different supplements, visit a drugstore and get a plastic pill organizer. A typical kind has a row of seven boxes, and some have separate compartments for up to four doses a day. If you can't remember whether you've taken a supplement, just snap open a box and have a look. You can tell at a glance which pills you missed. Plus, this method ensures that you don't take two doses when you should take only one. If you like beepers and gadgets, you can even get a pill box that has a programmable timer on top. Ask your pharmacist.

licky odor. If you take too much vitamin A, as people who are self-treating for acne sometimes do, you'll develop a headache, vomiting, hair loss, and dry mucous membranes.

If you take vitamins and minerals within their safe ranges, you'll get the benefits rather than the toxic effects. For each vitamin and mineral, however, the range is different, according to John Hathcock, Ph.D., director of nutrition and regulatory science for the Council for Responsible Nutrition in Washington, D.C. The DV for vitamin A, for instance, is 5,000 IU, but toxic effects have been reported at amounts above 10,000 IU.

With other nutrients, the range of safety is so broad that toxicity has never been reported. Chromium appears to be safe even at more than 1,000 micrograms, which is more than eight times its DV of 120 micrograms. Vitamin C has no reported adverse effects at doses of 1,000 milligrams, and except for causing occasional bouts of diarrhea, seems to be safe at any amount. Vitamin B_{12} does not appear to have any toxic effects, says Dr. Hathcock. "For most vitamins and minerals, the amounts that are safe and beneficial are far below the amounts that are toxic," he concludes.

Pushing the Limits

Given the careful guidelines that scientists have established, it may seem odd that some doctors prescribe doses that are much higher than what is usually considered safe. This is a considered risk, because large amounts—even amounts that could be toxic—may be needed to treat a particular condition.

If you're taking large, therapeutic doses of a vitamin or mineral for a long period of time, you need to be careful, says Dr. Hathcock. These large doses can have damaging effects on organs or tissues. The occasional liver-damaging side effects of large doses of niacin (nicotinic acid) (35 mg per day without a physician's supervision)—prescribed to reduce cholesterol—are well-documented, he notes, as are the nerve-damaging effects of huge doses of vitamin B_6 (upper limit is 100 mg per day without a physician's supervision).

In addition, there are limits that are simply unknown. No one knows the potential side effects of many vitamins and minerals when taken in large doses over the long term. While we know that large amounts of calcium can impair absorption of other minerals such as zinc and manganese, for example, what are the other possible side effects? A total calcium intake of 2,500 milligrams is safe, but we don't know what levels might cause long-term problems, says Dr. Hathcock.

Your best bet is to work with a doctor who's knowledgeable in nutrition. Confirm with your doctor that the amount of each nutrient you're taking is within a safe range. Don't take extra multivitamin/mineral pills to

Food in a Pill?

Why bother with real food if you can just pop a pill that provides all the nourishment you need? That's what the Jetsons did for breakfast in the cartoon series set in an imaginary twenty-first century, and they had more than enough energy.

If you're really into pill popping, it's true that you can get all the known essential nutrients from vitamin and mineral pills. You can also buy protein and carbohydrate powders and capsules of essential fatty acids. In fact, some people who are unable to eat food live on liquid versions of the same; it's called parenteral nutrition.

You won't want to live on synthetic food alone if you have a choice, though, says Scott Smith, Ph.D., research nutritionist for NASA at the Johnson Space Center in Houston. "The engineers would be happy if we could get to that point, but not the astronauts or the medical staff."

Why? For the astronauts, shared meals of real food provide a major psychological benefit, Dr. Smith says. "On long flights especially, with very few things that look like home, food reminds them of something they had back on Earth," he explains. The same sorts of foods that you may have found reassuring as a kid—such as pudding, for instance—provide some psychological comfort in outer space.

In addition to psychological benefits, real food also provides some distinct nutritional advantages over pills and powders. Your digestive system is accustomed to handling real food. It needs bulk. Even aromas and appearance play a role by stimulating your appetite and prompting some food-processing enzymes to jump into action, initiating the process of breaking down foods for absorption into the body. Real food also offers a sense of fullness and satiety that pills and powders just can't provide, Dr. Smith says.

So, even astronauts dine on meals that are as close to real food as they can get. The usual space shuttle fare is reconstituted freeze-dried, packaged food similar to the lightweight stuff that backpackers eat. These foods can provide all the energy, vitamins, and minerals the astronauts need.

In addition, astronauts may take along vitamin and/or mineral supplements if they like, Dr. Smith says. On longer missions, supplements may be required to compensate for potential deficiencies.

get more of one nutrient. Take single supplements of an individual nutrient if necessary, says Dr. Hathcock.

Doctors advise that you not mix different multinutrient pills unless you've confirmed that the totals are within a safe range. If you have been diagnosed with a chronic health condition or take prescription drugs regularly and want to use any of the remedies mentioned in this book, talk with your health-care practitioner first. Women who are pregnant or nursing or who are trying to become pregnant should always consult their doctors before using any home remedy, including vitamins and herbs. Also, if you have kidney, liver, or heart problems, it's best to check with your doctor before you take anything other than a standard multivitamin/mineral supplement that offers the DV of most nutrients.

Within individual chapters, you'll find dosage recommendations, contraindications, potential side effects, and other essential information about specific supplements. This information is based on advice from health-care professionals who have worked extensively with supplements and on guidelines from authoritative references. Remember, a remedy is most effective when used properly.

Watching the Clock

Is there a best—or worst—time to take a supplement? If you can benefit from taking a specific supplement at a certain time or in a certain manner, you'll find that advice in part 2. Meanwhile, here's some general information that can help you decide when to take your supplements.

When it comes to taking a multivitamin, your best bet is to keep it simple. "Just take the darn thing every day, and don't worry about where or when or with what," says Paul Saltman, Ph.D., professor of biology at the University of California at San Diego.

That said, most people take multivitamins with meals, and that's just fine, Dr. Saltman says. Digestive juices that flow when you eat help you digest the ingredients in the pill, too. Even if there are some elements in foods, such as fiber, that interfere somewhat with nutrient absorption, unless you have serious gastrointestinal problems, you'll still absorb plenty.

Here are some additional ways to optimize vitamin and mineral absorption.

• Take fat-soluble vitamins—E, D, A, and K—with a meal that contains a teaspoon or so of fat to aid absorption, says Dr. Saltman.

• Take these fat-soluble vitamins in small doses throughout the day rather than in one large dose. If you take a large, one-a-day dose, more of the vitamin is likely to be stored rather than utilized, he says.

• If you are taking a therapeutic amount of a water-soluble vitamin such as vitamin C, it's also best to divide the dose into three or more smaller doses, according to Dr. Saltman. This way, you absorb more of the vitamin, plus your blood levels of the vitamin will stay more steady throughout the day than if you take one large dose.

• Avoid taking minerals with meals that are mostly fiber, such as a high-fiber breakfast cereal, he says. As good as it is for you, fiber impairs mineral absorption.

• Minerals are also better absorbed in divided doses, says Richard Wood, Ph.D., associate professor at Tufts University School of Nutrition. If you're taking 750 milligrams a day of calcium, for instance, you might want to try dividing it into three 250-milligram doses taken at midmorning and midafternoon and before bed.

Minerals can compete for absorption as well. If you are taking a supplement containing many mineals, dividing it into three doses will increase absorption of all minerals.

In the next two parts of this book, you'll find everything that you need to know about vitamins and minerals. If you want details on a specific vitamin or mineral and how it works in your body, you can read about it in part 2. Along with each vitamin or mineral that's included, you'll also find specific information—what it's recommended for, the DV, cautions about its use, and other details. If you have a particular health problem, turn to part 3 for details on the vitamins and minerals that show promise for that condition.

herbs

our green allies in health and healing

Every culture on Earth has used plants to cure disease, ease pain, and heal the ills and discomforts of the human body. Herbal medicine undoubtedly predates written history. We can assume that at the same time that human beings were learning which plants were good to eat and which were poison, they also were discovering which plants could heal them.

People first started to keep records of herbal medicine some 5,000 to 7,000 years ago in China and Mesopotamia. Much later, in A.D. 78, a Greek physician named Discorides described some 700 healing plants in a comprehensive work called *De Materia Medica*. For several centuries afterward, this was the foundation text for practitioners of herbal medicine throughout Europe.

The New World added new pages to the growing book of herbal cures. When Europeans stepped ashore in North America, they found Native Americans who had a flourishing apothecary that drew on healing plants of the forests and prairies. As white settlers pushed farther into the interior, many turned to Native American plants and herbal practices when they needed frontier treatments for illness and infection.

Native American herbs were still used by North American doctors throughout the nineteenth century and well into the twentieth. Entrepreneurial pharmacists drew on Native American lore when they started marketing patent medicines. They would grind up some of the traditional ingredients and include them in cures for a wide range of ailments.

Today, the search continues for plants with healing properties. Ethnobotanists, who study how herbs are used in other cultures, continue to bring back new plants for study from places as remote as the South American rain forests. Even drug companies have gotten into the act, hoping through exploration and experimentation to discover sources of new chemicals for the development of possible drugs.

In other words, herbal healing is nothing new.

What Is an Herb?

Simply put, a healing herb is a plant, so the range of potential sources of medicines is just as diverse as the plant kingdom. Herbs range from the towering, rock-hard lapacho tree of the Brazilian rain forests, which has an inner bark that helps cure fungal infections, to the lowly, common feverfew, a weed found in roadside ditches that does a remarkable job of preventing migraine headaches.

Discovering that a plant or part of a plant has healing properties is only part of the challenge, however. Anyone who prescribes or uses herbs also would like to know how these plants can deliver the most healing benefit to our bodies. During the several millennia that humans have known about herbal healing, practitioners have used herbs in a wide range of forms, from teas and tinctures to poultices and compresses—and today, as supplements.

When medicines are derived from healing herbs, they're called phytomedicines, botanicals, or herbal supplements. The terms are interchangeable, and all mean medicines derived solely from plant material. Today, these botanicals are widely distributed. Many are available in drugstores, health food stores, grocery stores, and even department stores. Others may be provided by naturopathic doctors, Chinese doctors, or practitioners of alternative medicine who use herbs as important elements in their healing regimens.

In parts 2 and 3 of this book, you'll find details about what these herbal supplements can do for you, the most effective ways to use them for particular health conditions, and specific cautions that you'll want to observe. Before you turn there, though, it's helpful to know something about herbal supplements in general and why some are considered far more effective than others.

Isolating Medicinal Properties

Many of the medicines that we consider pharmaceuticals actually come from plant sources. It was in the early 1800s that scientists first began to isolate and extract healing compounds from plants. Poppies yielded morphine, the narcotic that can help to dispel pain but can also be addictive. From willow bark comes aspirin, perhaps the most universal of all pain relievers. Quinine, widely used to prevent and control malaria, comes from a plant species called cinchona. A wildflower, foxglove, yields digitalis, which is used as a medication for a wide range of heart problems. Taxol, an extract from the bark of the yew tree, is used as an anticancer drug.

Concentrating an active ingredient that's derived from a plant—or synthesizing that chemical in the lab—has its advantages. Drugs allow doctors to deliver a powerful dose of medicine that's intended to cure a specific ailment. The concentrated active ingredient delivers a well-aimed punch.

When ingredients are intensely concentrated in a small package, however, taking large doses can have unwanted effects. "Whenever you use an isolated ingredient, you're increasing the likelihood of side effects," says Eran Ben-Arye, M.D., a researcher at the natural medicine research unit at Hadassah University Hospital in Jerusalem. "That's one reason that you might want to try an herb," he says. "Herbs are not so concentrated and are almost always milder on your system."

Another reason is that you may not need the powerful punch of a pharmaceutical. A case in point: The herb St. John's wort can be very effective against mild to moderate depression and has some advantages over antidepressant medications. On the other hand, just because St. John's wort appears to be a very good treatment for mild depression doesn't mean that anyone with *severe* depression should ignore a doctor's prescription and take St. John's wort as a substitute.

"If you have a moderate to severe problem with depression, you probably should be taking one of the antidepressant drugs," says Dr. Ben-Arye. "If it's mild, St. John's wort may be all you need."

Making a Comeback

Botanical medicines are making a comeback in America. Before the 1940s, many doctors were still prescribing phytomedicines for health problems, but that all changed with the advent of antibiotics during World War II. Considered "wonder drugs" because of their remarkable ability to fight bacterial infections, antibiotics spawned a whole new generation of pharmaceuticals specifically targeted to mow down bacteria. Plant-based medicines quickly fell out of favor.

"People were looking for magic bullets," says Steven Dentali, Ph.D., a natural products chemist with Dentali Associates in Troutdale, Oregon, and a member of the advisory board of the American Botanical Council. "When we adopted these new medicines, we left behind herbs and a way of healing

Choosing an Herbal Supplement

They're sold under many brands, with a wide range of information on their labels. So what should you look for when you're choosing an herbal supplement? Here are some tips.

Buy the standardized extract. If you can find the supplement you want in the form of a standardized extract, it's your best assurance that the product contains a measured amount of a particular ingredient that's thought to be the active ingredient in the herb.

"A standardized extract gives you some guarantee that what's supposed to be in the product is probably in there. It's a good quality marker," says Alison Lee, M.D., a pain-management specialist and medical director of Barefoot Doctors, an alternative medicine practice in Ann Arbor, Michigan.

Remember, though, that a standardized extract contains many other beneficial substances besides the "primary" ingredient listed on the label.

Check the botanical name. Look for the genus and species names on the product label to make sure you're getting the right herb. (You'll find the correct Latin names of recommended herbs in the "Supplement Snapshots" in part 2.) That's important because a common name can sometimes refer to two or three different herbs. Ginseng, for instance, is a common name, but each of three bottles of ginseng might contain a

that had served many people well for a long time. Herbs just weren't in vogue anymore."

This was true only in the United States, however. In Europe, healing herbs continued to be recommended, prescribed, and used by mainstream medical doctors. European private companies, sometimes with government support, extended their research into plant-based medicine. In central Asia and China, where herbal traditions date back thousands of years, it was virtually unthinkable for plant medicines to be neglected as they had been in the United States. In these Asian countries, scientific methods of investigation continue side by side with traditional medicine. Hospitals and research institutions frequently analyze and find scientific evidence to support the use of many herbal cures, Dr. Dentali says.

As was almost inevitable, researchers and doctors in the United States are now looking more closely at phytomedicines, says William Page-Echols,

different species of the herb, and each species has different properties.

Stick with single herbs. Beware of herbal combinations and formulas, says Andrew Weil, M.D., clinical professor of internal medicine and director of the program in integrative medicine of the University of Arizona College of Medicine in Tucson, and author of *Eight Weeks to Optimum Health*.

Herbal medication formulas take a shotgun approach, says Dr. Weil. They may expose you to more medication than you need, which makes side effects more likely.

Check expiration dates. Herbal products age rapidly with light and heat. Buy the freshest supplements you can find, says Steven Dentali, Ph.D., a natural products chemist at Dentali Associates, in Troutdale Oregon, and a member of the advisory board of the American Botanical Council.

Keep it cool. Herbs generally stay potent longer if they're kept cool, says Dr. Dentali. Store them in the refrigerator.

Buy from the big guys. Large companies like Nature's Way, the Eclectic Institute, and Enzymatic Therapy, have established reputations for quality control, says Dr. Weil. Without federal regulation of herbal products, you have to rely on the manufacturer for quality control. Look for GMP-certified companies.

D.O., an assistant clinical professor of family medicine who teaches alternative medicine at the Michigan State University College of Osteopathic Medicine in East Lansing. People hear about herbal alternatives, and naturally they ask their doctors whether these herbs are effective.

People want medicines that are less invasive, easier on their systems, and readily available. They're learning that herbs offer another way of healing, a way to help the body help itself, says Dr. Page-Echols.

Saw palmetto, for example, is said to help shrink an enlarged prostate. "I have patients who come in and ask me about saw palmetto," says Dr. Page-Echols. "They've heard about it in the media or from other men who have the same problem."

Also, people who have had less-than-satisfactory experiences with conventional medications are likely to consider an herbal alternative. If you have insomnia, for instance, an M.D. might immediately prescribe a phar-

Food, Spirit, and Magic

Native Americans introduced several important phytomedicines to Western medicine, including cinchona, sarsaparilla, coca, black cohosh, sassafras, witch hazel, capsicum, goldenseal, and echinacea.

When Europeans first encountered the healing traditions of Native Americans, their perception was shaped by an entrenched attitude toward healing medicines. To the Europeans, herbs were medicines that you took when you were sick—and that was all. To Native Americans, herbs represented not only food and medicine but also spirit and magic, says David Winston, a professional member of the American Herbalists Guild and a practicing herbalist in Washington, New Jersey.

"North American Indians saw plants as living beings," says Winston. "They were used with great respect. Plants had life and power."

Religious and mystical overtones pervaded Indian herbal traditions. While the average Native American probably knew 100 to 200 useful plants, a medicine man or shaman might be learned in using some 800 plants, says Winston.

"Sometimes, there was a certain allure or quality associated with Native American medicine," says Winston. Frontier physicians who practiced native medicine often advertised themselves as Indian doctors. Hucksters of patent medicines boasted that their elixirs contained Indian herbs with wondrous healing properties. In fact, the *Pharmacopoeia of the United States of America*, first published in 1820, contained more than 200 indigenous drugs. Most of these were the herbs originally used by Native Americans.

maceutical sleeping pill. As many people have discovered, a sleeping pill is less than magic. While it may put you to sleep at night, you may find that you wake up the next morning feeling hung-over and spaced-out.

In the search for alternatives, you might turn to kava kava or valerian, the phytomedicines used for insomnia. Kava kava (root) must be used. Hepatotoxicity is associated with preparations made from above ground plant parts. Many people who have used these botanicals report that they relieve anxiety or take the nervous edge off enough to allow an easier transition to sleep and an awakening free of the typical side effects of pharmaceuticals. "A gentle herbal remedy may be much better," says Woodson Merrell, M.D., a specialist in alternative and complementary medicine and assistant clinical professor of medicine at the Columbia University College of Physicians and Surgeons in New York City.

There's another appeal as well. "Herbs fit in with self-healing and prevention," says Dr. Merrell. "That's one reason that you're seeing them out in the marketplace in such quantity."

A Regulatory Purgatory

Currently, herbal medicines sold in the United States are in limbo between regulation and free-market distribution. Since they are classified as dietary supplements, not drugs, they can be purchased without a prescription.

This policy raises doubts in the minds of many health practitioners. In Europe, where phytomedicines are common, people are accustomed to having herbs prescribed by doctors. In the United States, however, you can just walk into a health food store and buy them in quantity. Why should there be such a discrepancy in the way they're distributed?

"Just because they are readily available or advertised as so-called natural products does not mean that they are completely safe and free of side effects," warns Dr. Ben-Arye. "You really should treat herbs like drugs. They shouldn't be used indiscriminately or taken for fun."

The quality of the products is another concern. The U.S. government does not hold supplement manufacturers to the same standards as drug companies. The potency and quality of herbal products vary greatly. You can't always be sure you're getting the real thing. "Many of the products are overpriced and ineffective. Also, there's a great deal of promotion about health benefits by these companies that is pure baloney," says Andrew Weil, M.D., clinical professor of internal medicine and director of the program in integrative medicine of the University of Arizona College of Medicine in Tucson, and author of *Eight Weeks to Optimum Health*.

By law, manufacturers of herbal supplements aren't allowed to make specific health claims for their products, Dr. Weil says. They can instead make general statements about an herb's effect on the body's structure and function. Thus, a supplement label will not say "prevents atherosclerosis" or "relieves arthritis." Instead, the label is likely to say that it is "good for circulation" or "good for joint health."

Despite these limitations, there's a rich tradition and a long history of anecdotal evidence as well as a growing body of scientific references to support the use of herbs for overall, general good health and for specific health problems. Just because the landscape is confusing doesn't mean that you should ignore what you can find. It does mean, however, that if you're going to use herbs, it will help to have the guidance of a book like this one. Or you may want to go a step further as well and consult a health practitioner who has experience with herbal medicines.

If you do consult an experienced practitioner, you have a number of choices. One alternative is to find a certified herbalist who is a member of the American Herbalists Guild. Or you might want to see a *licensed* naturopathic doctor, who will integrate the use of herbs with other healing techniques. A doctor of oriental medicine will also prescribe herbs. Some chiropractors and some physicians—both M.D.'s and D.O.'s—have taken the time to learn about phytomedicines. In addition, you may find some pharmacists who are quite knowledgeable.

Unfortunately, it's impossible to say which practitioners are fully qualified to prescribe herbal medicines. Just as there are no set standards for botanicals, we have no government or professional organizations that oversee the standards of practitioners.

Word-of-mouth recommendations and professional reputation are important. In gathering the information on herbal supplements that you find in this book, we turned to herbalists and practitioners who are recommended by their peers or who have made significant contributions to the research on the subject. In addition, we have asked the opinions of many medical doctors and well-qualified naturopathic doctors who observe practical results in their daily practices. As you read about herbal supplements in parts 2 and 3, you'll find dosages and cautions that have been recommended by these experts. You'll also learn how to take these supplements for maximum effect and discover how other supplements can boost or reinforce their healing power.

Thinking about Herbs

Whether you visit an herbal practitioner or choose to self-medicate, there are two ways to consider herbal supplements.

One view is that botanicals are simply substitutes for drugs. If you have a tension headache, for instance, you want instant relief, so you reach for an over-the-counter pharmaceutical like aspirin, ibuprofen, or acetaminophen. If these are no longer effective or have undesirable side effects, you might consider taking an herbal supplement instead. In a case like that,

Look to Germany

In Germany, people seeking herbal medicine have access to nearly 700 plant-based remedies, and the cost of many of them is covered by health insurance. In fact, some 70 percent of German physicians routinely prescribe phytomedicines. Drugstores carry them, and pharmacists are knowledgeable about their many uses.

Germany has undertaken the most comprehensive science-based investigation of herbs of any Western country. In 1978, the German government established Commission E to evaluate herbal medicines and write a series of monographs, or scholarly works, on them. A team of physicians, toxicologists, pharmacologists, and other specialists set about to produce the most comprehensive study ever attempted.

The commission's series of monographs covers some 400 herbs. For each herbal medicine, Commission E sets certain guidelines for dosage and uses. Unlike the Food and Drug Administration in the United States, which uses a requirement of "absolute certainty" before licensing a drug, Commission E uses a criterion of "reasonable certainty" to determine if an herb is effective. To arrive at its conclusions, the commission took scientific studies into account, but it also considered historical use, anecdotal evidence, and information from field studies as well as other sources.

you're really looking for a one-to-one substitute—an herb to relieve a symptom instead of a drug to relieve a symptom.

Looking for quick, targeted relief is a mindset of Western medicine. The model is allopathic, which simply means trying to substitute a new, benign condition (no headache) for a condition that's causing a lot of discomfort (oh, that aching head). In the allopathic model of medicine, when you have a symptom or a disease, you expect to find some treatment that will produce a different effect and relieve whatever ails you as soon as possible.

Sometimes, the treatment addresses the underlying cause. If so, that treatment might get rid of the pain or discomfort and also keep it from coming back again. But what happens if you just treat the symptom without eliminating the cause? A tension headache is a good example of that. Aspirin or ibuprofen might beat the pain and help you get through the rest of the day, but it does nothing to prevent the headache from recurring a day or a week later.

Herbalists and naturopathic doctors tend to look beyond the allopathic model for just that reason. Why not address what's *causing* those headaches, they ask, on the chance that they can be prevented in the future? Symptoms are important clues to an underlying imbalance. A skilled herbalist can use herbs to treat hormone imbalances, stress, or allergies that cause a headache, not just provide anti-inflammatories that subdue the immediate pain. Yes, herbs can be used for particular problems, but they also provide nourishment for the whole body.

"Herbs can help the body achieve a healthier condition so it can better protect and heal itself," says Jennifer Brett, N.D., a naturopathic doctor at the Wilton Naturopathic Center in Stratford, Connecticut. "It's really a nutritive or positive cure viewpoint."

The second view of using herbs is a more holistic model, as opposed to the allopathic model, meaning that the body is viewed as a whole rather than a set of isolated parts. Instead of seeing a headache as an isolated problem that begins somewhere above your shoulders, a holistic practitioner wonders what's happening all over. Is digestion a contributing factor? Mood? Lifestyle factors? Posture? In the view of the holistic practitioner, if we understand how other body factors contribute to the problem, we can better address the causes.

In many cultures, it's not unusual to consume different healing herbs at different times of the year to keep the whole body healthier and prevent disease. When winter comes on, the Chinese often add astragalus to their soups and stews as a way to boost their immune systems and fight off seasonal colds and flu. People living on the Indian subcontinent use red pepper, curry, and garlic on their food all year round, not just as spices but also as medicines to aid digestion, improve liver health, or lower cholesterol, Dr. Brett says.

Balms and Cures

Of course, herbs wouldn't be your first choice if you had an acute-care situation, such as a heart attack, pneumonia, or a broken leg. In these cases, it's best to get yourself to the hospital, says Dr. Brett.

Herbal supplements are well-suited for preventing illness, building up the body's defenses, and easing the symptoms of long-term conditions such as heart disease, diabetes, migraines, and asthma. They can also make a big difference if you have elusive problems like insomnia, anxiety, depression, or lack of energy, she adds.

Unlike synthetic drugs designed to cure specific ills, herbs tend to have a wide range of applications. In fact, the very terms *drug* and *medicine* are inappropriate descriptions of what they actually do. Many herbalists use other terms, such as *tonic* and *adaptogen*. Tonic herbs restore, nourish, and support individual organs or the entire body. Adaptogens help restore balance in the body, particularly helping it to adapt to stress, be it physical, environmental, or emotional.

An adaptogen can make adjustments on the plus or the minus side. Let's say you're feeling run-down and sluggish—or just the opposite: stressed-out and wired. Although the symptoms seem totally different, the cause may be the same—adrenal glands that are not working optimally, says Dr. Brett. Maybe your adrenal glands are overactive, producing more hormones than they should, or perhaps they're not producing enough. Either way, an adaptogen might help.

By taking an adaptogenic herb that supports adrenal health, you can restore the balance of the adrenals and normalize function, says Dr. Brett. "An adaptogen really shunts in wherever it is needed. It just helps your body do what it should be doing."

Subtle Healing

In most instances, you'll find the work of herbs to be subtle and gentle, says Dr. Dentali. Sometimes, you really need to pay attention to notice whether they're working. Also, if they're causing a side effect, that might not be readily apparent.

Feverfew, for example, has been very successful in limiting migraines, but it may take weeks before the herb has an effect. If you start taking it, your headaches may ease so gradually that it may seem as if the herb has nothing to do with the relief you're getting. The cause-and-effect relationship isn't entirely clear.

"If you are going to self-medicate, you really need to pay attention, even take notes on your condition. That way, you can better tell if the herb is working," says Dr. Dentali.

Stanley W. Beyrle, N.D., a naturopathic doctor at the Kansas Clinic of

From Plant to Shelf

Making herbal supplements these days is a far cry from the traditional hunter-gatherer methods of yore. As with any complex manufacturing operation, supplement makers require a steady stream of raw materials, and there are many checkpoints for quality control throughout the process.

When you step inside the doors of Herbalist and Alchemist, an herbal medicine manufacturer in Washington, New Jersey, the complexity of the operation is immediately apparent. In the factory, which employs 13 people, technicians make herbal tinctures in a processing room that's the picture of scrupulous hygiene. People wear gowns, goggles, hair and beard nets, and rubber gloves. Some have respirators. In an area that resembles a very neat, well-organized chemistry lab, there are checklists and formulas, glass beakers, electronic scales, and a computer that assigns lot numbers and expiration dates to bottled products.

Herbs come from a wide range of sources. Nearby herb farms in New Jersey supply plants that are native to the region. Kava kava is imported from Hawaii and Vancouver. Botanical brokers on the West Coast link small farmers and organic growers to this hub of manufacturing activity in New Jersey. Other brokers represent the people who gather plants from fields and forests in the Carolinas.

All the herbs used by Herbalist and Alchemist are grown organically and gathered responsibly, according to Beth Lambert, the company's chief executive officer. Once delivered to the facility, the herb is ground, measured, and placed in five-gallon glass jars with a solution of ethanol and distilled water. The solution, called a menstruum, extracts the healing chemical compounds from the plant material. Most plants soak in the menstruum for about two weeks. A technician then strains and presses out the plant material. What's left behind is tincture, a colored liquid with a strange but earthy odor of alcohol and plants.

Depending on the herb, the manufacturing process can be more complicated. Herbs may be cooked or percolated in the menstruum. Plants are

Traditional Medicine in Wichita, says that after 18 years of practicing herbal medicine, he tends to prescribe much lower dosages than he once did. "A little bit can be enough. What you're looking to do is nudge the body in one direction or another so it can take care of itself," he says. "You don't want to overdo it."

sometimes shredded when wet. Processing times can be shortened or extended. Sometimes, several tinctures are mixed together in herbal combinations developed by David Winston, the company's founder.

The company makes only tinctures, even though the end product may be higher-priced than other popular forms of the herb. "We only make tinctures because we believe that once the active ingredients are extracted by the menstruum, the medicines are more easily assimilated into the body," Lambert says.

Despite the high-tech trappings, the sampling and selection of ingredients is a subjective process based upon the instincts and experience of the people who scan the raw material and maintain quality control. The key people in that selection process are Winston and Betzy Bancroft, both herbalists who are professional members of the American Herbalists Guild.

"We do our own grinding," says Bancroft. "We want our herbs as whole as possible because they stay fresher longer that way."

She and Winston subject every shipment to a detailed examination. It's the first hurdle that the product must pass before it can be approved by the two certified herbalists. They use sight, smell, taste, and feel to evaluate whether the raw materials pass muster. If a shipment of ginger arrives, Winston will taste it to make sure the plant meets his criteria for gingerols, the active ingredients that give ginger its pungent taste.

As for the rest of the process, the strict hygiene and quality-control practices are self-imposed rather than required by law, according to Lambert. She thinks that these careful processes will someday be required of everyone. The labeling of their products also follows strict guidelines. "We can trace a bottle of our tincture at a health food store right back to the herb supplier," she says.

Begun in 1982, the company sells most products wholesale to medical doctors, naturopathic doctors, homeopaths, herbalists, chiropractors, and health food stores.

Timing is also a factor. There are really very few herbs that you should be taking long-term unless it's to address a chronic condition, says Alison Lee, M.D., a pain-management specialist and medical director of Barefoot Doctors, an alternative medicine practice in Ann Arbor, Michigan. People should take breaks from herbal therapies.

A Few Studies, a Lot of Tradition

Determining the effectiveness of an herb is difficult. Many people who are enthusiastic about herbal remedies and have strong beliefs in alternative medicine may experience a so-called placebo effect when they take herbs. Yes, they feel better, but no one knows whether they feel better because the herb is effecting some kind of change in the body or because the positive messages about herbs are changing how they feel. Both count, of course. Any remedy that makes you feel better is worth taking, as long as it has no harmful side effects. In the interest of scientific curiosity, though, we'd all like to know how these things work and whether they can help everyone.

Some herbs, like hawthorn, garlic, and ginkgo, have quite a bit of scientific research behind them. Others, such as cat's claw, have almost none. If you take cat's claw, you're relying on anecdotal evidence and tradition—sometimes going back centuries.

Why aren't there more studies of herbal medicines? For one thing, testing a phytomedicine is difficult and expensive. In the United States, the Food and Drug Administration (FDA) relies on drug companies to finance research and development. If a drug wins approval from the FDA, the economic rewards can be enormous. Along with a patent for the medicine, the company gets exclusive rights to sell the drug to the public before it becomes public domain, explains Dr. Dentali.

Phytomedicines can't be patented. Hawthorn, echinacea, and thousands of other herbs belong to everyone, and the supplements derived from them are universally available. Without the expectation of a high-profit license to pay the costs of exhaustive research, drug companies have little incentive to make the exorbitant investment required to get FDA approval.

The other barrier to herb testing is the sheer volume of active ingredients that would have to be tested. The classic method of understanding the active compounds in a plant or drug is to isolate each chemical and test it for medicinal properties, using first cell-based, then animal, and finally human studies to supply evidence, says Dr. Dentali. That type of isolation and testing, applied to the scores of active ingredients in an herb, turns into a prohibitively expensive and time-consuming task. It may also be fruitless. Many scientists believe that the chemicals in healing herbs frequently act together. By singling out the "active" ones, they say, we'll neglect all the other ingredients that make herbs different from drugs.

That's why herbalists say that herbs are meant to be taken as a whole, including all of their chemical constituents, known and unknown, and they don't recommend extracting the active ingredients so that they become plant-derived chemicals that act independently. You might say that an herbal treatment is like the sound produced by an orchestra. Each instrument plays a separate part, but you don't get the orchestral sound until they're all playing together.

Dosage Dilemma

The lack of "scientific evidence" and research studies supporting the effectiveness of herbal preparations in humans has an impact on the medical community. Not many M.D.'s are writing prescriptions for herbs, and that's largely because of the lack of studies, says Jonathan Sporn, M.D., an oncologist and associate professor of medicine at the University of Connecticut Health Center in Farmington.

Eating more garlic or taking a garlic supplement is probably good for your heart and circulatory system. It may very well prevent stomach cancer as well, says Dr. Sporn. There are questions, however: How much garlic should a person take? How often? In what form? Doctors who want to answer these questions hear many opinions but few firm recommendations.

"We do know that garlic has some anti-cancer properties," says Dr. Sporn, "and there's evidence that eating more garlic or taking a garlic supplement may prevent gastrointestinal cancer. That's all that science can tell us right now, though. We can't tell you whether garlic should be generally recommended as an anti-cancer agent."

Instead, what doctors and herbalists have to rely upon is the clinical experience of herbal practitioners, the folklore of native healers, and centuries of traditional use.

"Up until 5 to 10 years ago, with many of these herbs we only had anecdotal or clinically based evidence—how they've been used in the past or within the doctor's own practice," says Dr. Merrell. "More recently, however, there have been hundreds of well-designed, published studies examining the scientific basis and clinical outcomes to help guide us on the safe and effective use of herbal medicines."

Evaluating herbs is like trying to pin down the benefits that we get from food, observes Dr. Dentali. "Sure, you could attempt exhaustive studies on these herbs, but is that any better than doing exhaustive studies on something like a carrot, so we know what every little chemical in a carrot does for us? What we already know is that carrots are good for you. Moreover, we know that about many of these herbs. Centuries of use by people tell us that."

Selecting a Supplement

Considering all the different kinds of herbs and the ways that we use them, what's the best way to take them? Should you eat the plant? Drink it as a tea? Extract its active ingredients? Or take it as a pill or capsule?

In years past, people simply added medicinal herbs to their foods, or they made some kind of brew using the dried and ground-up plant. Today, the large and small companies that distribute herbs have developed many ways to process them for consumption. Squeezing the herb into a pill or capsule certainly makes it convenient to take, but certain decisions are made by the producers when herbs are processed this way.

In an extraction process, it's possible to isolate specific chemicals from the plant. When those chemicals are included at a specific, guaranteed concentration, they're said to be standardized.

If you buy St. John's wort in supplement form, the label may tell you the amount of St. John's wort extract in each capsule. It will also say that the supplement is standardized for a certain percentage of hypericin, which is what some phytochemists think is the most important ingredient in the herb. This is the supplement maker's "guarantee"—without any regulatory verification—that each capsule contains a specific amount of the extract and a specific percentage of a primary ingredient.

Purists may say that the only way to take herbs is in their raw form, but there's a lot to be said for herbal supplements that come as capsules, pills, and liquid tinctures, especially if they're labeled as standardized extracts. The supplements offer convenience, uniform doses, and specific concentrations of certain ingredients.

They're also tasteless, which is sometimes a real plus, especially if you're taking an herb like valerian. When made into a tea, valerian smells and tastes downright obnoxious. Those familiar with its rank odor have dubbed it the gym-sock herb. Taken as a pill, however, it has no taste at all, so you can get the benefits without the challenge.

Putting the Genie in the Bottle

As their name implies, wildcrafted herbs are gathered in the wild. Cultivated herbs, however, ensure a constant supply with more consistent qualities. Nearly all ginseng, echinacea, and ginkgo, to name just three popular herbs, are now farmed as regular crops. Since some herbs, such as echinacea, are becoming scarce in the wild due to overharvesting, you should buy cultivated herbs whenever possible, says Jill Stansbury, N.D., assistant professor of botanical medicine, chair of the botanical medicine department at the National College of Naturopathic Medicine in Portland, Oregon.

Whether gathered in the field or in the wild, the herbs are dried before they're packaged. Throughout the growing, harvesting, drying, and packaging processes, reputable manufacturers will take steps to ensure that the final product has consistent, assured qualities. It's important that dried herbs be of consistent quality to yield a potent supplement.

Three kinds of herb supplements are most common. Here's a rundown.

Pills. The ground herb is pressed together and held by a binding substance. Some pills may have an enteric coating, a kind of second skin that's gradually dissolved by enzymes in the intestines. The coating ensures that the pill passes undisturbed through the stomach and starts to dissolve only when it reaches the intestines.

Capsules. These work in much the same way as pills, but they're constructed somewhat differently. The ground herb is inside a gelatin shell, where the ingredients are protected from light, moisture, and exposure to oxygen.

Extracts. These are concentrated preparations made from dried or fresh plant parts. The herb is soaked or cooked in a liquid to concentrate active ingredients or remove unwanted components. If the active ingredient is known or suspected, manufacturers may try to include or concentrate that ingredient in their products. The content of desired constituents is calculated and standardized.

A tincture is a type of liquid extract in which alcohol is used as a solvent to extract active constituents from dried or fresh plant material. If you have difficulty swallowing pills or capsules, tinctures are a good way to go. You can simply use an eyedropper to put drops of an alcohol-based solution on your tongue, in a cup of tea, or in water.

Glycerites are a type of liquid extract in which active constituents are held in glycerin, a sweet-tasting fatty compound with a syrupy consistency. Glycerin makes herbs taste better, which can help if the raw herb is bitter or has a disagreeable flavor.

Mostly Mild, Mostly Safe

The mild nature of many herbal supplements makes them relatively safe, but that's not true of every herb, and it's important to follow any directions from your health practitioner and the dosage recommendations on the product's label. Don't exceed the dosage, says David Winston, a professional member of the American Herbalists Guild and a practicing herbalist in Washington, New Jersey.

"A lot of folks have this idea that if a little is good, more is better. That's never a good idea, even with herbs," says Winston. "Just because herbs are natural does not necessarily mean that they are harmless."

Also, be cautious if you're already taking other medications. Side effects are possible when you mix pharmaceutical drugs and herbs. If you have concerns about possible side effects or interactions, be sure to consult a health practitioner who has experience with herbs. Also, to guard against potential drug interactions, tell your regular doctor about any herbs that you're taking.

emerging supplements

exploring the outer boundaries

Walk through the supplement section of your local health food store, supermarket, or drugstore, and you'll see many supplements that don't fit the category of either vitamins and minerals or herbal supplements. You'll see strange names like phosphatidylserine and chondroitin sulfate, mysterious abbreviations like DHEA, or headline-grabbing labels like melatonin and shark cartilage.

How do we classify these other supplements that are neither vitamins, minerals, nor herbs?

There are so many different kinds that they defy a single classification. Since all of them are in some stage of being tested, challenged, advertised, and marketed, however, it seems simplest to call them emerging supplements.

Many of the emerging supplements are almost literally new inventions. True, they may come from natural sources (shark cartilage is an obvious example) and be considered nonpharmaceuticals, but many of them are put together in laboratories. Before long, supplements that begin to show promise can fall into the hands of promoters who ascribe almost-miraculous powers and properties to the newly created compounds. While that doesn't necessarily mean that they're ineffective or even marginally unsafe, it does mean that you, the buyer, might need to beware of premature or exaggerated claims made by overzealous marketers.

Why are we so willing to try these emerging supplements, or any supplements, for that matter?

One reason is our growing desire to act preventively and steer our own health destinies, says Mark Stengler, N.D., a naturopathic doctor and author of *The Natural Physician: Your Health Guide for Common Ailments.* "People are taking more control over their own health, and supplements are a way of becoming proactive," he explains.

The Roads to Discovery

Sometimes, the discovery of a supplement begins with simple observation and a powerful sense of curiosity. In other cases, a new supplement is found when scientists look closely at existing data. Something as insignificant as pineapple juice is thought to be a digestive aid or the shell of a crab is suspected of being a possible arthritis cure.

There are many ways that supplements are discovered. Modern researchers may take clues from ancient medical texts or modern-day folk medicine. They may accidentally stumble across the next big supplement or test a hypothesis based on years of research.

Consider the strange case of fish oil.

Doctors working in the Arctic in the 1970s observed that the Eskimo people were rarely afflicted with heart disease, despite a high-fat, high-cholesterol diet of whale meat, seal meat, and fish.

Later, researchers in Japan in the early 1980s also noted a low death rate from heart disease in their country. Like the Eskimos, the Japanese people ate a lot of fish. Scientists began to wonder if fish was the common bond.

On closer examination of statistics, researchers found that this theory seemed to be reinforced. In Japan, the lowest death rates from heart disease were found on the island of Okinawa, where fish consumption was about twice as high as in mainland Japan. Another study compared a fishing village where residents ate as much as 250 grams of fish a day with a farming area where people ate about 90 grams of fish daily. Sure enough, the lower incidence of heart disease was in the fishing village.

These early observations led researchers to study whether some aspect of seafood was protective against heart disease. Much of the research zeroed in on omega-3 polyunsaturated fatty acids, which were found in fish oils.

Today, research points to the conclusion that the omega-3's in fish oil reduce the risk of heart disease by influencing blood clotting and blood pressure. They may also reduce the risk of irregular heartbeat. Beyond heart health, researchers are now considering how fish oil can help other conditions, including rheumatoid arthritis and other inflammatory diseases.

Given these promising findings, it was almost inevitable that supplement makers would begin to manufacture fish-oil supplements. In fact, if you check the shelves of almost any drugstore or health food store, you're likely to find a number of different brands and concentrations.

Gaining Respect

Nearly every week, it seems, we read about an emerging supplement that's going to reverse aging, help us sleep better, improve our sex lives, or boost our immune systems.

How does a supplement move from obscurity to acceptability?

The media is instrumental in fueling our interest in dietary supplements, says Stephen DeFelice, M.D., founder and chairman of the nonprofit Foundation for Innovation in Medicine in Cranford, New Jersey. It was Dr. DeFelice, in fact, who coined the term *nutraceutical* to describe food or dietary supplements that offer health benefits, including disease prevention and treatment.

According to Dr. DeFelice, our current appetite for supplements can be traced back to the 1980s, when the word began to spread—from researchers to physicians to reporters to consumers—that calcium helps to prevent osteoporosis. The sales of calcium supplements took off, opening the door for the increased popularity of other supplements like fiber and fish oil, says Dr. DeFelice.

What set calcium apart was solid clinical data, reviewed by medical experts and published in a medical journal, says Dr. DeFelice. During a clinical trial, researchers compare health outcomes of two separate groups of people who are randomly selected. One group receives a real supplement; the other gets a look-alike pill, or placebo, that has no active ingredients. Since no one knows whether they're getting the real treatment, any difference in health effects is more likely due to the pill than to attitudes about the pill. This is the simplest way to eliminate what researchers call the placebo effect, which occurs when people feel better because they think they're *supposed* to feel better.

Prior to publication of glowing reports about calcium, most nutritional research was in the form of epidemiological studies. In these studies of large groups of people, scientists are simply observers. Rather than setting up a controlled situation, they observe what kinds of foods a group of people eat and then assess how healthy those people are.

A third kind of nutritional research uses animals, or it's done in a laboratory using test tubes. Doctors far prefer clinical data to animal studies, lab studies, or epidemiological studies, though, because clinical data can demonstrate direct cause and effect, says Dr. DeFelice. "That's what doctors want to know: Has this particular product been evaluated? If so, they'll recommend it."

Man's Search for Power Surges

As one of the greatest home-run hitters ever to step up to the plate, the legendary Babe Ruth sent 714 balls over the fence and into the pages of history.

Impressive, yes. But imagine how many home runs he might have hit if only he had known about the supplement called creatine.

By the late 1990s, this popular dietary supplement was being used by untold numbers of amateur and professional athletes. Whether they intended to or not, some of these athletes became, in effect, promoters of creatine as they publicly acknowledged using it. They seemed to provide living proof that creatine does what it claims—increases strength and provides short-term explosive power.

While using the extra boost of creatine might seem like a form of not-so-subtle cheating, athletes throughout history have sought ways to gain the competitive edge. Our early ancestors ate deer liver and lion heart for strength and speed. Modern-day athletes and their trainers know volumes about the presumed ergogenic (performance-enhancing) effects of protein, amino acids, and common food components like caffeine. Now, creatine and a number of other so-called ergogenic supplements have joined the list.

Skeptics abound. Most of the concoctions being marketed to athletes have no scientific basis whatsoever, says Melvin Williams, Ph.D., professor emeritus in the department of exercise science, physical education, and recreation at Old Dominion University in Norfolk, Virginia, and author of *The Ergogenics Edge: Pushing the Limits of Sports Performance*. "Athletes today are getting better because of improved training, sophisticated coaching techniques, and new technologies. With a few exceptions, including possibly creatine, I don't really think these supplements have any impact on performance," says Dr. Williams.

Apart from the expense of some performance-enhancing supplements, there's also the question of how much harm they might do. Few long-term studies have been done on safety, and the more widely these supplements are used, the greater the risk for a large number of athletes.

Still, the market for ergogenic supplements is a billion-dollar business, Dr. Williams says. Athletes seem to be willing to try almost any new supplement, including those with known health risks.

Based on the explosion of scientific research in the past decade, doctors are now in a better position to know what they can recommend and for what, according to Dr. Stengler.

As studies begin to prove some of the claims that are made about popular supplements, universities and companies have become less reluctant to provide funding for research in the area of natural products, adds Terry Lemerond, president of Enzymatic Therapy, a supplement company in Green Bay, Wisconsin. Also, of course, consumer demand is a stimulus to companies that can afford to perform laboratory tests. Supplements make up a lucrative market, and more companies than ever before are entering that market.

Making Pills with Possibilities

With so much interest in emerging supplements, what does it take for a new discovery to make the grade and win acceptance?

To answer that question is to tell the story of how an emerging supplement, well, emerges.

Although the process may seem mysterious, it's actually a lot like a very big homework assignment. For instance, at Thorne Research, a supplement producer in Sandpoint, Idaho, scientists in the technical division regularly scour existing research for anything that looks promising. In many cases, some research already exists but has gone unnoticed. Often, the researchers run across dietary supplements that have been ignored by the pharmaceutical industry or the medical profession in favor of pharmaceutical drugs that can be patented, says Al Czap, president of Thorne Research.

"In many cases, things are out there, readily available. We just have to open our eyes to look for them," Czap says. "We look at virtually every journal in the world, from biochemical to phytochemical to obscure European journals. We find many things that have been overlooked or that show potential."

Just because a dietary supplement is new to researchers in the United States doesn't mean that it's been ignored worldwide. In some cases, a supplement is already being used in another country as an alternative to costly prescription medications, Czap says. Doctors here have little incentive to seek out alternative remedies because insurance usually covers the cost of prescription medications for their patients, he adds.

What Gives a New Supplement a Good Name

Often, the evidence and advocacy for a newly discovered supplement come from real-life stories of people who took it with phenomenal results. While such stories—what researchers call anecdotal evidence—can't be written off as fiction, they are not accepted as proof, either. After all, what helps one person may not help another. No matter how much proof we may demand, anecdotal evidence is still compelling.

Such is the case with Betty Dwyer, a woman who believes that her life was saved by a little-known supplement with an unusual name. Her doctor, too, is convinced.

Dwyer, of Dallas, and her doctor, Peter Langsjoen, M.D., agree that without coenzyme Q_{10} (also known as coQ_{10}), Dwyer's condition probably would have been fatal. CoQ_{10} is a naturally occurring compound that our cells need to produce energy. It's found in all cells but is most highly concentrated in heart muscle cells because they use the greatest amount of energy.

Dr. Langsjoen, a cardiologist in Tyler, Texas, believes that when taken as a supplement, coQ_{10} protects the heart, normalizes blood pressure, and strengthens the immune system, among other benefits.

In 1981, when Dwyer was 50 years old, she was diagnosed with dilated cardiomyopathy, a life-threatening condition in which the heart becomes enlarged and weak. Dwyer had asthma, and when she went to the hospital complaining of shortness of breath, she thought her respi-

Once the company has decided to manufacture a supplement, Czap says, the supplements are thoroughly tested to make sure that they contain the right mixture of ingredients and are free of contamination. Samples are run through a laboratory, where an analysis is done to ensure that the product is completely mixed. A state-of-the-art instrument takes an infrared "fingerprint" of a product sample, which is then compared with the verified standard for the product and compared by computer with the other batch samples to ensure complete mixing.

The next step is to get uniform amounts of the mixture into capsules, which are made from gelatin. To make sure that all of the capsules contain the right amount of materials, samples are taken randomly and weighed. If

ratory problem was out of control. Subsequent tests revealed the cardiomyopathy.

"My heart was increasing in size and wasn't able to do its job. The bigger it got, the less efficient it was," says Dwyer. "When I first went to the hospital, I was told that I could expect to live five to seven years." At that time, doctors also told her that she'd probably need a heart transplant.

After two weeks in the hospital, Dwyer returned home for some rest and recovery, but she barely improved. She was short of breath and unable to stay on her feet for very long, and she had "absolutely no energy," she recalls.

Her condition remained poor for about three years. Then she joined a research program that was using coQ_{10} to treat cardiomyopathy. "I didn't have anything to lose," Dwyer says. In 1984, she began taking supplemental coQ_{10} under her doctor's supervision.

Although previously she had taken a number of medications for her asthma and heart conditions, Dwyer was able to cut back to a single prescription drug that controls her heart rhythm. With that drug and coQ_{10}, she no longer considers her diagnosis of cardiomyopathy a death sentence.

"I still have the heart I was born with. And as long as it works as well as it works now, I'm going to leave it alone," says Dwyer.

Dr. Langsjoen, who has been Dwyer's doctor since 1992, agrees that were it not for coQ_{10}, she would have had to have a heart transplant. He also believes that she wouldn't be alive today without this supplement.

necessary, the capsuling machine is adjusted to make sure that each capsule falls within an acceptable weight range.

Your Selection Process

Given all of the companies offering supplements, how do you know which ones are most reliable? How can you be reasonably sure that the product you buy contains what it says it does?

"In general, I educate my patients to buy brands recommended by a trusted professional, either a nutritionally trained doctor or health food store owner or employees with training and a good reputation in the community," says Emily Kane, N.D., a naturopathic doctor in Juneau, Alaska, and senior editor of the *Journal of Naturopathic Medicine*.

For what she calls designer supplements, Dr. Kane recommends products from Thorne Research, Scientific Botanicals, PhytoPharmica, Eclectic, Naturopathic Formulations, and Tyler Encapsulations. Some of these companies sell to consumers, but products from others, such as Thorne, are available only through a physician.

Dr. Stengler offers the following tips for selecting a supplement.

Read the label. Look for any potentially allergenic substances such as Red Dye #4. If the product does not clearly state ingredients and their amounts, do not buy it.

Ask for proof. The supplement company should be able to provide you with a product analysis of potency and purity. That analysis (GMP certified) gives you some assurance that the product you choose is free of contaminants such as bacteria, pesticides, and heavy metals.

Choose a reputable company. Get as much background as you can on the company you're buying from. Consider their number of years of experience in the industry and the quality of their educational materials. The company should also be able to tell you where the raw materials for their products come from, such as organic herb farms. Other measurements are the quality of their product analysis and their commitment to research and scientific validation. Finally, you should also seek out companies that have strong medical advisory boards.

Visit your health food store. In general, supplements sold at health food stores tend to be of higher quality than those sold in grocery and chain stores.

Find a direct source. Shop for a company that manufactures its own products. There is better quality control and more responsibility to the product from such companies, says Czap.

Besides being knowledgeable about labels and manufacturers, of course, you need information about the newest supplements and the claims that have been made for them. In part 2, you'll find many emerging supplements along with the vitamins, minerals, and herbs that experts describe.

2

the powerhouse of nature's medicines

acidophilus

When we hear the word *bacteria*, we usually think of something unsanitary. After all, don't we worry about bacteria whenever we pierce our skin with a rusty nail, use a dirty public washroom, or eat at an all-night roadside diner?

Believe it or not, there are certain types of bacteria that are actually good for us. Constantly doing good work in our intestinal tracts are more than 400 species of microscopic organisms that help digest food and perform other functions. One of the stars among these so-called microflora is *Lactobacillus acidophilus*. And these beneficial bacteria get around. Not only are they in the intestinal tract and mouth, they may also show up in the vagina.

We are not born with a ready-made supply of acidophilus—or any other bacteria, for that matter—but we all begin gathering herds of microflora soon after we leave the womb. Mom can help, transferring some of the beneficial bacteria through breast milk. Later, as soon as we're introduced to a variety of foods, the good and bad bacteria begin to colonize our bodies. Throughout our lives, we need enough of the good microflora to help keep us healthy and to keep the bad kind in check. There are times, though, when those friendly bacteria can use some help.

Friendly Flora

Acidophilus and other lactobacilli are considered friendly because they produce nutrients such as B vitamins. They also produce enzymes that aid in the digestion of proteins, carbohydrates, and fats, says Khem Shahani, Ph.D., professor of food science and technology at the University of Nebraska in Lincoln.

Acidophilus also takes part in an important balancing act in the intestinal tract and vagina. Under ideal circumstances, it and other types of beneficial bacteria help to create an environment that prevents harmful bacteria from multiplying.

Many things can deplete the good guys, including stress, disease, poor digestion, processed foods, and too much sugar. Alcohol and tobacco are also culprits. When these factors come into play, bad bacteria can multiply and take over, leading to a variety of intestinal problems, urinary tract infections, and vaginal yeast infections. Then something must be done to help restore acidophilus to power.

There's another sneaky predator as well. Antibiotics are prescribed to clear up bacterial infections, but that's not all they clear up. In their haste to sweep away the bad bacteria, they can knock out beneficial bacteria, too.

Whatever the cause, as your natural supply of acidophilus goes into retreat, the need for reinforcements increases. "That's when it becomes important to take an acidophilus supplement," says Dr. Shahani. Commonly available in tablets, capsules, and powders, supplements help to combat these problems by restoring the balance of bacteria in the intestines and vagina.

How Much, and When?

Supplements aren't the only sources of L. acidophilus. You can also get it from foods such as yogurt and other cultured milk products. Supple-

---

SUPPLEMENTSNAPSHOT

▶Acidophilus

Scientific name: *Lactobacillus acidophilus.*

May help: Vaginal yeast infections, urinary tract infections, lactose intolerance, diarrhea, fibromyalgia, irritable bowel syndrome, lupus, high cholesterol, osteoporosis, indigestion, constipation, and gas.

Special instructions: Take with food.

Good food sources: Fermented milk products, including yogurt and kefir. High temperatures destroy acidophilus, so fermented milk products are not good sources if they've been warmed.

Cautions and possible side effects: If you have any serious gastrointestinal problems that require medical attention, check with your doctor before taking.

Amounts exceeding 10 billion viable L. acidophilus organisms daily may cause mild gastrointestinal distress.

ments, however, provide a more concentrated form of the beneficial bacteria, according to Dr. Shahani.

In addition to its well-known use as a home remedy for preventing and treating vaginal yeast infections, acidophilus can also ease gastrointestinal distress such as diarrhea, constipation, and flatulence. Researchers are looking into its ability to lower cholesterol levels, prevent colon cancer, and provide relief for skin problems such as contact dermatitis, according to Dr. Shahani. It can even be a modest help in warding off osteoporosis, since some strains of acidophilus aid the transformation of calcium from your diet into the bone-strengthening form that keeps your skeleton healthy, he says.

While some of these benefits are speculative, there's no doubt that we all need acidophilus bacteria for good health. Also, doctors sometimes recommend supplements for very specific conditions. "I recommend that anyone with any kind of gastrointestinal upset or chronic vaginal yeast infection, and anyone who's going to take a trip overseas and is therefore at risk for traveler's diarrhea, supplement with acidophilus in one form or another," says Jennifer Brett, N.D., a naturopathic doctor at the Wilton Naturopathic Center in Stratford, Connecticut.

Biting Back at the Bacteria Bashers

A prescription antibiotic might be just the thing to conquer a common sinus infection. While the antibiotic is killing the bacteria that haunt your sinuses, it's also moving throughout your body and clearing out bacteria of all types, good and bad.

When it does this cleaning work in the vaginal area, the result can be very counterproductive. Vaginal yeast is held in check by beneficial bacteria such as acidophilus, and once that barrier is removed by the antibiotic, yeast can multiply quickly. That's where acidophilus supplements can help, by restoring good bacteria to chase away the bad, says Dr. Brett.

While it's true that most acute yeast infections are treatable with safe, inexpensive, over-the-counter medications, these remedies don't offer much long-term protection. Acidophilus supplements, on the other hand, may provide a long-term solution to chronic problems.

At the Long Island Jewish Medical Center in New York, researchers tested the effects of acidophilus by giving eight ounces of acidophilus-containing yogurt daily to 13 women who had histories of recurring yeast in-

Better Bacteria?

Move over, acidophilus. Make room for lactobacillus strain GG (LGG), a kind of beneficial bacteria that has been available as a supplement in this country only since 1998. Some experts say that LGG is superior to acidophilus for the prevention and treatment of diarrhea and other gastrointestinal disturbances.

No other beneficial bacteria—not even acidophilus—have been so well supported by scientific tests, according to Barry Goldin, Ph.D., a biochemist and professor in community health at Tufts University School of Medicine in Boston. Dr. Goldin is the researcher who discovered the strain in 1985, along with Sherwood Gorbach, M.D., professor of community health and medicine at Tufts. Since that discovery, he says, more than 100 scientific papers have reported the effectiveness of LGG in treating a number of gastrointestinal problems.

Unlike acidophilus, which is derived from a dairy strain, LGG comes from a sterile form of the bacteria that grow in the human intestine. For this reason, it may be better equipped to survive in the gastrointestinal tract and vagina than acidophilus and other dairy strains of lactobacilli, Dr. Goldin says.

fections. After six months, the incidence of yeast infections dropped nearly 74 percent.

Acidophilus also shows promise for lowering cholesterol levels. High cholesterol is a major risk factor in atherosclerosis (hardening of the arteries), which can lead to heart problems. According to Dr. Shahani, human and animal studies have shown significant decreases in LDL cholesterol—the bad kind—when diets were supplemented with certain strains of acidophilus. Other studies have shown acidophilus to increase HDL cholesterol.

Acidophilus supplements have also been shown to ease the symptoms of lactose intolerance, including bloating, gas, and diarrhea. This condition occurs when the body doesn't produce enough of an enzyme called lactase, which breaks down lactose, the sugar found in milk and other dairy products. Acidophilus can help because it produces large amounts of lactase, says Dr. Shahani.

Looking for Living Cells

If we never got sick, ate only nutritious, wholesome foods, and lived an enormously healthy and stress-free life, we probably wouldn't need to take acidophilus supplements, says Dr. Shahani. But "our lifestyles are such that supplements become necessary from time to time," he observes. "I think the capsules may be more reliable because you're swallowing living micro-organisms. You can't always tell how potent yogurt and other dairy products are," he says.

To get the supplements that are most effective, you have to choose very carefully, according to Dr. Shahani. In order to get one that's full of viable organisms, you can ask your pharmacist to recommend a brand. Prices vary. "Paying more is no guarantee that you'll get a quality product, but it does seem to improve your chances," says Dr. Shahani. In other words, it's no bargain if it doesn't contain living acidophilus.

Here's some additional advice from experts to help you choose your supplement.

• Look for a product that contains a mixture of bacteria strains and has a count of at least one billion organisms per capsule.

• Make sure the supplement you buy has been refrigerated prior to purchase, especially if the label recommends it. And keep it in the refrigerator after you buy it, with the lid on tightly, suggests Dr. Brett. Heat, light, humidity, and oxygen can rob supplements of their live bacteria.

• Check the label for an expiration date. If it doesn't have one, don't buy it, advises Dr. Brett.

• If you're ordering by mail, have the product sent overnight or second-day mail, suggests Dr. Shahani.

• Consider enteric-coated capsules, especially for more severe symptoms, says Dr. Brett. The coating allows the supplement to pass through the stomach in its entirety before breaking down in the intestines.

• Some brands of acidophilus contain fructo-oligosaccharides, food components that are intended to increase good bacteria such as acidophilus while reducing bad bacteria. According to Dr. Shahani, however, there's no solid research to back up this claim and justify the extra expense of these supplements.

• Search for products with a strain name that indicates that this specific strain has been researched, including LGG, DDS-1, and NCFM.

amino acids

Thumb through a muscle magazine, and you're likely to see advertisements for amino acid supplements that offer the promise of bigger, stronger muscles.

As it turns out, these claims are more than somewhat exaggerated. The key to a better bod can't be found in any pill. But that doesn't mean that you should forget about amino acids. They play critical roles in our day-to-day lives.

Amino acids are the building blocks of protein. Twenty of them combine to form the 50,000 to 100,000 different proteins in the body. Nine amino acids are classified as essential because your body is unable to produce them and you must get them by eating foods that supply them. They are histidine, isoleucine, leucine, lysine, methionine, phenylalanine, threonine, tryptophan, and valine. Meat, poultry, fish, eggs, milk, cheese, yogurt, and soy are considered complete proteins because they provide us with all nine aminos.

The other 11 amino acids that scientists have studied are considered nonessential. That doesn't mean that they are unnecessary, only that we don't need to get them from foods because most people's bodies can produce them as needed. Our bodies use the essential amino acids to make the nonessential ones—alanine, arginine, asparagine, aspartic acid, cysteine, glutamic acid, glutamine, glycine, proline, serine, and tyrosine.

Just as your right hand is the mirror image of your left, amino acids occur as mirror image forms. The left-hand forms are known as "l" and the right-hand forms are known as "d." You get l-amino acids from food, since they're part of proteins, and they are the ones that are packaged as supplements. If you look at the label of an amino acid supplement and it doesn't indicate "l" or "d," you can't assume it's the "l" form, however. Choose only supplements that are labeled as the "l" form, says Joanne Larsen, R.D., of Nutritional Data Services in Minneapolis, author of *Edmund's Food Ratings for Doctors*.

Amino Activities

Amino acids play several vital roles in keeping us healthy, says James Heffley, Ph.D., director of clinical nutrition for the Nutrition Counseling Service in Austin, Texas. Their main function is to build the protein that gives structure to such body components as skin, membranes, muscles, organs, and bones.

Some amino acids also act as neurotransmitters, the chemicals that ferry information from one nerve cell to another, says Dr. Heffley. Others are precursors of neurotransmitters, which means that they're involved in creating

SUPPLEMENTSNAPSHOT

▶Amino Acids

May help: Heart disease, high blood pressure, low immunity, indigestion, heartburn, diarrhoa, diverticulitis, prostate problems, intermittent claudication, infertility, wound healing, depression, and ADHD.

Good food sources: Meat, poultry, fish, eggs, milk, cheese, yogurt, and soy, and quinoa supply all nine essential amino acids; other good sources are beans, peas, seeds, and nuts.

Cautions and possible side effects: Don't take amino acids without a doctor's guidance. The use of individual amino acids in large doses is considered experimental, and the long-term effects on health are unknown.

High doses of arginine may cause nausea and diarrhea. People who have genital herpes should not take arginine because it may increase herpes outbreaks. Also, don't take arginine and lysine at the same time, as they can interfere with each other.

Cysteine in high doses can cause kidney stones in people who have cystinuria, and it can inactivate insulin, so use caution if you have diabetes. Taking cysteine may deplete zinc and copper, so if you plan to use cysteine or n-acetylcysteine for more than a few weeks, take it with a multi-vitamin/mineral supplement that supplies the Daily Value of these minerals.

Tyrosine and phenylalanine supplements can raise blood pressure to dangerous levels, especially in people taking MAO inhibitors as antidepressants. Do not take phenylalanine if you have phenylketonuria.

the compounds that do the transmitting. Tryptophan, for example, is a precursor of the neurotransmitter serotonin, which in turn is a precursor of melatonin, a hormone that's important in sleep and sensory perception. So, if you don't get enough of the tryptophan that helps produce serotonin, you may end up with a shortage of that neurotransmitter. You may also have some sleep problems because you're short on melatonin.

Amino acids are also the foundation for certain hormones such as insulin, and they help vitamins and minerals do their jobs. Taurine, for example, is used to transport magnesium and potassium from the bloodstream into the cells.

Protein and amino acids are so abundant in the foods we eat that very few people in the United States are deficient. If anything, we consume too much protein, says Larsen.

The only people who might be low in a particular amino acid are those with genetic defects that prevent them from making or using certain amino acids, she says. People with a hereditary condition called phenylketonuria, for example, can't metabolize phenylalanine properly. If they get this amino acid in their food, their bodies can't process it, and if the condition is left untreated, mental retardation and poor muscle coordination can result.

Zooming In on Specifics

Amino acid supplements come in many forms. Some are combinations of many different kinds of amino acids, but you can also get individual supplements.

Since most of us don't have an amino acid deficiency, you may wonder why you would take any supplements at all. In Dr. Heffley's view, it really doesn't make much sense to take a supplement that includes a mixture of amino acids, but it might be a good idea to take a single kind of amino acid, as long as you take it for a limited time with some guidance from a doctor.

Here's why Dr. Heffley makes that distinction. If we get all the protein—and therefore, amino acids—we need from food, there's no reason to take a combination supplement. Our bodies break down these supplements into protein and use them in the same way as they would use protein from soybeans or eggs, he says. "It makes more economic sense to increase the amount of protein in your diet than to buy a mixture of amino acids in a supplement."

It's a different matter, however, when you supplement with individual amino acids that might play very specific roles in the body. Sometimes, people can benefit from these, says Dr. Heffley. "If you take a single amino acid by itself, there's a tendency for it to do its nonprotein functions. You increase the level of that amino acid without competition from other amino acids."

You shouldn't take individual amino acids for more than two to three months at a time, but in his practice, Dr. Heffley has observed that the benefits of taking a single amino acid can persist long after supplementation has ended.

His explanation for the extended benefits of supplementation is based on his own theory that "once you open up pathways by using rather large amounts of amino acids, those pathways will stay open, and the end product will be made even without the extra amino acid—assuming it was what the body needed."

Keep in mind that the long-term effects and safe doses of most amino acids are unknown. Although you'll find supplements on the shelves of drugstores and health food stores, that doesn't mean that it's all right to take large doses for as long as you want.

Individual amino acid supplements should be used only for a specific reason and only under the supervision of a medical professional who's familiar with amino acids, says J. Alexander Bralley, Ph.D., director and CEO of Metametrix Clinical Laboratory in Atlanta.

As for the kinds of supplements to take, Dr. Bralley advises doctors and their patients to stick with amino acids labeled "free-form." These types of amino acids are easily abosrbed into the bloodstream and don't have to be digested, according to Dr. Bralley.

Here is what some of the specific amino acid supplements might be able to do for you, if taken with a doctor's guidance.

Alanine, glutamic acid, and glycine. Some studies have shown that these three amino acids may help relieve the symptoms of one kind of prostate problem in men. Called benign prostatic hyperplasia (BPH) , the problem occurs when the prostate gland swells and presses against one part of the urinary tract, the urethra. BPH is especially prevalent among older men and is characterized by an increased frequency of urination, waking at night to empty the bladder, and a reduced flow of urine. Many amino acids are present in the prostate, but alanine, glutamic acid, and glycine seem to be the ones that can help control BPH symptoms.

Arginine. This supplement is commonly used by body builders who want to put on weight by increasing body mass—but they just might be wasting their time. Although arginine may release a growth hormone, there's little evidence that this action actually improves muscle growth or strength, says Michael Janson, M.D., president of the American College for Advancement in Medicine, based in Laguna Hills, California, and author of *The Vitamin Revolution in Health Care.*

This nonessential amino acid is involved in nitric oxide production, and it may be this action that makes it helpful to our bodies. Nitric oxide relaxes the muscles of the arterial walls and helps to open up the arteries, says Dr. Janson. Studies suggest that arginine supplements may help with high blood pressure and coronary heart disease. It is also thought to help boost immunity and speed wound healing.

Branched-chain amino acids (BCAAs). This is a group that includes three essential amino acids—leucine, isoleucine, and valine—branched-chain amino acids are a favorite with body builders and other athletes. Dr. Bralley says they may improve performance and help prevent the muscle breakdown that occurs during endurance training.

BCAAs are found mostly in muscle, and they break down and are used up for energy during prolonged exercise. If there isn't a readily available pool of amino acids to draw upon, the protein synthesis doesn't remake muscle as quickly and efficiently. BCAAs help to boost the muscle-building process. "From what we've seen, branched-chain amino acids do tend to conserve muscle mass," says Dr. Bralley.

Carnitine. Carnitine is an amino acid made in the liver from two other amino acid building blocks—lysine and methionine. It's not one of the 20 amino acids that are used in protein synthesis, says Dr. Bralley, but it helps transport fat into the mitochondria within cells, where fat is burned for energy.

Carnitine has been found to lower serum cholesterol and triglycerides, build muscle tissue, and increase stamina. A deficiency may cause muscle weakness, confusion, or angina. A deficiency can also lead to an increase of fats in your bloodstream, especially a harmful type called triglycerides. Your doctor can spot a deficiency of carnitine with a blood or urine test.

Studies have shown that l-carnitine increases exercise capacity in people with some kinds of artery disease, and improves muscle function and exercise capacity in people with kidney disease. Acetyl-l-carnitine, a closely related amino acid, has been found to slow memory loss. A third form, d-carnitine, is synthetic and does not have any beneficial effect in the body. There is no reason to take d-carnitine or dl-carnitine.

Cysteine. Cysteine is needed to make another amino acid, taurine, which is a good anti-inflammatory, says Dr. Bralley. According to studies, cysteine can remove heavy metal toxins from the body, including mercury, cadmium, lead, and arsenic.

In the form of n-acetylcysteine, cysteine has been used to stimulate the synthesis of another amino acid, glutathione. Glutathione has antioxidant properties, so it helps to block free radicals, the free-roaming unstable molecules that harm cells.

N-acetylcysteine may also help combat the side effects of chemotherapy and radiation therapy as well as help to clear mucus out of the lungs of smokers and cystic fibrosis patients.

Glutamine. Under normal circumstances, glutamine is not considered an essential amino acid, but some people do need supplements in certain situations, says Dr. Heffley. Cancer cells like an acidic environment, and glutamine helps to shift the body chemistry in the other direction—that is, creating a less acidic, more alkaline environment. This happens even when cancer is present.

Glutamine has also been used for its calming effects. Once in the body, it's made into gamma-aminobutyric acid (GABA), a neurotransmitter in the central nervous system. But the calming effect is not universal. In fact, Dr. Heffley says that in 1 person in 10, glutamine can act as a stimulant. That's because it can also be made into glutamic acid, which sends signals that excite the nerves rather than calming them. There's no real danger, however, even if you happen to experience stimulating effects from glutamine, he adds. The worst that can happen is a restless night's sleep.

Glutamine is also used for wound healing, to repair the small intestine, to boost depressed immunity, and to break addictions to caffeine and other stimulants. It may also help treat diarrhea that's caused by gluten intolerance, Crohn's disease, AIDS, and other conditions, adds Larsen. If you take it for this purpose, you'll know within three days if it's working.

Lysine. This essential amino acid can decrease outbreaks of the herpes simplex virus, which is responsible for cold sores and genital herpes. With either kind of outbreak, a lysine supplement can help the infection heal more quickly.

If you're low in lysine, you might end up with a deficiency of carnitine.

A lysine deficiency may also lead to calcium loss, which could increase your risk of developing osteoporosis. Lysine deficiencies occur more often in people who do not consume any animal products than in those who do, says Dr. Heffley. The best way to tell if you are lysine deficient is to have your doctor perform a urine or blood test.

Lysine competes with arginine for absorption and use by the body, so if you're taking lysine, you'll get less-than-optimal results from arginine, and vice versa.

Phenylalanine and tyrosine. Phenylalanine is an essential amino acid that is used to make another amino acid, tyrosine. Tyrosine in turn is transformed into three kinds of neurotransmitters, the nerve-related chemicals that help messages travel through your body. Since phenylalanine and tyrosine have an energizing effect, studies suggest that they are useful in treating depression and lethargy.

There's a synthetic form of phenylalanine called d-phenylalanine. It's not used by the body in the same way that the naturally occurring l-form is, but it may be beneficial as a treatment for chronic pain, especially lower back pain and dental pain.

A combined form, called dl-phenylalanine, however, does have some separate benefits. Some studies suggest that it may be useful in treating the chronic pain of osteoarthritis and rheumatoid arthritis, lower back pain, menstrual cramps, and migraine, among other conditions. It's thought that it blocks certain enzymes in the central nervous system that are responsible for breaking down the brain's own painkillers. If it interferes with those enzymes, the theory is that the natural painkillers in your brain will be free to do their work of suppressing pain.

Taurine. This amino acid is important for the normal functioning of the heart, brain, gallbladder, eyes, and vascular system. It's the most abundant free amino acid found in the heart. In Japan, it's widely used to treat heart disease.

In the brain, taurine acts as a neurotransmitter that, among other things, inhibits anxiety. Preliminary trials suggest that it may be useful in treating some forms of epilepsy.

astragalus

Chinese folks are as likely as Americans to have soup or stew simmering on the stovetop for the evening meal. Unlike beef stew or tomato soup, though, that Chinese broth probably contains a medicinal element—a few sticks or slices of astragalus root to keep away the colds and flu that come with the winter season.

Astragalus is a member of the pea family whose name was derived from an ancient Greek word meaning "ankle bone." These bones were once used as dice, and it's thought that the name originated because the rattling seed pods of the Mediterranean variety of the plant sounded like rolling dice.

Western herbalists classify astragalus as a tonic herb, meaning that it helps strengthen the body return to a condition of normal functioning. In China, this popular herb is believed to strengthen *chi*, the body's defensive energy that protects against invading pathogens such as bacteria and viruses.

The root is the medicinal part of the plant, a perennial that can grow to about two feet tall. There are 2,000 species of astragalus worldwide—400 of them in North America—but the medicinal variety is found only in central and western Asia. Also known as *huang qi*, it was used in China for at least 2,000 years before European botanists wrote about its medicinal qualities in the 1700s.

"For the Chinese, astragalus is really a classic healing herb. It's thought to have a warm tonic action on chi, the protective energy," says Jennifer Brett, N.D., a naturopathic doctor at the Wilton Naturopathic Center in Stratford, Connecticut. "A lot of elderly people make it a part of their diets."

Defense, Defense

In Western terms, strengthening chi translates to bolstering the immune system, and astragalus appears to have a positive effect on resistance to diseases and infections, says Dr. Brett. It's like food or nourishment for your immune system, essentially giving it more vitality and "muscle" so it can ward off disease on its own. Some studies in China have shown that it can prevent or shorten the duration of colds.

Chinese doctors usually mix this chi tonic with other herbs, depending on a person's complaint. It's been used to combat shortness of breath, weakness, night sweats, respiratory diseases, lingering diarrhea, uterine and rectal prolapse, boils and sores, and other maladies, but its main use is to make the body's defenses a little tougher, says Dr. Brett.

"It's an herb that helps you cope with the physical and emotional stress that can make you more susceptible to getting sick," she says. "It doesn't so much stimulate the body as tone it."

Arming the Body

Astragalus has been used for centuries in fu-zheng therapy, an herbal treatment used by practitioners of Traditional Chinese Medicine to promote or bolster the immune system. In trying to strengthen their patients' natural defense mechanisms, doctors of oriental medicine have even begun to use fu-zheng therapy to help treat cancer patients. They use astragalus to boost immune function during and after radiation or chemotherapy treatments.

When cancer invades your body, your immune system naturally weakens. In the advanced stages of the disease or after rounds of chemotherapy or radiation—which are lifesaving but very toxic treatments—your immune system can be devastated. Shamelessly opportunistic,

---

SUPPLEMENTSNAPSHOT

▶Astragalus

Botanical name: *Astragalus membranaceus;* also known as *huang qi.*

May help: Low immunity due to disease, including cancer; fibromyalgia; stress; chronic fatigue syndrome; and poor appetite. Has been used in Traditional Chinese Medicine to treat shortness of breath, weakness, colds and flu, night sweats, respiratory diseases, lingering diarrhea, uterine and rectal prolapse, boils, and sores.

Origin: Medicinal species grows only in Asia.

Cautions and possible side effects: Generally regarded as safe.

a routine cold can turn into a deadly infection.

The effectiveness of astragalus and the fu-zheng treatment was put to the test in a study of cancer patients undertaken at the M.D. Anderson Cancer Center in Houston in the early 1980s. After giving a specially prepared astragalus extract to 19 cancer patients and 15 healthy people, doctors found that the treatment restored immune system functioning in the majority of the patients. In some cases, it made the cancer patients' immune systems resemble those of the healthy subjects. The researchers concluded that astragalus contains a potent immune stimulant.

"Those kinds of results really fit with the traditional use of astragalus," says Steven Dentali, Ph.D., a natural products chemist with Dentali Associates in Troutdale, Oregon, and a member of the advisory board of the American Botanical Council. "It's an herb that supports the immune system."

Down to the Marrow

Astragalus appears to influence the bone marrow, where immune cells are manufactured, says Dr. Dentali. Compounds called polysaccharides seem to stimulate white blood cell production and increase the activity of killer T cells, the body's defenders that hunt down and destroy invaders.

Astragalus also increases the production of interferon, a natural protein that adheres to the surfaces of cells and stimulates production of other proteins that prevent viral infection. In other words, it makes your cells more thick-skinned so viruses have a harder time getting in.

Dr. Brett recommends astragalus—usually in combination with other herbs—to people who feel run-down or stressed, have poor appetites, or can't shake colds. "It's an energy tonic that can do a lot to increase your stamina," she says.

Astragalus can also be useful if you're making a lot of trips to the bathroom at night. Dr. Brett sometimes recommends it for its diuretic effect. It can temporarily increase urination and clean out the urinary tract, she notes, so if you take it well before bedtime, the diuretic effect kicks in before the lights go out. "The astragalus tends to normalize urination so you don't have to get up so often," she explains.

In health food stores, you'll probably find bins of sliced and whole root, sometimes labeled as huang-qi. Either form is good for a tea. You can also take a tincture or capsule. It can be cooked into soups and stews where it is removed before eating the dish.

vitamin B₆

Make up a list of health problems that each vitamin or mineral is supposed to help, and there's a good chance that the list for vitamin B_6 will be the longest. This essential B vitamin has been recommended for everything from kidney stones and morning sickness to diabetes and PMS.

While it may actually help some of these conditions, there's just not enough scientific evidence yet to nail down many of its benefits, says James Leklem, Ph.D., professor of nutrition and food management at Oregon State University in Corvallis.

Like other vitamins and minerals, B_6 works with enzymes, the chemical spark plugs that start reactions in the body. It is an essential part of more than 100 enzymes that are involved in the production of energy and protein. B_6 has to be on hand when your body breaks down stored sugar for energy, when it creates the building blocks that will become protein, and when it makes the brain and nervous system of a developing fetus. Research also suggests that B_6 can help reduce the risk of heart disease and complications of diabetes.

Generating Energy

If we eat more food than we need for immediate energy, some of the excess calories are converted to a form of glucose (blood sugar) called glycogen, which is stored in the liver and muscles. When blood sugar drops, glycogen is broken down into glucose and used for fuel. The enzyme that does this requires B_6.

People start to use glycogen for energy if they've been exercising for an hour or longer or if they're dieting to lose weight. "But you'd have to be extremely deficient in vitamin B_6 to have a problem breaking down glycogen," Dr. Leklem says. "Most people just don't have this problem."

Vitamin B_6 also helps link the molecules that make up certain amino acids, Dr. Leklem explains. Strung together like pearls, amino acids are

68

the "bits" that make proteins. So B$_6$ indirectly aids protein production in the body.

This vitamin also helps link the molecules of nucleic acids, which make up our cells' genetic material. Low B$_6$ levels can slow down amino acid or nucleic acid production enough to lead to impaired immunity. In extreme cases, the deficiency can lead to a rare condition called sideroblastic anemia, Dr. Leklem says.

Good for the Heart and Brain

Our bodies need vitamin B$_6$, along with vitamin B$_{12}$ and folic acid, to be able to break down a potentially toxic amino acid by-product called homocysteine. "High levels of homocysteine have been associated with in-

---

SUPPLEMENT SNAPSHOT

▶ Vitamin B$_6$

Also known as: Pyridoxine.

May help: Morning sickness, PMS, menstrual problems, binge-eating disorder, depression, canker sores, endometriosis, diabetes, angina, heart disease, HIV, and kidney stones. With vitamins B$_{12}$ and folic acid, can also lower blood levels of homocysteine to reduce risk of heart attack and prevent intermittent claudication, phlebitis, Alzheimer's disease, angina, and high blood pressure.

Daily Value: 2 milligrams.

Special instructions: If you're supplementing with 50 milligrams or more, take in divided doses two or three times a day.

Who's at risk for deficiency: Alcoholics, elderly people with poor diets, people taking drugs that interfere with B$_6$ absorption, and people with intestinal absorption problems.

Good food sources: Chicken, fish, pork, and eggs; spinach, broccoli, tomato juice, bananas, watermelon, acorn squash, and fortified cornflakes are good nonmeat sources.

Cautions and possible side effects: Doses of 100 milligrams a day or more for several months may cause nerve damage.

creased risk of heart disease and stroke," says Alan Gaby, M.D., currently a specialist in nutrition and preventive medicine in Pikesville, Maryland. Compared with B_{12} and folic acid, however, B_6 seems to play a lesser role, according to Dr. Gaby. "Only about 15 percent of people with high homocysteine levels respond to B_6," he says.

A study from the Harvard School of Public Health showed that women who got at least 3 milligrams a day of B_6 had half the risk of having heart attacks compared with women who got 1.5 milligrams. This is still more than a woman's average daily intake of B_6, which is about 1.2 milligrams.

Vitamin B_6 also helps out neurotransmitters, the chemicals that our nervous systems produce in order to send out messages. It is needed to make an impressive array of neurotransmitters that help to activate and speed up communication among nerve cells. These include serotonin, taurine, dopamine, norepinephrine, and histamine.

"Unfortunately, there's not much research to tell us what all this may mean in terms of actual mental performance," Dr. Gaby says. But there is some. Higher blood concentrations of B_6 were associated with better performance on two tests of memory in a study by researchers at Tufts University in Boston.

Helping Hormones and Blood Sugar

Vitamin B_6 plays a role in maintaining normal hormone balance. When B_6 levels are low, hormones may have a stronger-than-normal action on specific cells or organs, Dr. Leklem says. In animals, the vitamin inhibits the way a hormone hooks up or binds within a cell, which is a step in the cell's activation. "In humans, however, we don't know for sure how it works," Dr. Leklem says.

Still, B_6 is known to help regulate a number of specific hormones, including estrogen, progesterone, androgens (male hormones), and glucocorticoid (a stress hormone.) This may be a reason that the vitamin sometimes seems to be an effective treatment for PMS and morning sickness, says Dr. Leklem.

For different reasons, vitamin B_6 may also be able to help people who have diabetes. One result of this disease is that blood sugar has the ability to stick to proteins, a process called glycosylation. "It's fairly well accepted that glycosylation of proteins is one of the things that causes the complications of diabetes, such as kidney and nerve damage and cataracts," Dr. Gaby says.

In a study at Yale University, researchers found that people with diabetes got some benefits from taking a B$_6$ supplement because of its apparent effect on glycosylation. When they took 50 milligrams of B$_6$ three times a day for six weeks, the participants had significant drops in the glycosylation of hemoglobin, a protein found in red blood cells.

Vitamin B$_6$ deficiency has been linked to glucose intolerance, a condition in which blood sugar rises sharply after eating. It has also been implicated in impaired secretion of insulin and glucagon, both hormones that are essential in regulating blood sugar levels.

Blood levels of B$_6$ are low in 20 to 25 percent of people with diabetes, and in some, levels fall abruptly when they are given sugar, Dr. Leklem says. "We don't know why this happens, but we do know that there are several good reasons that people with diabetes should make sure they are getting enough B$_6$. Preventing diabetes-related organ damage is apparently one of them."

Interactions with Others

Vitamin B$_6$ interacts with magnesium, an essential mineral used in more than 300 biochemical reactions in the body. In some cases, both the vitamin and the mineral are needed to activate the enzymes that start biochemical reactions such as breaking down sugar for energy. Some research also suggests that B$_6$ depends on magnesium to help it get inside cells, where it can do its work. "One thing we do know is that an extremely low intake of magnesium will compromise the body's ability to use B$_6$ properly," Dr. Leklem says.

The vitamin also interacts with oxalate, a by-product of metabolism that plays an important role in the formation of kidney stones.

Some people who develop kidney stones have a genetic abnormality that leads to a buildup of oxalate, and high concentrations in the kidneys cause it to form stones. Taking B$_6$ at doses of 10 to 50 milligrams a day can help, Dr. Gaby says. "And taking magnesium along with the B$_6$ is probably warranted," he adds. In his view, the magnesium helps prevent oxalate from crystallizing into stones. Your doctor should determine whether taking B$_6$ and magnesium would be beneficial if you've been diagnosed with kidney stones.

The Bottom Line

The more protein you eat, the more vitamin B_6 you need, because this vitamin assists in protein metabolism. Some protein foods contain good amounts of B_6, but you can't count on all protein-rich foods as super suppliers. Good sources include meats, fish, poultry, shellfish, legumes, fruits, egg yolks, whole grains, and leafy green vegetables. Dairy products, on the other hand, are relatively poor sources, and processed luncheon meats like sliced ham or turkey lose 50 to 70 percent of their B_6 in processing.

Alcoholics are most likely to be deficient, because alcohol actually promotes the destruction of B_6 and its loss from the body. If you're elderly and don't eat well for any reason, you're more likely than a younger person to have a deficiency. Others who might have a problem are people with absorption problems such as celiac disease and those who take drugs that interfere with the body's use of B_6.

More than 40 drugs can compromise absorption, including isoniazid (Laniazid, Nydrazid), a tuberculosis drug, and penicillamine (Cuprimine, Depen), used to treat Wilson's disease and rheumatoid arthritis and to prevent kidney stones. "Birth control pills used to be on the list of possible B_6 antagonists, but low-estrogen pills don't cause this problem," Dr. Leklem says.

People who are short on B_6 are likely to be weak and irritable and have trouble sleeping. They may also develop depression, impaired glucose tolerance, convulsions, cracking of the lips and tongue, and skin problems such as seborrhea or eczema.

vitamin B₁₂

Imagine having a disease that will very likely kill you—unless you can somehow choke down ⅔ pound of raw liver a day. Awful? Yes. But that was once the cure offered to people with pernicious anemia.

The researchers who discovered this cure won the Nobel Prize for medicine in 1934. It wasn't until 1948 that researchers isolated from raw liver the small red crystals of the nutrient that we now call vitamin B_{12}.

Unless you're a vegan (strict vegetarian), pernicious anemia is not often due to a lack of this essential vitamin. It's actually a problem with absorption. B_{12} differs from other vitamins in that before it can be absorbed into the cells lining the intestines, it has to hook up with a protein called intrinsic factor that is secreted as part of the stomach's digestive juices.

Some people, especially when they're older and on low-protein diets, don't make enough intrinsic factor to absorb all the B_{12} they need. Since intrinsic factor is provided by the body, not by food, when the body doesn't make enough, we can be at risk for B_{12}-related health risks.

Only about 1 percent of people develop the classic symptoms of B_{12} deficiency—anemia and nerve damage. About 30 percent of older people show signs of deficiency when their blood is tested, says Robert Allen, M.D., professor of medicine and biochemistry and director of hematology at the University of Colorado Health Sciences Center in Denver.

Even a low-level deficiency can have negative health effects. People may have depression, forgetfulness, trouble walking, and even incontinence. Sometimes, though, these are problems of old age rather than an outcome of vitamin deficiency. That's why proper testing is so important.

B_{12} Basics

This vitamin is essential to every cell in your body. It must be on hand for DNA synthesis, the process by which your body makes the genetic material that comprises the cell nucleus. Vitamin B_{12} is far more than a cheerleader in this process. It rolls up its sleeves and goes to work, helping to make the nucleic acids that are strung together like pearls to form DNA, the genetic e-mail system. It also helps make RNA, the copy of DNA that's sent along to each cell.

When cells are rapidly dividing, as they do during growth and development, more B_{12} is needed for this process, according to John Pinto, Ph.D., associate professor of biochemistry at Weill Medical College of Cornell University and director of the nutrition research laboratory at Memorial Sloan-Kettering Cancer Center, both in New York City. Extra B_{12} is also necessary in areas where cells normally have rapid turnover, such as the intestines and blood, he says.

When B_{12} is in short supply, DNA and RNA synthesis slows, and cells can no longer divide and multiply. This can show up in several ways. In the

SUPPLEMENT SNAPSHOT

▶Vitamin B$_{12}$

Also known as: Cobalamin, cyanocobalamin, hydroxocobalamin, and methyl cobalamin

May help: Pernicious anemia and nerve problems related to B_{12} deficiency; sometimes used for shingles, multiple sclerosis, canker sores, diabetes, depression, and binge-eating disorder and to help delay progression of HIV to AIDS. With vitamins B_6 and folic acid, can lower blood levels of homocysteine to reduce risk of heart attack and prevent intermittent claudication, phlebitis, Alzheimer's disease, angina, and high blood pressure.

Daily Value: 6 micrograms.

Special instructions: People with B_{12} deficiencies might not be able to rely on oral supplements and should see a doctor, who may recommend B_{12} injections as well as other supplementation.

Who's at risk for deficiency: People age 60 or older who have a condition that causes low stomach acid, people with problems related to intrinsic factor, people with Crohn's disease, strict vegetarians, and breastfed babies of strict vegetarians.

Good food sources: Cooked oysters and clams and all meats.

Cautions and possible side effects: Generally regarded as safe.

blood, it can mean anemia—a shortage of red blood cells—since the cells in the bone marrow that make red blood cells normally crank them out at the rate of at least 200 million a minute. In the intestines, it can mean absorption problems that create a domino effect, accelerating nutrient deficiencies as cells are deprived of the supplies that are delivered like groceries by the red blood cells.

In some places in the body, such as the cervix and intestines, a shortage of vitamin B$_{12}$ can begin to interfere with cell growth; the resulting cell abnormalities can lead to cancer. Your ability to fight infection may slow down because your body can't crank out enough infection-fighting white blood cells. In fact, one study showed that people with HIV, the virus that causes AIDS, were able to hold off full-blown AIDS longer if they had high levels of B$_{12}$. "The bottom line is, how fast can your system adapt to an adverse situation, such as infection, by making more DNA?" Dr. Pinto says. "When B$_{12}$ is in short supply, your body slows down and can't defend itself as well."

Friend of Folic

Vitamin B$_{12}$ works hand in hand with folic acid, which also helps to make DNA. One form of folic acid circulates throughout the body. When B$_{12}$ removes a piece of the molecule from this circulating form, the folic acid becomes available for other reactions. As it goes about its business, B$_{12}$ uses the stolen piece of molecule for some of its own important functions.

Since B$_{12}$ and folic acid are so closely linked, a deficiency of one can leave the other in cold storage. You may be getting plenty of folate (the food form of folic acid) in your diet, for instance, but if you're coming up short on B$_{12}$, the folate stays inside cells, trapped in its inactive form.

The Amino Acid Shuffle

Vitamin B$_{12}$ and folic acid are also necessary for amino acid synthesis, meaning that they need to be there when your body sends the wrecking ball up against the proteins in food and then reassembles those proteins to create new structures.

This demolition and reconstruction work is going on all the time. If your body wants to take those scrambled eggs you had this morning and turn them into useful energy and hearty body cells, B$_{12}$ and folic acid have

Should You Have a B$_{12}$ Test?

Doctors are usually pretty good about checking blood levels of B$_{12}$ when a patient shows signs of anemia or severe nerve damage, but sometimes the early signs of deficiency can escape a doctor's notice. Among the less noticeable symptoms of vitamin B$_{12}$ deficiency are numbness and tingling in the feet or hands, loss of balance, and memory loss or disorientation.

"Doctors should be testing people when they have these symptoms," says Robert Allen, M.D., professor of medicine and biochemistry and director of hematology at the University of Colorado Health Sciences Center in Denver. "And if B$_{12}$ is in the low-normal range, they should do a follow-up test that measures two additional things, methylmalonic acid and homocysteine. This test is very useful because it helps us accurately diagnose a deficiency and distinguish between a deficiency of B$_{12}$ and one of folic acid.

"Too many doctors still follow the old textbook rule from 15 years ago," Dr. Allen says. "They don't give their patients B$_{12}$ injections unless their blood levels are below 100, and that's clearly a mistake. It is now clear that many people who have levels in the 200- to 300-range require treatment or further evaluation."

to be on hand to do their part. They help to ensure that the protein parts—amino acids—are in the proper amounts to make new proteins.

As the redevelopment authority inside your body, B$_{12}$ can make trouble for your heart if it goes on strike. Along with folic acid and B$_6$, it is needed to break down an amino acid by-product called homocysteine. When you don't have enough, blood levels of homocysteine rise, "and high levels of homocysteine seem to increase your risk for heart disease and stroke even more than high cholesterol," Dr. Pinto says.

Homocysteine damages the cells lining the blood vessels, creating rough spots that attract cholesterol deposits and issue invitations for blood to start clotting. Exactly how much of the three B vitamins you need to prevent this problem isn't known. In one study where people received daily doses of 400 micrograms of B$_{12}$, 1 milligram of folic acid, and 10 milligrams of B$_6$, homocysteine levels dropped significantly.

So far, researchers have found that high levels of homocysteine are associated with heart disease and that B vitamins can help lower homocysteine levels. They are trying to complete the circle by showing that lowering homocysteine levels with B vitamins can also lower heart disease risk, says Dr. Allen.

Nerves of Steel

Vitamin B$_{12}$ also maintains the fatty sheath, called myelin, that surrounds and protects nerve fibers and promotes their normal growth, Dr. Pinto says. Like insulation around copper wires, this sheath allows your radiating network of nerves to send their electrical messages without short-circuiting. When B$_{12}$ is missing, the myelin sheath breaks down, which eventually leads to nerve damage.

Researchers used to think that since B$_{12}$ was needed to put together the fatty acids that make up the myelin sheath, a fatty acid problem caused nerve damage. "Now it looks more like this, too, is a problem with high homocysteine levels," Dr. Pinto says. "Homocysteine seems to be directly toxic to nerve cells."

This may partly explain the symptoms of B$_{12}$ deficiency—numbness, tingling feet or hands, trouble walking, memory loss, and personality and mood changes. It doesn't explain everything, though, since only about one-third of B$_{12}$-deficient people develop these symptoms, Dr. Allen says. "My feeling is that these symptoms are caused by a combination of deficiency and some environmental or genetic factor."

bee pollen

Whoever came up with the expression "busy as a bee" sure knew what they were talking about. This amazing insect makes an average of 10 pollen runs a day, flying from hive to flower and flower to hive as it gathers its bounty. In good weather, the combined efforts of a colony of worker bees can result in as many as 54,000 pollen loads a day.

Bee pollen is the male reproductive part of a flower that the worker bees collect. They pack the microscopically fine powder into granules by adding nectar or honey from their honey sacs, then they take it back to the hive, where they add an enzyme to prevent germination and metabolize it for food.

Pollen supplies all the nutrients a bee needs for growth and development. Without an adequate supply of pollen, a colony of bees would perish. Its nutrient content is about 24 percent protein, 27 percent carbohydrates (mainly the natural sugars fructose and glucose), and about 5 percent fat. It contains many minerals, including remarkably high levels of iron, zinc, manganese, and copper as well as potassium, calcium, and magnesium. It's also rich in most of the B vitamins and carotenes, the precursors of vitamin A.

The question is whether what's good for bees is also good for humans. Despite a glaring lack of scientific evidence, many people take bee pollen supplements for a range of health problems, including allergies, low energy, and prostate disease. It's also used to combat aging, indigestion, sore throat, acne, sexual problems, fatigue, and depression.

The Buzz about It

Bee pollen does appear to be helpful for some people with allergies, says Theodore Cherbuliez, M.D., a physician in Scarsdale, New York, and president of the American Apitherapy Society, a nonprofit organization that advances the investigation of the healing use of products from the beehive. But why would something like pollen, which causes allergies in some people, be used to treat those very same allergics? The reasoning is similar to what's used for immunization: Take a small dose of what ails you, and your body builds up its defenses to fight it off.

There are two types of pollen, says Dr. Cherbuliez: pollen carried by the wind, and pollen carried by insects. "If you take small doses of pollen carried by insects—for example, bee pollen—it builds up your immunity and protects you from having a reaction when you breathe airborne pollen," he says.

Anyone who takes bee pollen should do so with caution, because it can cause adverse allergic reactions in some people. In rare cases, it can cause a life-threatening anaphylactic reaction in which the throat swells shut and inhibits breathing. Do not take bee pollen if you have a history of anaphylactic reactions, says Steve Nenninger, N.D., a naturopathic doctor in New York City.

SUPPLEMENT SNAPSHOT

▶ Bee Pollen

May help: Allergies, asthma, indigestion, sore throat, acne, sexual problems, fatigue, and depression. May increase energy and stamina, promote prostate health, and possibly slow aging.

Special instructions: Take with meals. Begin with three pollen granules (they're small, but you can separate them with your fingernail) and double the dose each day until you're taking a teaspoon. If you have no adverse reaction, you can take pollen in other forms—capsules, tablets, powder, or liquid.

Cautions and possible side effects: Rarely, may cause life-threatening anaphylactic shock in sensitive people; do not take if you have a history of anaphylactic reactions. May cause stomach pain, diarrhea, irritation and itching in the mouth and throat, and less commonly, headache, fatigue, asthma attacks and general feelings of poor health. If you have asthma or diabetes, check with your doctor before taking. Bee pollen contains allergens that can worsen asthma, and it contains natural sugars.

Another reason that people take bee pollen supplements is to improve physical stamina. In fact, both ancient and modern Olympians have used it for energy, says Dr. Nenninger.

Collecting Pollen

Bee pollen supplements are available as capsules, tablets, granules, powder, and liquids. Extracts of bee pollen are also ingredients in facial and hand creams and lotions. Look for supplements free of preservatives, artificial colors, and artificial flavors, says Dr. Nenninger.

Dr. Cherbuliez, who has kept up to 30 hives of his own, prefers granules over other commercial preparations because they are closest to the original product from the hive. "As with all natural products, I believe that the less you touch it, the less you damage it. That's why I steer clear of pollen that has been pressed into tablets or otherwise modified or mixed with things like honey," he says.

If you decide to buy pollen granules, select the ones with the widest range of colors, which reflects a variety of plant sources and therefore nutrients.

Because bee pollen is not readily digestible, Dr. Cherbuliez suggests soaking pollen granules for 12 hours in water or orange juice to "crack" the shells of the individual grains of pollen. Without soaking, only 2 to 7 percent of the pollen is absorbed by the digestive system, he says. After soaking, as much as 90 percent may be absorbed.

Whatever form you prefer, Dr. Cherbuliez suggests contacting the producer to make sure that the pollen comes from healthy, unstressed colonies that are located away from fields contaminated with pesticides. Beekeepers typically collect pollen by setting traps outside the colony to remove some of the pollen from the hind legs of the worker bees. Then debris, insect fragments, and floral parts are manually removed before the pollen is made available for human consumption.

Some commercial supplements contain pollen collected directly from flowers, so check the label before you buy the product to make sure that you are getting bee pollen.

bee propolis

Whenever we go to work, make a trip to the supermarket, or just step outside to smell the roses, we risk picking up germs and bringing them back to the nest. It's darn near impossible to avoid.

The same goes for bees. As tens of thousands of bees traipse in and out of the hive each day, they pick up germs along the way and take them back to the colony. Thanks to a sticky brown substance called propolis, however, bees keep the insides of their hives germ-free.

Bee propolis is the resin that bees collect from the buds and wounds of trees and other plants and mix with beeswax. In warm weather, propolis is sticky and soft and can be used to fill holes or spread over surfaces like a shellac. In cool weather, the propolis hardens and becomes brittle. The bees use it to caulk, seal, line, and strengthen the hive, but they also use it to ward off contamination and germs in the hive. That's because propolis, also known as Russian penicillin, has antibacterial properties.

It's this ability to fight bacteria that makes it an intriguing supplement for humans. The use of propolis as medicine dates back to the time of Aristotle, about 350 B.C.

The Greeks used propolis for abscesses, while the Assyrians used it to heal wounds and tumors, according to Steve Nenninger, N.D., a naturopathic doctor in New York City.

The Egyptians used it for mummification—and so do bees, says Theodore Cherbuliez, M.D., a physician in Scarsdale, New York, and president of the American Apitherapy Society, a nonprofit organization that advances the investigation of the healing use of products from the beehive. If a mouse crawls into the hive for warmth in the winter, bees will sting it to death. Then, since they can't physically remove the mouse, they will mummify it with propolis to protect the health of the hive. "Imagine the inside of a beehive, says Dr. Cherbuliez. "It's hot, humid, and an ideal milieu to grow bacteria on that dead mouse. Propolis prevents this from happening."

Proponents today use propolis to treat a variety of illnesses, including colds, flu, and sore throats; skin problems; wounds and bruises; stomach ulcers; burns; hemorrhoids; gum disease; high blood pressure; bad breath; and tonsillitis. They also promote it for boosting immunity. But even the strongest supporters rely on stories of healing, rather than on statistical studies, when they claim that it's a nutritional supplement. No carefully controlled studies exist to back these claims.

Stoked-Up Sticky Stuff

There are more than 300 components in propolis, including bioflavonoids, says Dr. Cherbuliez. Because propolis comes from a variety of plants, the amount and type of these components can vary by season and region.

Collecting propolis for human use is an arduous task. To get the purest product, beekeepers place small inserts into the hives. To bees, the inserts look like cracks. Thinking that their hive needs repair, the bees fill the inserts with propolis. Propolis can also be scraped out of the hive, but this yields an inferior product that may contain unwanted by-products.

Bee propolis is available in tablets, throat lozenges, chewable tablets with vitamin C, cough syrup, toothpaste, mouthwash, skin lotions, lipstick, throat spray, salve, and tincture. It's best to buy propolis from a supplement manufacturer that specializes in bee products.

SUPPLEMENTSNAPSHOT

▶Bee Propolis

May help: Wounds, infections, colds, sore throats, skin problems, stomach ulcers, burns, hemorrhoids, gum disease, bad breath, and tonsillitis.

Special instructions: Take with food.

Cautions and possible side effects: Do not take if you have asthma; it contains allergens that can worsen asthma. May also cause a rash when handled.

beta-carotene and vitamin A

Carrots. Squash. Broccoli. Kale. Orange and yellow vegetables. Dark leafy greens. They all contain beta-carotene.

Liver. Milk. Eggs. They all contain vitamin A.

At first glance, these two sources of nutrients seem far, far apart. One source is the plant world, the other is all animal. Once the beta-carotene from plant sources gets inside the body, however, it undergoes a transformation. Through a number of chemical processes, it can be converted into vitamin A. Not only that, but once the transformation is complete and the body has all the vitamin A it can use, any excess beta-carotene goes on to do some other good works.

As for the supplement forms of these nutrients, they're often separate, but not equal. The problem is that the pure form of vitamin A, called preformed vitamin A, can create a number of nasty toxic effects if you take too much of it. Although beta-carotene isn't without its problems, low doses may be taken in supplement form.

The best source of vitamin A is a beta-carotene supplement or a multivitamin that contains a nontoxic amount of vitamin A along with an ample amount of beta-carotene. Both are readily available in drugstores and health food stores. And here's why you might want to pick some up—along with carrots, squash, broccoli, and dark green, leafy vegetables.

All the Roles of A

Vitamin A plays vital roles throughout the body. In our eyes, it helps maintain a crystal-clear outer window, the cornea. Without enough vitamin A, the cornea clouds over. "At the back of the eye, in the retina, vitamin A is part of the pigment that reacts chemically when struck by light and helps create the nerve impulse that goes to the brain and creates a visual message," says James Allen Olson, Ph.D., professor of biochemistry and director of the vitamin A research group at Iowa State University in Ames. For this reason, vitamin A can help with the condition known as night blindness.

Without adequate vitamin A, your eyes recover very slowly after flashes of bright light at night, or you're unable to see in dim light. In Indonesia, where vitamin A deficiency is common, this condition is called chicken eyes because chickens can't see at night and go to sleep when the sun goes down.

SUPPLEMENT SNAPSHOT

▶ Beta-Carotene and Vitamin A

May help: Cancer of the lung, stomach, esophagus, mouth, cervix, and colon; angina; genital herpes; colds and flu; osteoarthritis; and low immunity in people with HIV.

Daily Value: Beta-carotene—no DV; vitamin A—5,000 international units (IU), or 1,500 retinol equivalents (RE).

Special instructions: For maximum absorption, take supplements with meals that contain some fat. Do not take with meals or supplements that contain large amounts of pectin, a type of soluble fiber found in citrus fruits.

Who's at risk for deficiency: Cigarette smokers, alcoholics, and people who eat fewer than three servings a day of fruits or vegetables.

Good food sources: Beta-carotene—dark green, leafy vegetables, orange and yellow vegetables, and yellow fruits. (One large carrot—one of the best food sources—has about 10,600 IU.) Vitamin A—fortified milk and milk products, such as cheese, cream, and butter, and fortified margarine.

Cautions and possible side effects: Avoid taking more than 25,000 IU of beta-carotene as supplements. There is evidence that it causes lung cancer in smokers taking 50,000 IU in supplement form.

Do not take preformed vitamin A supplements unless you are under a doctor's supervision. Taking more than 50,000 IU (15,000 RE) of preformed, animal-source vitamin A a day over a long period of time can lead to headaches, blurred vision, hair loss, joint pain, dry skin, drowsiness, diarrhea, and enlargement of the liver and spleen. Symptoms slowly disappear once the dosage is reduced. Do not take more than 5,000 IU if you are pregnant or trying to conceive.

Vitamin A also has another basic function. "It helps cells to mature and develop certain definite characteristics and properties, a process called cell differentiation," Dr. Olson says. It acts as a kind of traffic cop for cells in a developing embryo. As the cells start to divide and multiply, vitamin A helps guide them in the direction they need to go, putting this one on its way to becoming a muscle cell, steering another one toward becoming a liver cell, and so on.

Vitamin A helps maintain the surfaces of the skin, the mucous membranes lining the nose and throat, and the tissues lining the intestines, bladder, and other internal cavities. All of these benefits can help boost immunity, since mucous membranes help prevent invasion by bacteria and viruses.

The vitamin also plays a direct role in immunity by helping the immune cells change into the special forms necessary to fight off infection. "One special kind of cell, called a T-helper cell, which helps to direct other immune cells, is very sensitive to vitamin A status," Dr. Olson says. "There's no question that the immune system doesn't function very well with inadequate vitamin A, and you don't necessarily need to be clearly deficient for this to happen."

Vitamin A even helps bones. It's involved in the dismantling and reforming of bone, an important part of making new bone.

The Many Beta Benefits

Given the many roles of vitamin A in the body, it's fortunate that we can get it from so many sources—plant as well as animal. While the transformation from beta-carotene into vitamin A is chemically complex, it doesn't take long to happen.

Beta-carotene is what's known as a precursor of vitamin A, which means that it's an essential part of the production process. As your body needs vitamin A, it can split beta-carotene in half, producing two molecules of vitamin A. Alternatively, the beta-carotene might split other ways, leaving one molecule of vitamin A.

In either case, the presence of beta-carotene leads to the production of vitamin A when it's needed. "When the body is lacking vitamin A, more beta-carotene is converted to vitamin A by an enzyme in the intestines as well as elsewhere, in other tissues in the body," says Susan Taylor Mayne, Ph.D., director of cancer prevention and control research at the cancer center at Yale University School of Medicine.

Apart from the role it plays in vitamin A production, beta-carotene gives you other benefits that have been studied by researchers. Studies often involve other forms of plant chemicals, including beta-carotene, that are known as carotenoids.

For years, researchers have seen a growing body of evidence to suggest that the more foods we eat that contain beta-carotene, the less likely we are to develop certain types of cancer. It looks as if beta-carotene may help prevent cancers of the lung, stomach, and esophagus. There's also been some evidence that beta-carotene might lower the risk of developing cancer of the cervix and colon as well. Mouth and throat cancers may also be on the hit list.

"A reduction in the risk of lung cancer really stood out, followed by mouth and throat cancer," says Dr. Mayne, summing up some studies. "Again, beta-carotene and other carotenoids showed very strong preventive activity. In fact, an international group of researchers reviewed this data, and the evidence of a protective effect remains very compelling."

Given these results, scientists have tried to find some evidence of how beta-carotene can produce a protective effect in our bodies. What they've found is that beta-carotene acts as an antioxidant. Like vitamins E and C, it can neutralize free radicals, the free-roaming, unstable molecules that can damage cells. Vitamin A is a staunch cell protector. Once incorporated into the fatty membranes around a cell, it also guards structures inside it. Among its protectorates is the very heart of the cell, the nucleus, which houses essential genetic material.

With beta-carotene—along with other antioxidants—fortifying the cell membrane from attack by free radicals, the cell is still vulnerable, but it's far better protected. Since cancer seems to get rolling when cell damage is at its peak, any form of protection is likely to reduce risk. At least, that's the theory—one that would explain why beta-carotene seems to play a cancer-protective role.

Making Good Neighbors

Beta-carotene may also help to regulate the proteins that enable cell-to-cell communication. "Every cell in the body has the ability to communicate with its neighbors, as though it were calling out across the backyard fence,"

Dr. Mayne says. This ability to communicate is thought to play a role in inhibiting cancer.

When normal cells are grown in the laboratory, they won't pile up on top of one another, she says. "Once they have filled up the top of a layer in a cell culture system, they send messages to each other that say, in effect, 'We are done growing.' This makes all the cells stop."

To cancer researchers, that's a fascinating effect, because cancer cells *don't* stop growing, and that's the problem. "In cancer cells, that communication goes awry, and they just continue to grow and grow," says Dr. Mayne.

In their frenetic growing process, the cancer cells eventually pile up, forming tumors. As the pile-up continues, the cells eventually invade the space of normal, healthy cells and generally take over the neighborhood. If beta-carotene is really a key link in cell-to-cell communication, maybe it can help to keep cells from overgrowing. At least, that's what researchers are hoping.

Starting with some studies in the 1980s and 1990s, however, doctors began to see that the scenario is even more complex. While some doses of beta-carotene in certain forms may have the cancer-preventive effect that we want, there are many variables. In fact, in certain high-risk groups, certain kinds of beta-carotene in high doses may tilt the balance the other way and actually increase the risk of one kind of cancer.

The Carotene Conundrum

A study conducted in Finland showed an unexpected outcome among heavy smokers, ages 50 to 69, who took 20 milligrams (33,200 international units, or IU) a day of beta-carotene for five to eight years. Compared with other smokers who had similar lifestyles but took no beta-carotene, the people who took the supplements seemed to have an increased rate of cancer. In fact, they had an 18 percent higher incidence of lung cancer than the heavy smokers who did not take supplements. This study also found an 11 percent increase in deaths from heart disease or stroke among the smokers who were taking beta-carotene.

Another study, called the Carotene and Retinol Efficacy Trial, was conducted at a number of U.S. medical centers that specialize in the prevention of lung cancer. Again, the study focused on very high-risk groups—in this case, heavy smokers and asbestos workers who were also smokers. But scientists had to end the study almost two years earlier than planned because the supplement seemed to *increase* health risks. The supplemented group, who were taking 30 milligrams (50,000 IU) a day of beta-carotene in combination with 25,000 IU of vitamin A (five times the Daily Value), were showing a 28 percent greater risk of developing lung cancer. They also had a 25 percent higher risk of death from heart disease. "It's hard to draw conclusions from this study, since it was stopped early and used a combination of nutrients," Dr. Mayne says. "But the data did indicate that there was the possibility of harm from beta-carotene, and little likelihood of benefit."

In a third study, the Physicians' Health Study, participants took 50 milligrams (83,000 IU) of beta-carotene every other day. Although the study went on for 12 years, the researchers found that beta-carotene had no effect—either beneficial or harmful—on the risk of cancer or cardiovascular disease. This study included relatively fewer smokers, however.

These results have researchers puzzled because they're so contrary to what scientists would expect, given the positive results of earlier studies with people involving foods rich in beta-carotene and animal studies involving supplements. "There's no doubt that now there are more questions than answers about beta-carotene," says Dr. Mayne.

What's the Right Dose?

What does the uncertainty about beta-carotene mean to you if you are wondering whether to take a supplement?

Well, if you don't smoke, you probably shouldn't worry. Those who were adversely affected were heavy smokers, and they were taking large amounts of supplements. "The only evidence of possible harm we have is in people who smoke more than one pack a day of cigarettes," Dr. Mayne says.

Researchers still don't know why harm occurs in this select group, but the very large doses are certainly a factor. "Antioxidants can promote free radical formation rather than inhibit it under certain circumstances, which could perhaps occur in someone with lots of oxidative damage going on in their body," Dr. Mayne says. "In smokers, there's a lot of oxidative damage."

A heavy smoker's mouth, throat, lungs, and blood are constantly being exposed to chemical reactions that involve oxygen, Dr. Mayne points out.

When oxygen is involved, trouble can follow. "These compounds can damage the cell membranes, which hinders the cell's ability to function properly. And they can go right through the cell membrane and chemically react with the cell's genetic material, setting the stage for cancer."

"It's possible that one dose of beta-carotene might offer protection from oxidative damage, while a higher dose could promote it, especially in already-damaged cells," Dr. Mayne says.

Judicious Approaches

People at risk for vitamin A deficiency can benefit from beta-carotene supplements. In the United States, most people get enough vitamin A from food; worldwide, vitamin A deficiency is a common cause of blindness. Those most likely to have low supplies are children from poor families, who may not get enough vitamin A–fortified milk or beta-carotene–rich fruits and vegetables. In some areas of Africa and Asia, both children and adults die as a result of lack of vitamin A, usually from infections.

Others who may suffer from vitamin A deficiency are alcoholics, people who can't absorb fat properly, and people with liver disease (vitamin A is stored in the liver). If you don't get enough zinc, an essential trace mineral, you can also become deficient, because your body needs zinc to make a protein that carries vitamin A in your bloodstream from the liver to other organs. If zinc's not there, vitamin A is not used effectively.

bioflavonoids

Hidden inside vegetables, fruits, flowers, herbs, and grains are certain pigments that seem to do a lot more than add color to the scene. Once thought to be lacking in nutritional value, the compounds called bioflavonoids are now in the spotlight and are being given new consideration for a lot of their colorful activities. Among their other powers, research has shown, these hidden stars may have anti-inflammatory, anti-allergic, antiviral, and anti-cancer properties.

Bioflavonoids were discovered in the 1930s by Albert Szent-Györgyi, a Hungarian-born American chemist who won a Nobel Prize in medicine for his work with vitamin C. He found that when combined with vitamin C in his animal studies, a substance in the rinds of citrus fruits, which he named citrin, helped strengthen the small blood vessels called capillaries. When he traced the active ingredients in citrin, Szent-Györgyi discovered a group of compounds that he named vitamin P, later to be called bioflavonoids.

Subsequently, doctors began using these compounds to treat various bleeding problems such as bruising. In 1950, though, a committee of experts decided that they were not actually vitamins, since no studies could prove that they are essential to our health. And in the late 1960s, the Food and Drug Administration determined not only that bioflavonoids were not vitamins but also that they had no nutritional value whatsoever.

Back by Popular Demand

With the publication of new research, some medical experts regard these substances as powerful antioxidants, providing protection against the free-roaming, unstable molecules called free radicals. That's a significant contribution because free radicals have been linked to cancer, heart disease, arthritis, and other ailments. Supplements are now being used to prevent and treat fragile capillaries, bleeding gums, varicose veins, hemorrhoids, bruises, diabetes, heavy menstrual bleeding, glaucoma and other vision problems, and many other conditions.

Between the date of Szent-Györgyi's original discovery and today, a lot of laboratory work has been done. Nearly 4,000 bioflavonoids have been identified. Selected from this vast array, a much smaller number are commonly found in supplements.

One that has been studied is quercetin, found in grapes, green tea, tomatoes, onions, kale, green beans, and strawberries. Other supplements contain rutin, which comes from buckwheat and a number of other plants. A third widely available bioflavonoid is hesperidin, derived from the rinds of oranges, lemons, and other citrus fruits.

You'll also see supplements called proanthocyanidins, or PCOs, which are primarily from red wines and grapeseed extract. In the United States, Pycnogenol is a registered trademark name for a PCO from a different source—the bark of the French maritime pine tree.

Some bioflavonoid supplements contain both hesperidin and rutin. A combination of rutin and vitamin C is sold as vitamin C complex, says Michael Janson, M.D., president of the American College for Advancement

SUPPLEMENT SNAPSHOT

▶ Bioflavonoids

Individual names: Quercetin, rutin, hesperidin, and proanthocyanidins, among others.

May help: Allergies, asthma, carpal tunnel syndrome, bruises, gout, high cholesterol, varicose veins, hemorrhoids, low immunity, arthritis, and sciatica. With vitamin C, used for gingivitis, colds and flu, canker sores, cold sores, menopausal discomforts, heavy menstrual bleeding, vaginitis, and genital herpes. May also strengthen capillaries, enhance connective tissue repair, decrease risk of heart disease and stroke, and help prevent cancer.

Special instructions: Take with food.

Good food sources: Rinds of oranges, lemons, and other citrus fruits; blueberries, blackberries, blackcherries, onions, kale, green beans, broccoli, endive, celery, cranberries, tomatoes, red bell peppers, apples, green and black tea, grapes, and red wine.

Cautions and possible side effects: Generally regarded as safe.

in Medicine, based in Laguna Hills, California, and author of *The Vitamin Revolution in Health Care*. The combination makes sense because bioflavonoids and vitamin C work together to provide protection from free radicals, says Dr. Janson. He adds, however, that it's usually less expensive to take vitamin C and bioflavonoid supplements separately.

A Case for Quercetin

Among the bioflavonoids, quercetin is perhaps the most highly regarded as a supplement to reduce inflammation and relieve asthma and allergies.

The main causes of run-of-the-mill allergy symptoms are histamine and leukotrienes, biochemicals that are released by your immune system to defend your body against invading allergens. For many allergies, antihistamine drugs do just what their name implies: They help prevent histamines from getting into your cells and causing symptoms such as congestion and sneezing, says Elliott Middleton Jr., M.D., professor emeritus of medicine at the State University of New York at Buffalo.

In preventing allergy symptoms, quercetin and other bioflavonoids act somewhat differently. Instead of blocking the pathways into the cells, they inhibit the manufacture and release of histamine and leukotrienes in the first place, explains Dr. Middleton. Plus, it seems that they can inhibit the action of these allergy-causing chemicals even after they've been released.

Because of quercetin's anti-allergy properties, some naturopathic doctors regularly prescribe supplements. During hay fever season, Jennifer Brett, N.D., a naturopathic doctor at the Wilton Naturopathic Center in Stratford, Connecticut, recommends quercetin for many of her patients, particularly those who are allergic to ragweed and leaf mold. According to Dr. Brett, quercetin helps reduce her patients' allergy symptoms, including itchy eyes, runny noses, and scratchy throats. She's found that it's also effective for people who have asthma, which is sometimes touched off by allergic reactions. If they take the bioflavonoid, Dr. Brett says, they don't need to rely as much on inhalers for relief.

Something for the Heart . . . and More

Quercetin and other bioflavonoids have also been targeted for biodetective work because of their ability to prevent heart disease and strokes. When Dutch scientists studied the eating patterns of 805 men ages 65 to 84, they discovered that those who consumed the most bioflavonoids—specifically from tea, onions, and apples—were less likely to die from a heart attack than those who ate less. The more bioflavonoids the men consumed, the lower their risk of heart attack. Those who got the most preventive paybacks were consuming the equivalent of 4 cups of tea, an apple, and ⅛ cup of onions a day.

In another study from the Netherlands, researchers gathered health and dietary information from 552 men ages 50 to 69. Fifteen years later, during follow-up examinations, the researchers found that those who consumed a high amount of bioflavonoids—mostly from black tea—had a 73 percent lower risk of stroke than those with a low intake.

Bioflavonoids appear to reduce the risk of cardiovascular disease by making small blood cells called platelets less sticky, explains Joe Vinson, Ph.D., professor of chemistry at the University of Scranton in Pennsylvania. Sticky platelets can cause blood clots that ultimately result in heart attacks.

Bioflavonoids also act as antioxidants and may prevent the oxidation of LDL cholesterol, which is believed to be a leading cause of atherosclerosis (hardening of the arteries).

Preventing Cancer and Cataracts

These multitalented pigments also show some promise in cancer prevention, according to Dr. Middleton. So far, the evidence comes from animal and laboratory studies in which bioflavonoids were used. "They have some remarkable effects," says Dr. Middleton, "but the one that especially fascinates me is that certain bioflavonoids can convert malignant cells into normal cells. It's extraordinary."

Cataract prevention is another area where bioflavonoids, particularly quercetin, may help. When cataracts develop, obscuring normal vision, substances called sugar-protein complexes are deposited on the lens of the eye. According to Dr. Janson, quercetin reduces the activity of an enzyme that leads to these deposits. When the deposits are reduced, there's less risk of developing cataracts.

Finally, bioflavonoids are believed by some to enhance vitamin C activity in situations where the vitamin alone is ineffective and to improve the strength of blood vessels and connective tissue. You can get the benefit of those actions in a number of ways. Stronger blood vessels mean less bruising and offer some protection against the development of varicose veins and hemorrhoids. There's also less chance of developing bleeding gums.

Bioflavonoids may strengthen and repair connective tissue by stimulating the synthesis of collagen, the fibrous protein that helps hold cells together. They also inhibit the breakdown of collagen, which means that connective tissue between your cells is more likely to stay strong and unbroken. This benefits the nervous system and may reduce allergy symptoms, such as inflammation.

The Pluses of Getting Enough

While the many benefits of bioflavonoids are being explored, experts are still trying to decide whether most of us can benefit from supplementation. Some say that we get all the bioflavonoids we need from our diets and that supplementing provides no additional benefits. Others argue that supplements provide extra protection and help fill the gaps when our diets are lacking.

"There are many good things in your food that you can't isolate in a supplement," says Dr. Vinson, who believes that bioflavonoid supplements aren't usually necessary.

Dr. Janson agrees that food is the preferred source of bioflavonoids, but he recommends supplementation as well. "Therapeutic doses for allergies, for example, are higher than you can get from diet. If people eat a wide variety of plant-based foods, they'll probably get a good supply of bioflavonoids. But I still believe there are benefits to supplementation." Based on this view, Dr. Janson regularly prescribes bioflavonoids to his patients.

biotin

You may regard biotin merely as a cure for your brittle nails—it's been shown to thicken fingernails as well as the hooves of horses and pigs—but this B vitamin means more to our bodies than simple beauty care.

Biotin has a daily job that it does with great reliability in our bodies: It helps us use carbohydrate, fat, and protein to produce the energy that allows us to stay alive. It also helps to make the tissues that form our bodies. Biotin may be especially beneficial to newborns and people with diabetes.

One of the major roles of this vitamin is very simple. It helps to attach a carbon and two oxygen molecules, called a carboxyl group, to other molecules. "This is a basic step in a lot of the chemical reactions that go on in our bodies," says Donald McCormick, Ph.D., chairman of the department of biochemistry at Emory University in Atlanta. "It happens when we break down carbohydrates for energy, when we use amino acids that come from protein, and when we use fats for energy. So biotin is working all over our bodies, all the time. It is critical for good health.

Are You Absorbing This?

Luckily, most people never become deficient in biotin. Among adults, people who are most likely to be deficient are those with absorption problems. People who have Crohn's disease, an intestinal disorder, may be deficient because they don't absorb enough biotin from food. Anticonvulsant medications can promote biotin deficiency.

Some infants have a genetic inability to use biotin. Lacking the support of this hardworking vitamin, they develop skin problems, such as an oily, flaky rash around their ears, noses, and mouths and on their buttocks. Eventually, they may also develop muscle weakness and potentially fatal nerve damage.

"Evidence of a biotin deficiency is most likely to be seen first where there are rapidly regenerating cells, such as those that lead to the formation of skin and hair," Dr. McCormick says. Even if you don't have a biotin deficiency that affects your health, the lack of this vitamin might be evident in some parts of your body. One study found that an additional 2,500 micrograms a day of biotin helped to strengthen and thicken brittle fingernails.

"Hair and nails contain a lot of a type of protein called keratin, which gives them their hard structure, and keratin production indirectly requires biotin," Dr. McCormick says. Certain fatty acids that our bodies use to make hair and nails can't be utilized unless biotin is on hand.

In fact, all animals need biotin. In furred animals such as mink and fox, a deficiency leads to a condition called spectacle eyes—baldness around the eyes. Horses and cattle that are short on biotin have hoof problems.

A Diabetes Connection?

In several studies, biotin supplementation has been shown to enhance the performance of insulin, the hormone that plays a critical role in helping your body incorporate blood sugar. The supplements can also increase the activity of an enzyme, glucokinase, which the liver uses early in the process of utilizing blood sugar, says Michael Murray, N.D., a naturopathic doctor and co-author of *The Encyclopedia of Natural Medicine.*

One study that looked at biotin supplementation in people with type 1

SUPPLEMENT SNAPSHOT

▶ Biotin

May help: Thin, brittle nails and seborrheic dermatitis; may also help lower blood sugar in some people with diabetes.

Daily Value: 30 micrograms.

Special instructions: Take in divided doses throughout the day.

Who's at risk for deficiency: People with intestinal absorption problems and babies with problems metabolizing biotin.

Good food sources: Brewer's yeast, molasses, egg yolks, milk, liver, soybeans, walnuts, peanuts, wheat bran, and cauliflower.

Cautions and possible side effects: Generally regarded as safe.

(insulin-dependent) diabetes found significant improvements in blood sugar control. Another study looked at the potential benefits of biotin supplements in people with type 2 (non-insulin-dependent) diabetes.

Every day for a month, Japanese researchers gave nine milligrams of biotin to 18 people with type 2 diabetes. After 30 days, the participants' blood sugar fell to nearly half its original levels. Researchers have also shown high-dose biotin to be very helpful in the treatment of severe diabetic nerve disease, Dr. Murray reports.

A Little Goes a Long Way

Two things make biotin deficiency rare. For starters, you need only a small amount—300 micrograms, or about one-third of a milligram. Second, many foods contain some biotin, although only a few, such as egg yolks, molasses, and soybeans, are rich sources. Ounce for ounce, the very top sources are two old-time "health foods"—royal jelly, a substance secreted by bees, and brewer's yeast.

Bacteria in our intestines also make biotin, although just how much they make—and how much of it we absorb—remains a mystery, according to Dr. McCormick. "Most of these bacteria are in the colon, and we just don't absorb much biotin in that part of our intestines."

black cohosh

In the late 1800s, when many women were embarrassed to consult male doctors about "female problems," they found comfort in Lydia Pinkham's Vegetable Compound, a patent medicine advertised to cure everything from nervous prostration to a prolapsed uterus.

Pinkham, a grandmotherly type from Lynn, Massachusetts, first shared her mixture of ground herbs and alcohol with neighbor women. Her son urged her to market the formula with her picture on the bottle, and within a few years, the compound was the best-selling medicine of the era. Pinkham was exalted as the "savior of her sex."

One of her principal herbs was black cohosh, a native American plant with a long folk history of relieving menstrual cramps and easing childbirth. Whether women found relief from the herb or from the 18 percent alcohol content in the compound is a matter of debate.

Not for Women Only

Pinkham's wasn't all hooch and no medicine, however. Black cohosh is a powerful relaxant and antispasmodic for both nerves and muscles. It is especially good at relieving cramping in smooth muscles, which include the uterus.

All of these properties are helpful to women who have problems with their reproductive systems: excessive bleeding, irregular periods, delayed menstruation, severe menstrual cramps, and the hot flashes of menopause. Black cohosh works as a regulator or normalizer of the female reproductive system by helping to restore hormone balance, says Stanley W. Beyrle, N.D., a naturopathic doctor at the Kansas Clinic of Traditional Medicine in Wichita.

"When it comes to gynecological complaints, there isn't a better herb than black cohosh," says Dr. Beyrle. "It's always one of my base herbs in any herbal formula for females."

Although it has a reputation as a woman's herb, black cohosh may have therapeutic benefits for both sexes. As an anti-inflammatory, it has been used to reduce pain and swelling in people who have rheumatoid arthritis, sciatica, osteoarthritis, neuralgia, or inflammation as a result of joint and muscle injuries.

"Anything that reduces inflammation, cramping, and swelling can reduce pain," says Dr. Beyrle. "That makes black cohosh useful for many conditions."

A Forest Herb

A member of the buttercup family, black cohosh is a native plant found in eastern deciduous forests from Ontario to Georgia. In North America, most black cohosh root is still harvested from the wild. In Europe, supplies come from herb farmers.

Native American women made a tea from the plant's resinous roots and rhizome to soothe menstrual cramps and promote menstruation. Black cohosh was also important in folk medicine as a childbirth aid that eased delivery by stimulating the uterus. Native Americans and American colonists also valued it as a treatment for rheumatism and sore throats.

SUPPLEMENT SNAPSHOT

▶ Black Cohosh

Botanical name: *Cimicifuga racemosa.*

May help: Bronchial, stomach, and muscle spasms; rheumatoid arthritis; osteoarthritis; sciatica; neuralgia; muscle and joint injuries; breast cancer; premenstrual syndrome; leg cramps, endometriosis; menstrual cramps; heavy menstrual bleeding; irregular periods; and hot flashes and other menopausal discomforts.

Origin: Found in eastern deciduous forests from Ontario to Georgia.

Cautions and possible side effects: Do not take while pregnant. Do not take while breastfeeding or for longer than six consecutive months without a doctor's supervision. May cause occasional stomach upset, diarrhea, abdominal pain, headache, and lowered heart rate and blood pressure.

As early as 1787, the plant attracted the interest of Europeans. Eclectic physicians, a nineteenth-century branch of early American medicine, made black cohosh one of their central healing botanicals for women. From 1820 to 1926, the herb was listed as an official drug in the *United States Pharmacopoeia*.

Like many phytomedicines, however, it eventually fell out of favor with the American medical community. It continued to be used in Europe, and today, in Germany, it is a government-approved treatment for premenstrual syndrome, painful menstruation, and nervous conditions connected to menopause.

Hormone Harmony

The herb has many active ingredients, but an isoflavone called formononetin is the critical one for women. Formononetin and other compounds in the root and rhizome are able to bind to estrogen receptors in the uterus and other tissues, particularly the brain (pituitary).

If you have fluctuations in estrogen—as is the case in menopause—the herb acts like a hormone modulator. If you have too much estrogen, which is frequently the case when menstruation is painful and cramping is severe, the phyto-estrogens block estrogen from binding at those receptor sites, says Kathleen Head, N.D., a naturopathic doctor in Sandpoint, Idaho, and senior editor of *Alternative Medicine Review*.

Besides replacing estrogen, black cohosh also eases the symptoms of menopause by inhibiting the production of luteinizing hormone (LH). LH levels tend to increase in the body at the same time that estrogen levels plummet. Hot flashes may be linked to high levels of this hormone.

The results of one clinical study seem to reinforce black cohosh's effectiveness in menopause. Researchers studied 60 women under age 40, all of whom had had hysterectomies. Because their uteruses had been removed, these women experienced premature menopause-like symptoms. Some were given black cohosh extract, while others were treated with various estrogen replacements.

The study found no difference between the two treatments. The black cohosh appeared to be equally as effective as its pharmaceutical counterparts. As with most herbs, however, the beneficial effects took longer to appear—as much as four weeks. The pharmaceutical drugs tended to work much faster.

"It's really a useful treatment during menopause," says Dr. Head, "but it's mild, and it may take time before it starts to work."

Quash That Cramp

The antispasmodic effect of black cohosh is much more immediate. Dr. Beyrle recommends the herb for patients who've sprained their backs, strained muscles, or have cramping and pain from arthritis. Pain from an injury often comes from tightness and soreness in a muscle, he says.

"I routinely use black cohosh in an herbal pain formula," he says. "If you can get those muscles to loosen up and relax, you can give someone relief from pain."

The herb has also been used to relieve stomach cramps as well as to quell coughing and relax constricted blood vessels in cases of whooping cough, bronchitis, and asthma. Sometimes, herbalists combine black cohosh with valerian or other sedative herbs to create a botanical tranquilizer for the central nervous system.

As a single supplement, black cohosh is available in tablets, capsules, and tincture.

brewer's yeast

Wouldn't it be wonderful news for beer-lovin' adults if a nice cold brew turned out to be the answer to all of their health problems? We can just hear the doctor now: "Got a cold? Have a Bud," or "Allergies acting up? Try a Heineken."

A beer drinker's dream—but not true of the brew. There's no beer that will fulfill our nutritional needs. But there is a related substance, brewer's yeast, that can help some of what "ales" us.

Available as a powder, flakes, or tablets, brewer's yeast is a slightly bitter-tasting ingredient that's used in brewing beer. It's also a by-product of beer-making. The yeast itself—a tiny fungus—is grown on grain, usually barley.

Brewer's yeast is a rich source of many nutrients, including protein, some B vitamins, phosphorus, and chromium. The protein content of yeast accounts for slightly more than half of its weight.

It's this variety and abundance of nutrients that have made brewer's yeast such an enduring supplement, says Michael Janson, M.D., president of the American College for Advancement in Medicine, based in Laguna Hills, California, and author of *The Vitamin Revolution in Health Care*.

A Big Sweet Tooth

Yeast is a living, single-cell organism. It's grown on anything sugary, including sugarcane sap, yeast extract, malt extract, or just a handful of salt and sugar, says Richard M. Walmsley, Ph.D., senior lecturer in the department of biomolecular sciences at the University of Manchester Institute of Science and Technology in England.

Like humans, a single yeast cell has a life span, but it will divide about 20 times before it dies. Within days, these 20 divisions and the divisions of all of the offspring give rise to millions of yeast cells.

There are many kinds of yeast. They all acquire their nutrients the hard way, says Michael J. Conboy, a researcher in the department of biological sciences at Stanford University. They require many of the same vitamins and amino acids that humans need, but because they often grow on foods that are lacking in certain nutrients, like grains and fruit, they are forced to manufacture their own amino acids and vitamins biochemically. In doing so, the yeast cells become a much more complete food for anyone who eats them, Conboy explains.

Among the many varieties of yeast are baker's, brewer's, and nutritional yeast. Baker's yeast, the secret ingredient that makes bread rise, contains living cells and is also a good source of vitamins and minerals. The live cells are killed during the baking process, but the B vitamins that are accumulated by them are still present in the baked bread. The live cells in brewer's yeast are also destroyed during the brewing process, but the dead cells still have nutrient value.

The terms *brewer's yeast* and *nutritional yeast* are sometimes used interchangeably, but they are not exactly the same. Basically, nutritional yeast is any yeast grown for the specific purpose of being a food supplement, Conboy explains. While it might be a brewer's yeast, it could also be yeast from another species.

Brewer's yeast is used as a nutritional yeast when it's grown in the presence of vitamin B_{12} and other nutrients. It can have a wide range of nutritional values, depending on the species of yeast and on what medium it

SUPPLEMENT SNAPSHOT

▶Brewer's Yeast

May help: Diabetes, hypoglycemia, high cholesterol, eczema, nervousness, fatigue, and constipation.

Special instructions: Take on an empty stomach unless indigestion occurs; then take with food.

Cautions and possible side effects: If you have diabetes or hypoglycemia, consult your doctor before taking. Do not take if you have candidiasis, gout, or high blood levels of uric acid. Use with caution if you have a known allergy to molds. Rarely, may cause occasional flatulence or digestive upset.

was grown in, such as grain or sugarcane sap. Some yeasts are grown with a high chromium content, for example, while others have a high selenium content.

Brewing Up Healthy Benefits

If we get most of the vitamins and minerals we need from our diets, is there any reason to make brewer's yeast a regular supplement? Possibly not, says Dr. Janson. "But I like my nutrients to come from a variety of sources," he adds, noting that foods such as brewer's yeast may contain undiscovered nutrients that do have some benefits. "Think of brewer's yeast as an additional supplement, not as a replacement for whole foods and a comprehensive supplement program."

When it's grown with vitamin B_{12}, brewer's yeast is the supplement of choice for some vegetarians, especially vegans (strict vegetarians who eat no meat, fish, poultry, eggs, or dairy products). "There are very few natural vegan sources of B_{12} except certain forms of brewer's yeast," says Jennifer Brett, N.D., a naturopathic doctor at the Wilton Naturopathic Center in Stratford, Connecticut.

Many vegetarians take vitamin and mineral supplements rather than brewer's yeast, Dr. Brett says. The doses contained in these supplements are known, while the amounts of specific nutrients found in yeast will vary. Each type of yeast has varying amounts, and the variations are also affected by how old the yeast is, she says.

Brewer's yeast also has been used to prevent and reduce the symptoms of diabetes. That's because it contains chromium, a mineral that has been shown to regulate blood sugar (glucose), says Richard Anderson, Ph.D., lead scientist in the nutrient requirements and functions laboratory at the U.S. Department of Agriculture Beltsville Human Nutrition Research Center in Maryland. Chromium works together with insulin to help transport blood sugar across cell membranes and into cells, where it can be burned for energy.

The chromium in brewer's yeast may also help raise HDL cholesterol, the "good" kind, and reduce LDL, the "bad" cholesterol, says Dr. Anderson. Some of the chromium found in brewer's yeast is thought to be glucose tolerance factor, a combination of chromium, nicotinic acid (a form of niacin), and amino acids.

If you're supplementing with brewer's yeast simply because of its chromium content, though, you might want to take a chromium supplement instead, suggests Dr. Anderson. "With brewer's yeast, you don't know what you're getting, because the nutritional quality varies from batch to batch and supplier to supplier," he cautions.

Dr. Brett, however, has had success with prescribing brewer's yeast to her patients who have a personal or family history of diabetes or hypoglycemia (low blood sugar). She has found that her patients get much better long-term control of their symptoms when they take brewer's yeast than when they take a chromium supplement. Why? "It's possible that the nutrient is more bioavailable from the yeast, and therefore more effective," she says.

Since chromium may affect blood glucose and insulin levels, people with diabetes or hypoglycemia should consult their doctors before supplementing their diets with brewer's yeast.

Brewer's yeast has also been used to treat eczema, nervousness, fatigue, and constipation. Interestingly, some pet owners believe that brewer's yeast somehow helps their four-legged friends repel fleas and ticks, although there is no scientific evidence that it works.

In general, brewer's yeast has the strong taste of yeasty bread or sweet bread dough. Some people find that brewer's yeast grown on sugar beets is sweeter and more appealing, says Dr. Brett. As flakes or powder, it can be stirred into juice, especially grape juice, and soups; sprinkled over salads, popcorn, cottage cheese, or yogurt; or added to casseroles and any dish made with tomato sauce. Heating makes the flavor of brewer's yeast stronger, so it's best to add it to foods as they are being served, advises Dr. Brett.

If you find the taste unpleasant, try taking the tablets instead, says Dr. Anderson.

bromelain

Kitchen wizards know that you can't make a gelatin dessert with fresh pineapple. The natural enzymes in this prickly fruit prevent the gelatin from setting, leaving the amateur cook with a runny mess.

What's bad for Jell-O may be good for you, however. Bromelain, the enzyme found in pineapple, has been credited with a number of health benefits, including aiding digestion, speeding wound healing, and reducing inflammation.

Bromelain is found in both the fruit and stem of the pineapple, but the enzyme in supplements comes from the stem.

An Inflammation Tamer

More than 200 scientific papers have been written about bromelain since it was first introduced as a health-boosting substance in 1957. Much of the research has focused on its anti-inflammatory effects. Whether you have a sprained ankle, a nasty bruise, sinusitis, or any other type of inflammation, bromelain may help you heal faster, says Greg Kelly, N.D., a naturopathic doctor in Stamford, Connecticut. In fact, he routinely recommends that his patients take bromelain before and after surgery to speed the healing process. "I would consider using bromelain for any type of inflammation for which you might use aspirin," he says.

Bromelain inhibits the release of certain inflammation-causing chemicals, explains Alan L. Miller, N.D., technical advisor for Thorne Research in Sandpoint, Idaho, and senior editor of *Alternative Medicine Review*. It also activates a chemical in the blood and tissues that breaks down fibrin, a protein-sugar complex that is partly responsible for blood clotting.

By breaking down fibrin, bromelain produces another benefit: It reduces swelling. That's because fibrin prevents injured tissues from draining, and when they can't drain, they swell. "Bromelain is most beneficial when used after trauma such as surgery or injury," says Dr. Miller. "I also prescribe it for colds, flu, and ear infections to loosen thick mucus so it can drain or be coughed up."

Bromelain may also keep platelets from sticking to each other and to blood vessel walls, which is a major factor in atherosclerosis (hardening of the arteries). Bromelain helps prevent platelet clumping by decreasing the release of a chemical that causes them to stick together.

Treating Troubled Tummies

If you overestimated the size of tonight's dinner and ate more steak and potatoes than your stomach was prepared to digest, you might want to try a bromelain supplement to quell the discomfort. It is a digestive enzyme that helps break down protein, thus aiding digestion, says Dr. Kelly.

Bromelain also appears to be helpful for people with food allergies, especially allergies to wheat and other grains, says Dr. Kelly. In one Japanese study, bromelain was added to wheat flour, which was then used to make bread. The enzyme changed the structure of a protein in the wheat and allowed people with wheat allergies to eat the bread without having an allergic response.

Some research has shown that bromelain also holds promise for in-

SUPPLEMENT SNAPSHOT

▶Bromelain

May help: Digestive disorders, inflammation, wound healing, colds and flu, ear infections, atherosclerosis, food allergies, muscle soreness, phlebitis, lupus, gout, intermittent claudication, osteoarthritis, and rheumatoid arthritis; may also increase the effectiveness of some antibiotics.

Special instructions: As a digestive aid, take with meals; for all other uses, take on an empty stomach.

Good food source: Pineapple.

Cautions and possible side effects: May cause nausea, vomiting, diarrhea, skin rash, and heavy menstrual bleeding; may increase the risk of bleeding in people taking aspirin or anticoagulants (blood thinners). Do not take if you are allergic to pineapple.

creasing the potency of antibiotics, and it is used that way in several countries outside the United States. In one study, combined bromelain and antibiotic therapy was given to 53 hospitalized patients with a variety of infectious ailments. For every disease studied, there was a significant reduction in disease symptoms when the patients received the combined therapy as compared to antibiotics alone.

Dr. Kelly concedes that the studies are dated, but he reviewed the evidence and found it convincing. Since bacteria have become increasingly resistant to antibiotics, using bromelain to increase a drug's potency makes sense, he says.

Doing Your Homework

Manufacturers of bromelain supplements really make you do your math, because the supplements are measured in milk-clotting units (mcu) or gelatin-dissolving units (gdu); 1,200 gdu equal roughly 2,000 mcu per gram. Check the label carefully. Some brands list the mcu by the pill and others by the amount per gram. If the label lists only the weight in milligrams, it may be an inferior product.

Dosages for bromelain vary, depending on the reason that you're taking it. Look for standardized supplements so you know that you are getting the same potency from batch to batch. You can buy either capsules—which do not contain any binders or fillers—or tablets.

If you're lactose intolerant, read the labels or check with the manufacturer to find out whether a particular product is mixed with lactose. Manufacturers are not required to list lactose with other ingredients on the label, says Dr. Miller, but some products offer the information or specify that the product is lactose-free.

vitamin C

During the days of Columbus, sailors who joined the crew of a seagoing ship knew that they had only a 50 percent chance of coming home alive. The danger wasn't that they might fall off the edge of the Earth or be eaten by sea monsters. Instead, it was that they might contract a dreadful disease, unnamed at the time, that would make their gums bleed, loosen their teeth, cause bruises and bleeding under their skin, and ultimately, kill them. Only men on short voyages, especially around the Mediterranean Sea, seemed able to avoid these symptoms.

At that time, no one knew that the disease was scurvy, caused by a deficiency of vitamin C. On long ocean voyages, the cook used up the fresh fruits and vegetables first, then served only cereals and meats, which contained no vitamin C, until the ship returned to port. That sometimes meant that the crew went for months without this essential vitamin.

Even though James Lind, a British physician, showed in 1747 that oranges and lemons could prevent scurvy, it was another 50 years before the British navy mandated a daily ration of lime juice on all vessels (thus giving British sailors the traditional nickname, limeys). And it took another 200 years before the component of citrus that protected against scurvy, vitamin C, was isolated. Its scientific name, ascorbic acid, reflects its anti-scurvy past.

Our C Rations

These days, we get so much vitamin C from foods that we never have to worry about scurvy or lime juice rations. A lot of us even keep bottles of vitamin C on hand so we can down a couple of hundred extra milligrams if we feel a cold coming on. In fact, vitamin C is the most popular vitamin supplement in the United States. And while it may be best known for its cold-fighting powers, that's just one of its vital roles in the body.

Body Building

Vitamin C helps to form the fibrous structural protein known as collagen, the single most important protein of connective tissue and literally, the stuff that holds us together.

SUPPLEMENT SNAPSHOT

▶Vitamin C

Also known as: Ascorbic acid.

May help: Bacterial and viral infections, including colds and flu, HIV, and urinary tract infections; cancer; gingivitis; genital herpes; asthma; emphysema; angina; cataracts; sunburn; bedsores; diabetes-related organ damage; depression; impotence; intermittent claudication; phlebitis; infertility; high cholesterol; heavy menstrual bleeding; muscle soreness; osteoarthritis; menopausal discomforts; chronic inflammatory diseases such as lupus and rheumatoid arthritis; recovery from surgery or injury; and exposure to toxins.

Daily Value: 60 milligrams; for smokers, 100 milligrams.

Special instructions: Take larger doses in several spaced doses of less than 1,000 milligrams each throughout the day. Take with adequate amounts of water.

Who's at risk for deficiency: Smokers and people exposed to cigarette smoke; people with viral or bacterial infections, diabetes, high cholesterol, cardiovascular disease, cancer, or chronic inflammation; and people who take aspirin or barbiturates regularly.

Good food sources: Broccoli, brussels sprouts, cabbage, all peppers, citrus fruits, collard and turnip greens, guavas, kale, parsley, red and green bell peppers, and strawberries.

Cautions and possible side effects: Safe at a wide range of doses, although more than 3,000 milligrams a day can cause diarrhea; if this occurs, cut back until the diarrhea stops. If you're taking high doses, cut back to 100 milligrams at least three days before a physical exam or tests, as high amounts can interfere with some tests, including those for blood in the stool and sugar in urine. Large doses may interfere with anticoagulants (blood thinners). Supplements made from a corn base may cause a reaction in people allergic to corn.

"Vitamin C lets these fibers cross-link, or weave together, to make them strong," explains Robert Jacob, Ph.D., a research chemist in micronutrients at the U.S. Department of Agriculture Western Human Nutrition Research Center in San Francisco.

When these fibers don't cross-link, we get the symptoms typical of scurvy. We start to fall apart. Our teeth loosen because our gums can't hold them in anymore; our gums bleed, and we develop little pinpoints of blood under our skin as blood vessels break down and release blood. If we get hurt, we don't heal, because the body relies on collagen to fill the gaps in wounds. If we break a bone, it doesn't heal either, because bones regenerate by depositing minerals such as calcium on a matrix of collagen.

Some doctors believe that a low intake of vitamin C does more than aggravate the symptoms of scurvy, says Balz Frei, Ph.D., professor of biochemistry and biophysics and director of the Linus Pauling Institute at Oregon State University in Corvallis. A shortage may also worsen symptoms of osteoporosis, cancer, and heart disease.

Fat for Fuel

One of the first symptoms of vitamin C deficiency is fatigue, and one reason for that may be an often-overlooked function of this vitamin, says Dr. Frei. "Vitamin C is required for the synthesis of a compound called carnitine, which transports fatty acids into the mitochondria, the tiny powerhouses that generate energy inside cells," he explains. "If you don't have enough vitamin C, you can't synthesize enough carnitine, so you can't convert all the fatty acids into usable energy."

While it's true that carbohydrates are the main source of energy for most of our body parts, fatty acids are the major sources for the production of energy in the heart and skeletal muscles. These areas are particularly vulnerable to a carnitine shortage, Dr. Frei says.

Vitamin C also helps your body convert the amino acid tyrosine into two important hormones, epinephrine and norepinephrine. Both are released by the body in response to stress.

"These hormones are responsible for mobilizing energy and activating a lot of metabolic pathways so that you can respond to stressful situations in a physical way," Dr. Frei explains. "They produce the fight-or-flight response."

In fact, our adrenal glands, which produce these two hormones, have a higher concentration of vitamin C than any other organ in the body. "It's well-established that if you're under physical stress, such as during an in-

The Rationale behind Megadosing

Some doctors recommend so-called megadoses of vitamin C, amounts far higher than the Daily Value, to literally flood the body with the vitamin during certain illnesses.

The thinking is this: Many illnesses involve damage from free radicals, unstable molecules that affect healthy cells. Once it gets started, the damage can cause a chain reaction that quickly depletes areas of inflamed tissue of vitamin C and allows the damage to spread even more.

"I am trying to literally pickle the tissues involved in the disease in order to neutralize all the free radicals," says Robert Cathcart, M.D., a physician in Los Altos, California, who is a long-time practitioner of megadosing. "I want to push the vitamin into cells and flood the tissue to stop the chain reaction of free radical damage. This is not a nutritional effect. Rather, it is a pharmacological effect."

Dr. Cathcart recommends and has successfully used large doses of vitamin C in the form of ascorbic acid. In this form, the vitamin isn't buffered—that is, no chemicals have been added to help the body absorb it. The ascorbic acid, he says, can help with many kinds of health conditions, from the common cold to life-threatening viral hepatitis.

Normally, he recommends that his patients take the vitamin to bowel tolerance (meaning until it begins to produce loose stools), and then back off a bit until the loose stools stop. His reasoning: When people are sick, they tend to tolerate a lot more ascorbic acid than they do when they are healthy. The one exception is people with bowel problems, who may not be able to take much ascorbic acid orally. In these cases, Dr. Cathcart administers a form of the vitamin intravenously.

fection or after surgery, you need more vitamin C," Dr. Jacob says. "There's less evidence to indicate that psychological stress also raises vitamin C needs, but since psychological stress also makes the adrenal glands crank up production, it makes sense that you would need more vitamin C."

Stopping the Thieves

In the annals of research, vitamin C has won considerable renown as an antioxidant. That means that it helps keep a lid on chemical reactions

For a bad cold or the flu, for instance, Dr. Cathcart might recommend that someone take 2 to 12 grams of ascorbic acid every 15 minutes until they reach bowel tolerance. The time frame varies from person to person, but tolerance could occur within four to eight hours, Dr. Cathcart says. For a condition like severe mononucleosis, he says, one woman was able to tolerate 200 grams of ascorbic acid before she reached bowel tolerance.

"When you reach that point," Dr. Cathcart says, "generally, your symptoms quickly vanish." How long you need to take high amounts to keep your symptoms at bay depends on many variables and could range from a few days to months. Some people take several grams a day indefinitely.

While there is some research to indicate that taking additional vitamin C can help shorten the duration of a cold, there is little evidence to support the use of large amounts for illnesses such as mononucleosis, hepatitis, cancer, or AIDS, says Balz Frei, Ph.D., professor of biochemistry and biophysics and director of the Linus Pauling Institute at Oregon State University in Corvallis. "I'm not saying that it doesn't work or that the theory behind this isn't sound. I'm saying that there is currently not enough scientific evidence to conclude that megadoses of vitamin C provide health benefits beyond those of more moderate doses of the vitamin," he says.

As for everyday, or anti-aging, use of vitamin C, Dr. Cathcart believes that the amount an individual needs is based on their own "free radical load." "If you have a chronic illness or inflammation, if you've abused your body with alcohol or smoking, or if you look old for your age, you probably can use more than someone who's healthier," he says. For a vitamin regimen tailored to your needs, see your doctor.

that involve oxygen, explains Dr. Frei—reactions that go on all the time, all over our bodies. We have oxygen in our lungs, but blood carries it to every cell, where it is used as part of the process of energy metabolism. These chemical reactions have the potential to create molecular particles called free radicals. A free radical lacks an electron, which makes it unstable, so it tries to "steal" an electron from some other molecule. Then that molecule is minus an electron and becomes a free radical, causing a kind of free radical domino effect.

Vitamin C breaks up this cycle of larceny. "It can give up one of its electrons without becoming a dangerous free radical, so every time a molecule of vitamin C does that, it helps to stop a whole string of electron pilfering," Dr. Frei explains. That's important because free radical damage is thought to be involved in many diseases and conditions, including inflammation, viral infections, cancer, heart disease, and even aging.

Vitamin C can also regenerate vitamin E, another important free radical scavenger, by giving it an electron.

As an antioxidant, vitamin C helps many parts of the body function better. When immune cells are called into action, for instance, they use a lot of oxygen and produce free radicals and oxidants that can damage cells and surrounding tissue. Vitamin C helps protect these cells.

In your lungs, this versatile vitamin helps you breathe more easily by fighting off the onslaught of oxidants you inhale, says Dr. Frei, especially if you are a smoker. In your liver, it helps to protect the cells as they break down toxins. And in your stomach, vitamin C is secreted in gastric juices and helps to neutralize potential cancer-causing substances called nitrosamines, which are found in some lunch meats and smoked foods. However, vitamin C combined with iron should be avoided in people with stomach inflammation.

How Much Is Enough?

Only about one out of every four Americans gets less than the Daily Value for vitamin C, which is 60 milligrams. They are people who simply don't eat fruits and vegetables, Dr. Frei says.

The bigger question today is how much vitamin C is optimum for good health. Dr. Frei believes that everyone should get a minimum of 200 milligrams, and in fact, studies show that in healthy people, 200 milligrams daily produces tissue saturation. It's about as much as most parts of your body can hold.

There are some decent arguments that can be made for some people's need for higher amounts, however. Smokers and people exposed to cigarette smoke; people with viral or bacterial infections, diabetes, high cholesterol, cardiovascular disease, cancer, or chronic inflammation; and people who take certain drugs such as aspirin or barbiturates on a regular basis may need more vitamin C, Dr. Frei says.

calcium

Chalk, eggshells, milk, and bones have something in common. All get their dense white color from calcium—they're loaded with it.

Sharing this natural resource sometimes leads to some strange lend-lease arrangements. Bones and eggshells are often ground up for calcium supplements that go into livestock feed; then, from milk and other dairy products, we pick up some of the calcium that we need for better bones and other body-building biology projects. If we don't get quite enough, we can turn to supplements that are often made from the basic geological substrata—the same mineral deposits that are sometimes used to make chalk.

We have more calcium than any other mineral in our bodies, and we're right to associate it with bones because that's where 99 percent of it is found. It's vital throughout our lifetimes for building strong bones and teeth.

Calcium is used for much more, however. It's also dissolved in the fluids in the body, those inside cells and those that bathe cells. There, it helps muscles spring into action and aids proper blood clotting. It assists nerves in transmitting impulses and helps launch hormones and enzymes on their journeys to inner organs.

Usually, the dissolved calcium in our bodies never gets so low that these important functions are impaired, but our bodies sometimes behave like poachers during lean times. Robbing Peter to pay Paul, they take calcium from bones as needed to make sure that the vital functions go on.

Like a Rock . . . Not

Bones aren't the inert, rocklike objects that we might imagine them to be. They are in a constant state of flux, dissolving and forming new bone all the time.

As bones begin to form, calcium salts form crystals on a gridwork of strands of a protein called collagen. These crystals invade the collagen and gradually lend more and more strength and rigidity to the developing bone.

This happens with the speed of Federal Express deliveries when bones grow fastest, during childhood and adolescence; when a fractured bone is healing; and, indeed, throughout your lifetime. Bones reach their peak mass—when they're strongest and most dense—in your late twenties. That's why it's so

SUPPLEMENT SNAPSHOT

▶ Calcium

Supplement forms: Calcium carbonate, citrate, citrate-malate, lactate, gluconate, and aspartate; dicalcium phosphate; bone meal; oyster shell; and dolomite.

May help: Osteoporosis, high blood pressure, insomnia, menstrual cramps, muscle cramps, pregnancy-related high blood pressure, and restless legs syndrome.

Daily Value: 1,000 to 1,300 milligrams.

Special instructions: Divide your daily dose into two smaller doses, no more than 500 milligrams each. If you use calcium citrate, lactate, or gluconate, you can take it between meals without absorption problems, and it also won't interfere with absorption of iron and other trace minerals. All other forms of supplemental calcium are best absorbed when taken with food. Avoid taking supplements at the same time as large amounts of wheat bran. To further aid absorption, get 400 international units of vitamin D daily from sunlight, fortified foods, or supplements; it's not necessary to take the supplements together.

Who's at risk for deficiency: People who don't eat many dairy products, those who don't get adequate vitamin D, women who are pregnant or breastfeeding, and people over age 50.

Good food sources: Milk and milk products, sardines (with bones), kale, calcium-fortified orange juice, sea vegetables, and sesame seeds.

Cautions and possible side effects: If you have had calcium oxalate kidney stones, check with your doctor before taking calcium. The supplements may slightly increase your risk of getting stones again. Supplements from natural sources—oyster shells, dolomite, or bone meal—may be contaminated with lead or other toxic metals; check labels for refined or purified sources. High doses may cause constipation.

What's in the Bottles?

Calcium comes in so many forms, even as a supplement, that choosing among the varieties may be confusing. Here's a clue: When you're reading labels, look for the "elemental calcium" listing to tell you how much you're really getting, says Robert E. C. Wildman, Ph.D., professor of nutrition at the University of Delaware in Newark. Most labels include this listing, he adds.

If the label does not indicate how much elemental calcium is in each tablet, you can use the table below. If you're taking a 500-milligram tablet of calcium carbonate, for example, you can see that it contains 40 percent elemental calcium—which translates into 200 milligrams of calcium from each tablet. Here are the typical percentages of actual calcium in supplement products.

Supplement	Elemental Calcium (%)
Calcium carbonate	40
Dicalcium phosphate	38
Bone meal	31
Oyster shell	28
Dolomite	22
Calcium citrate	21
Calcium lactate	13
Calcium gluconate	9

You don't absorb all of the elemental calcium that's in a tablet, Dr. Wildman points out—only about 30 to 40 percent (in fact, calcium citrate-malate, which is available mostly in fortified orange juice, is perhaps the best-absorbed form). If you take a supplement with food, a tablet of calcium carbonate is the most efficient way to get what you need. With supplements like calcium citrate, lactate, or gluconate, you'll need to take more tablets to equal the amount of calcium in a single dose of calcium carbonate.

important to get enough calcium early on: The denser your bones are at their peak, the longer they'll stay strong.

The shipments of calcium need to continue well beyond that peak, however. "After that time, continuing to get enough calcium will help to reduce the rate of bone loss that occurs with aging," says Richard Wood, Ph.D., chief of the mineral bioavailability laboratory at the Jean Mayer USDA Human Nutrition Research Center on Aging at Tufts University in Boston.

For Muscles and Nerves

Calcium is also vitally important when it comes to properly functioning muscles, explains Lisa Ruml, M.D., a physician in Wharton, New Jersey. To contract and then relax, a muscle depends on the presence of calcium. "Calcium ions in the cell move from one spot to another very quickly, and that changes the electrical charge of certain proteins in the muscle cell so that the proteins change shape," she explains. These proteins tighten up and, in effect, pass along the tightening action to increase the tension.

As proteins shorten the muscle cells, the muscle contracts. When the calcium ions move back to their former positions, the proteins ratchet down from their state of peak tension, and the muscle relaxes. If you have too little calcium in your cells, however, the muscle cells tend to stay in the tightened position. You'll become more prone to muscle cramps.

Along with other electrically aggressive minerals like potassium, calcium also allows our nerves to transmit messages. Because the electrically charged calcium ions in cells rapidly shift position, an electrical charge is handed along the chain of nerve cells. The result is that a small electrical current travels along the nerve. Once the current reaches the end of the nerve, it triggers the release of a neurotransmitter, a chemical that allows the message to be relayed to another cell.

In the heart, calcium's role in both muscle contraction and nerve transmission comes into play. Calcium interacts with potassium and sodium over and over again in a carefully orchestrated sequence to produce a heartbeat. You would have to be seriously ill to be so low on calcium that it affects your heart, but it does happen. Doctors sometimes use drugs called calcium channel blockers to slow down and regulate heartbeat in people with high blood pressure, Dr. Ruml says. "These drugs temper the shift of calcium in and out of cells," she explains. Normally, however, getting more calcium isn't going to help—or hurt—your heart.

Bowel Binder

In the intestines, calcium can combine with other nutrients and foods—such as saturated fat—to create compounds that cannot be ab-

Calculate Your Calcium Needs

Although calcium calculations may seem like higher math, there's a simple way to figure out what you need. As a starting point, let's say you get about 500 milligrams, which is the equivalent of about two cups of milk, and you're aiming for the 1,200 milligrams that are recommended for many people. You'll need to make up the shortfall with 700 milligrams of supplemental calcium each day, says Robert E. C. Wildman, Ph.D., professor of nutrition at the University of Delaware in Newark.

If you know that your intake isn't average—or you just like to play with figures—take the custom-tailored route.

1. Add up your daily servings of calcium champs—foods that you eat every day that supply substantial calcium. The champs most likely to be consumed daily (in single-serving amounts) are eight ounces (one cup) of 1 percent or fat-free milk, eight ounces of low-fat or nonfat yogurt, eight ounces of calcium-fortified orange juice, eight ounces of low-fat or nonfat calcium-fortified soy or rice milk, and two one-ounce slices of reduced-fat or fat-free cheese.

After you've determined which of these you eat regularly, count 300 milligrams of calcium for each serving (or check labels, since calcium content can vary by brand).

2. To this number, add 200 milligrams for women and 300 milligrams for men, which is an estimated calcium total for all the other foods you eat throughout the day.

3. If you take a multivitamin/mineral supplement, add the amount of calcium that you get from that. (Don't assume that a multi will cover your needs; most have too little calcium to make up average shortfalls.)

4. Subtract the total of steps 1, 2, and 3 from your daily requirement, 1,200 milligrams. Anything over zero is your daily shortfall and is the amount you should take in a supplement, says Dr. Wildman.

sorbed into the body. In one study, a group of people getting 1,000 milligrams or so of calcium a day from fortified foods and 1,000 milligrams from supplements excreted twice as much saturated fat as people getting normal amounts of calcium. They also had an 11 percent drop in harmful LDL cholesterol.

Calcium may also play a role in preventing colon cancer by binding with cancer-promoting fats and bile acids, the digestive fluids secreted by the liver, says Dr. Wood. This neutralizes the toxic effects of the fats and acids, and if all goes well, they are excreted more rapidly, along with intestinal cells that might be cancer generators. But don't count on miracles, he says. "The effects are fairly modest and occur only at amounts well above normal intake."

Calcium also helps to prevent the absorption of toxic minerals such as lead by interfering with cellular transport, says Dr. Wood. Unfortunately, it can interfere with minerals that we may need more of, such as iron, zinc, copper, and manganese. That's why some doctors recommend that you not take calcium supplements with meals.

Coming Up Short

Women in the United States average between 700 and 800 milligrams a day of calcium. Men get nearly 1,000 milligrams, which is the DV. Some experts recommend higher amounts to protect against a deficiency, which results in more calcium being withdrawn from bones than is deposited.

Usually, you don't know how frail your bones have become until you develop a condition called osteoporosis (the term means "porous bones"). At worst, your bones can become as riddled with holes as a termite-infested log and so fragile that simply bearing your own weight causes them to break.

Even if it's not that bad, invisible damage can take its toll, eventually producing evidence that your bone skeleton has been starved of calcium. If you develop tiny fractures in your spine, you also end up with the bent-over stance called dowager's hump, which many women accept as a sign of old age. Moreover, with osteoporosis, one fall can produce complicated and serious fractures. These are all good reasons to take calcium seriously and make sure that you're getting enough.

cat's claw

When you hear about all of the potential medicinal plants in a tropical rain forest, you probably picture an inconspicuous fern beneath the damp forest canopy or a dainty water lily floating in a steamy swamp.

How about a tree-climbing, 100-foot vine that's 12 inches around, with thorns as sharp and tenacious as a jaguar's claws?

Cat's claw is one of the newly discovered herbs of the Amazon. It's actually new, however, only to Western civilization, since the Peruvian Indians of the region have used the vine medicinally for centuries.

If you follow the news on cat's claw, you might think it's the cat's meow. It's been called a superb immune system booster, a vigorous antioxidant, a plant able to flush chemical toxins from the body, and a kind of scrubber that removes plaque buildup in clogged arteries.

Health food stores in North America brim with products that contain cat's claw, but there really isn't much known about this herb. The labels make many claims that may be exaggerated, warns Eran Ben-Arye, M.D., a researcher at the natural medicine research unit at Hadassah University Hospital in Jerusalem.

"Right now, all we have are anecdotal reports and very preliminary findings regarding the herb's immunological and antifungal properties," Dr. Ben-Arye says. "Cat's claw may have very good potential as a medicine, or it may not. We just don't know yet."

Putting Teeth into Immunity

In the burgeoning marketplace of herbal products and nutritional supplements, cat's claw has gained a reputation as a cure-all for conditions such as lupus, arthritis, bursitis, fibromyalgia, chronic fatigue syndrome, and chemical and environmental allergies.

Although there are many theories about how it fights these conditions, the one most often cited is stimulation of the immune system, says Tirun

121

Gopal, M.D., an obstetrician and gynecologist who practices holistic and Ayurvedic medicine in Allentown, Pennsylvania.

"It's used mostly for degenerative diseases where there is a significant loss of immunity," says Dr. Gopal. When people have diseases like cancer, lupus, or rheumatoid arthritis, their immune systems take a hard knock, leaving them open to secondary infections from colds and flu. Such infections—manageable for healthy people—can be life-threatening for people battling a chronic illness, he says.

"I've found that cat's claw can make the body more tolerant and better able to fight an infection, especially at its initial onset," he says. "You can use cat's claw by itself or with echinacea and astragalus—two other immune system stimulators—to boost its effectiveness."

The Jaguar's Claw

Historically, the Peruvian Indians made a tea from the root and inner bark of the plant to treat arthritis, tumors, ulcers, and inflammation. But since the Indians have an oral rather than a written tradition, the methodologies and uses of the plant remain obscure.

The first references in literature to this woody vine date back to the late 1700s, but it wasn't until the 1970s that an Austrian doctor drew attention to the herb in the West. The name cat's claw, or *uña de gato* in Spanish, comes from the vine's sharp, curved thorns that resemble the claws of a jaguar or cat.

SUPPLEMENT SNAPSHOT

▶Cat's Claw

Botanical names: *Uncaria tomentosa*, *U. guianensis*; also known as *uña de gato*.

May help: Heart disease, low immunity, bursitis, rheumatoid arthritis, chemical poisoning, fibromyalgia, chronic fatigue syndrome, and lupus.

Origin: Found in the Peruvian rain forest.

Cautions and possible side effects: Don't use if you have hemophilia or are pregnant. May cause headache, stomachache, or difficulty breathing; also has contraceptive properties.

Chemical analysis has revealed that the plant contains several important medicinal ingredients. Some of its alkaloids are known to be immune stimulants, and the plant appears to stimulate the activity of T cells, a type of white blood cells, says Dr. Gopal. These blood cells hunt down and act against virus-infected cells and tumor cells.

One alkaloid in particular seems to reduce blood pressure and may reduce the risk of stroke and heart attack.

The herb also contains compounds called glycosides that exhibit antiviral and anti-inflammatory activity. Some researchers suggest that cat's claw is effective at relieving swelling. "Because of this anti-inflammatory effect, some people have advocated its use with rheumatoid arthritis," comments Dr. Gopal.

Three of the glycosides in the herb have antioxidant activity, meaning that they have the ability to scavenge free radicals, the free-roaming, unstable molecules that cause aging and cell damage. An Italian study in 1992 suggested that cat's claw can also stop cells from mutating, which may mean that it could have value as a cancer treatment.

As good as all of this sounds, it's important to remember that these analyses and studies have been done using laboratory tests. No published study has looked at how the herb works in the human body, says Dr. Ben-Arye.

"Even though there have been some important ingredients found, we have no idea if the herb and those ingredients are actually beneficial to people," says Dr. Ben-Arye. "That has to be studied in a clinical setting, and those studies have not been published to date."

In other words, looking at the individual active ingredients can only partially explain why cat's claw works as well as it does. The healing power may actually come from a combination of these chemicals working together, says Dr. Ben-Arye.

Soap for Your Innards

Although the science may still be inconclusive on cat's claw, many herbalists and health professionals believe that this Amazonian plant has healing properties. Julie Clemens, N.D., a naturopathic doctor in Sagle, Idaho, says cat's claw is one of her workhorse herbs. She uses it frequently, usually as part of detoxifying therapy.

Dr. Clemens believes that many lifestyle diseases—arthritis, diabetes, headaches, and chronic constipation—are a result of chemical toxicity. The chemicals come from the environment, diet, or a person's lifestyle choices, such as smoking and drinking, she says.

"What eventually happens is that your body is unable to process and eliminate the toxins at the same rate they are coming in," she explains. "That can cause all types of problems."

Cat's claw has a reputation for diminishing a person's chemical sensitivity. It's also been used to cleanse and detoxify the intestinal tract, says Dr. Clemens. Typically, she prescribes cat's claw to an overweight person who has high blood pressure, problems with digestion and stomach acidity, and an unhealthy lifestyle. Her aim is to lower the toxic load, start cleaning plaque out of the arteries, and convince the person to make healthier lifestyle choices, she says.

"Cat's claw works on the entire system of the body. I like to call it an internal scrubber. Think of it as soap for your insides," she says.

Get the Real Cat

Cat's claw has grown so quickly in popularity that supplies of the herb are not consistent. Only the inner bark and root have medicinal value, but analysis of some cat's claw products have found outer bark, stems, and twigs mixed in.

The popularity of the herb has caused the Peruvian government to declare it a threatened species and to ban the harvesting of the root. Today, people are leaving the root, taking only the inner bark, and allowing the plant to recover.

In North America, cat's claw is available as a tincture, in capsules, and in raw bark form for brewing tea. Cat's claw tea tends to be very bitter, so most people prefer capsules. "I'd look for a product that contains at least a 0.3 percent alkaloid content," says Dr. Clemens.

Although you may hear cat's claw referred to as *uña de gato*, that can be a generic name for more than 20 herbs from Peru, some of which are toxic. Cat's claw belongs to the genus *Uncaria*, of which there are some 60 species in the world. Only 2, however—*U. tomentosa* and *U. guianensis*—from Peru are known to have the medicinal value discussed here.

cayenne

Capsicum is a pure, energetic, permanent stimulant, producing in large doses vomiting, purging, pains in the stomach and bowels, heat and inflammation of the stomach, giddiness, a species of intoxication, and an enfeebled condition of the nervous power.

—King's American Dispensatory, *a nineteenth-century herbal medical text*

When a medicinal herb makes your gut growl like that, it brings new clarity to the old adage "The cure is worse than the disease."

Of course, dosage matters. Who knows how much capsicum, better known as cayenne pepper, brought on such a purging?

In the case of cayenne, a little is good, but more isn't usually better, says Priscilla Evans, N.D., a naturopathic doctor at the Community Wholistic Health Center in Chapel Hill, North Carolina. "In small amounts, it is often beneficial, but by its very nature, cayenne is an irritating herb," she says.

Whether eaten as a food or taken as medicine, cayenne pepper has been used for centuries to treat asthma, fevers, sore throats, respiratory infections, and digestive problems. It can relieve flatulence and stimulate the stomach and gastrointestinal tract, and it may also reduce blood cholesterol and decrease a tendency to form blood clots.

Many of these actions stem from the ability of cayenne to stimulate the circulation and generate heat, says Dr. Evans. "Cayenne is found in many herbal formulas to get the blood moving."

Stops a Charging Bear

Cayenne is native to tropical America. Also called chile pepper or red pepper, it comes from the dried fruit of several species and hybrids of plants in the Solanaceae family.

The main active ingredient in cayenne is capsaicin, the stuff that makes hot peppers hot. In concentrated form, cayenne is so irritating that it's bottled in self-defense sprays that are advertised as being strong enough to stop a charging grizzly bear. Other constituents in cayenne include carotenoids, vitamins A and C, and volatile oils. The carotene molecules are potent antioxidants.

In 1552, an Aztec herbal text recommended cayenne as a treatment for toothaches and scabies, a skin disease caused by parasites. Subsequently, it was introduced to Europe, where it was used to reduce swollen lymph glands caused by tuberculosis, which was then known as the king's evil.

By the nineteenth century, doctors and herbalists prescribed cayenne as a general stimulant, believing that it "made the blood go round" and restored "internal heat." In the early twentieth century, it was used as part of the cure for alcohol and opium withdrawal. Doctors reasoned that the quickened action of the circulation increased the rate of blood cleansing and purification.

Mucus Mover

Because cayenne acts as a diaphoretic (which means that it makes you sweat), it was an herbal mainstay for general cleansing of the body, breaking fevers, and fighting infection.

"When you eat something hot like cayenne, your nose runs, you sweat, and all your fluids get moving," says Dr. Evans. That's a good thing when

---

SUPPLEMENT SNAPSHOT

▶ Cayenne

Botanical names: *Capsicum frutescens*, *C. annuum*, and other species.

May help: Blood clots, asthma, fever, sore throat, respiratory infections, flatulence, and high cholesterol and triglycerides.

Special instructions: Take with food.

Origin: Native to tropical America.

Cautions and possible side effects: May cause a burning sensation in the gastrointestinal tract in high doses or for some sensitive people.

you have a cold or flu and your mucous membranes are swollen and inflamed. Breaking up stagnant and congested mucus brings some relief from cold symptoms, says Dr. Evans, but even better, it brings fresh blood to the site of the infection. Fresh blood contains infection fighters from the immune system—white blood cells and leukocytes—that fight viruses and other foreign invaders.

Cayenne is frequently found in herbal cold and flu combinations, especially those with immune stimulants like echinacea and goldenseal, says Dr. Evans. "Cayenne helps the action of these other herbs by stimulating circulation and therefore the delivery of the herbs," she adds.

Its stimulating effects may also be good for your heart, says Pamela Herring, N.D., a naturopathic doctor at the Naturopathic Clinic of Concord in New Hampshire.

People in cultures that consume large amounts of cayenne appear to have lower rates of cardiovascular disease. There's evidence that frequent consumption of cayenne reduces levels of cholesterol and triglycerides (another type of blood fat) in the bloodstream. High levels of either can lead to atherosclerosis (hardening of the arteries) and blockages in the blood vessels.

Cayenne also appears to decrease the tendency to form blood clots and reduces the bunching up of blood platelets around plaque buildups in the vessels.

Dr. Herring believes that the herb's antioxidant properties and circulation-enhancing effects benefit the heart muscle. "Cayenne really stimulates the whole cardiovascular system," she says.

Fire Down Below

Cayenne is available in pills, capsules, and tincture. You can take it by itself or in combination with other herbs. You can also add it to foods as a spice.

When you take a capsule, you're likely to feel a bit of heat in your belly. For that reason, it's best to take it with food and start out with just one or two capsules a day, advises Dr. Herring. Sensitivity to cayenne varies from one person to the next.

chromium

No question, it's been overhyped. The headline of one supermarket tabloid proclaimed "Chromium Pill Will Add 25 Years to Your Life."

With dubious promotion like that, chromium's shine has definitely been somewhat tarnished. In fact, advertisements that touted chromium's weight-loss and muscle-building talents were exaggerated to the point where several big companies had their hands slapped for false advertising.

Still, this essential trace mineral is vital to health. In fact, the evidence is stronger than ever that chromium deficiency plays a fundamental role in the development of type 2 (non-insulin-dependent) diabetes. Type 2 is the kind of diabetes that typically affects people in their forties, fifties, or sixties rather than being a lifelong problem. Supplementation, experts say, may partly reverse some of type 2's effects.

Getting to Insulin and Arteries

In our bodies, chromium improves insulin effectiveness, says Richard Anderson, Ph.D., lead scientist in the nutrient requirements and functions laboratory at the U.S. Department of Agriculture Beltsville Human Nutrition Research Center in Maryland. Insulin is a hormone secreted by the pancreas that helps our bodies use blood sugar (glucose) by binding to receptor sites on the membranes of cells. This primes the cell in a way that allows it to take in blood sugar.

Chromium improves insulin function in two ways: It increases the sensitivity of receptor sites so that when insulin binds with the site, the cell is strongly activated and takes in lots of blood sugar. Plus, it increases the available number of insulin receptor sites on cells.

Keeping insulin and blood sugar levels normal is important because high levels of either—or both—can cause circulation problems that may lead to clogged arteries.

In studies, supplemental chromium has helped people with glucose intolerance, or insulin resistance, an early sign of diabetes for many people. A study conducted by Dr. Anderson in China showed that chromium supplements can reduce blood sugar and insulin levels in people with full-blown type 2 diabetes.

People with diabetes have a high risk of developing heart disease, but chromium may help reduce that risk as well, says Dr. Anderson. "High insulin levels have a direct damaging effect on the cells lining the arteries, so anything that keeps the level of insulin normal is helpful," he says. Also, since chromium is needed for your body to use fats just as it's needed to help your cells incorporate blood sugar, it helps clear fats out of your blood-

SUPPLEMENTSNAPSHOT

▶Chromium

Supplement forms: Chromium picolinate, nicotinate, aspartate, and chloride.

May help: Glucose intolerance, type 2 diabetes, binge-eating disorder, and high cholesterol.

Daily Value: 120 micrograms.

Special instructions: Take chromium picolinate, nicotinate, or aspartate; chromium chloride is the least absorbable form. Avoid the form called glucose tolerance factor (GTF), a combination of chromium, nicotinic acid, and amino acids, which may vary so much in composition that it is not a reliable source.

Who's at risk for deficiency: People who eat large amounts of refined sugar and carbohydrates and those who have diabetes, are insulin resistant, or are fighting infection or recovering from injuries.

Good food sources: Broccoli, turkey, ham, and grape juice.

Cautions and possible side effects: Don't take more than 200 micrograms a day without medical supervision, although doses up to 1,000 micrograms daily seem to be safe. If you have diabetes or hypoglycemia, consult your doctor before taking. If you have diabetes, the upper limits are 400 to 600 micrograms a day, but have your doctor carefully monitor your blood sugar levels.

stream. In several studies, people who were given supplemental chromium had drops in total cholesterol and "bad" LDL cholesterol and increases in "good" HDL cholesterol.

Chrome-Plated Muscles?

Promotions for chromium supplements often imply that chromium can help you lose fat and gain muscle. The reasoning behind this claim is based on chromium's insulin-enhancing effect. Insulin builds up muscles and other tissues, promotes utilization of amino acids and production of protein, and retards protein breakdown. In theory, at least, this would mean that people getting optimal amounts of chromium would be able to build more muscle than people whose chromium intake was low.

In reality, though, the truth is a little harder to pin down. In some studies—mostly of young, hard-training athletes—those taking chromium supplements sometimes saw some favorable changes in body composition. They had less fat and more muscle than comparable athletes not taking supplements. In a number of other studies, however, supplementation appeared to offer no advantage.

"Now that several of these studies have been done, it seems that the real gains in body composition don't start to appear until the fourth month," Dr. Anderson says. And even the "real gains" aren't what the ads might have you expect. You might see 1 to 2 percent more muscle and 1 to 2 percent less fat, with no change in body weight. "For highly trained athletes, that edge may make the difference," Dr. Anderson says.

If you don't exercise hard, Dr. Anderson adds, chances are that you'll see less of an effect. "Don't expect chromium supplements to do as much for your body as exercise," he says. "Don't think that chromium alone is going to take you from a size 16 to a size 8 dress."

The Short Story

It's clear that few people are getting the Daily Value of 120 micrograms of chromium. In fact, studies show that the average diet contains about 25 micrograms of this important mineral, and even balanced diets designed by dietitians contain less than 50 micrograms.

Some nutritionists argue that people simply don't need more chromium than they get from foods—that 25 micrograms a day may be sufficient.

Others, including Dr. Anderson, believe that people are less likely to develop diabetes and heart disease if they get 200 micrograms or more—the amounts that were found helpful in his studies. Moreover, he recommends as much as 400 to 600 micrograms for people who have diabetes.

If you are taking insulin for diabetes and you want to start taking high doses of chromium, check with your doctor and make sure that he keeps close tabs on your blood sugar levels, because your insulin needs will probably drop, Dr. Anderson says.

What about trying to help *prevent* diabetes by monitoring your chromium levels?

Unfortunately, says Dr. Anderson, there's no good way to test for chromium deficiency. "The only way to find out if supplemental chromium is going to be helpful to you is to try it under a doctor's supervision and see if it improves your blood sugar, insulin, and cholesterol levels," he says.

Your doctor can get a reading of these levels before you start taking supplements. After you've been taking the supplement for a while, the doctor can take a second reading for comparison.

coenzyme Q$_{10}$

When a 19-year-old college student from Houston experienced short-ness of breath and a racing heartbeat, his doctors diagnosed dilated car-diomyopathy, a condition characterized by an enlarged and weakened heart. They also told him that he would someday need a heart transplant.

Then he went to see Peter Langsjoen, M.D., a cardiologist in Tyler, Texas, who recommended a little-known substance called coenzyme Q$_{10}$ (coQ$_{10}$). Within a few weeks of starting to take coQ$_{10}$, the student required fewer prescription heart medications. Eventually, his heart size and function returned to normal.

"This is someone who, before coQ$_{10}$ came along, would most certainly have gone downhill," says Dr. Langsjoen. "It's clearly lifesaving."

Similar stories, coming directly from medical practitioners, have drawn public attention to this naturally occurring compound that our cells need to produce energy. Proponents credit coQ$_{10}$ with protecting the heart, strengthening the immune system, boosting energy and endurance, nor-malizing blood pressure, and healing periodontal disease.

Before you spend as much as $60 for a bottle of supplements, though, consider this: Many cardiologists have never even heard of coQ$_{10}$, much less recommended it to their patients.

Getting to the Heart of the Matter

CoQ$_{10}$ is made by the body and stored in the liver, kidneys, pancreas, and heart. We also get it from a variety of foods, especially liver and other organ meats. It is found in all cells, but it's most highly concentrated in heart muscle cells because they use the greatest amount of energy.

Most of us have plenty of coQ$_{10}$ in our bodies until around the age of 30. About then, our bodies lose the ability to manufacture it at the same levels, so the natural supply begins to diminish.

Apart from the decline in production that accompanies aging, there are other reasons for a shortage of coQ$_{10}$. Certain conditions, such as viral illnesses and shock, can rob us of this compound, says Dr. Langsjoen.

CoQ$_{10}$ deficiency is especially common in people with various types of heart disease. In fact, the more severe the heart disease, the lower the levels of coQ$_{10}$ found in heart muscle cells. Doctors don't know, though, whether the deficiency is one of the contributing causes or whether the reduced level of coQ$_{10}$ is the result of heart disease, says Dr. Langsjoen.

"CoQ$_{10}$ is definitely a factor in heart health because we know without a doubt that when you replenish it and restore levels to where they should be, heart function improves. If you let levels slide down again, heart function worsens," he explains.

This substance may improve the function of the heart by enhancing energy production, improving the ability of the heart to contract, and providing powerful antioxidant protection. The activity of coQ$_{10}$ helps prevent the buildup of oxidized LDL cholesterol, the "bad" kind of cholesterol that starts to block arteries when it's exposed to certain kinds of oxygen molecules. Because coQ$_{10}$ provides antioxidant protection, it helps prevent this

SUPPLEMENT SNAPSHOT

▶ Coenzyme Q$_{10}$

Also known as: CoQ$_{10}$.

May help: Gingivitis, chronic fatigue syndrome, Parkinson's disease, heart disease, high blood pressure, high cholesterol, congestive heart failure, mitral valve prolapse, angina, and arrhythmia; may provide some protection during heart surgery; may boost immunity and improve physical performance.

Special Instructions: Take supplements, preferably gelcaps, with food. Take tablets or capsules with a little peanut butter or other food that contains fat to aid absorption.

Good food sources: Liver and organ meats are possible sources but are not recommended because of their high fat and cholesterol content.

Cautions and possible side effects: Rarely, a slight decrease in the effectiveness of the blood thinner warfarin (Coumadin) has been observed. No other known side effects.

oxidizing process, and in so doing, it helps keep LDL cholesterol from blocking your blood vessels.

It may also speed recovery after heart surgery. When patients take coQ_{10} for several days prior to surgery, they recover faster and better, with fewer complications, according to Dr. Langsjoen.

Unfortunately, some of the medications that are beneficial for heart disease patients actually deplete the body's supply of coQ_{10}. Among the thieves are cholesterol-lowering statin drugs and beta-blockers such as propranolol (Inderal) and metoprolol (Toprol XI).

For prevention and recovery—and to counteract the depletion due to heart drugs—a number of doctors are now advocating the many benefits of coQ_{10}. It can help almost any disease related to the heart muscle, they say, including such problems as recurrent chest pain (angina) or irregular heart rate (arrhythmia). Some studies also suggest that it may enhance the benefits of cholesterol-lowering drugs, help lower blood pressure, and improve heart health for those with congestive heart failure, a condition in which the heart is unable to maintain normal blood circulation.

The Q_{10} Controversy

Critics and skeptics argue that many studies of coQ_{10} have been flawed or poorly controlled. Many of them have not been double-blind, for example. Considered the definitive form of medical research, a double-blind study is one in which neither the researchers nor the subjects know who is receiving the actual treatment. That's ideal because neither of them can influence the outcome by wishing for a positive result.

In experiments that don't use the double-blind method—like the coQ_{10} studies—there's a lot of room for bias. Another criticism of the research is that some study periods have been too short to be conclusive.

"The information about coQ_{10} is purely anecdotal," says Robert Di-Bianco, M.D., director of cardiology research at Washington Adventist Hospital in Takoma Park, Maryland, and associate professor at Georgetown University in Washington, D.C. "To date, I have not seen any convincing scientific data that suggest a benefit with coQ_{10} in a clinical situation. And I have honestly kept my eyes and ears open to this." More than 10 years ago, Dr. DiBianco took part in a study investigating whether coQ_{10} relieved angina. "We turned up very little," he says.

One popular use for the supplement is as a booster for aerobic endurance, especially among younger adults. It actually provides little in the way of benefit to athletes. If you're young and healthy, chances are that your body already has all the coQ$_{10}$ it needs, says Dr. Langsjoen.

On the other hand, there's no question that your body's supply of coQ$_{10}$ is depleted with aging. It seems to make sense that—all other things being equal—you would continue to have a "younger" heart if you used a supplement that provides some of the missing ingredient. It's prohibitively expensive, however, so it may not be widely available to many people.

How to Get Your CoQ$_{10}$

If you decide to give coQ$_{10}$ a try, stick with the gel caps that come mixed with oil for better absorption. If you do buy tablets or capsules, taking them with a small amount of peanut butter or other food that contains fat will help absorption, suggests Dr. Langsjoen.

As for the recommended dosage, Dr. Langsjoen says that most people have a good response with 60 to 120 milligrams twice a day. The appropriate individual dosage can best be determined by measuring blood levels of coQ$_{10}$, although there are currently few commercial laboratories that offer this test. To determine your dosage, ask your physician, who should also test your heart function at least twice a year if you're taking coQ$_{10}$.

copper

Shiny new pennies remind us of copper's value as currency, but it would take many bagfuls to buy a week's worth of groceries. In our bodies, however, a little copper goes a long way. It's an essential part of many enzymes, which spark the chemical reactions that sustain life.

Copper-containing enzymes have diverse roles. They help us form strong, flexible connective tissue; produce energy; use iron; and manufacture cholesterol. "Copper has a direct effect on our bones, skin, heart, liver, blood, kidneys, thyroid, immune system, and just about every part in between," says Judith Turnlund, R.D., Ph.D., a trace mineral specialist at the U.S. Department of Agriculture (USDA) Western Human Nutrition Research Center in San Francisco.

Like a Chain-Link Fence

If you examine a chain-link fence, you'll see that each strand of wire knits with the adjacent one, forming a strong mesh. In our bodies, copper helps link the long strands of proteins that make up the connective tissues throughout our bodies. It literally helps to hold us together.

"A copper-containing enzyme cross-links collagen, the body's most important connective tissue, which is used to make skin, bones, lungs, and many other tissues," says Leslie Klevay, M.D., a doctor of hygiene and research medical officer at the USDA Human Nutrition Research Center in Grand Forks, North Dakota. Copper also cross-links elastin, a fiber that can stretch and rebound. It is found mostly in the skin and blood vessels.

Copper-deficient animals have weakened hearts and blood vessels and may die of heart failure. Lacking copper, the heart or the aorta, the main artery from the heart, may burst, Dr. Klevay says. Also, copper-deficient animals have bone defects that are very similar to osteoporosis. These dangers may lie in wait for humans, too. That's one reason why nutritionists keep an eye on this significant trace mineral.

Enzymes That Lean on Copper

Two copper-containing enzymes are essential for our bodies to be able to use another important mineral—iron. These enzymes help move iron out of storage in cells lining the intestines or liver and transport it to the bone marrow, where it becomes part of the red blood cells produced there.

"If you don't have enough copper, your body simply can't use iron," Dr. Klevay says. Babies born with the inability to use copper and people who are copper-deficient develop anemia (insufficient red blood cells) because the copper shortage creates an iron shortage. When iron's in short supply,

SUPPLEMENT SNAPSHOT

▶Copper

May help: Bacterial, viral, and fungal infections and high cholesterol.

Daily Value: 2 milligrams.

Special instructions: Take as part of a multivitamin/mineral supplement that contains up to 2 milligrams of copper and less than 100 milligrams of vitamin C. If you want to take more vitamin C, take it separately; vitamin C interferes with copper absorption and utilization. Iron and zinc can interfere with absorption if taken in amounts greater than the Daily Value.

Who's at risk for deficiency: People who take more than 30 milligrams a day of zinc, because zinc may be absorbed instead of copper; people who take more than 100 milligrams of vitamin C at the same time as copper supplements; people who don't eat copper-rich foods or take non-steroidal anti-inaflammatory drugs; and those who consume large amounts of fructose, a component of both fruit and table sugar that can interfere with copper absorption.

Good food sources: Chocolate, legumes, mushrooms, nuts, peanut butter, seeds, shellfish (especially cooked oysters), and whole grains.

Cautions and possible side effects: Excess copper from supplements or from water from copper pipes can cause health problems. Signs include vomiting and diarrhea. Taking less than 10 milligrams occasionally is considered safe, but do not take more than 2 milligrams on a regular basis. Consult your doctor before taking higher amounts.

What Are Trace Minerals?

If you check the label on your multivitamin/mineral bottle, you may find some unfamiliar ingredients that seem somewhat suspicious, including such items as nickel, molybdenum, manganese, and vanadium. Some high-priced "designer" multis even contain silver or gold.

These are all trace minerals. Like iron and copper, some of them, such as molybdenum and manganese, are essential to human health in tiny amounts. "Both are enzyme activators," says Forrest Nielsen, Ph.D., director of the U.S. Department of Agriculture Human Nutrition Research Center in Grand Forks, North Dakota. These minerals are necessary for certain vital chemical reactions that take place in your body.

Molybdenum is important because it activates the enzyme that produces uric acid—the substance that helps carry excess nitrogen out of your body when you urinate. Manganese is a component of an enzyme that plays a role in preventing degenerative disease.

Lots of other trace minerals, even those found in multivitamins or sold singly, haven't been proven essential. There's some evidence that nickel, silicon, boron, and vanadium might be, but scientists still don't know for sure. And the jury's still out on minerals like germanium.

We get more than enough of certain trace minerals such as molybdenum and silicon in our diets, Dr. Nielsen says. Others, such as man-

the body doesn't produce enough hemoglobin, the protein in red blood cells that carries oxygen.

Along with iron, copper is also needed for many reactions that transform the food we eat into energy that our bodies can use. In a series of chemical reactions, the food is broken down and transported to cells. Inside the cells, tiny powerhouses called mitochondria change the food into energy-containing molecules that can either be stored or hacked apart to release energy. This process involves a kind of assembly line of proteins, Dr. Klevay explains, and "the final protein in this line must contain two or three molecules of copper or the job of energy production stops before it is completed."

The activity of the copper-containing enzyme lysyl oxidase and prolyl-oxidase, which cross-links collagen, is highest in cells that use the most energy—those in the heart, brain, liver, and kidneys.

Another copper-dependent enzyme, superoxide dismutase, plays a role

ganese and boron, may be in short supply. Either way, it's okay to take the 10 to 25 micrograms of any of these that you might find in a multi-vitamin/mineral tablet, he says. They won't hurt you, and they may even be helpful. Some trace minerals come from unprocessed foods like whole grains and certain vegetables and fruits, but if you're not likely to eat these foods, the supplements can easily make up any deficit.

What's not safe is using large amounts of trace mineral supplements for druglike effects. Vanadium, which supposedly builds muscle or prevents diabetes, and germanium, which has been said to prevent cancer and build the immune system, are sold singly. These supplements have shown little evidence of benefit, Dr. Nielsen says, and no studies have assessed the long-term effects of high amounts.

"I am concerned because vanadium is toxic if you build up to a high enough quantity in your body," says Dr. Nielsen. Furthermore, germanium might be contaminated with germanium dioxide, an inorganic form that can cause kidney damage. Worldwide, some 20 to 30 people have died from kidney damage caused by inorganic germanium. While it's true that you can order it from the Internet, that doesn't mean that you should. "This is not something to take lightly," Dr. Nielsen says.

as an antioxidant. Like vitamin E, it can neutralize the free-roaming, unstable molecules called free radicals. It circulates inside cells, soaking up free radicals that are produced as the cells break down waste products. Or it rushes to help immune cells called phagocytes, which "digest" bacteria that they swallow whole. With copper as an essential part of its wiring, superoxide dismutase helps cells stay young and protect themselves from bacterial, viral, fungal, and free radical onslaughts.

The Cholesterol Connection

Copper research has led to some close scrutiny of cholesterol metabolism. "Over 20 independent laboratories around the world now show that copper deficiency raises cholesterol levels in animals," says Dr. Klevay. When people are deprived of copper, their cholesterol levels shoot upward, similar to what happens in animals that are deprived of the mineral.

At least three enzymes seem to be involved, but the most important is HMG-coA reductase, found in the liver. Studies have found that this enzyme is overactive in copper-deficient animals. "What's so interesting about this is that the newest cholesterol-lowering drugs, called statins, also act on HMG-coA reductase," Dr Klevay explains. "They are specifically designed to inhibit its activity, which lowers cholesterol very efficiently."

Does that mean that people with high cholesterol aren't getting enough copper in their diets? "I think it's certainly a possibility for some people, but it has yet to be studied," Dr. Klevay says.

A Penny Short?

Severe copper deficiency is extremely rare, and it takes more than a poor diet to cause it. Still, some researchers believe that marginal copper deficiency is more common than we know and that people may develop chronic illnesses such as heart disease and osteoporosis as a result. Supporting the connection to osteoporosis are two studies that were done with women who took copper supplements. Both showed that the women's bone density improved when they had supplementation.

Most people get less than 1.5 milligrams a day of copper from foods, which is less than the Daily Value of 2 milligrams. You can increase your copper intake to recommended amounts by making appropriate food choices, Dr. Klevay says. Copper from foods is tolerated better than supplemental copper, so "you don't want to go overboard with supplements," he cautions.

creatine

After the Denver Broncos trounced the Green Bay Packers in Super Bowl XXXII, Broncos tight end Shannon Sharpe shared a little "secret" with ESPN and its large viewing audience. One of the team's smartest strategies wasn't drawn up beforehand on a chalkboard or whispered in a huddle. Instead, it came in the form of a powdery substance called creatine.

This nutritional supplement has become as common in locker rooms as sweaty gym socks and Right Guard. Olympians are taking it. High school athletes are taking it. Even weekend warriors pumping iron in their basements are taking it. So what is creatine, and why do so many athletes think it's the best thing to come along since barbells?

Creatine is an amino acid that our bodies make in the liver, pancreas, and kidneys. We also consume up to two grams of it each day in our food, especially when we eat red meat and fish. In the form of phosphocreatine, it's an important storehouse of energy in muscle, according to Richard Kreider, Ph.D., associate professor and assistant chair of the department of human movement sciences and education at the University of Memphis in Tennessee.

When we perform short bursts of intense exercise, phosphocreatine breaks down into its two components, creatine and phosphate, and the resulting energy is used to form a high-energy molecule called adenosine triphosphate (ATP).

ATP fuels muscles when they need a quick source of energy for activities such as sprinting, but only a small amount of ATP is stored in muscle cells. In fact, the total amount of ATP in the body provides just enough energy to perform at a maximum exercise level for several seconds. This is the level that athletes attain when they deliver a serve in tennis, leap over a high jump, or throw a shot-put, not the everyday exertion of walking fast or climbing stairs at normal speed.

By regenerating ATP, phosphocreatine lets you create even more energy. As phosphocreatine is depleted, energy levels and output drop because ATP can't be regenerated fast enough to meet the body's demands.

That's where creatine enters the picture. Its proponents say that by taking in extra creatine, you can make more phosphocreatine, maintain ATP levels for longer periods of time, and thereby generate more energy for sprinting, weight lifting, playing football, or any other sport that requires quick bursts of power.

A Boon for Athletes

Because creatine helps regenerate ATP more quickly, athletes need less rest and can recover faster. This helps them return to hard exercise sooner with fewer rests between sets, says Melvin Williams, Ph.D., professor emeritus in the department of exercise science, physical education, and recreation at Old Dominion University in Norfolk, Virginia, and author of *The Ergogenics Edge: Pushing the Limits of Sports Performance.*

To look at it another way, athletes who use this supplement are basically doing the same thing with creatine that marathoners have been doing with carbohydrates for years, namely, fueling up before exercising to top off their energy stores.

Creatine also may help delay the buildup of lactic acid that occurs in muscles during intense exercise. Lactic acid can limit the amount of intense exercise you can do because it causes a burning sensation in the muscles that makes you want to stop, especially if you haven't exercised at that level before.

SUPPLEMENT SNAPSHOT

▶Creatine

May help: Enhance athletic performance and allow athletes to recover faster and increase muscle mass.

Good food sources: Red meat and fish.

Cautions and possible side effects: There are no long-term studies of creatine's impact on human health; may cause cramping, muscle pulls, dehydration, and stress on the kidneys.

Weighty Evidence

Many studies back up proponents' claims that creatine improves the body's ability to explode with energy. Research also shows that creatine boosts short-term muscle strength.

In one of Dr. Kreider's studies, 25 NCAA division 1A football players were divided into two groups. One group took creatine and the other took a supplement that looked like creatine but wasn't (a placebo). Neither the researchers nor the players knew who was receiving creatine and who was receiving the placebo. During a four-week supplementation period, the athletes participated in a standardized training program that included weight lifting, high-intensity sprinting, and football agility drills. At the end of the study, the creatine group had greater gains in weight-lifting volume, sprint performance, and weight gain.

In another study, researchers at Pennsylvania State University investigated the influence of creatine supplementation on muscle performance during repeated sets of high intensity resistance exercise. In this study, 14 men were randomly assigned to a creatine or a placebo group. Both groups performed bench presses and jump squats before and after taking either 25 grams of creatine or a placebo.

At the end of the test period, researchers found that performance was unchanged for the men in the placebo group. The creatine group, however, had significant improvement in peak power output during jump squats and bench presses after only one week on the supplement.

Ergogenic Factors

Not all studies have shown that people gain from creatine supplementation. In a study in which Dr. Williams looked at 60-meter sprint times for highly trained athletes, he found no improvement in a creatine group when compared with a placebo group.

Despite those findings, Dr. Williams thinks that creatine is still in the running as an energy booster. He points to studies that specifically focus on ergogenic factors—that is, the ability of the supplement to boost energy production. "With any studies using ergogenic aids such as creatine, you will have variability in performance on a day-to-day basis," he says.

Also, not all types of athletic efforts can be enhanced by creatine, adds Dr. Kreider. Taking creatine for short periods of time will have little or no benefit for endurance athletes such as marathoners, for example. In fact, it may even hamper performance because creatine leads to an increase in body mass that could slow down these athletes.

Is It Safe?

Although scientists first discovered creatine more than 100 years ago, it's only been marketed as a nutritional supplement since 1992, so there's no way to know its long-term effects. Although proponents claim that creatine is a harmless dietary supplement, no one knows what will happen if people continue to take it for many years at the recommended dose of 5 to 25 grams daily.

"Creatine is relatively safe, and it's a biological material that's normally found in the body anyway. The question is, what happens if you take a lot of it over a long period of time? We don't know that yet," says Ara Der-Marderosian, Ph.D., professor of pharmacognosy and medicinal chemistry at the University of the Sciences in Philadelphia.

Dr. Kreider, however, puts a time limit on its use, noting that it's safe for up to two years in athletes.

Some Downsides

One known potential hazard is that too much creatine can stress the kidneys, says Dr. DerMarderosian. For that reason, he recommends that anyone with kidney problems avoid the supplement altogether. Product purity is also a concern for some researchers, who claim that minor impurities could be harmful at the daily doses that athletes are taking.

Bill Bryan, M.D., clinical associate professor at the Baylor Sports Medicine Institute in Houston, says short-term creatine use leads to muscle strains, cramping, and dehydration and to weight gain that's mostly the result of water retention. "I think it works, but there are adverse effects. Maybe not when you run tests in a laboratory or a university setting, but when you get into field conditions, there are some problems," says Dr. Bryan, who is also director of medical services for the Houston Astros baseball team.

Dr. Bryan voices another concern—that athletes will neglect good nutritional habits while taking creatine. He also doesn't trust the influx of new products that contain not only creatine but also other unproven ingredients such as chromium.

He is not alone in his opposition to creatine. In a survey of members of the Association of Professional Team Physicians, 85 percent of respondents said they would not recommend using the supplement until more research has been completed.

Loading Up

Athletes typically take creatine in two phases, beginning with the "loading" phase. A typical loading program is a five-gram dose four times a day for a week. After that, the dose is reduced to two to five grams daily as "maintenance." This regimen can be expensive, with a one-month supply costing as much as $60.

It's best to leave creatine to competitive athletes, says Dr. Williams. "The only reason to supplement is to enhance performance. If you're not competitive, there's really no reason to take it."

It's possible, though, that in the future, creatine could be found in other places besides sweat-soaked workout rooms. According to Dr. Kreider, researchers are looking into its therapeutic value for people who experience skeletal muscle weakness due to conditions such as chronic heart failure. Researchers are also investigating whether it can help slow bone loss in the elderly. "If you can prevent the loss of lean muscle mass, perhaps you can slow down bone loss," he suggests. Finally, at least two studies have shown that creatine lowers total cholesterol. More research is expected.

vitamin D

Vitamin D is an essential nutrient that our bodies can make on any reasonably sunny day. In fact, it's called the sunshine vitamin because we can make all we need if we have enough sunlight hitting our skin.

Ultraviolet rays from the sun convert one type of chemical compound in our skin to a substance called previtamin D_3, which is then converted to vitamin D_3. This in turn is converted twice more, in the liver and kidneys, into active vitamin D. While either liver or kidney disease may cause a shortage, people who have liver disease can usually make enough to get by. People with kidney disease, on the other hand, often need to take the active form of vitamin D, which is available only by prescription, to prevent deficiency.

In the body, vitamin D acts more like a hormone than a vitamin. In other words, it has a direct effect on organs such as the intestines, kidneys, and bones. The cells of these organs have receptor sites, similar to docking platforms, just for vitamin D. All of these organs respond to the vitamin by making calcium available for bone growth.

Harden Up and Grow Right

Open just about any nutrition textbook to the pages on vitamin D and you'll see haunting photographs of children with rickets, a deficiency condition. Their heads are large because their skull bones haven't fused properly, and their legs are bowed because their bones are too soft to support their weight.

Rickets is no longer common in the United States, but "vitamin D deficiency may play a contributing role in two common conditions that affect older adults," says Hector DeLuca, Ph.D., chairman of biochemistry at the University of Wisconsin in Madison and a leading vitamin D researcher. One of these conditions is osteomalacia, or softening of the bones, and the other is osteoporosis, or bone loss. "Low blood levels of vitamin D make both of

146

these conditions worse," he says. In fact, just a few weeks' worth of the Daily Value, which is 400 international units (IU), or 10 micrograms, will improve some symptoms of these conditions if vitamin D levels are low. "People improve dramatically once they start getting enough vitamin D," Dr. DeLuca says.

Vitamin D helps to make calcium and phosphorus available in the blood that bathes the bones. As these essential minerals are deposited, the bones mineralize, or harden.

It makes calcium and phosphorus available in three ways. In the intestines, it sends cells the message, "Absorb more calcium and phosphorus." In the kidneys, the instruction is "Don't pee out that calcium and phosphorus—recirculate it." And when blood levels of calcium begin to drop, vitamin D sends bone cells the message, "Start breaking down bone and get that calcium into the bloodstream."

That final message is important because calcium is needed throughout our bodies to maintain normal muscle and nerve function. Low levels can lead to fatal convulsions. And if you have only calcium in circulation—without the vitamin D that's necessary to help incorporate it—you could

SUPPLEMENT SNAPSHOT

▶ Vitamin D

May help: Osteomalacia, osteoporosis, and multiple sclerosis.

Daily Value: 400 international units (10 micrograms).

Who's at risk for deficiency: People who have chronic intestinal absorption problems or chronic liver or kidney disease, people who don't eat many dairy products and aren't exposed to sunlight, and those who use sunscreen at all times.

Good food sources: Fatty fish such as mackerel and salmon and fortified milk and milk products. (The best nonfood source of vitamin D is the sun.)

Cautions and possible side effects: Large doses (more than 2,000 IU daily) over several months can cause high blood levels of calcium, kidney stones, and calcium deposits in heart and kidney tissues, which can be fatal.

end up with a calcium deficiency. You need that calcium, and you also need vitamin D to help it do its job.

Why D Is a Big Deal

Bones aren't the only parts of our bodies that vitamin D befriends. Researchers are finding more and more places where it's active.

Forms of vitamin D are being studied in the laboratory for the treatment of breast, prostate, and colon cancer, plus a deadly skin cancer, melanoma. One form of vitamin D, as a topical cream named calcipotriene (Dovonex), has shown marked improvement of psoriasis for up to 70 percent of the people who used it.

Researchers don't know exactly how vitamin D works in these cases, but like vitamin A, it promotes a process called cell differentiation. Like a traffic cop, it directs developing cells in the right direction, toward their proper, mature form. In the skin, for example, it normalizes the growth rate of cells called keratinocytes. In psoriasis, these cells proliferate like crazy without going through their normal growth process. That's what causes the snowstorm of flaky skin.

Also, a deficiency of vitamin D "almost certainly plays a role in the development of type 1 (insulin-dependent) diabetes," Dr. DeLuca adds. The vitamin is needed for cells in the pancreas, called islet cells, to produce insulin, the hormone that allows cells to take up blood sugar. Without adequate vitamin D, islet cells don't produce insulin.

In animals with an inherited tendency to develop type 1 diabetes, the active vitamin D hormone helps prevent the disease, Dr. DeLuca says. While studies have not yet been done in humans, researchers speculate whether it might prove to have a similar effect.

Help for T-Helpers

Vitamin D also helps to regulate some of the white blood cells that make up the immune system. In animals, it helps one kind of "supervisor" (T-helper) cell release biochemicals that stop another kind of T-helper cell from attacking the body's own tissues. Thus, in animals at least, this vitamin helps block the destructive assault that occurs in autoimmune diseases such as rheumatoid arthritis, lupus, and multiple sclerosis, Dr. DeLuca says.

Researchers at the University of Wisconsin may soon learn whether fairly small doses of the active form of vitamin D can help stop nerve-damaging lesions in people who are newly diagnosed with multiple sclerosis.

Milk May Let You Down

Vitamin D deficiency is a real problem in the United States, and it becomes increasingly likely in people age 50 and older, says Michael Holick, M.D., Ph.D., chief of the section on endocrinology, nutrition, and diabetes at Boston University Medical Center. People just don't get enough of the few foods that contain vitamin D—milk and fatty fish such as mackerel and salmon.

"In fact, milk may not be as reliable a source as people think it is," Dr. Holick says. In the United States, milk is generally fortified with 400 IU of vitamin D per quart. When Dr. Holick's laboratory analyzed samples of milk in all regions of the United States and western Canada, however, researchers found that many didn't contain as much vitamin D as they were supposed to. Fat-free milk was worst: One out of every six samples contained no vitamin D at all.

"Most older people, especially those who use sunscreen, probably don't get enough sun to meet their vitamin D requirements," Dr. Holick says. Nevertheless it is possible to get an adequate amount of vitamin D from sunlight, he says. Dr. Holick recommends that you expose your hands, face, and arms to sunlight in the midmorning or afternoon. If you live in the north—about the latitude of Boston—you'll have enough exposure if you get 5 to 15 minutes of sunlight three times a week in spring, summer, and fall. Winter sun isn't strong enough to meet your needs for vitamin D unless you live in Florida or a similar clime.

Supplements are another reliable way to get what you need if you're not getting enough vitamin D from dairy sources or sunlight. You can take a multivitamin/mineral supplement that offers the Daily Value of 400 IU.

The National Research Council, which sets standard, official guidelines for U.S. health agencies, has recommended a daily dose of 600 IU for people over 70. Some studies show that people over 65 benefit from getting up to 800 IU a day, especially during the winter months.

DHEA

"Boosts sex drive!" "Restores memory!" "Fights cancer!" "Prevents heart disease!" "Helps erase wrinkles!" "Strengthens immunity!" "Fights fat!" These are just a few of the claims being made for a popular dietary supplement known as DHEA (short for dehydroepiandrosterone).

In the body, this hormone is made by the adrenal glands. In the form of DHEA sulfate, it is shipped to various tissues, including the breasts, endometrium (lining of the uterus), prostate, and muscles.

DHEA is a precursor of other hormones, which means that upon arrival, it sets off a chain reaction that produces another kind of hormone. Once in the tissues, it is converted to the appropriate sex hormone for that tissue.

For some tissues, the male hormone testosterone is required. Other tissues receive the principal female sex hormone, estrogen, and still others get both types of hormones.

When a woman gets DHEA, for example, it's converted to estrogen in the ovaries. In a man, it's converted to testosterone in the prostate. In both sexes, DHEA is transformed into testosterone and estrogen in the muscles.

Add together these hormonal effects, and it becomes apparent why proponents are making so many claims for DHEA. This hormone supplement, they say, should stop or even reverse the aging process and the diseases that can occur in our later years.

There is a danger in taking DHEA supplements, though, because a number of tumors are hormone-dependent, says Richard L. Sprott, Ph.D., executive director of the Ellison Medical Foundation, an organization that funds research on the biology of aging, in Bethesda, Maryland.

If you have an existing hormone-dependent tumor such as a testicular or prostate tumor, DHEA could be sent directly to the tumor, where it would be converted into the testosterone that the tumor needs to grow. "The tumor will kill you sooner than it would have otherwise," Dr. Sprott explains. The same may be true for endometrial, ovarian, and breast tumors in women.

For elderly men, there could be a significant risk. Among men ages 70 to 74 in the United States, more than 1 in 100 will be diagnosed with prostate cancer each year. But that doesn't mean that it's the leading cause of death among this group.

According to Dr. Sprott, "It's a very slow-growing cancer that won't kill them before they die of other causes. But if you were to feed DHEA to the tumor and accelerate its rate of growth, the cancer might become significant and life-threatening."

DHEA production peaks between the ages of 25 and 30, then declines with age. This decline is the reason that some suggest that aging may be linked to DHEA deficiency. Replenish DHEA, they argue, and you'll slow the effects of aging. But diminishing DHEA levels could also mean that elderly people simply don't need as much, says Dr. Sprott.

"Many things decline with advancing age," he adds. "Whether DHEA is important in that decline is unknown, although the dietary supplement industry suggests that it's a causal relationship. We don't know that it is. We're not trying to say that DHEA has no effect, but we do think that there is significant risk that has not been explained to the consumer."

SUPPLEMENT SNAPSHOT

▶ DHEA

Also known as: Dehydroepiandrosterone.

May help: Lupus; may slow or reverse aging, but any beneficial effect of DHEA use in humans has not been established by scientific studies.

Cautions and possible side effects: Do not take without your doctor's knowledge; may cause liver damage, acne, irritability, irregular heart rhythms, accelerated growth of existing tumors, loss of scalp hair in men and women, and growth of facial hair and deepening of the voice in women. Men and women under 35 should avoid supplements because they could suppress the body's natural production of DHEA; deficiencies in this group are rare.

Future Promise

Taking these risks into account, researchers are still exploring the possible benefits of DHEA. As studies continue, doctors may find that DHEA, taken judiciously, has other promising uses.

Dr. Sprott says that the most encouraging DHEA data he's seen was a study of systemic lupus. In this type of lupus, the immune system seems to attack normally healthy cells and tissue. There are many long-lasting symptoms that involve the skin, joints, kidneys, and other tissues and organs.

In a study of women with mild to moderate systemic lupus, 14 received 200 milligrams of DHEA daily for three months, while a second group of 14 women received a look-alike pill (placebo) that contained no DHEA. At the end of the study, two-thirds of those receiving DHEA showed marked improvement. Women in the placebo group showed almost no improvement.

There is also preliminary evidence that DHEA may boost immunity, enhance memory, and improve mood, energy, and libido in the elderly. It may reduce the risk of type 2 (non-insulin-dependent) diabetes. One study even suggested that DHEA may have a future role as an adjunct to hormone replacement therapy, helping out the estrogen that's a standard element in this treatment for postmenopausal women.

It's important to note that much of the DHEA research is based on animal data, says Arthur G. Schwartz, Ph.D., researcher and microbiologist at Temple University Medical School in Philadelphia, who has been studying DHEA for over 20 years.

Many supplement manufacturers are picking up on the results of animal studies and applying them to humans—an irresponsible practice, as Dr. Schwartz sees it. One of his studies reporting anti-obesity effects of DHEA on laboratory animals was widely touted by manufacturers as proof that DHEA could promote weight loss in humans, but it's not true, he says.

Doses found in supplements are based on the doses given to animals in laboratory experiments—from 25 to 50 milligrams daily, says Dr. Schwartz. When you convert that amount to what a human would need to get the same or similar effects for weight loss, though, you'd have to increase the dose to up to 2,000 milligrams a day.

Working with the National Cancer Institute, Dr. Schwartz has also tested a modified compound of DHEA. It may have some of the positive benefits of DHEA, but at a lower dose and without producing the hormonal side effects. Even if the results continue to be promising and the DHEA passes tests for approval, however, don't expect to find modified DHEA on store shelves, Dr. Schwartz says. For this form of DHEA, you will probably need a prescription.

Tinkering with Mother Nature

Most people who take DHEA are overdosing, says Ray Sahelian, M.D., a physician in Marina del Rey, California, and author of *DHEA: A Practical Guide.* Although he's a proponent of DHEA, he's concerned that many people are taking doses of 25 milligrams or more daily, an amount that can lead to side effects he's seen in his patients, including acne, growth of facial hair on women, irritability, accelerated scalp hair loss in both men and women, and even irregular heart rhythms. A less measurable effect may be the possibility of accelerating tumor growth, according to Dr. Sprott.

Dr. Sahelian says that he has lowered his recommended dose significantly, to 1 to 5 milligrams daily, since he first started prescribing DHEA to his patients. The problem is that many supplements are sold in 25-milligram or 50-milligram capsules.

Almost nothing is known about DHEA's interactions with other drugs or its long-term effects. "This doesn't work fast, like poison. You're not going to take DHEA for a week, develop a testicular tumor, and die. This is something whose effects you might not see for 5 to 10 years. And by then, it's too late, because you've been accumulating a risk over a long period of time," warns Dr. Sprott.

The Food and Drug Administration (FDA) banned over-the-counter sales of DHEA in 1985, but the ban was lifted with the passage of the Dietary Supplement Health and Education Act of 1994. This law allows certain substances to be sold for human consumption without FDA approval, as long as they are marketed as "dietary supplements" and not labeled for a particular use like prescription or over-the-counter drugs.

To make DHEA supplements, vitamin and pharmaceutical companies extract sterols, most commonly diosgenin, from wild yams. Some supplements, however, are extracts of wild yams that haven't been processed into DHEA. These are marketed as containing natural precursors for the body's production of DHEA, but they have not been found to boost DHEA levels.

vitamin E

Vitamin E got itself a reputation as a "sex vitamin" early on. When it was being tested on laboratory animals, it gave every sign of deserving that reputation.

When male animals were deprived of vitamin E, their testicles shrank. In pregnant female animals with vitamin E deficiency, the fetuses were reabsorbed into the uterus, preventing the animals from bearing young. Giving the animals even a single drop of vitamin E–rich wheat germ oil restored their fertility. In fact, vitamin E got its scientific name, tocopherol, from this particular ability. It means "to bring forth offspring."

Today, most vitamin E research focuses on much broader roles, such as preventing heart disease and cancer. And since most people don't get enough vitamin E from foods to protect themselves from these diseases, it wasn't long before favorable reports on vitamin E began to affect sales of the supplements. Soon, sales of vitamin E were catching up with those of vitamin C, the biggest-selling single supplement nutrient in the United States.

A Heart Helper

In the case of heart disease, two studies from Harvard University involving a total of about 135,000 health professionals found that those who took daily supplements of vitamin E were one-fourth to one-third less likely to develop heart disease than those who didn't take supplements. They took at least 100 international units (IU) over a period of at least two years.

A study done in England, called the Cambridge Heart Antioxidant Study, showed that people with heart disease who took at least 400 IU of vitamin E had about one-quarter the risk of having nonfatal heart attacks compared with people who took look-alike pills (placebos) that didn't contain any vitamin E.

Researchers in another study found that among male smokers who took 50 to 75 IU a day of vitamin E, the incidence of prostate cancer was reduced by about one-third. There were 41 percent fewer deaths from prostate cancer among the men who took vitamin E as opposed to those who didn't.

Many other studies point to areas in which vitamin E looks promising. In Boston, for instance, Tufts University researchers discovered that 200 IU a day of supplemental vitamin E could reverse age-related declines in immune function. Researchers at Columbia University in New York City

SUPPLEMENTSNAPSHOT

▶Vitamin E

Supplement forms: D-alpha-tocopherol, d-alpha tocopheryl acetate, and d-alpha tocopheryl succinate.

May help: Heart disease, angina, cancer, multiple sclerosis, diabetes, Alzheimer's disease, cataracts, emphysema, high cholesterol, intermittent claudication, infertility, impotence, genital herpes, bedsores, leg cramps, muscle soreness, phlebitis, menopausal discomforts, HIV, osteoarthritis, and chronic inflammatory diseases such as lupus and rheumatoid arthritis.

Daily Value: 30 international units.

Special instructions: For doses higher than the Daily Value, take in divided doses with meals that contain some fat. Take a natural form (d-alpha tocopherol or d-alpha tocopheryl acetate or succinate).

Who's at risk for deficiency: People who can't absorb fat properly and those with Crohn's disease or cystic fibrosis.

Good food sources: Almonds, spinach, turnip greens, mustard greens, kohlrabi, kale, dandelion greens, margarine, peanut oil, safflower oil, soybean oil, sunflower oil and seeds, wheat germ, and wheat-germ oil.

Cautions and possible side effects: Use only with medical supervision if you are taking anticoagulants (blood thinners), ginkgo, or fish-oil supplements; if you take aspirin regularly to help prevent heart disease; if you have high blood pressure, heart disease, or cancer; if you smoke; if you have had a stroke; or if you are at high risk for stroke. Although vitamin E is commonly sold in doses of 400 IU, one small study showed a possible risk of stroke in doses over 200 IU.

found that people with Alzheimer's disease who took 2,000 IU a day were able to delay certain problems associated with the disease. Those who took the supplement were able to go longer (by seven months) before they lost their ability to groom or feed themselves or had to make a switch from their own homes to nursing homes.

For treatment of rheumatoid arthritis, vitamin E also has shown promise. European researchers have found that people with rheumatoid arthritis who take 800 IU a day of vitamin E report less pain than those who go without it.

Playground Supervisor

Vitamin E apparently has only one major role in the body, but that one is a whopper. "It functions as our bodies' major fat-soluble antioxidant," says Maret Traber, Ph.D., principal investigator at the Linus Pauling Institute and associate professor of nutrition at Oregon State University in Corvallis. Vitamin E is found throughout our bodies in the tissues that contain fat, including the protective membranes surrounding cells and their nuclei, which contain the genetic material.

This all-important vitamin is also found in the fatty sheaths that wrap around and insulate nerves and in molecules called lipoproteins, which circulate in our blood. "In these places, vitamin E helps to neutralize molecular particles called free radicals that are produced as a normal part of reactions that involve oxygen," Dr. Traber says.

These reactions, called oxidation-reduction reactions, go on all the time. Problems occur, though, when a chemical reaction generates a free radical. "A free radical is a molecule that has an unpaired electron, making it unstable," Dr. Traber says. Because the imbalance makes it hungry for an electron, it steals one from some other molecule.

Stopping a Chain Reaction

Unfortunately, that means that another molecule is short an electron, so it becomes a free radical that in turn strives to pluck an electron from some other unlucky molecule nearby. The effect is a chain reaction of free radical damage, kind of like a game of tag that's gotten out of control.

This innocent game leads to trouble. Cell membranes are damaged, sometimes beyond repair. Cell contents leak out, and the cell dies. Or, if the damage occurs in the membranes inside a cell, the cell's genetic material is harmed.

If the damage occurs in the membrane of the cell's power plant, the mitochondria, trouble multiplies like a breakout fight at a hockey game. Free radicals normally generated inside the mitochondria leak out into the cell. Cellular unrest spreads like wildfire.

Vitamin E can stop all this by donating one of its own electrons to a free radical. When that happens, there's no chain reaction. Vitamin E stops the outbreak of electron-grabbing dead in its tracks. You could think of it as a playground supervisor for that rowdy game of tag.

High-Speed Chase

Vitamin E moves with uncanny speed throughout the fluid cell membrane. Because it moves so quickly, it can help protect about 1,000 of the molecules that make up the membrane, Dr. Traber says. Once it neutralizes a free radical, the vitamin E twists within the membrane so that its free radical part is exposed to the watery solution surrounding the cell. There, it meets up with any vitamin C that's available, and vitamin C is an award-winning ally in this process. It regenerates vitamin E by giving up one of its own electrons, allowing vitamin E to go right back to work.

Many diseases, and even aging, seem to be associated with free radical oxidative damage, Dr. Traber says. Cancer, for instance, may be started by free radical damage to a cell's genetic material. Heart disease may begin when free radicals oxidize LDL cholesterol, the artery-clogging kind of free-floating fat that doctors monitor most closely. In effect, the free radicals turn this fat rancid. In so doing, they initiate what is thought to be an early step in heart disease.

Also, it seems that inflammation anywhere in the body—joints, nerves, or connective tissues—may well involve out-of-control free radical damage, Dr. Traber says. That's why vitamin E and other antioxidants, such as vitamin C, are being studied for their effects on such a variety of conditions.

Supplements Are Essential

The amounts of vitamin E that studies suggest provide protection from heart disease or enhance immunity can't be gotten from even an exemplary diet. The Daily Value for vitamin E is 30 IU, but estimates of an optimal dose really start at around 100 IU. You'd have to eat 58 cups of boiled spinach, 6 cups of peanuts, 1½ cups of corn oil, or three tablespoons of wheat germ oil to get close to that amount.

If you are watching your weight and reducing the amount of fat in your diet, you are even less likely to get close to the DV for vitamin E. In one study of people who had cut their fat intake below 30 percent of calories, daily vitamin E intake dropped from 14.5 to 9.5 IU.

Even the DV, however, is only a measure of what it takes to prevent a deficiency, while most of us, and most doctors, are interested in how much we might need to significantly improve health. There's a huge gap between the DV and what researchers call the optimal value. And when it comes to discussing optimal value, there's even more divergence of opinions and recommended amounts.

While some researchers recommend from 100 to 400 IU a day, a number of clinicians recommend even higher amounts for people age 45 and older or for those with chronic diseases. One study, from researchers at the University of Texas Southwestern Medical Center in Dallas, found that the minimum dose of vitamin E required to significantly reduce LDL oxidation was 400 IU a day. Doses up to 1,200 IU—which is 40 times the DV—provided additional benefits. Taking 200 IU a day did not significantly reduce LDL oxidation, they found. Given this wide range of results, Dr. Traber and other experts are involved in ongoing discussions about new guidelines for recommending vitamin E.

Is E for You?

Certainly, it's worth discussing with your doctor whether you should take vitamin E supplements, and of course, you'll want to ask about risks. One concern is that large doses of vitamin E might elevate the risk of bleeding problems and lead to hemorrhagic stroke, a fairly uncommon type. Unlike other strokes, it's caused not by a blood clot but by a bleeding or broken blood vessel in the brain.

The same study that saw a reduction in the risk of prostate cancer in men taking 50 to 75 IU of vitamin E also saw an increase in the number of hemorrhagic strokes in the vitamin E takers. The percentage of men in the study who actually had strokes, though, remained fairly small.

"This is a finding that poses additional questions and requires further study," says Demetrius Albanes, M.D., a senior investigator in the cancer prevention studies branch of the National Cancer Institute.

The link with hemorrhagic stroke is directly related to the way vitamin E works. One reason that vitamin E helps to reduce heart attack risk is that it interferes with little particles in the blood called platelets, which play a role in blood clotting. Platelets can clump together or stick to artery walls when they shouldn't, which can cause a clot that closes off an artery. Vitamin E helps to prevent that, but it could also prevent the platelets from sticking and clumping when they need to.

Until there are answers about vitamin E's real effects on the risk of bleeding problems, and until additional research supports vitamin E's beneficial effects on cancer and cardiovascular disease, Dr. Albanes suggests caution when you consider taking more than the Daily Value. Before giving you the go-ahead for large doses of vitamin E, your doctor can do a test that checks your bleeding time. With that test in hand, you're better able to discuss the benefits versus possible risks.

Choosing the Right Form

As for what form of vitamin E to take, several studies support the use of vitamin E in its natural form, d-alpha tocopherol, over its synthetic form, dl-alpha tocopheryl acetate. The natural form is twice as active, so manufacturers make up for that by putting more of the synthetic form into capsules. But natural vitamin E is also retained twice as long in the body as synthetic vitamin E, which means that it can build up and stay at higher levels.

Natural vitamin E also contains more than just d-alpha tocopherol. It is typically combined with other forms, such as gamma tocopherol, that appear to offer added protection. Researchers at the University of California at Berkeley, for example, discovered that gamma tocopherol also has powerful antioxidant properties. These other tocopherols are not present in synthetic vitamin E, although they are found in foods rich in the vitamin.

Multivitamins usually contain vitamin E in one of its water-soluble forms, d-alpha tocopheryl acetate or d-alpha tocopheryl succinate. These forms are just as good as d-alpha tocopherol, Dr. Traber says.

Most multivitamins don't offer enough vitamin E for optimal protection from chronic disease, however. If you want to take more than 100 IU of vitamin E a day, you need to take either an antioxidant formula or supplements that contain only vitamin E (usually d-alpha tocopherol), she says.

echinacea

When you catch a cold or wince with the pain of an ear infection, your body is like a neighborhood invaded by unsavory characters.

In your body, viruses and bacteria are the bad guys. The cops are your white blood cells, and the S.W.A.T. team is made up of snuff-out cells called phagocytes. These specialized cells roam through your circulatory system on a special mission, ingesting and destroying specific substances, like viruses and bacteria, that could do harm to your body. This process is called phagocytosis, and by the time it's complete, few foreign invaders are left in the neighborhood.

If you want to take out a cold virus or prevent an ear infection, you need the body's equivalent of a beefed-up police force. It's time to send out the call for more phagocytes—and echinacea can help you do that.

In the Trenches of Germ Warfare

There are several herbs that act as immunostimulants—botanical medicines that help your body fight off illness by bolstering its natural defenses. Echinacea is the best-known of these herbs and the one with the most scientific evidence behind it.

This North American plant kicks your immune system into high gear. Echinacea can stop a cold, influenza, or bacterial infection before it can spread in the body. It can also shorten the duration and lessen the symptoms of the infection, says Alison Lee, M.D., a pain-management specialist and medical director of Barefoot Doctors, an alternative medicine practice in Ann Arbor, Michigan.

"I recommend that people carry a tincture of echinacea with them and start taking it as the package directs at the first sign of a cold. It's really effective right at the beginning of an infection," says Dr. Lee.

Echinacea may kill some viruses and bacteria directly, but it is also known to arm the immune system to do the dirty work, she says.

Your Immune System on Mocha Java

When you take echinacea, your immune system responds as if it had just downed several cups of strong Colombian coffee. It can't sit still. Echinacea speeds up the process of phagocytosis and increases the number of white blood cells—natural killer cells—hunting down foreign particles such as viruses and bacteria in your body.

"Your natural killer cells are the cops who come and say, 'Who's in the neighborhood that doesn't belong here? Let's get rid of them,'" explains Steven Dentali, Ph.D., a natural products chemist with Dentali Associates in Troutdale, Oregon, and a member of the advisory board of the American Botanical Council.

Echinacea works on another level of the immune system as well. It seems to prevent the action of an enzyme called hyaluronidase. When you're sick, this enzyme breaks down the walls of healthy cells, allowing the invaders to get inside. By interfering with this enzyme, echinacea helps the body maintain its lines of defense in the deadly game of germ warfare, says Dr. Dentali.

"There's still some debate over the actual mechanism. Maybe it inhibits the enzyme, or perhaps it supports the cell wall so it's a more formidable

---

SUPPLEMENTSNAPSHOT

▶ Echinacea

Botanical names: *Echinacea purpurea*, *E. angustifolia*, and *E. pallida*.

May help: Low immunity, celiac disease, diverticulitis, chronic fatigue syndrome, colds and flu, genital herpes, bronchitis, ear infections, laryngitis, and cystitis.

Special instructions: Use at the first signs of a cold or other infection, not as a long-term preventive.

Origin: Native to the Great Plains and southern United States; currently scarce in the wild but cultivated in the United States and Europe.

Cautions and possible side effects: Not recommended for people with autoimmune diseases such as lupus, rheumatoid arthritis, or multiple sclerosis. Do not use if you are allergic to plants in the daisy family, such as chamomile and marigold. Consult your doctor before using for longer than eight weeks.

barrier and harder to penetrate. No one really knows," he says, "but the result is that it seems to slow down the spread of infection in the body."

Echinacea has antiviral, antifungal, anti-inflammatory, and antibacterial properties. Although taken internally, it can also be used topically on wounds or inflamed skin. It has been used to treat candida, a maddening yeast infection, and in some cases used as a mouthwash to treat gingivitis.

Handy for Bites and Stings

There are several medicinal species of echinacea. All are native to the Great Plains and southern United States, but they are becoming scarce in the wild today due to overharvesting by paid gatherers. Some medicinal supplies come from cultivated fields in the United States and Europe.

One species, *Echinacea purpurea*, is a herbaceous plant three to four feet in height with reddish, purple, or pinkish flowers. It is commonly called purple coneflower, black Sampson, or Kansas snakeroot. The leaves, roots, and flowers are the medicinal parts of this plant.

North American Indians were the first to use another species, *E. angustifolia*, as a medicine to treat snakebite, toothache, sore throats, respiratory ailments, and skin wounds. In the 1700s, European settlers applied it to saddle sores on their horses.

It wasn't until a century later on the Great Plains that echinacea became better known as medicine. In Nebraska, Dr. H. C. F. Meyer created Meyer's Blood Purifier, a concoction of echinacea root extract, hops, and wormwood. Dr. Meyer touted his patent medicine as being "valuable for the bites of serpents and insect stings," and it became quite popular. Within a few decades, echinacea became the most widely used medicinal plant in the country. It got an unlooked-for marketing boost when Louis Pasteur discovered that many diseases and conditions were caused by germs. Then its advocates could say that echinacea was a germ killer.

In that era, echinacea was thought by physicians to be a treatment for many infectious diseases. By the 1930s, however, it fell out of favor, partly because some of its supporters linked it with the outdated idea that germs were generated spontaneously within the blood.

Meanwhile, in Germany . . .

While Americans' interest waned, however, Europeans' continued. Researchers from one German company started to import echinacea seeds from North America. Eventually, they discovered that they were growing and testing *E. purpurea* rather than *E. angustifolia*, which was the most widely used species. As a result, nearly all of the scientific research conducted with echinacea in the last 50 years has been on that species. Most of those studies use a formulated ethanol extract—that is, an extract mixed with alcohol. The medicinal extract is made from the aerial parts (leaves and flowers) of the plant.

In Germany in 1994, there were more than 300 echinacea preparations on the market, and doctors wrote 2.5 million prescriptions for this herb alone.

"It's funny how, in the early part of this century, echinacea was widely used by Americans. It was in most people's medicine cabinets, and then it fell out of fashion," says Dr. Dentali. "Now, it's back, partly because it's been proven safe and effective in Germany."

Special Effects

Although dozens of studies prove echinacea's effectiveness as an immune stimulator, scientists still aren't certain which active ingredients are responsible. Some evidence, however, points to a group of polysaccharides, a combination of different kinds of sugar molecules. By conducting lab tests and injecting the plant sugars directly into humans, researchers have found that polysaccharides increase phagocytosis.

In addition, echinacea contains many other compounds that seem to have antiviral properties and a gearing-up effect on the immune system. "With herbs, it not always possible to isolate all of the active ingredients," says Dr. Dentali. But the research on echinacea is leading to a better understanding of how it works, he points out.

As for which species of echinacea is the more powerful medicine for your immune system, that isn't known yet. Suffice it to say that the major medicinal species of echinacea appear to have similar benefits. Perhaps the species of the future will be a hybrid.

Picking Your Fighters

In health food stores, you'll probably find dozens of echinacea products. The herb comes as a tincture, a freeze-dried extract in capsules or tablets, and a simple herb powder packaged in capsules.

Look at the labels carefully, says Jennifer Brett, N.D., a naturopathic doctor at the Wilton Naturopathic Center in Stratford, Connecticut. There have been problems with adulteration—that is, replacing echinacea with less potent herbs. The ground-up roots of Missouri snakeroot are sometimes passed off as echinacea.

Your best bet is to look for a label that says explicitly that the product contains the leaves and flowers of *E. purpurea* or the roots of *E. angustifolia*. Sometimes, you'll find products containing both varieties as well as *E. pallida*. If you do, that's fine.

"Echinacea tincture also has a distinctive buzz to it. The more root in the mixture, the stronger the sting," says Dr. Dentali. "It ought to make your tongue tingle and numb your mouth."

A Dose Will Do You

At the onset of a cold or flu, you may want to take an extra amount to kick your immune system into overdrive, says Dr. Brett. In the first 24 hours of an illness, she recommends two capsules every 4 hours or 30 drops of tincture every 3 hours.

The revved-up effect, however, may be short-lived. Research suggests that echinacea loses its effectiveness with continuous use. Consequently, you will want to use it only when you feel a cold coming on or when your immune system is weakened by stress, says Dr. Brett.

"It's not a good idea to take this on a daily basis. If everyone in your office is sick, however, and you have no doubt that you're going to get sick, you can take it as a prophylactic," she says. "Just remember that it's most potent in those first few days that you take it."

If you have an autoimmune disease such as lupus or rheumatoid arthritis, you should be cautious, says Dr. Lee. "These diseases are partly due to an already overactive immune system. Anything that stimulates the immune system may, in theory, be harmful," she says. "You may be able to use echinacea really short-term, but I'd consider other choices, such as zinc."

enzymes

Driving from New York to Los Angeles takes several long days, even if you keep driving at a steady rate of speed. Hop on a jet, however, and you'll make the transcontinental trip in less than six hours.

Enzymes are the jet engines in our bodies. They take some plodding chemical processes and add considerable zip so our bodies get the job done, and fast. Enzymes accelerate nearly every chemical reaction.

In fact, high-speed action is written into the definition of an enzyme. It's any protein that increases the rate at which a chemical reaction occurs. Many of these chemical reactions happen in the mouth, stomach, and intestine, where enzymes immediately go to work on your morning toast and cereal and continue to assail every food that you put in your mouth all day long. Other enzymes speed up nerve impulses that make your heart pump, your head turn, and your hand pull away from a hot stove.

At a less obvious level, enzymes help form cell structures such as the genetic code, DNA, that determines everything from your eye color and height to the number of gray hairs you're getting—or losing. In fact, without enzymes to speed along the process, very few chemical reactions would proceed at a meaningful rate.

A lot of enzymes are needed to crack these many whips, and our bodies are home to an estimated 10,000 different ones. Each has a specific, nontransferable role. The enzyme that speeds digestion won't do a thing to help your nerves, and one that's dedicated to forming new cell structures is useless when it comes to driving nerve impulses.

Given their many intricate roles, however, there are good reasons to respect the enzymes that we have—and also give them a helping hand from time to time. If any are missing or not doing their jobs, an appropriate enzyme supplement may be useful, says David B. Roll, Ph.D., professor of medicinal chemistry at the University of Utah College of Pharmacy in Salt Lake City.

Gut-Level Aid

The enzymes that seem to need the most assistance are those in our intestines. These digestive enzymes break down the food we eat so it can be stored in the liver and muscles, where it is acted upon by other enzymes to produce energy. Digestive enzymes also make sure that the nutrients in our food are absorbed.

In the stomach and intestines, a variety of these digestive enzymes goes to work on carbohydrates, fats, and proteins, breaking them into pieces that can be absorbed through the lining of the small intestine. The more food that's digested, the better, since your body relies on that energy supply.

If food is allowed to pass undigested through the small intestine into the large intestine, bacteria will prey upon it, causing bloating and other intestinal problems, says Dr. Roll.

One food that many people have trouble digesting is milk. That might seem odd, since most of us grew up thinking that we had to drink three glasses a day. But a surprising number of adults have a condition called lactose intolerance, which means that they have trouble digesting a natural sugar that's in all milk as well as other dairy products such as ice cream.

Help for Intolerance

If you're lactose intolerant, you're actually short on an enzyme called lactase. Without that worker-bee enzyme in your intestines, you can't handle the lactose that accompanies the milk on your morning cereal. You need that enzyme to break down lactose into smaller sugars that are easier to digest.

Without lactase, lactose sits around too long in your small intestine. Left undigested, it is fermented by bacteria, causing gas, cramping, and bloating.

When people discover that they're lactose intolerant, it's usually because they have such symptoms. Once you know what the problem is, you can usually deal with it by avoiding dairy products or taking an enzyme supplement that can ease the symptoms. Available in tablets, liquid drops, or dairy-treated milk and sold under brand names such as Lactaid, lactase enzymes take over the exact function of the missing natural lactase. The supplemental enzyme cracks the lactose sugars into smaller, more easily digestible components.

Bean Busters

As soon as intestinal gas is mentioned, you can be sure that the conversation will quickly deteriorate to mention of the lowly bean. Surely, this is a food—if ever there was one—that needs some firm coaching in the digestive process.

The fact is that, yes, most of us do have a hard time digesting beans. Here again, an enzyme supplement can come to our aid. It's an easy-to-take supplement that can also help with other gas producers such as broccoli, cabbage, and onions. These foods contain certain complex sugars that we cannot digest. The sugars ferment in the large intestine, causing gas and abdominal distress.

Alpha-galactosidase to the rescue. This supplement is highly effective and has been known to save many from social embarrassment. Products containing alpha-galactosidase include Beano, The Ultimate Florazyme, and Prevail Bean/Vegi Enzyme Formula.

In the small intestine, alpha-galactosidase supplements help break down the indigestible sugars found in certain foods. This benign action helps to stop gas before it starts.

The supplements come as drops or tablets, and dosage instructions are right on the bottle. If you get the drops, however, don't add them to foods

SUPPLEMENT SNAPSHOT

▶ Enzymes

Individual names: Lactase, alpha-galactosidase, bromelain, papain, pancreatin, and other digestive enzymes.

May help: Digestive problems such as irritable bowel syndrome and indigestion; lupus; and chronic fatigue syndrome.

Who's at risk for deficiency: The elderly, people with digestive disorders such as chronic pancreatitis, and those with cystic fibrosis.

Cautions and possible side effects: Alpha-galactosidase supplements alter the way you process sugar; if you have diabetes, check with your doctor before using. Do not use if you have galactosemia, a rare condition that causes an adverse reaction to all foods containing the sugar galactose. Do not take if you are sensitive to mold or penicillin; these supplements are often made from a type of mold.

during cooking, since high temperatures kill the active enzymes. Instead, add drops to your first bite of food.

Other Enzymes to Watch

While many of us don't need enzyme supplements to aid normal digestion, the situation may change as we age. "As we get older, we don't produce adequate amounts of some enzymes," says Dr. Roll. "In that case, supplements may be helpful for digestion."

Enzymes that deal with the gut-wrenching effects of lactose and beans are just two of many that can help with digestion and are available in supplement form.

Many supplements contain pancreatin, a combination of enzymes derived from the pancreas of a hog or an ox; some are made up entirely of pancreatin.

You can also find supplements made from natural enzymes that are extracted from tropical fruits—bromelain from pineapple and papain from papaya. Both help your body digest protein if you are lacking digestive enzymes. Some people who get bloating and cramps after eating high-protein foods like steak may benefit from these supplements.

Enzyme supplements designed to aid protein digestion must be enteric-coated to allow them to pass safely through the stomach and into the intestinal tract, where they perform their function, says Dr. Roll. Without the coating, the supplements would be digested in your stomach and therefore be useless.

Some enzyme supplements contain ox bile, pancreatin, or a mixture of other enzymes. These may help people whose bodies don't produce enough enzymes to digest food properly, such as those with pancreatitis or cystic fibrosis.

feverfew

Feverfew, a common perennial known to gardeners for its feathery foliage and aromatic blossoms, has been used as a botanical medicine since A.D. 78. The herb earned its name because it was commonly used to lower fever, but today, it's more likely to be used by herbalists as a headache cure.

Some good evidence of feverfew's headache-healing powers emerged in the mid-1980s during a study at the City of London Migraine Clinic. All of the people included in the study were accustomed to taking crushed feverfew leaves for their headaches, but researchers wanted to find out scientifically whether the cure worked as well as people claimed.

To test its effectiveness, one group was given capsules of pulverized feverfew leaves and another was given capsules that looked exactly the same but contained no feverfew (placebos). Neither group knew what they were taking. The people in the placebo group experienced a return of their headaches, while those taking the real thing did not. The feverfew was apparently doing its job.

After the study was published in 1985, feverfew emerged from the obscurity of the garden and into the limelight of botanical healing.

"I use it 100 percent of the time with my patients for migraines because it usually works," says Jennifer Brett, N.D., a naturopathic doctor in Stratford, Connecticut. "It's a good alternative for people who have tried everything else."

An Herb for the Head

The modern view of this herb is fairly close to that of sixteenth-century herbalist John Gerard. In 1597, Gerard recommended this member of the chrysanthemum family to "them that are giddie in the head" and suggested placing a poultice of the leaves on an aching noggin.

Ingesting rather than wearing the herb is the recommended course of treatment today, but it's clear that the early healers were on to something, says Steven Dentali, Ph.D., a natural products chemist with Dentali Associates in Troutdale, Oregon, and a member of the advisory board of the American Botanical Council. "This is really a case where the folk use coincided with the science," he says. "Feverfew appears to be a good alternative to the drugs now being used for migraines."

In previous centuries, feverfew wasn't just for headaches. Herbalists recommended it to relieve menstrual pain, expel the placenta after birth, treat arthritis, and break fevers. The common name is derived from *febrifugia*, which is Latin for "fever reducer."

"It does work for reducing fevers, but probably no one really uses it for that anymore," says Dr. Brett.

A Spasm Stopper

Just how feverfew works, scientists aren't certain. The leaves—the medicinal parts of the plant—are rich in parthenolide, a compound that makes the walls of the blood vessels in the brain less reactive to substances that cause them to contract and dilate. That's how migraines begin. The opening and closing of blood vessels may set off pain nerves and inflame the smooth muscles that line the blood vessels, says Alison Lee, M.D., a pain-management specialist and medical director of Barefoot Doctors, an alternative medicine practice in Ann Arbor, Michigan.

SUPPLEMENT SNAPSHOT

▶ Feverfew

Botanical name: *Tanacetum parthenium*.

May help: Migraines, menstrual pain, osteoarthritis, and rheumatoid arthritis.

Special instructions: For migraine prevention, take regularly; you may not see benefits for several months.

Origin: Native to central and southern Europe.

Cautions and possible side effects: Do not take if pregnant or breast-feeding. Chewing fresh leaves may cause mouth sores; take capsules containing powdered leaves instead.

"Feverfew has a pronounced regulatory effect on these vascular muscles," she explains. "It seems to calm them down."

The herb may also inhibit the release of two inflammatory substances that cause the vessels to go into spasm in the first place—serotonin from blood platelets and prostaglandin from white blood cells. Because prostaglandin and other related substances are also culprits in the inflammation that occurs during painful bouts of rheumatoid arthritis, feverfew has been used in its treatment as well, says Dr. Lee. "If I have a patient who isn't a candidate for other anti-inflammatory treatments, I might recommend feverfew."

Since the herb can lessen or regulate the spasms of smooth muscles, it's not surprising that it also has a reputation for easing menstrual cramps. It also seems to prevent migraines that coincide with menstruation, adds Dr. Brett.

Give It a Chance

As a migraine preventive, feverfew is effective for 70 to 80 percent of the people who use it, says Dr. Brett. It takes time to work, however, and you may need to take it daily for two to five months before it has any effect.

"You can't just take a feverfew pill when you feel a migraine coming on. It won't do any good," she explains. "You have to take it over a long period."

You'll find capsules of powdered leaves in health food stores and drugstores. Make sure there's an expiration date on the bottle, and always store the herb in the refrigerator, says Dr. Dentali, since some of the plant's chemical constituents are sensitive to warm temperatures.

Look for a product with a parthenolide concentration of 0.2 percent or higher, says Dr. Dentali. These are the criteria recommended by the Canadian government, which has recently allowed manufacturers to specifically label feverfew as a treatment for migraines.

fiber

Think about what you ate yesterday. How many high-fiber foods did you have? If you're like most Americans, probably not enough. Our typical diets include only about 10 to 15 grams of dietary fiber a day, but the Daily Value is 25 grams. For many of us, that means doubling our current intakes.

For more than two decades, scientists have been taking a close look at fiber and its potential health benefits. What they've found is that high-fiber diets may decrease the risk of colon and breast cancer, ease constipation and irritable bowel syndrome, and help prevent diverticulosis, hemorrhoids, high cholesterol, and diabetes.

Nature's Glue, Nature's Sponge

Fiber is the indigestible part of all plant foods, including fruits, vegetables, grains, and beans. It is not found in meat or any other animal foods. Most fiber-rich foods contain both soluble and insoluble fiber. Soluble fiber dissolves in water in your intestinal tract, forming a gluelike gel. It softens stools and slows down stomach emptying, allowing for better digestion and helping you feel fuller longer, an effect that may aid weight loss.

Soluble fiber has been credited with lowering blood cholesterol. It may also help people with diabetes by lowering the amount of insulin necessary to process blood sugar after a meal. When taken with plenty of water before meals, a soluble fiber supplement binds with water in the stomach and forms a gummy mass—and that's what makes us feel full.

Insoluble fiber is the champion of the gastrointestinal tract. It's a good natural laxative because it holds onto water and moves waste quickly through the intestines, says David Beck, M.D., chairman of colon and rectal surgery at the Ochsner Clinic in New Orleans. It also adds bulk and softens stools.

In general, soluble fibers are found in higher concentrations in fruits, oats, barley, and beans. When shopping for soluble fiber supplements, you can choose from psyllium, gums, mucilages, glucomannan, or pectins, says

Dr. Beck. Insoluble fibers are more abundant in vegetables, wheat, and cereals; supplements include wheat bran and flaxseed.

Although it's helpful to classify fiber as either soluble or insoluble, we need both kinds in our diets. And fibers don't always fit neatly into categories. Psyllium, for example, which is a soluble fiber, promotes bowel movements, a benefit usually associated with insoluble fiber. And rice bran, an insoluble fiber, lowers blood cholesterol, which is a trait of some soluble fibers.

Moving Things Along

Some studies have shown a link between high-fiber diets and a decreased risk of colon cancer, says Dr. Beck. Since fiber increases the bulk of the stool, it may dilute cancer-causing substances there. It also moves waste

SUPPLEMENT SNAPSHOT

▶Fiber

Supplement forms: Psyllium, gums, mucilages, glucomannan, pectins, methylcellulose, calcium polycarbophil, flaxseed, and brans.

May help: Colon cancer, breast cancer, heart disease, diverticulosis, hemorrhoids, constipation, diabetes, overweight, Parkinson's disease, irritable bowel syndrome, indigestion, high blood pressure, and high cholesterol.

Daily Value: 25 grams.

Special instructions: Do not take with food; always drink at least eight ounces of water for each tablespoon of fiber that you take.

Who's at risk for deficiency: Many Americans; average consumption is only 10 to 15 grams a day.

Good food sources: All plant foods. The best sources include wheat-bran cereals, beans, dried figs, peas, raspberries, bulgur, oatmeal, pears, sweet potatoes, oranges, apples, and barley.

Cautions and possible side effects: Do not take if you have trouble swallowing. Talk to your doctor before taking any fiber supplement, especially if you have diverticulitis, ulcerative colitis, Crohn's disease, bowel obstruction, or any other serious gastrointestinal disorder, or if you are taking any medications because it blocks absorption. May cause bloating or constipation.

faster through the digestive tract, leaving less time for potentially harmful or even cancerous substances in your stool to have contact with the lining of the bowel, he says.

Fiber, particularly insoluble fiber, is also thought to help prevent hemorrhoids and diverticulosis, a condition in which small sacs develop in weak areas of the intestinal wall. It does so by softening stools and speeding up the movement of waste through the intestinal tract.

Fiber may also help ease the symptoms of irritable bowel syndrome, a condition characterized by alternating constipation and diarrhea, gas, and cramps.

While much research has focused on the link between fiber and gastrointestinal health, studies also show that dietary fiber may protect against breast cancer, according to David P. Rose, M.D., Ph.D., D.Sc., chief of the division of nutrition and endocrinology for the American Health Foundation in Valhalla, New York. High intakes of fiber have been shown to reduce estrogen levels in the blood, he says. That's important because high levels of estrogen are associated with increased breast cancer risk.

Fiber may reduce estrogen by binding with it in the intestine before carrying it out of the body in the stool. Fiber may also help prevent the reabsorption of estrogen in the blood.

Help for the Heart

Studies have shown that people who get the most fiber in their diets are less likely to have heart disease.

In a Finnish study of nearly 22,000 male smokers ages 50 to 69, men who ate the most fiber, averaging 35 grams daily, suffered one-third fewer heart attacks than those who ate the least fiber. To look at it another way, each 10 grams of fiber added to the diet decreased the risk of death from heart disease by 17 percent.

In a study of 44,000 male health professionals, those who ate more than 25 grams of fiber a day had a 36 percent lower risk of developing heart disease than those who ate less than 15 grams daily.

Soluble fiber gets a big chunk of credit for helping the heart because it's repeatedly been shown to lower blood cholesterol levels. It does so in several ways, says Tom Wolever, M.D., Ph.D., professor of nutritional sciences and medicine at the University of Toronto. When we fill up on fiber, there is less room for high-fat, high-cholesterol foods. In fact, a growing number of studies show that a diet rich in soluble fiber will lower blood cholesterol levels by 6 to 8 percent, he says.

Soluble fiber has another cholesterol-lowering effect, Dr. Wolever says. It binds with bile acids, which affects the way the liver handles blood cholesterol. As a net result of this process, cholesterol levels go down.

This cholesterol-lowering effect of fiber seems to be limited to specific foods and supplements that contain a generous amount of soluble fiber, including pectin, guar gum, psyllium, oat bran, oatmeal, and legumes.

Do You Need a Fiber Supplement?

Health experts generally recommend that you get your fiber from food, not supplements, because food contains nutrients that supplements don't.

"I don't often prescribe fiber supplements, because I want people to change to a whole-foods diet," says William D. Nelson, N.D., a naturopathic doctor at the Docere Naturopathic Centre in Colorado Springs. Patients who switch from processed and fast foods to whole foods, including whole grains, fresh vegetables, fruits, and beans, usually don't need supplemental fiber, he says.

Sometimes, though, we can't or won't get all the fiber we need. That's when supplements can help, says Dr. Beck. "Most of us are very busy. Fiber supplements allow us to worry less about what we're eating."

Whether you're adding more fiber-rich foods to your diet or taking fiber supplements, you need to increase your intake gradually. Since fiber isn't absorbed, it can ferment in the intestine, causing gas, bloating, cramps, and diarrhea.

Always drink at least eight ounces of water with a fiber supplement, advises Dr. Beck. Fiber acts like a sponge, and if you don't drink plenty of fluids, it can swell and block part of the gastrointestinal tract. It can also block the esophagus, so experts recommend avoiding fiber supplements if you have trouble swallowing.

Too much fiber can block the absorption of minerals such as iron, calcium, and zinc. It could also cause calcium losses.

If you supplement, try to get your fiber from a variety of sources in addition to a high-fiber diet. Look for products like psyllium, apple and grapefruit pectin, guar gum, methylcellulose, and calcium polycarbophil. At your local health food store, you may also find wheat and oat bran tablets and multifiber tablets with ingredients like beet and carrot fibers.

Psyllium is a popular and inexpensive fiber supplement with a laxative as well as a cholesterol-lowering effect, says Dr. Nelson. This supplement is available in pill, capsule, or powder form. All forms are equally effective, but fiber capsules and tablets are more expensive than powders.

If you're taking a tablet or capsule, you have to take as many as 10 to get the same amount of fiber you'd find in a tablespoon of psyllium seed powder, says Jennifer Brett, N.D., a naturopathic doctor at the Wilton Naturopathic Center in Stratford, Connecticut. With so many pills to take, people tend to abandon them more quickly than they do powder supplements.

Psyllium causes gas and bloating in some people. If that happens to you, try flaxseed, which is easiest to take in capsules or in powdered form. In addition to fiber, flaxseed contains lignans, compounds that may have anti-cancer, antibacterial, antifungal, and antiviral effects, says Dr. Nelson.

Be leery of marketing claims that fiber supplements containing chitosan (a form of chitin, which is a component of the shells of shellfish) promote weight loss, says Dr. Brett. "I've never seen any evidence that it works for weight loss," she says. Even if chitosan did remove fat from the body as its proponents claim, it would also bind with and remove fat-soluble vitamins that your body needs, she says.

Animal studies have shown that chitosan can absorb LDL cholesterol (the bad type) and reduce lipid concentrations, but further studies are needed to confirm any cholesterol-lowering action. As for a weight-loss effect, some animals in the studies actually gained weight when they were fed chitosan, while others lost.

fish oil

Imagine going to your favorite fast-food restaurant and ordering a blubber-packed whaleburger on a sesame seed bun instead of a flame-broiled burger. Sound unhealthy?

Maybe not.

Like some types of fish, whales and other marine mammals are high in a type of fat called omega-3 polyunsaturated fatty acids. Physicians working in the Arctic first began to uncover the heart-healthy benefits of omega-3's when they puzzled over why the Inuit Eskimos—who regularly dined on a high-fat, high-cholesterol diet of whale, seal, and fish—rarely developed heart disease.

Later, studies in Greenland confirmed that the rate of heart disease among the Inuits was much lower than that of Westerners, even though both diets provided similar amounts of fat.

The difference, scientists concluded, was due to the source of fat in the two diets. Whereas Westerners get their fat from land animals and plants, the Inuits get most of theirs from marine mammals and fish. Since this discovery, much research has focused on the role of the omega-3's and their impact on heart disease and other ailments.

Not All Fats Are Created Equal

Our bodies make most of the fat they need from the carbon, hydrogen, and oxygen atoms that are found in food. But they don't have any way to create omega-3's and another type of fatty acids, omega-6's. Both of these belong to a category called essential fats, and they come only from certain foods.

There are two varieties of omega-3's. The first is made up of eicosapentaenoic acid (EPA) and docosahexaenoic acid (DHA). To get your fill of these, feast on fatty fish such as salmon and mackerel.

The second type of omega-3's is alpha-linolenic acid (ALA), which is

177

provided by plant foods. Once it's inside your body, some ALA can be converted into EPA and DHA. Sources high in ALA include flaxseed oil, black currant oil, walnut oil, perilla seed oil, and canola oil.

The other essential fat that the body can't manufacture is known as omega-6, or linoleic acid. While omega-6 oils are vital to our health, we may be getting too much in our diets. Most vegetable oils today have very high amounts of omega-6's but not enough omega-3's, and that kind of imbalance could turn into risky business for our bodies.

Scientists think that in the diets of our ancestors, the ratio of the two types was nearly 1 to 1. Today, the omega-6/omega-3 ratio is about 15 to 1. When linoleic acid dominates too heavily over omega-3's, it may jeopardize our health. A ratio of 4.5 omega-6 to 10 omega-3 is considered balanced.

Fish Oils to the Rescue

The body uses both types of omegas to create a variety of short-lived, hormonelike substances called eicosanoids. These substances perform many functions, such as regulating blood pressure, controlling important aspects

SUPPLEMENT SNAPSHOT

▶ Fish Oil

Supplement forms: Omega-3 fatty acids, eicosapentaenoic acid (EPA), and docosahexaenoic acid (DHA).

May help: Heart disease, angina, high blood pressure, high cholesterol, asthma, breast cancer, colon cancer, lupus, multiple sclerosis, arthritis, gout, migraines, prostate problems, eczema, ADHD, and inflammation.

Good food sources: Mackerel, salmon, herring, bluefish, albacore tuna, rainbow trout, and swordfish.

Cautions and possible side effects: Increases bleeding time, possibly resulting in nosebleeds and easy bruising, and may cause upset stomach. Do not take if you have a bleeding disorder or uncontrolled high blood pressure, take anticoagulants (blood thinners) or use aspirin regularly, or are allergic to any kind of fish. Take fish oil, not fish-liver oil, which is high in vitamins A and D—vitamins that may be toxic in high amounts. People with diabetes should not take fish oil because of its high fat content.

of the reproductive cycle, and inducing blood clotting, among other things.

Prostaglandins, one of the better-known types of eicosanoids, have an effect on the brain, blood vessel walls, certain blood cells, and blood platelets. They are involved in regulating almost every body function, including those of the digestive, nervous, and reproductive systems. Prostaglandins also influence the ways in which blood vessels expand and contract, and they help manage blood clotting.

When an overabundance of prostaglandins and other eicosanoids is set loose in the body, the result may be excessive blood clotting and narrowing of the arteries. That's where fish oils may act. EPA and DHA decrease the stickiness of the blood platelets involved in clotting, thus reducing the risk of a clot that could lead to a heart attack.

If omega-6's dominate and omega-3's are in short supply, eicosanoids can provoke inflammation, blood clots, and other problems. If omega-3's are plentiful, if there are more omega-3's in diet more anti-inflamatory messengers are made.

Heart-Healthy News

Let's return to the Eskimos. Studies have revealed that their omega-3–rich diet results in lower blood cholesterol, lower triglycerides (another type of blood fat), lower LDL cholesterol (the "bad" type), increased HDL cholesterol (the "good" type), and lower rates of heart disease. These Eskimos also have prolonged bleeding times. Ominous though that sounds, it is actually something that heart disease researchers like to see, because it means that blood is thinner and therefore flows more smoothly.

There's also evidence that fish consumption may make heart attacks less dangerous if they do happen. In one study, a number of men who had survived heart attacks went on a diet that was high in fish. Compared to male heart attack patients who just had normal diets, those in the fish-eating group were more likely to live longer.

How does fish oil help the heart? The omega-3's in fish oil may reduce the risk or even the severity of heart disease by influencing several factors, including blood clotting and blood pressure. They may also reduce the risk that a person will have cardiac arrhythmia (irregular heartbeat).

When you eat foods that are high in omega-3's, that valuable fish oil becomes incorporated into the cell membranes of platelets, making them less likely to clump together. In a way, fish oil acts like a very weak form of aspirin, which also has a good reputation as a heart disease preventive and, like fish oil, is believed to decrease the clumping of platelets.

Aid for Arthritis

Various studies have tested fish-oil treatments for the symptoms of rheumatoid arthritis, the kind of joint-attacking arthritis that can begin as early as childhood. Analyzing data from the 10 best-conducted trials to date, researchers concluded that taking fish-oil supplements for at least three months resulted in modest but positive improvements, mainly less morning stiffness and tender joints.

The amounts of fish-oil supplements used in most clinical studies are high—about 3,000 to 5,000 milligrams of omega-3's daily. To get this much from your diet, you would have to eat at least 10 ounces of cooked rainbow trout. Most fish-oil supplements contain about 500 milligrams of omega-3 fatty acids in each 1,000-milligram capsule.

Benefits may come from smaller amounts of fish oil as well. In one study, women who ate two or more servings of broiled or baked fish a week had about half the risk of developing rheumatoid arthritis as women who ate only one serving.

Fish oil appears to ease rheumatoid arthritis and a variety of other inflammatory diseases by suppressing inflammation. While no one seems ready to proclaim fish oil a cure, at least one study has shown that it helps reduce or even eliminate the need for the nonsteroidal anti-inflammatory drugs that are most commonly prescribed for the disease.

An Ocean of Uses

Fish oil may even prove beneficial in preventing and treating certain cancers. In one study, researchers had 25 women with breast cancer eat a low-fat, high-fiber diet and take 10,000 milligrams of fish-oil supplements daily—far more than anyone would think of taking under normal circumstances. After three months, the omega-3 fatty acids stored in the women's breasts increased. This is significant because animal studies have shown that omega-3's delay the development of cancer and can inhibit tumor growth.

Despite the implications of this study, you should not try to take this large dosage of fish oil every day to combat breast cancer or the risk

What's in a Name?

Fish-oil supplements are sold under many names, from the obvious, such as fish oil or omega-3, to the not-so-obvious, including supplements that feature docosahexaenoic acid (DHA) or eicosapentaenoic acid (EPA) prominently in the name. Chances are, most fish-oil supplements include a mixture of EPA and DHA, no matter what they're called. Usually, a closer look at the label will tell you.

It's not yet clear whether DHA and EPA have health benefits independent of each other, says William S. Harris, Ph.D., professor of medicine at the University of Missouri in Kansas City. EPA, which has been marketed as promoting heart health, is more likely to be beneficial for that purpose than DHA. On the other hand, DHA, which has been touted as a brain food by marketers, may be more likely to promote the proper functioning of brain and nerve tissues than EPA.

Dr. Harris recommends striving to get 500 to 1,000 milligrams daily of omega-3 fatty acids, including both EPA and DHA.

of it. Such high amounts should be taken only under a doctor's direction.

When it comes to reducing risk of colon cancer, there's evidence that far lower doses of fish oil might help with prevention. In one study, researchers selected people with a history of precancerous growths to see how they responded to fish-oil supplements. The study showed that doses of as little as 2,500 milligrams of fish oil a day could prevent the abnormal cell proliferation that's associated with the risk of polyps and of colon cancer.

Researchers are also looking into the links between fish oil and reducing childhood asthma, helping women have healthier pregnancies and healthier babies, improving bone growth, and lengthening remission for patients with Crohn's disease (a chronic inflammatory gastrointestinal disorder) who are already in prolonged remission.

Fish oil might even have an influence on the nervous system. For years, researchers have linked depression with low intake of fish oils. New research shows that supplementing with omega-3 fatty acids may alleviate symptoms of disorders such as schizophrenia.

Easy Does It

Although eating more omega-3–rich fish is beneficial to our health, many experts advise against taking fish-oil supplements.

"I know of no compelling reason to supplement," says Gary J. Nelson, Ph.D., research chemist for the U.S. Department of Agriculture Western Human Nutrition Research Center in San Francisco. "If you eat a good variety of foods, you should be getting plenty of fatty acids in your diet." The only caveat is to make sure that diet includes more of the omega-3 fatty acids and less of the omega-6 fatty acids, he adds.

If you decide to supplement with fish-oil capsules, it's important to remember that the amount of fish oil used in research studies is extremely high. Patients who take fish oil at the therapeutic levels used in many studies may require 15 to 30 capsules to derive similar benefits.

You can benefit from smaller doses, however, says William S. Harris, Ph.D., professor of medicine at the University of Missouri in Kansas City. "You probably get good health benefits from taking one or two fish-oil capsules a day if you don't want to eat fish," he says. "But the evidence that fish-oil supplements do this or that at one to two grams (1,000 to 2,000 milligrams) a day is very tenuous." The American Heart Association currently recommends 1 gram daily for people with existing heart disease and note that people with elevated triglycerides may need 2 to 4 grams per day.

While both fish-oil capsules and fish have been shown to improve health, fish produces a greater effect on reducing platelet stickiness. Also, fish-oil capsules are high in fat and put stress on our antioxidant defense mechanisms.

Some experts also worry that fish-oil supplements may be contaminated with the same agricultural and industrial pollutants found in fish. For that reason, Andrew Weil, M.D., clinical professor of internal medicine and director of the program in integrative medicine of the University of Arizona College of Medicine in Tucson and author of *Eight Weeks to Optimum Health*, says that he cannot recommend fish oil in capsule form.

flaxseed

You've probably worn and touched more flax than you've eaten. Linen, that cool staple of summer wardrobes, is made from flax, as is linseed oil, which is used in paint and varnish. But the blue-flowered flax plant is cultivated for more than cloth and paint. Researchers have turned up some pretty convincing evidence that flaxseed and flaxseed oil may improve heart health, fight breast and colon cancers, boost the immune system, ease rheumatoid arthritis, cool down hot flashes, and provide other healthy benefits.

Flaxseed is one of the richest source of alpha-linolenic acid (ALA), a plant source of omega-3 fatty acids. As mentioned in the fish oils chapter, the omega-3's are one of two families of essential fatty acids, which are necessary for growth and development and cannot be made by the body. Omega-3's are the building blocks of eicosanoids, hormonelike compounds that regulate blood pressure, clotting, and other body functions.

Other fatty acids, omega-6's, are abundant in vegetable oils such as corn, soybean, safflower, and sunflower oils as well as in the many processed foods made from these oils. They're also available in the meat from grain-fed livestock.

The discoveries about omega-3's and omega-6's are relevant to flaxseed as well as to fish oil. Our bodies function best when our diets contain a well-balanced ratio of these fatty acids, meaning no more than 4 times as much omega-6 as omega-3. But we typically eat 10 to 30 times more omega-6's than omega-3's, which is a prescription for trouble, says Artemis Simopoulos, M.D., president of the Center for Genetics, Nutrition, and Health in Washington, D.C., and author of *The Omega Plan*. This imbalance puts us at greater risk for a number of serious illnesses, including heart disease, cancer, stroke, and arthritis, he says.

As we've noted, an excess of omega-6 fatty acids, when not checked by a complementary amount of omega-3's, can lead to the overproduction of potentially inflammatory biochemicals called prostaglandins and leukotrienes.

A deficiency of omega-3's is linked to various skin disorders, arthritis and joint stiffness, irritable bowel syndrome, premenstrual syndrome, immune dysfunction, and depression, says Michael Janson, M.D., president of the American College for Advancement in Medicine, based in Laguna Hills, California, and author of *The Vitamin Revolution in Health Care*. As the most abundant plant source of omega-3 fatty acids, flaxseed helps restore balance and lets omega-3's do what they're best at—balancing the immune system, decreasing inflammation, and lowering some of the risk factors for heart disease.

Seeds of Hope

These small brown seeds hold some big promise for combating breast and colon cancer. In animal studies, flaxseed has significantly reduced existing breast and colon tumors while stopping new ones from getting started. In one study, researchers at the University of Toronto were able to reduce tumor size by more than half in animals that were fed flaxseed over a seven-week period. Flaxseed and flaxseed oil reduced the growth of existing tumors, but another component of flaxseed, called lignans, appeared to help prevent the development of new ones.

Lignans are plant-based compounds that can block excessive estrogen

SUPPLEMENT SNAPSHOT

▶ Flaxseed

Botanical name: *Linum usitatissimum*.

May help: Heart disease, heart arrhythmia, high cholesterol, angina, breast cancer, colon cancer, diabetes, stroke, lupus-related kidney damage, low immunity, irritable bowel syndrome, high blood pressure, fingernail problems, constipation, diarrhea, hot flashes, gout, migraines, asthma, osteoarthritis, rheumatoid arthritis, dermatitis, sunburn, and sciatica.

Special instructions: Take with food.

Origin: Consumed in Europe and Asia since around 8,000 B.C.; introduced to North America during Colonial days but not widely used as food until the 1960s.

Cautions and possible side effects: Generally regarded as safe.

activity in cells, reducing the risk of certain cancers. Many plants have some lignans, but flaxseed has at least 75 times more than almost any other plant.

Lignans are phytoestrogens, meaning that they are similar to but weaker than the estrogen that a woman's body produces naturally. Therefore, they may also help alleviate menopausal discomforts such as hot flashes and vaginal dryness. They are also antibacterial, antifungal, and antiviral.

Flaxseed also appears to reduce the risk of heart disease and stroke. One way that ALA helps the heart is by decreasing the ability of platelets to clump together, a reaction involved in the development of atherosclerosis (hardening of the arteries), says Dr. Janson. ALA also lowers levels of dangerous LDL cholesterol and helps the body rid itself of blood fats called triglycerides, which, at high levels, can also be harmful to heart health.

Need more convincing? The ALA in flaxseed oil has an anti-inflammatory effect that can benefit a number of illnesses, says Emily Kane, N.D., a naturopathic doctor in Juneau, Alaska, and senior editor of the *Journal of Naturopathic Medicine*. In her practice, she recommends flaxseed oil for inflammatory diseases such as arthritis, irritable bowel syndrome, and asthma.

Flaxseed oil and lignans have also been credited with reducing inflammation of the kidneys experienced by some people with a condition known as lupus nephritis. Lupus is an autoimmune disease that affects the skin and other organs.

Flax Facts

Flaxseed oil comes in liquid and gelatin capsules, but you may want to skip the oil and just add flaxseed to your diet. The oil contains only trace amounts of the cancer-protective lignans because they are removed during processing, says Diane Morris, R.D., Ph.D., a nutritionist in Winnipeg, Manitoba.

Flaxseed is also an excellent source of fiber, whereas the oil has virtually none. As little as ¼ cup of ground flaxseed contains six grams of fiber—as much as 1½ cups of cooked oatmeal. The fiber is beneficial for treating constipation and diarrhea, says Dr. Janson.

Experts like Dr. Morris don't discourage the use of the oil. It's just that they would like to see you get all the benefits of flaxseed, not just the omega-3's.

"As a dietitian and nutritionist, I would prefer that people use the ground or whole seed, either sprinkled on their toast or cereal or incorporated into breads and other baked goods," says Dr. Morris.

Whether you decide to go with the seeds or the oil, keep the following tips in mind.

• Skip the gelatin capsules. Oil is less processed, more practical, and less expensive than capsules. With 1,000-milligram capsules, for example, you'd have to swallow about 10 capsules a day to equal one tablespoon of the oil. A typical daily dose for overall health is one tablespoon; therapeutic doses range from one to three tablespoons, depending on the severity of your condition and your weight, says Dr. Kane.

• Stick with flaxseed oil from the refrigerated section of your health food store. Buy only oil that comes in an opaque bottle, and store it in the refrigerator as soon as you get home. Or, if you don't plan to use it right away, keep it in the freezer. Flaxseed oil degrades quickly when exposed to heat and light.

• Look for oils certified as organic by a third party. Also, quality oils have a "pressing date" listed on the bottles. If the oil was pressed more than six months ago, don't buy it, says Dr. Kane.

• Use flaxseed oil for salad dressings instead of vegetable, olive, or other oils. The oil has a nutty taste, and some people don't like the flavor at first, says Dr. Kane. She recommends the following salad dressing recipe: Combine ½ cup olive oil, ½ cup flaxseed oil, ⅓ cup freshly squeezed lemon juice, and 1 heaping tablespoon of mustard. Shake well for a few minutes before serving. Refrigerate between uses.

• Never cook with flaxseed oil, since it's sensitive to heat.

• To avoid weight gain, be sure to take the high calorie content of oil into account when figuring your daily calorie intake.

• Grind whole seeds in your electric coffee grinder and sprinkle them on cereal, add them to smoothies, or mix them with yogurt or oatmeal, says Dr. Morris.

• You can store whole seeds in a cool, dry pantry for up to one year. Use any ground flaxseed immediately or keep it in the freezer, says Dr. Morris.

folic acid

Here's an easy way to remember the best sources of this essential B vitamin: think "foliage." Folic acid and its food form, folate, were discovered by researchers who waded through *four tons* of spinach to isolate enough of it to study.

You don't need to eat four tons of spinach to get all the folate you need in a day. If you have a yen for spinach, about four cups of the raw greens will provide the Daily Value of 400 micrograms. (Like your spinach cooked? You'll have to eat twice that amount, since up to half of the folate in foods is lost in cooking.) Or you can get a spinach-bowl's-worth of this nutrient in capsule form.

Genetic Engineering

Folic acid is essential for DNA and RNA synthesis. That means it has to be on hand for your body to make the genetic material—the blueprint—that allows a cell to grow and divide to make more cells. "Folic acid actually helps to make the building blocks, called bases, that are strung together like pearls to form the DNA," says Barry Shane, Ph.D., professor of nutrition and chair of the department of nutritional sciences at the University of California at Berkeley.

RNA is kind of a "working copy" of DNA. Parts of DNA can be copied to RNA when a cell has to make a certain kind of protein, for instance. The RNA then travels to the part of the cell where the protein can be made and hands over the instructions.

"More folic acid is needed for this process when cells are rapidly dividing, as they do during growth and development, and in areas where cells normally have a relatively short life, such as the intestines and blood cells," Dr. Shane says. When folic acid is in short supply, DNA synthesis slows, and cells lose their ability to divide and multiply. That has the potential to create major, body-wide problems. In the blood, for instance, it can cause anemia, a lack of red blood cells. In the intestines, it can create absorption problems. Folic acid deficiency can also be a factor in heart disease. Also, in some cases, when your body is short on this nutrient, it could produce abnormal cells, a condition called dysplasia that can lead to cancer. Low folic acid levels during pregnancy can set the stage for birth defects.

Tired Blood

If folic acid intake is low enough for long enough, you'll develop megaloblastic anemia. In this form of anemia, "your red blood cells are unable to fully mature, and if you look at them under a microscope, they're large

SUPPLEMENT SNAPSHOT

▶Folic Acid

Also known as: Folate; folacin.

May help: Prevent birth defects, including defects of the neural tube, cleft palate, and cleft lip; reverse precancerous cell changes (dysplasia) in the cervix, lungs, or colon; treat megaloblastic anemia, canker sores, depression, gout, and gingivitis. With vitamins B_6 and B_{12} can also lower blood levels of homocysteine to reduce risk of heart attack and prevent intermittent claudication, phlebitis, Alzheimer's disease, angina, and high blood pressure.

Special Instructions: Best taken on an empty stomach.

Daily Value: 400 micrograms.

Who's at risk for deficiency: People who use the cholesterol-lowering drug cholestryramine (Questran); people with cancer; the elderly, especially if their diets are nutritionally deficient; pregnant women; people recovering from burns; those who have had blood loss, gastrointestinal tract damage, chicken pox, or measles; alcoholics; and smokers.

Good food sources: Spinach, lentils, navy beans, pinto beans, and sunflower seeds. Heat and oxidation during cooking and storage can destroy as much as half of the folate in foods, so many food sources don't provide very much.

Cautions and possible side effects: Do not take doses above 1,000 micrograms a day without medical supervision.

and egg-shaped," Dr. Shane explains. Your body also produces fewer red blood cells than you need for good health. Normally, cells in the bone marrow crank out red blood cells at the rate of 200 million a minute, but in this case, there's just not enough folic acid to maintain this pace without producing a lot of duds.

Megaloblastic anemia is most likely to occur during pregnancy, when there is an increased requirement for growth, and in people taking drugs that deplete the body of folic acid, Dr. Shane says. "Most people who develop this sort of anemia have been low on folic acid for months. It is also a fairly common problem in the elderly," he adds.

Cancer Cop

Cancer results from an accumulation, over time, of damage to the DNA. Smoking, exposure to harmful chemicals, frequent exposure to x-rays, and certain viruses can damage a cell's genetic material. Add the injury of a folic acid shortage to any one of these insults, and "you are turning up the speed of the damage several-fold," explains Patrick Stover, Ph.D., assistant professor of nutritional biochemistry and cell biology at Cornell University in Ithaca, New York.

Folic acid deficiency has been strongly linked to DNA damage in several studies. In one, researchers at the University of California at Berkeley found that even a mild deficiency caused a large increase in the amount of damaged DNA. Other studies have shown a link between folic acid deficiency and dysplasia in the cervix, colon, and lungs.

Healthy Heart Helper

What happens to that steak you devour? In your body, protein from the steak is broken down into bits—amino acids—that your body can disassemble even further, then reassemble to make some urgently needed new amino acids. The amino acids may be strung together again to form new proteins, so that steak may eventually help form cells in your nose. Folic acid helps that happen because it helps to metabolize—break down and reassemble—several amino acids.

In that role, folic acid deficiency may play a part in the development of heart disease. It is needed to transform homocysteine—an amino acid byproduct that in high concentrations is toxic to the body—to a more useful form called methionine. "When you don't have enough folic acid, blood levels of homocysteine rise, and those higher levels are linked with an increased risk of heart disease and stroke," says John Pinto, Ph.D., associate professor of biochemistry at Weill Medical College of Cornell University and director of the nutrition research laboratory at Memorial Sloan-Kettering Cancer Center, both in New York City. "In fact," he says, "the connection seems to be as strong as, if not stronger than, the connection between high cholesterol and heart disease. So this isn't a mere curiosity. It's something to pay attention to."

High levels of homocysteine contribute to heart disease in a couple of nasty ways, Dr. Pinto says. They damage the cells lining the blood vessels, creating rough spots that attract cholesterol deposits. Plus, they cause blood to clot more readily at those rough spots. When that happens, the artery-clogging clots begin to set the stage for heart attack or stroke.

"One problem being investigated right now is how much folic acid you need to protect against heart disease," Dr. Pinto says. In one study, people who got five milligrams a day for two weeks had significant drops in homocysteine, especially those whose initial levels were high.

Building Better Babies

To "construct" a baby, a woman's body has to turn a single fertilized egg into billions of cells, all in nine months. That takes a lot of DNA and RNA—and so it takes a lot of folic acid. "Requirements for folic acid increase in a pregnant woman, both because of the rapid rate of cell growth and division in the fetus and because the woman is making more cells herself," says Joseph Mulinare, M.D., chief of the prevention branch at the birth defects division of the Centers for Disease Control and Prevention in Atlanta. During pregnancy, a woman's blood volume may increase by as much as 50 percent.

Pregnant women sometimes don't get enough folic acid. If the shortage isn't detected and corrected, these moms can have children with birth defects, especially spinal cord and brain problems called neural tube defects. These defects are initiated very early in fetal development, often before a woman knows she is pregnant. "That's why it's important to start taking folic acid before you get pregnant," Dr. Mulinare says.

Of course, pregnancy isn't exactly a preprogrammed event. If you're a woman who is trying to conceive, though, it's definitely a smart move to get all you need of this important nutrient. If you're using a contraceptive and decide to go off it, doctors recommend that you start taking 400 micrograms daily of folic acid three months before you stop using contraception. Then continue the same daily dose for at least three months into the pregnancy.

Figure Out How to Fill Up

Most people get about 200 micrograms of folate a day, about half the Daily Value. With folic acid–fortified foods such as breads and breakfast cereals now on the market, daily intake could increase on average to about 300 micrograms a day, Dr. Mulinare says, possibly leaving a 100-microgram daily deficit. Most over-the-counter multivitamins contain 400 micrograms, and a few super-potency vitamins provide 800 micrograms. "It's also possible to get supplements that contain only folic acid, usually 400 micrograms," he says.

gamma-linolenic acid

In the Middle Ages, people used borage, an herb with bright blue flowers, to treat heart disease and rheumatism and to reduce inflammation. Today, it's making a comeback for some of the same medicinal uses.

Borage oil is one of three major supplemental sources of gamma-linolenic acid (GLA), a polyunsaturated omega-6 fat that is used to treat a number of conditions, including rheumatoid arthritis, eczema, and premenstrual syndrome (PMS).

Besides borage oil, GLA comes from the seeds of the evening primrose plant and from black currants. The human body also manufactures its own supply of GLA from linoleic acid, which is abundant in vegetable oils and meats, according to Elson Haas, M.D., director of the Preventive Medical Center of Marin in San Rafael, California, and author of *Staying Healthy Shoppers Guide*.

In the body, linoleic acid is converted first to GLA and then to di-homo-gamma-linolenic acid (DGLA), a chemical that does wonders for our health. DGLA is essential for the production of prostaglandin E1, an important hormonelike chemical that reduces inflammation, boosts immunity, lowers blood pressure, keeps platelets from sticking together, and improves blood vessel tone, says Michael Janson, M.D., president of the American College for Advancement in Medicine, based in Laguna Hills, California, and author of *The Vitamin Revolution in Health Care*.

As we age, our bodies become less efficient at converting linoleic acid to GLA and therefore less efficient at producing the beneficial prostaglandins, says Dr. Janson. Several diseases, including cancer, eczema, multiple sclerosis, and diabetes, also make the conversion less efficient.

This doesn't necessarily mean that supplementing with GLA will cure or prevent these diseases. In fact, some experts warn that GLA supplements have the potential to aggravate symptoms because GLA and DGLA can actually help promote inflammation, by being shunted into a pathway that makes arachidonic acid, the precursor to inflammatory eicosanoids.

"With GLA, an omega-6 fatty acid, the very strategy that you're using to help yourself might actually be putting gasoline on the fire, unless you balance it with an adequate intake of omega-3's," says William E. Lands, Ph.D., a long-time researcher in the field of essential fatty acid nutrition in Bethesda, Maryland.

Aiding the Achy and Itchy

In his practice, Dr. Janson commonly prescribes GLA supplements for cardiovascular health, PMS, menstrual cramps, rheumatoid arthritis, and eczema. For the last two—rheumatoid arthritis and eczema—there are numerous scientific articles supporting the value of GLA.

In one promising study, 56 patients with rheumatoid arthritis were randomly assigned to take 2,800 milligrams a day of either GLA or a sunflower oil placebo for six months. Researchers discovered that the patients taking GLA were more than six times more likely to have significant improvement in their symptoms, especially tender joints. Patients who weren't getting GLA did not show any significant improvement. In fact, they were more than three times more likely to have their symptoms worsen.

For another six-month period, all of the patients in the study received GLA, and all showed improvement in their symptoms. For those who re-

SUPPLEMENT SNAPSHOT

▶Gamma-Linolenic Acid

Also known as: GLA.

May help: Heart disease, lupus, osteoarthritis, rheumatoid arthritis, diabetes, eczema, fingernail problems, endometriosis, menstrual cramps, premenstrual syndrome, and sunburn.

Special instructions: Take after a meal.

Cautions and possible side effects: Do not use supplements without the supervision of a physician if you are taking aspirin or anticoagulants (blood thinners) regularly, have a seizure disorder, or are taking epilepsy medication such as phenothiazines. Do not take borage oil if you are pregnant or breastfeeding. May cause headaches, indigestion, nausea, and softening of stools.

ceived GLA throughout the study, that improvement was progressive, and seven in this group reduced their reliance on nonsteroidal anti-inflammatory drugs or prednisone.

There was just one hitch: Most patients who finished the study found that their swelling and joint pain returned within three months of its conclusion, indicating that they would have to continue to take GLA to suppress their symptoms.

Before you try GLA for yourself, keep in mind that the doses used in this study were much higher than the typical daily dosage of up to 320 milligrams.

Proponents of GLA also believe the oil can help treat inflammatory skin disorders such as eczema. Research has come up with conflicting evidence: Two large studies have shown no benefit at all, but others have found improvement, particularly for patients with mild to moderate eczema.

One study involved 60 patients with atopic dermatitis, a chronic, recurring, inflammatory disease marked by eczema and itching. Researchers divided the patients into two groups. One group received 274 milligrams of GLA from borage oil twice a day, and the second group took a placebo. After 12 weeks, patients in the GLA group reported significantly less itching, redness, oozing, and blistering than patients in the placebo group. They were also able to reduce the use of drugs commonly used to treat the disease, such as antihistamines and topical steroids.

Time-Honored Cure for Monthly Woes

Evening primrose oil, an herbal supplement that's high in GLA, has also been examined for its healing properties. Woodson Merrell, M.D., a specialist in alternative and complementary medicine and assistant clinical professor of medicine at the Columbia University College of Physicians and Surgeons in New York City, says that women he's treated with evening primrose oil often get relief from the symptoms of PMS. They have less breast pain, cramping, and discomfort, he says.

"In my experience, it does seem to work for some women," he says. "I think it's definitely worth trying."

Native American women apparently thought so, too. They chewed the seeds of evening primrose to combat menstrual problems. The Indians and early European settlers also used the plants to treat asthmatic coughs and stomach disorders. Beginning in the early nineteenth century, the leaves were applied as a poultice for skin conditions like ulcers and scabies.

Evening primrose is a hardy, biannual, native American flower. The plant found its way to Europe when the highly fertile seeds apparently hitched rides in the ballast tanks of ships sailing the Atlantic between the new world and the old one.

During the seventeenth and eighteenth centuries, evening primrose gained a reputation for relieving symptoms of gout, rheumatism, and headaches. In England, it earned the nickname King's Cure-All because of its ability to heal skin diseases. Today, it is cultivated in more than 30 countries.

Is GLA for You?

Of the three oils, evening primrose has been the most studied, primarily in England, where it is an approved medical treatment for breast pain and eczema. Borage oil is the most concentrated source of GLA, however, which means that you have to take fewer capsules to get the same therapeutic benefits, says Dr. Janson.

Borage oil can come in 1,000-milligram capsules containing 240 milligrams of GLA, which falls within the range of the standard therapeutic daily dose of 180 to 320 milligrams, according to Dr. Janson.

The next most concentrated source is black currant oil, which has about 80 milligrams of GLA in each 500-milligram capsule. Three of these capsules give you the amount of GLA in one borage-oil supplement.

Each 500-milligram capsule of evening primrose oil contains 45 milligrams of GLA, so taking five a day would give you almost the amount provided in one capsule of borage oil.

garlic

No other medicinal herb is more universally recognized and consumed by people worldwide than garlic. It is valued in every major culture in the world as a food, condiment, culinary herb, and botanical medicine.

Garlic has been part of the human experience for so long that it's considered a cultigen, meaning that the plant is known only in cultivation, not in the wild. The original herb may have come from the high plains of a west-central Asian desert, but it evolved to its current form under the husbandry of humans.

For at least 5,000 years, since the time of the Egyptian pharaohs and even before the earliest Chinese dynasties, people have used garlic as medicine. In central Europe in ancient and medieval times, peasants wore necklaces of garlic cloves to keep away vampires and other evils. It is used in China as a preventive for colds and a folk remedy for dysentery. It is even administered as a juice in enemas to kill intestinal parasites.

"I find it fascinating that people have been aware of garlic's medicinal properties for thousands of years," says William Page-Echols, D.O., an assistant clinical professor of family medicine who teaches alternative medicine at the Michigan State University College of Osteopathic Medicine in East Lansing. "People weren't just using it in flights of fancy. They knew it was beneficial."

The Taste of Medicine

In the last few decades, more than 1,000 scientific papers have been published on garlic and related herbs of the Allium family. These studies provide strong—although not conclusive—scientific evidence that garlic has extraordinary medicinal powers.

Garlic seems to reduce blood pressure and cholesterol levels, dilate blood vessels, and thin the blood, all of which lowers the risk of heart attack and stroke. It's believed to kill harmful bacteria in the stomach and protect against gastric cancer. It appears to be a potent antioxidant and may boost the response of your immune system. It also works as an anti-inflammatory.

"When you think about the health problems that most people suffer from today, such as heart disease, cancer, and pain, they usually have as a component some type of inflammation," says Alison Lee, M.D., a pain-management specialist and medical director of Barefoot Doctors, an alternative medicine practice in Ann Arbor, Michigan.

Across cultures, garlic has been used to treat colds, flu, sore throats, high cholesterol, high blood pressure, atherosclerosis (hardening of the arteries), digestive disorders, bladder infections, and liver and gallbladder problems.

"Garlic is an inexpensive, easy-to-obtain medicine," says Dr. Page-Echols. "You can incorporate it into your diet and get its benefits through food. Or, if you don't like the taste or odor of garlic, you can take it as a supplement."

A Healing Burn

The stinking rose, as garlic was called by the Greeks and Romans, is a member of the genus *Allium*, which also includes onions, leeks, shallots,

SUPPLEMENT SNAPSHOT

▶ Garlic

Botanical name: *Allium sativum.*

May help: Heart disease, stomach cancer, high blood pressure, infections, colds and flu, sore throat, chronic fatigue syndrome, high cholesterol, atherosclerosis, digestive disorders, diarrhea, bladder infections, liver problems, and gallbladder problems.

Special instructions: Try to get your quota of garlic in food, as it may be more easily absorbed into your system.

Origin: May have originated in a west-central Asian desert; most garlic used today comes from widely cultivated modern hybrids.

Cautions and possible side effects: Don't use garlic supplements if you're taking anticoagulants (blood thinners) or hypoglycemics (a type of diabetes drug). Do not take if breastfeeding. Rarely, may cause allergic reactions.

and chives. Allium, the ancient Latin name for garlic, is believed to come from an ancient Celtic word—*all*, meaning "hot" or "burning."

The volatile oil of garlic gives the herb its distinctive smell and taste. The oil contains more than 30 sulfur compounds, including allicin and a number of others that are biologically active.

The most important of these is allicin, which is produced only when you crush, bruise, or cut a garlic clove. As the membranes of the garlic cells break down, alliin, a sulfur-containing amino acid, comes into contact with an enzyme called allinase. The resulting chemical reaction produces allicin, a pungent and strongly antibiotic compound.

Allicin is highly unstable and quickly degrades into a number of other chemical compounds. Some of these have therapeutic properties, but exactly how they work in the body as medicines has not been determined. Since the process begins with the formation of allicin, researchers believe the allicin content of garlic is the best indication of its medicinal value.

Killing Bad Bacteria

Louis Pasteur, who invented the process of milk pasteurization and developed the germ theory of disease, first demonstrated back in 1858 that allicin is a strong antibacterial. Before the advent of modern antibiotics in the 1930s, cuts and abrasions were treated by expressing garlic juice into a wound. On the Russian front in World War II, the Soviet army relied on garlic to treat the wounded when penicillin and sulfa drugs weren't available.

This proven antibacterial action may have profound implications in the prevention of one of the world's most commonly fatal cancers: stomach cancer.

Scientists have found that *Helicobacter pylori*, a type of bacteria sometimes found in the stomach, appears to be involved in the development of stomach cancer and peptic ulcers, says Jonathan Sporn, M.D., an oncologist and associate professor of medicine at the University of Connecticut Health Center in Farmington. There may be other factors as well, but the link to *H. pylori* is strong.

"We're not sure where these bacteria come from, but they're probably very common in the environment," explains Dr. Sporn. In fact, *H. pylori* infects half of the people on the planet and up to 90 percent of the populations of some developing countries.

In cultures with diets high in allium vegetables such as garlic and onions, the risk of stomach cancer is low, says Dr. Sporn. And in laboratory tests conducted at the Fred Hutchinson Cancer Research Center and University of Washington Medical Center in Seattle, scientists were able to kill *H. pylori* using a garlic extract. This study and others have found that garlic is toxic to many "bad" bacterial strains, even some that resist standard antibiotic treatment.

"It's very provocative evidence, and it fits with the folk wisdom surrounding the use of garlic," says Dr. Sporn. "These studies suggest that there may be something very valuable in garlic."

According to studies in India, garlic may actually benefit the good bacteria in the intestine, thereby improving digestion and enhancing the absorption of minerals. It has been used to re-establish good bacteria in the gut after an infection or antibiotic treatment.

Does all this mean that you should be eating garlic or taking garlic supplements every day? Perhaps, says Dr. Sporn. But how much? And how often? "That's the problem," he adds. "Although we have evidence that garlic may be preventive against cancer, we don't have enough information yet to make any specific recommendations."

Have a Heart for Garlic

Garlic may prevent two other major killers, heart disease and stroke, says Dr. Page-Echols. According to several studies, if you make garlic part of your diet or if you take it as a supplement, you may lower your risk of heart disease and atherosclerosis.

When fatty plaque builds up in arteries, blood flow to the heart and brain may be impeded. Clots can form, or chunks of plaque may break loose and form blockages. That sets the stage for a heart attack or stroke.

Garlic benefits the circulatory system in several ways. It lowers levels of cholesterol and triglycerides, another type of blood fat. It also has an antispasmodic action, meaning that it dilates blood vessels and increases blood flow to the heart and brain.

One especially important group of chemicals, called ajoenes, thin the blood and make clotting less likely. So even if you have plaque-filled arteries, the blood platelets are less likely to bunch up behind blockages. Essentially, they slide by a little more easily, says Dr. Page-Echols.

"Garlic can do a lot for your circulatory system. Just keeping the blood vessels more open can have a significant effect on hypertension. Your blood pressure drops," he says.

One study found that after just four weeks of taking garlic supplements, participants had a 5 to 6 percent reduction in total cholesterol. In another study, researchers at the University of California, Irvine, gave 40 men with elevated cholesterol levels either a combination garlic/fish-oil supplement or a look-alike, inactive capsule (placebo). During the study, the men maintained their normal, Western-style diets and kept up their usual activities.

After four weeks, cholesterol levels in the group taking supplements dropped by 11 percent. The placebo group showed no significant change. The researchers concluded that the combination of garlic and fish oil significantly reduces risk potential in people with elevated levels of cholesterol.

"The good thing is that garlic doesn't tamper with the good cholesterol, only the bad stuff," observes Dr. Page-Echols. "And for someone who wants to do a natural approach to taking care of their heart—in addition to better diet and more exercise—garlic can be very beneficial."

Spice Up Your Immune System

At least one component of garlic, alliin, is also an antioxidant. Some nutrients, such as selenium, vitamin C, vitamin E, and in particular alliin, scavenge free radicals, the free-roaming, unstable molecules that lead to cell damage and premature aging. Free radicals have also been implicated in the growth of tumors. In laboratory animals, garlic extracts have actually inhibited the growth of cancer cells.

Garlic is effective against bacterial, fungal, viral, and parasitic infections. The volatile oil is excreted by way of the lungs—hence garlic breath—and can fight infections in the upper airway. Some Chinese studies have shown that garlic has a beneficial effect in helping to battle colds and flu.

Because of garlic's antibacterial properties, it can help prevent secondary infections in people who have lowered immunity. An American study in 1989 found that protective natural killer cell activity was restored in some AIDS patients after they took garlic supplements for six weeks.

A Pill Will Do You

You don't have to eat garlic to get the medicinal benefits. If you find the flavor repulsive or you don't want to walk around all day with dragon breath, you can take powdered supplements, which are widely available in health food stores and drugstores.

"I prefer that people take garlic in their food because I think it is more easily absorbed into the system. The truth is, however, that most patients can't get raw garlic down because of the taste," Dr. Lee says. "In that case, taking a garlic supplement is appropriate."

Supplements are available as tablets, capsules, and tinctures. Although oil-based garlic preparations are widely available, their effectiveness is questionable, since allicin is unstable in oil. Moreover, since allicin is formed only when the cells of garlic are crushed to create the enzyme reaction, dried garlic doesn't contain this important component.

Dried garlic does contain alliin and alliinase, the enzyme that converts alliin to allicin. Look for enteric-coated tablets or capsules, which are designed to pass through the stomach and degrade in the alkaline environment of the intestine, where the beneficial conversion takes place. You'll get the medicinal benefits without the odor or taste.

ginger

In ancient Rome, most spices were expensive because they were so scarce. Ginger was costly for just the opposite reason—because it was plentiful. It was so common and in such demand that the government taxed it.

After the fall of the Roman Empire, ginger almost disappeared from Europe, until Marco Polo rediscovered it in China and India in the thirteenth century. Once again, the European taste for spices made it a treasured and expensive ingredient. In fourteenth-century Britain, a pound of ginger could cost you an entire sheep.

Columbus was trying to find another way to bring ginger and other spices home when he stumbled upon North America, but he didn't find ginger in the New World. It wasn't until the English introduced it to the colonies that it became a popular spice in the Americas.

Once introduced, ginger didn't go away. Today, this lowly root enhances a wide variety of food and drink, from the flavoring in ginger ale to the thin-sliced pickled ginger that's served alongside sushi. It's also been appreciated for its medicinal properties for thousands of years and employed by many cultures, including India's Ayurvedic medicine, Traditional Chinese Medicine, and Western herbalism. People have used ginger to treat indigestion, nausea, gout, flu, fever, headache, and flatulence.

Good for the Gut

The medicinal part of ginger is the rhizome, an underground stem that most people mistakenly refer to as a root. In Chinese and Ayurvedic medicine, the rhizome has a long-standing reputation as a digestive aid. It is ground up and used in numerous Chinese herbal prescriptions. Ayurvedic practitioners refer to ginger as the universal medicine because it aids the body's digestive function by relieving gas, bloating, and cramps, says Joseph Selvester, an Ayurvedic herbalist in Gainesville, Florida.

Western herbalists classify ginger as a carminative, an anti-inflammatory, and a diaphoretic, among other things. A carminative is an herbal remedy that settles the intestine and eases pain by removing gas from the digestive tract. Most herbs high in volatile oils have the ability to dispel gas and reduce bloating in the intestine, and ginger is rich in such oils.

As an anti-inflammatory, ginger is known to reduce the production of inflammatory compounds, which makes it useful for some types of headaches, for body aches caused by flu, and for arthritis.

A diaphoretic is capable of slightly raising body temperature and promoting sweating. "I use ginger for my patients who are unable to develop a fever to recover from a cold or flu," says Jill Stansbury, N.D., assistant professor of botanical medicine, chair of the botanical medicine department at the National College of Naturopathic Medicine in Portland, Oregon, and a naturopathic doctor in Battle Ground, Washington. She recommends boiling sliced gingerroot in water, then adding honey and lemon to taste. "A cup or two of hot ginger tea, drunk while in a hot bath, can help induce a brief fever and speed recovery from an infection," she adds.

Lose the Woozies

If it's just an upset stomach or a woozy feeling that's unsettling your gut, you may want to turn to ginger. Two of the herb's active ingredients, gingerol and shogaol, help combat nausea, whether it's caused by flu, motion sickness, or the surging hormones of early pregnancy, says William

SUPPLEMENT SNAPSHOT

▶ Ginger

Botanical name: *Zingiber officinale*.

May help: Arthritis, indigestion, intermittent claudication, phlebitis, muscle soreness, heartburn, diarrhea, and nausea, including morning sickness and motion sickness.

Origin: Unknown; probably Southeast Asia; cultivated in India and China for thousands of years.

Cautions and possible side effects: Fresh ginger is safe when used to season food. Do not use the dried root or powder if you have gallstones.

Page-Echols, D.O., an assistant clinical professor of family medicine who teaches alternative medicine at the Michigan State University College of Osteopathic Medicine in East Lansing.

Ginger appears to have no side effects, while many motion sickness drugs, such as dimenhydrinate (Dramamine), cause drowsiness. This makes it a safe alternative for pregnant women battling morning sickness. In a Danish study of pregnant women, 1,000 milligrams of ginger powder daily, divided into four doses, was effective. But you may need to experiment to find a dosage that works for you, says Dr. Page-Echols.

"It is safe to take during pregnancy, but as with any drug, I'd still recommend that you use it only when necessary or for short periods of time," he adds. Be sure to talk to your doctor first.

Motion sickness drugs act on the central nervous system, so some researchers believe that gingerol and shogaol work in the same way. Others believe that the medicinal action takes place in the stomach itself.

Saying No to Nausea

No one knows exactly how ginger helps to quell nausea, says Alison Lee, M.D., a pain-management specialist and medical director of Barefoot Doctors, an alternative medicine practice in Ann Arbor, Michigan. You can't rule out some effect on the brain, she says, because a ginger tincture seems to work as well as a powdered supplement.

"Sometimes it just takes a drop or two on the tongue to stop nausea," she says. "It apparently gets into your bloodstream and inhibits the vomiting center in your brain."

If the mechanism isn't certain, the results are. A study involving 80 Danish naval cadets found that ginger is an effective treatment for seasickness. While the cadets were learning the ropes of seamanship aboard a training vessel in heavy seas, half the group was given 1,000 milligrams of ginger powder, while the other cadets received an inactive substance that looked the same (a placebo).

The cadets, ages 16 to 19, were good test cases because none had experience on the open seas, nor were any of them overly susceptible to becoming seasick. They were, so to speak, fresh fish. Over the following few hours, the ginger group had "remarkably" fewer symptoms of vertigo and nausea, according to the researchers. Ginger reduced vomiting and cold sweats better than the placebo. The placebo group presumably spent more time retching over the side or running to the head (that's ship talk for bathroom).

Hot Spice for Heart and Joints

Ginger is good for your heart as well as your stomach. Among its other benefits, it seems to have a blood-thinning effect. In a study conducted in India, powdered ginger significantly reduced the clumping of blood platelets in people with coronary artery disease.

If platelets clump up, they can cause rough spots on artery walls, which then attract fat molecules that build up to form a dense, clogging substance called plaque. When enough plaque builds up, the arteries narrow, causing blockages that can lead to heart attack and stroke.

"The Chinese use dry ginger in many heart and kidney treatments, and in Ayurvedic medicine, ginger is considered a heart tonic," says Selvester.

In limited test-tube studies, ginger has also shown anti-inflammatory action. Research has shown that it can reduce pain and swelling in people with rheumatoid arthritis, osteoarthritis, and muscle pain.

Common over-the-counter anti-inflammatories like aspirin and ibuprofen work in a similar manner, but long-term use of anti-inflammatory drugs can have serious consequences. These drugs sometimes reduce the beneficial enzymes that maintain the protective mucous lining of the stomach. If that happens, the corrosive gastric juices that help digestion may irritate the stomach and cause an ulcer, says Dr. Page-Echols.

Easy Relief

Ginger appears to regulate two types of chemicals that are responsible for inflammation and to do it in a safer way than anti-inflammatory medications, without the stomach-irritating side effects.

Dr. Page-Echols recommends ginger—often in combination with the herb turmeric—to many elderly patients who have a history of using anti-inflammatories for chronic pain and arthritis. "They are at risk for developing bleeding ulcers from the typical drugs taken for inflammation," he says. "Ginger is easier on the system."

As with most herbal anti-inflammatories, if you take ginger for pain, it takes time to have the desired effect. You can't just pop a ginger supplement as you might an aspirin and get immediate relief, says Dr. Lee.

"Herbs do take time to work, but if you're in a situation where you have a chronic, recurring problem like arthritis, you need something that you can take often and safely," she says. "Eventually, the ginger will have an effect."

Food or Pill?

Ginger is readily available in several forms. Most pharmacies and health food stores sell ginger powder in pills or capsules. Look for an extract standardized to 5 percent gingerols when trying to treat arthritis or motion sickness, suggests Dr. Stansbury.

Candied ginger sticks are sold at many health food stores and may do in a pinch, especially for nausea, but they are probably less valuable for arthritic problems, says Dr. Stansbury. You can also incorporate ginger into your food as a flavoring to help lower cholesterol. "Use fresh sliced or grated gingerroot in soups, stir-fries, rice, and salad dressings," she suggests.

Dr. Page-Echols recommends that his patients cook with ginger at least twice a week to help with arthritis, heart health, and general health. Many people in India use 8,000 to 10,000 milligrams of fresh ginger a day in cooking, he says. "A lot of people aren't accustomed to thinking of food as a medicine, but in this case, it really is. Ginger is something that most people have used in their food. I try to encourage them to use more and use it more often."

ginkgo

In 1945, a few months after the A-bomb leveled Hiroshima, the blackened, apparently lifeless stubs of ginkgo trees near ground zero sprouted new leaves. Although in its 200 million years on Earth, the ginkgo tree had never before encountered a nuclear blast, it was well-equipped to survive the devastation.

Ginkgo is indifferent to fire, resists bug infestation, and thrives in dirty, polluted air; some individual trees have been known to live for up to 1,000 years. Such tenacity has made the ginkgo the oldest living tree species on Earth, a living fossil preserved from days when dinosaurs plodded the terrain.

Delaying Fossilhood

The medicinal compounds found in this ancient and remarkable tree may enable you to avoid turning into a fossil yourself—or at least keep you from doing so prematurely. A concentrated extract of ginkgo leaves can intensify blood circulation, avert heart attacks and strokes, rev up the brain, and even delay the progress of dementia and Alzheimer's disease. Thus, this mighty herb can help deter many of the afflictions associated with growing old.

Ginkgo biloba is *the* herb for an aging population, says Jennifer Brett, N.D., a naturopathic doctor at the Wilton Naturopathic Center in Stratford, Connecticut. Most of Dr. Brett's older patients—those over 65—are taking supplements of ginkgo.

"People who are getting old worry about two things: Is my heart going to fail? Is my brain going to fail?" she explains. "In terms of prevention, this is an herb that people can take every day for the rest of their lives. It improves their general circulation and mental acuity."

In Europe, where botanical healing is common, many older people routinely take a ginkgo extract to improve their mental fitness. It is the most widely prescribed herb in Germany and has been approved in that country as a treatment for dementias, afflictions (including the type caused by Alzheimer's disease) that are associated with loss of memory in older people.

It's in the Leaf

Ginkgo is native to China, where the fruit and seeds have been used for 4,000 years to treat everything from asthma to problems with frequent urination and nocturnal emissions. The seeds and fruit are highly toxic, always require careful preparation, and need to be given in carefully measured doses to avoid poisoning. The leaves were rarely used as a medicine until a few decades ago, when European researchers concentrated dried leaves into an extract and discovered their remarkable medicinal properties.

Working with the extract, the researchers isolated two groups of active chemicals: flavone glycosides and a unique set of terpenoids that the scientists called ginkgolides. Over the years, an extract of 24 percent flavone glycosides and 6 percent ginkgolides became the standard used in scientific

SUPPLEMENT SNAPSHOT

▶ Ginkgo

Botanical name: *Ginkgo biloba.*

May help: Heart disease, angina, stroke, intermittent claudication, depression, dementia, Alzheimer's disease, Raynaud's disease, Parkinson's disease, head injuries, leg cramps, macular degeneration, tinnitus, impotence due to poor blood flow, clogged arteries, and diabetes-related nerve damage.

Origin: Native to China; the oldest living tree species on Earth.

Cautions and possible side effects: Avoid ginkgo if you are taking anticoagulants (blood thinners), aspirin or other nonsteroidal anti-inflammatory drugs, or antidepressant MAO inhibitor drugs such as phenelzine sulfate (Nardil) or tranylcypromine (Parnate). Taking more than 240 milligrams of concentrated extract may cause vomiting, diarrhea, or rash. Rarely, gingko may cause headache, stomachache, or other allergic reactions.

studies. Today, this formula, known as EGb 761, is used throughout Europe to treat heart disease, eye ailments, impotence due to low blood flow, tinnitus (ringing in the ears), poor circulation to the extremities, and head injuries and other brain-related conditions.

Although doctors and scientists don't fully understand how the chemicals in ginkgo work in the human body, the effects and benefits are pretty well known, says Alison Lee, M.D., a pain-management specialist and medical director of Barefoot Doctors, an alternative medicine practice in Ann Arbor, Michigan. "Ginkgo is really an important herb because there's a lot of good research behind it," she says. "It works for many conditions."

Blood Flows like Water

Ginkgo is mostly known as a circulatory herb, or what doctors call a vasodilator. It widens blood vessels and holds them open so blood flow increases. While enlarging arteries and large veins, a vasodilator also expands capillaries, the tiny vessels webbed into your body tissues and organs.

This effect makes ginkgo especially useful for people who have cold hands and feet due to poor circulation. Dr. Brett routinely uses the herb to treat Raynaud's disease, a severe constriction of blood vessels in response to cold. Raynaud's sufferers literally can't get blood to their fingers and toes, she says, but with the active chemicals in ginkgo, the blood vessels expand, allowing more warming blood to flow to the extremities.

Dr. Brett also prescribes ginkgo to people with diabetes who have lost feeling in their feet due to inflamed nerves and high blood sugar levels. Ginkgo stabilizes the blood flow, and its glycosides have strong anti-inflammatory properties. "I use it for any circulatory disorder," she says. If you have diabetes and want to consider using ginkgo, discuss it with your doctor.

Thinning Action

Increasing blood flow isn't ginkgo's only action. The ginkgolides apparently thin the blood by counteracting the effects of platelet activating factor (PAF), a chemical that causes blood platelets to stick together and clot.

Clotting, as you might imagine, is pretty important when you've sliced yourself with the potato peeler. But PAF also forms clots when there's an irregularity in an artery, such as a chunk of fatty plaque sticking to the vessel wall, says Dr. Lee. "You want your platelets sticky when you get a wound, but you don't want them bunching up around plaque in a blood vessel," she explains. "That's going to create a blockage and reduce the flow of blood."

By thinning the blood, ginkgo may protect you from a stroke or heart attack, which can be triggered by a blocked artery or a blood clot that has broken away from an artery wall. In the same way, it may ease or prevent angina attacks—heart pain caused by constricted vessels—and pain due to cholesterol buildup in the vessels of your legs.

Thin blood will still clot, but it may take longer, says Dr. Lee. If you're already on an anticoagulant (blood-thinning) medication or taking aspirin to reduce your risk of heart attack or stroke, you should be careful about using ginkgo. "If you're already on a blood thinner, talk to your doctor," she cautions. "Two of my patients got nosebleeds after they started the ginkgo."

Platelets are not the only blood cells modified by ginkgo, adds Dr. Lee. There's evidence that after several weeks, the herb eventually makes the membranes of red blood cells bend and stretch more easily. This effect may be important in increasing blood flow to the brain.

"If the membrane is more pliable, the cells can actually squeeze their way into tighter places, past blocked or partially blocked arteries and vessels," she says. "That may be very important in increasing blood flow, particularly in the small vessels in the brain."

Feed Your Head

The benefit of any increased blood flow is that your tissues and vital organs receive additional nutrients and oxygen. Increased blood flow to the brain has been shown to improve alertness, short-term memory, and the ability to concentrate. It may also relieve tinnitus, improve mood, and counteract depression.

Ginkgo not only feeds your head, it also improves the action of substances called neurotransmitters, which help carry signals between nerve cells. Influenced by the herb, these substances work more efficiently, so that messages travel from cell to cell more quickly. "This is an herb that can make you think better. It directly stimulates the brain," says Dr. Brett.

Ginkgo also apparently holds off or slows down the destructive consequences of an aging brain. Free radicals—the free-roaming, unstable molecules that invade cells and damage them—are natural metabolic by-products of aging. When someone has Alzheimer's disease, the damaging effect of free radicals leads to more fat being deposited in brain cells. As that happens, those cells quickly become inoperative. Substances in ginkgo help to scavenge free radicals and slow down the rate at which fat is deposited, so the whole deterioration process is slowed.

Some research in Europe and the United States has shown that ginkgo can be helpful to people who have Alzheimer's. For years, European studies have indicated that dementia patients taking ginkgo show signs of improvement. A few years ago, a U.S. study appeared to confirm these findings.

American researchers gave people with mild to moderately severe dementia 120 milligrams of EGb 761, the European ginkgo extract, each day for one year. Meanwhile, another group received an extract with no ginkgo (a placebo). After looking at the comparative results of treatment, researchers concluded that the ginkgo extract appeared to stabilize or, in some cases, improve mental functioning.

The researchers estimated that the ginkgo may have bought the patients a delay in the disease of between six months and a year. They note, however, that the treatment appears to work best in the early stages of the disease.

A Slow Process

For treating any condition, ginkgo takes time to build up in your system. You may have to take the herb for weeks before you begin noticing the benefits, says Dr. Lee. "I tell people to give it about six weeks," she says.

For long-term use, ginkgo is considered a relatively safe herb. Except at very high levels—more than 240 milligrams of concentrated extract—it usually produces no side effects.

Ginkgo is available in tablets and capsules, but the best way to take it is in tablets, says Dr. Lee. A standard dose is 120 milligrams a day. To avoid possible gastrointestinal discomfort, take one 40-milligram tablet three times a day.

At the drugstore or health food store, look for a supplement that contains 24 percent ginkgoflavoglycosides and 6 percent terpenelactones, says Dr. Brett. "Then you have the same concentration of the active ingredients that has been used in all the studies."

As for using ginkgo leaves, there's no practical way to get a dose equivalent to what was used in studies. It takes about 50 pounds of leaves to get 1 pound of the extract in the appropriate percentages, says Dr. Brett.

ginseng

If you drive through north-central Wisconsin on your way from Minneapolis to Green Bay, no doubt you'll notice some odd-looking farm fields along the way: one- to two-acre plots of knee-high, red-berried bushes growing beneath canopies of fabric.

You're in the ginseng capital of the United States. Those fabric canopies cut the light by about 80 percent, artificially reproducing the muted light of a hardwood forest, which was the original home of American ginseng.

Wild ginseng, once found east of the Mississippi River, is rather rare these days due to overharvesting. Cultivating the herb remains a difficult endeavor, but Wisconsin's cool weather and glacial soils, along with growing techniques that have been passed down through many generations, permit the region to produce 95 percent of America's ginseng crop. Most American ginseng root—the medicinal part of the plant—is exported to the Orient, where herbalists and doctors of oriental medicine value it as an overall body tonic or energy tonic.

American ginseng (*Panax quinquefolius*) is only one type. There are two other plants that are commonly called ginseng. Asian ginseng (*P. ginseng*) is also used in the Orient.

For over 2,000 years, American ginseng has been a mainstay of oriental medicine, used as a revitalizing agent for general weakness, lack of appetite, anemia, forgetfulness, and deficiency of the "vital energy" known as *chi*. But oriental doctors often use American ginseng instead of the Asian species because it is said to be milder, less stimulating, and better suited for older patients and long-term use.

In recent years, many herbalists and herbal companies have begun using Siberian ginseng (*Eleutherococcus senticosus*), the third type. This plant isn't a true member of the ginseng family, but it's less expensive. Although it's a bit weaker than the true ginsengs, it has many of the same properties. Siberian ginseng is most often found as part of herbal formulas.

The medicinal properties and active ingredients of the three types are similar, and all can accurately be called energy herbs. Take them when you're fatigued, run-down, worn out, or dealing with stress, suggests Alison Lee, M.D., a pain-management specialist and medical director of Barefoot Doctors, an alternative medicine practice in Ann Arbor, Michigan.

Herbalists credit ginseng with elevating mood and reducing fatigue. It won't make you leap tall buildings or run a four-minute mile, but it does seem to restore energy and improve performance—both physical and mental—says Julie Clemens, N.D., a naturopathic doctor in Sagle, Idaho.

"I use it primarily as a tonic, mostly to improve people's vitality when they've been experiencing times of weakness," says Dr. Clemens. "That could be after the flu, after a funeral, or during times of great mental stress. I tell patients to use it for a short period of time, until they start feeling better."

Dr. Lee notes that the herb is not an instant stimulant. You might have to take it for a while before you begin to feel its effects.

SUPPLEMENT SNAPSHOT

▶Ginseng

Botanical names: *Panax quinquefolius* (American ginseng), *P. ginseng* (Asian ginseng), and *Eleutherococcus senticosus* (Siberian ginseng).

May help: Fibromyalgia, chronic fatigue syndrome, genital herpes, impotence, stress, muscle soreness, low immunity, and depression; may improve stamina, breathing, and coordination; normalize blood sugar levels; strengthen appetite; and increase alertness and reaction time.

Special instructions: Avoid coffee while taking.

Origin: Grows only in eastern Asia and parts of North America; plants may be remnants of ancient forest that covered much of the Northern Hemisphere some 70 million years ago.

Cautions and possible side effects: If you have a heart condition, high blood pressure, or an anxiety disorder, consult your doctor before taking ginseng. May cause insomnia, nervousness, diarrhea, headaches, and sometimes high blood pressure. Has been reported to cause menstrual bleeding in post-menopausal women.

The Friskiness Factor

Ginseng comes from the Chinese words *jen shen*, meaning "man root." The branches of the root resemble arms and legs, and the Chinese felt that the human appearance was a clue to its effectiveness as a whole-body tonic. Many Native Americans viewed the herb in the same way. The Penobscots believed that native ginseng increased female fertility, while the Fox of Wisconsin considered the plant a universal remedy. The plant genus, *Panax*, actually comes from the Greek word *panacea*, or cure-all.

Although there is a lack of scientific evidence, ginseng also has a reputation as an aphrodisiac. In the early 1800s, Appalachian folks gathered the plant in the wild to use when "old-timers used to go a'courting." The Ginseng Board of Wisconsin publishes an herbal recipe for baked goods called Sex Muffins, although they do acknowledge that any increase in sexual activity among ginseng users is probably related to a boost in energy rather than any direct elevation of the libido. In other words, if you feel more energetic, maybe you'll feel more frisky.

Despite all of this folk use and titillating talk of aphrodisiac qualities, ginseng never became a very important herb in American medicine, and it was never a favorite among old-time practitioners. One reason may be that ginseng really isn't a panacea, and many of the claims for it are exaggerated, says Tirun Gopal, M.D., an obstetrician and gynecologist who practices holistic and Ayurvedic medicine in Allentown, Pennsylvania.

"Ginseng is one of the most abused herbal medications that I know of. If you look in any lay literature or magazine, it's still being touted as therapeutic for everything from cancer to an ingrown toenail," he says. "It certainly has its uses, but it is not a panacea."

Despite these reservations, though, there are still some things that ginseng seems to do quite well.

Adapting to Conditions

The Chinese think of ginseng as a normalizing or restorative agent. Western herbalists classify it as an adaptogen, an herb that has the ability to normalize function. It can be a stimulant, increasing alertness, reaction time, respiratory output, and motor coordination, or it can have a milder tonic action, lowering blood pressure, regulating blood sugar (glucose) levels, maintaining the immune system, and helping the body deal with the effects of stress.

"An adaptogen just sort of goes where it's needed, putting your body into a more balanced state," says William Page-Echols, D.O., an assistant clinical professor of family medicine who teaches alternative medicine at the Michigan State University College of Osteopathic Medicine in East Lansing.

Ginseng's dual nature as both a calming influence and an energy booster can be traced to a group of active ingredients called panaxosides or ginsenosides. There are at least 13 types of ginsenosides in ginseng. Some stimulate the central nervous system, while others apparently act as pain relievers and tranquilizers, calming the stomach and nervous system.

Asian ginseng may be more stimulating than its American cousin because it contains a different balance of ginsenosides. No one is really sure, however, because there may be as many as 30 active ingredients in ginseng.

"I prefer American ginseng, because less stimulation is usually better," says Dr. Lee.

Energizing Agent

Ginseng has been used for thousands of years as a tonic to elevate mood and reduce fatigue. Some of the first scientific studies to gauge the herb's effectiveness included a study of mice that were able to swim longer distances after being given ginseng. A Russian study showing that soldiers who were given an extract of ginseng ran faster in a three-kilometer race than those given a look-alike substance (a placebo).

Ginseng may give you an extra push in several ways. It temporarily increases the amount of oxygen uptake by the body and causes the muscles to use glycogen, the body's stored sugar, more efficiently, says Dr. Page-Echols. Also, ginseng augments the number of insulin receptors in the body, thus driving the sugar in foods into your cells, where it can be burned, he says.

"Not only does that give you more energy, it also lowers or regulates your blood sugar," says Dr. Page-Echols. "Ginseng improves the glucose balance in the body and improves its sensitivity to insulin." That's important to people who have high blood sugar, because insulin is the chemical released by the body to "escort" glucose into the cells, where it becomes a useful energy source.

A Finnish study found that people newly diagnosed with type 2 (non-insulin-dependent) diabetes who took 200-milligrams of ginseng extract daily for eight weeks experienced improved blood glucose levels, enhanced mood, and better psychological and physical performance. When first diagnosed, these people were fatigued and depressed by their illnesses. Ginseng gave many of them the energy lift they needed to change lifestyles and to cope better with their conditions, the researchers concluded.

Ginseng's stimulating properties have also been helpful in treating people with chronic fatigue syndrome. It can also help with depression when fatigue and stress are contributing factors.

Withstanding Stress

Adaptogens like ginseng have a unique capacity to strengthen the body's resistance to stress and limit damage caused by stress, says Dr. Lee.

Stress can make you irritable, weaken your immune system, and accentuate any pain or discomfort you may be feeling, she says. She sometimes prescribes ginseng to her chronic pain patients, especially if they work in stressful environments like noisy offices or construction sites or have high-pressure jobs. "Pain is a stress, too, so I use ginseng to help people tolerate pain and not be so run down by it," says Dr. Lee.

Apparently, ginseng helps inhibit the output of chemicals and hormones that stress you out, says Dr. Page-Echols. An increased capacity to withstand stress keeps your immune system strong and makes you less susceptible to colds and other illnesses, he adds.

Ginseng also stimulates the immune system directly, increasing the function of natural killer cells and accelerating phagocytosis, the process in which white blood cells eat up invading bacteria or viruses. Although ginseng is not as powerful an herb as echinacea in this regard, it can help you fight off an infection, says Dr. Page-Echols.

"In the wintertime, some people take an immune stimulant, like echinacea or astragalus, daily, but you don't want to take the same one all the time because eventually, the herb loses its effect," says Dr. Page-Echols. "You can use ginseng as a substitute for a couple of weeks."

Spotting the Disguises

Because ginseng is reputed to be a cure-all, many herbal formulas contain it. At the typical health food store, you'll confront a bewildering array of ginseng-type products—everything from candy to teas and soft drinks.

Yet, many of these herbal combinations or products contain either little ginseng at all or ginseng of questionable quality, says Dr. Lee.

"I like the assurance of seeing the whole root," she says, but adds that purchasing a standardized extract of ginseng root from a reputable manufacturer is another option. A list of Wisconsin ginseng producers is available by writing to the Ginseng Board of Wisconsin, 16H Menard Plaza, Wausau, WI 54401. The board has also developed a seal to identify Wisconsin-grown ginseng products; look for it on the ginseng products at drugstores or health food stores.

Your best bet is to look for capsules or pills standardized to 7 percent ginsenosides. Most clinical studies of ginseng use this standard, and the supplement gives you some assurance that you're getting the real thing, says Dr. Page-Echols. You'll also find ginseng as a tea, tincture, or root powder.

Both American and Asian ginseng tend to be very expensive, and American ginseng is in short supply because it's often shipped overseas. Consequently, much of the ginseng found in the U.S. market is Siberian.

goldenseal

At the beginning of the twentieth century, between the demise of old folk remedies and the emergence of professional medicine, came the hucksters of patent medicines—an odd breed of shady entrepreneurs, self-appointed doctors, and bona fide quacks.

One of the most successful was Dr. Roy Pierce, a physician who made a mint hawking Dr. Pierce's Golden Medical Discovery: The Only Guaranteed Liver, Blood, and Lung Remedy.

Dr. Pierce, who created an entire line of popular patent medicines, never discovered anything beyond the power of mass advertising and the public's gullibility in believing in a so-called magic elixir. His "discovery" consisted mostly of alcohol and sugars, but it did get its distinctive amber color from goldenseal, a medicinal herb long used by Native Americans.

Bacteria Batterer

The Cherokees used the roots and rhizomes of the plant to treat skin diseases and relieve sore eyes. Today, goldenseal is still used as an external wash for canker sores and skin wounds, but most people take it internally, usually in capsule form, to soothe inflamed mucous membranes, stop or slow down infections, and stimulate digestion, says Jennifer Brett, N.D., a naturopathic doctor at the Wilton Naturopathic Center in Stratford, Connecticut. It is frequently recommended for ulcers in the upper intestine and especially advocated for respiratory infections, she says.

"It seems to be really effective for upper respiratory infections like sore throats and sinus infections," says Dr. Brett. "It has the ability to stimulate your immune system and slow down the rate at which bacteria invade your cells and tissues."

If used early, goldenseal is effective against nearly any kind of infection, from a sore throat to a cut on the hand, says Dr. Brett. Its antibacterial and antiseptic properties can help fight off bacteria. While that doesn't mean that goldenseal should be used in place of an antibiotic when one is needed, "it can help keep an infection from spreading long enough so that your immune system can take care of it," she says. "If the infection has really set in, though, you may need more help than goldenseal can give you."

Goldenseal can make the symptoms of an infection less bothersome. It's especially effective in reducing phlegm and drying up secretions from inflamed mucous membranes, the tissues that make up the inner lining of the body, explains Dr. Brett.

When you have an irritated sinus or a sore throat from postnasal drip, the herb can bring great relief, Dr. Brett says. "It works best when you can get the goldenseal right on the infection. I tell people to gargle with a tea of goldenseal when they have a sore throat."

Tastes Like Medicine

In olden days, people generally put goldenseal root into water and brewed a tea, but it was a bitter tonic to swallow. Even rinsing out your mouth with goldenseal can be a memorably unpleasant experience. Herbalists classify it as a potent, bitter, astringent herb, and it simply tastes terrible, says Alison Lee, M.D., a pain-management specialist and medical

---

SUPPLEMENTSNAPSHOT

▶Goldenseal

Botanical name: *Hydrastis canadensis*.

May help: Upper respiratory infections, inflamed mucous membranes, diverticulitis, colds and flu, heartburn, diarrhea, canker sores, chronic fatigue syndrome, urinary tract infections, celiac disease, and skin infections; also used for ulcers and as a blood purifier and digestive stimulant.

Origin: United States; was introduced to European settlers by Native Americans.

Cautions and possible side effects: Do not take while pregnant. Do not use if you have high blood pressure or an autoimmune disease such as multiple sclerosis or lupus or if you are allergic to plants in the daisy family such as chamomile and marigold. Do not take for more than a week.

director of Barefoot Doctors, an alternative medicine practice in Ann Arbor, Michigan.

Traditionally, bitter herbs were used as stomach medicines, and goldenseal has a well-deserved reputation for stimulating the digestive system to secrete more bile and salivary and gastric juices, says Dr. Brett.

Whenever you produce more digestive juices, you also produce more digestive enzymes, which aid in digestion and can normalize bowel movements, she says. She often prescribes goldenseal as a cure for diarrhea caused by either a bacterial or viral infection.

"It's also a good treatment for stomach ulcers. Since we now know that most ulcers are caused by bacteria, it makes sense that it would be effective," she adds.

Flush the Toxins

Goldenseal has long been touted as a blood purifier, an herb that normalizes liver function. Some herbalists believe that the blood and liver can become congested with toxins when there's too much poison in the body for the liver and endocrine system to process, metabolize, and purify, says Dr. Lee.

By stimulating the digestive system, a bitter herb like goldenseal can increase the actions of the liver and spleen, pump out more bile from the gallbladder, and, in the process, expel more toxins through sweating and the excretion of waste. "It's a way to clean out the system. That's what bitters are said to do," says Dr. Lee.

'Seal Hunting

Many health food stores and drugstores carry goldenseal capsules and tinctures. Look for a standardized extract that concentrates berberine, the active ingredient, suggests Dr. Lee.

In comparison with other herbs with similar infection-fighting actions, such as echinacea and astragalus, goldenseal is expensive. Today, it is rare in the wild because of overcollecting. In fact, Dr. Lee cautions against its overuse because the plant is becoming endangered. Herb growers are just beginning to domesticate and cultivate it.

gotu kola

Commonly called Indian pennywort, gotu kola grows abundantly in the wetlands of India, Sri Lanka, and other parts of the Southern Hemisphere. When people in Sri Lanka observed elephants feeding extensively on the slender, creeping plant, they suspected that the herb was responsible for the elephants' long life span—up to 75 years. A Sri Lankan proverb advises, "Two leaves a day will keep old age away."

If this elephant tale sounds fanciful, consider the legend of Li Ching Yun, a Chinese herbalist who supposedly lived to be 256 years old because he regularly consumed gotu kola.

These stories clearly show one thing—people on the Indian subcontinent and in the surrounding region plainly believed that gotu kola promoted longevity and a healthier life.

Clear Thinking

Medicinal use of gotu kola comes from the Chinese and Indian (Ayurvedic) herbal traditions. The herb normalizes the nervous system, improving mental activity and well-being, says Priscilla Evans, N.D., a naturopathic doctor at the Community Wholistic Health Center in Chapel Hill, North Carolina.

Gotu kola appears to have steroidlike properties, and in a number of studies, it also improved circulation. Either action could have a beneficial effect on the chemistry of the brain, says Dr. Evans. "We're not really clear about the herb's mechanism in the body, but we know it relaxes people and increases their mental clarity," she says.

Naturopathic doctors frequently mix gotu kola into their herbal formulas to help their patients relieve stress and rejuvenate the mind and body, says Irene Catania, N.D., a naturopathic doctor and homeopathic practitioner in Ho-Ho-Kus, New Jersey. Gotu kola tends to balance out the function of the adrenal glands, which secrete hormones in response to stress, she says.

"When you're exhausted or burnt out, your adrenals are often fatigued," says Dr. Catania. "Gotu kola is a nice rejuvenating herb."

Studies have also shown that gotu kola works as a botanical treatment for high blood pressure, varicose veins, burns, and circulatory problems. In Ayurvedic medicine, it was a popular treatment for healing skin ulcers and treating leprosy.

A Wound Healer

In Sri Lanka, people eat the leaves in salads or use them to brew a medicinal tea. The entire plant, however, has healing properties.

The most active compounds in the herb are triterpenes and saponin glycosides. The glycosides are particularly important. Animal studies have shown that large doses of two kinds of glycosides have a sedative or calming quality, while another type has anti-inflammatory properties. A fourth type seems to stimulate wound healing.

When researchers injected gotu kola extract into animals, they found that one of the glycosides seemed to increase the development and maintenance of blood vessels in connective tissue. That mechanism relates directly to its healing properties, because any time more blood is delivered to the site of a wound, the healing process is enhanced, says Dr. Catania.

In addition to helping the blood arrive where it's needed, gotu kola is like a food or balm for the connective tissues, says Dr. Catania. It contains

SUPPLEMENT SNAPSHOT

▶ Gotu Kola

Botanical name: *Centella asiatica*.

May help: Varicose veins, poor circulation, wounds, scarring, keloids, stress-related high blood pressure, exhaustion, and burnout.

Special instructions: Take on an empty stomach.

Origin: India, Sri Lanka, and other countries in the Southern Hemisphere.

Cautions and possible side effects: Do not take if you are pregnant or breastfeeding. Talk to your doctor if you are thinking of taking it for an extended period of time. Rarely, may cause rash or headache.

many important raw materials such as flavonoids that help build healthy tissues. "Although you get some of these building blocks in your food, they're more concentrated in the herb," says Dr. Catania. "Gotu kola helps the structure of connective tissues develop normally."

Dr. Catania recommends gotu kola for people with skin conditions and for those who are about to have surgery or are recovering from an injury. It's also helpful for anyone who tends to heal poorly, a condition sometimes caused by diabetes.

Making Scars Scarce

Because gotu kola works well for skin conditions, it can be helpful in the treatment of cellulite and keloids, says Dr Evans.

Cellulite is caused by a hardening of connective tissue cells below the skin's surface. Gotu kola seems to be able to reduce or slow down this process.

"But you can't just take a few capsules of gotu kola and expect cellulite to go away," Dr. Evans warns. "The herb is beneficial because it has a general strengthening and toning effect on connective tissue. It should be just one part of a therapy that includes diet, exercise, and massage."

For keloids, gotu kola's action is much more direct. Keloids are raised, irregularly shaped, progressively growing scars. They form when healing fails to proceed as it should, resulting in an excessive formation of collagen. In other words, the scar continues to grow until it eventually turns into a type of benign tumor.

Gotu kola makes scars mature faster by enhancing the later stages of the healing process. In a study, researchers gave an extract of gotu kola to 139 patients with keloids or hypertrophic scars—scars in which the cells had grown dramatically in size. After 2 to 18 months of treatment, 82 percent of the study participants showed signs of improved healing as a result of taking gotu kola.

Vein Vitality

Beneath the skin, gotu kola has long been an important herbal therapy for varicose veins. These lumpy purple veins form when the blood vessel walls weaken and blood flow is sluggish, particularly in the legs. Tiny valves within the veins no longer work efficiently, so instead of flowing steadily upward toward the heart, blood slips down through the weakened valves. As a result, the veins bulge and swell with stagnated blood.

Gotu kola strengthens the epithelium, the layer of cells that line the outside and inside of blood vessels and arteries, says Dr. Evans. It also strengthens the connective tissue sheath surrounding the vein, which makes it beneficial for preventing varicose veins.

"Gotu kola is an ideal tonic for the elderly," says Dr. Evans. Older people, she notes, are more likely to have problems with weakened blood vessels, particularly their veins. Also, it may take longer for their skin to heal after cuts, scratches, bruises, or similar injuries. Gotu kola helps with both of these problems—plus, it helps to improve mental clarity.

Gotu kola isn't difficult to find in health food stores, and it's also available in some drugstores. It's sold as a tincture, in capsules, and in bulk herb form.

hawthorn

Long before anyone installed barbed wire and split-rail fences, German farmers kept their animals penned in with natural fences or hedges of hawthorn. The bushes had thorns so sharp and dense that they created a nearly impenetrable barrier to livestock.

Although hawthorn is a sturdy, tenacious plant, it also has a gentler side. In spring, hawthorn flowers (also called mayflowers; remember the tiny ship that brought the Pilgrims to America?) sweetly scent fields throughout Europe. When country folk had colds, they used to pick and eat the herb's reddish blue berries because the tart taste relieved the scratchiness of sore throats.

Old-time herbalists sometimes used hawthorn to treat heart ailments, but they apparently never knew what a treasure they had in this hedgerow plant. Hawthorn is probably one of the best heart tonics in the plant kingdom, according to Irene Catania, N.D., a naturopathic doctor and homeopathic practitioner in Ho-Ho-Kus, New Jersey.

Whether you have angina, arrhythmia, an enlarged heart, or congestive heart failure, you can benefit from taking hawthorn. It's helpful anytime that there is deterioration of the heart muscle, says Dr. Catania.

"That's not to say that hawthorn can reverse severe damage done by heart disease. If you have an enlarged heart, hawthorn won't make it smaller," she says, "but it will probably ease some of the symptoms and increase the function and strength of your heart."

Hawthorn assists healthy hearts, too. It's been shown to lower blood pressure, reduce levels of blood cholesterol, and prevent cholesterol buildup on artery walls—actions that help prevent heart disease.

A study by the German Federal Ministry of Health found that hawthorn gently increases the strength of the heart, normalizes rhythm, and benefits circulation within the heart itself by dilating the coronary arteries. In Germany, many extracts and medicinal preparations use hawthorn alone or in combination with other herbs.

A Tonic for the Ticker

In herbal parlance, hawthorn is known as a tonic. Tonic herbs typically strengthen and normalize function and, depending on the problem, they have different actions in the body.

In the case of congestive heart failure, hawthorn helps make the heart muscle contract more forcefully and pump more blood. If your heart beats erratically or too fast but medication is not yet required, hawthorn can help restore your heartbeat to normal and might keep the condition from getting worse.

Hawthorn is a potent antioxidant that scavenges free radicals, the free-roaming, unstable molecules that damage cells and cause premature aging. It also protects and regulates collagen, a fibrous protein that is essential for healthy tendons, ligaments, and other connective tissues in the body, says Pamela Herring, N.D., a naturopathic doctor at the Naturopathic Clinic of Concord in New Hampshire.

Any type of inflammation destroys collagen, so hawthorn can be a good treatment for people with an inflammatory disease like arthritis, she says. "I recommend hawthorn to a lot of patients who are getting up in years and have heart problems and arthritis. It's an herb that addresses all of these conditions."

SUPPLEMENTSNAPSHOT

▶Hawthorn

Botanical name: *Crataegus oxycantha*.

May help: High blood pressure, atherosclerosis, heart arrhythmia, enlarged heart, angina, congestive heart failure, mitral valve prolapse, high cholesterol, degeneration of collagen, and inflammation.

Special instructions: Take capsules with food; take a tincture 15 to 20 minutes before a meal.

Origin: Native to Europe; some species are grown in the United States.

Cautions and possible side effects: Safe for long-term use but may cause health problems at very high doses. Do not take without a doctor's supervision, especially if you are taking heart medications.

Many Medicinal Species

The genus name, *Crataegus*, refers to the plant's hard wood and sharp thorns. Hawthorn can be termed either a small tree or a large shrub because it can reach 30 feet in height. Many people commonly called the plant haw.

Haw's healing properties were known as far back as the first century A.D. In the sixteenth century, it shows up in herbalists' texts as a remedy to stem the flow of blood, because the berries were so astringent. It apparently wasn't widely used for heart problems until the beginning of the twentieth century, when some American drug companies began manufacturing a hawthorn extract as a cardiac tonic. Some American physicians still prescribed the extract in the 1940s to treat high blood pressure.

Herbalists long considered the berries the medicinal part of the plant, but the flowers and leaves also contain active ingredients. As with most herbs, hawthorn probably has several active ingredients that work in harmony.

Some of the more important ingredients include a mixture of pigment chemicals known as flavonoids. These compounds give the hawthorn berry its distinctive reddish blue color. Flavonoids scavenge free radicals and lessen the bad effects of inflammation. They also seem to reduce cholesterol in the bloodstream.

Proanthocyanidins, another large group of chemicals, seem to be largely responsible for its beneficial actions on the heart. These chemicals relax smooth muscles in blood vessels so they won't suddenly constrict and shut off blood flow, which can happen when emotional and physical stress taxes the heart muscle so it demands more blood and oxygen.

Get the Drop on Dropsy

When ancient physicians used hawthorn as a heart herb, they usually were treating congestive heart failure, which they loosely termed dropsy. *Dropsy* actually describes the symptoms of edema, an accumulation of fluid in the tissues. When the heart is weak and can't pump enough blood, fluid often accumulates around the ankles. Because hawthorn works as a mild diuretic and purges excess fluid from the tissues, it gives relief from this symptom of heart failure.

Hawthorn also has an extraordinary effect on the heart itself. In some cases, it improves the heart's mechanical pumping action and increases the force of its contractions, says Eran Ben-Arye, M.D., a researcher at the national medicine research unit at Hadassah University Hospital in Jerusalem.

In some cases of congestive heart failure, hawthorn seems to work well. In a German study, researchers studied 78 patients between the ages of 45 and 73 who had mild to moderate congestive heart failure. Over an eight-week period, some of the patients received 600 milligrams of hawthorn extract daily, while others were given a liquid that looked and tasted the same but contained no hawthorn (a placebo). During the study, patients were not allowed to take any other types of heart medication except diuretics. Their fitness levels were measured using a type of stationary bicycle.

At the end of the study, those treated with hawthorn significantly improved their performance on the bicycle. They also had lower systolic blood pressures (the upper number in a blood pressure reading) and lower heart rates, both of which indicate improved pumping action.

"It was a good, well-controlled study with results that seemed to reinforce the folk use of the herb," says Dr. Ben-Arye. "In the case of mild congestive heart failure, I think hawthorn may be an efficient medication."

In more advanced cases, hawthorn can be used in combination with digitalis or other herbs and medicines containing compounds called cardiac glycosides. Studies show that hawthorn appears to enhance the action of these compounds.

Open the Flow

Hawthorn also acts as a vasodilator, meaning that it opens blood vessels and increases blood flow. This is especially important in the coronary blood vessels that supply the heart with oxygen.

The herb dilates the vessels by relaxing smooth muscles in the artery walls. Through the use of a natural chemical that acts much like synthetic drugs that are widely used to treat high blood pressure and heart disease, it also inhibits an enzyme that makes blood vessels constrict.

Because of this action, it probably improves the mechanical function of the heart. A better-functioning heart is better able to utilize oxygen, which has a beneficial effect in cases of angina, a crushing chest pain that occurs when blood supply to the heart decreases.

"I've used hawthorn to treat angina and eventually have been able to take people off their nitroglycerin medications," says Dr. Herring. "But I'd recommend that you do it only with the help of a physician."

The flavonoids in hawthorn may help keep you from ever having angina pain because they appear to strengthen the structure of collagen, which makes up arteries and blood vessels. When the collagen is stronger, the blood vessels are less susceptible to plaque buildup.

A Protective Connection

The power to help build collagen is useful in other parts of the body as well. Collagen can be destroyed if you have inflammation caused by rheumatoid arthritis or other types of autoimmune diseases. The consequences can be painful. When collagen in cartilage decays, the connective tissues between bones may disintegrate, and you may end up with bone rubbing against bone, says Dr. Herring. "Collagen is important for all kinds of structures in the body, so you want to hang on to it and protect it," she says.

Hawthorn has a chemical action that helps tone down inflammation. While helping to protect collagen, it may be able to slow down the progression of chronic inflammatory disease, says Dr. Herring. It also helps protect cells from premature aging.

Lick the Spoon

Hawthorn comes in several forms: freeze-dried berries, tincture, capsules, and a concentrated extract that resembles a tarlike syrup. "You can lick the extract off a spoon or make a tea with it. It actually tastes pretty good," says Dr. Herring.

Don't expect instant results, however. The therapeutic effects take time to develop, usually a period of weeks or months. If you think you might have a heart or blood pressure problem, first get an accurate diagnosis, says Dr. Ben-Arye. After you know what the problem is, you can make your choices about medications and supplements.

iron

Considering how much iron surrounds us (it's the fourth most abundant element on Earth) and how little we need in our bodies (less than a teaspoon), it's surprising that iron deficiency is the most common nutritional shortcoming both in the United States and worldwide.

Iron problems may hit infants, especially between the ages of six months and two years, if they're weaned from breast milk, which contains sufficient iron, to cow's milk, which doesn't. For them, iron-fortified formula and cereals are the solution.

Adults also need iron, and sometimes, we just plain come up short. A woman's iron needs are especially great. During her childbearing years, she needs one-and-a-half times as much iron as a man. Liver and red meat—both loaded with iron—are considered health foods in parts of the world where meat is scarce, and that's just what they are to tired women and irritable, listless babies. The form of iron found in meat is also more easily absorbed than iron from, say, vegetables or soy.

Men rarely become iron-deficient unless they've lost blood. Because getting too much can increase a man's risk for other conditions, doctors say that men should not take supplements unless a deficiency is diagnosed.

Show Me the Oxygen

It takes only about 30 seconds, maybe a minute at most, for us to realize how vital oxygen is to our well-being. Stop breathing, and in 10 minutes or so, you're dead. Every cell in our bodies requires oxygen to make the energy that keeps it going.

Iron delivers the oxygen. "It's kind of like the breeze that fans the flames," explains Janet Hunt, R.D., Ph.D., a researcher with the U.S. Department of Agriculture Human Nutrition Research Center in Grand Forks, North Dakota.

This mineral looms large in oxygen delivery because it's a vital part of hemoglobin, a protein that's found in red blood cells. Each hemoglobin molecule can carry four molecules of oxygen. A particular kind of iron, called heme iron, plays an integral role in this process of toting oxygen molecules from the lungs to other parts of the body. As red blood cells pass through the lungs, the heme iron, which is indirectly bound to the hemoglobin in a special way, readily picks up oxygen. Then, as the red blood cells pass through other tissues in the body, they release their oxygen freight wherever it's needed.

Iron is also a crucial part of another protein, myoglobin, found in mus-

SUPPLEMENT SNAPSHOT

▶Iron

Supplement forms: Ferrous gluconate, sulfate, and glycinate.

May help: Iron-deficiency anemia, heavy menstrual bleeding, and canker sores.

Daily Value: 18 milligrams.

Special instructions: For maximum absorption, take on an empty stomach unless indigestion occurs; then take with food. A meal containing 25 to 30 milligrams of vitamin C can enhance absorption by as much as 85 percent. Avoid using over-the-counter preparations such as enteric-coated tablets or capsules containing slow-release granules. Don't take iron and calcium supplements, prescription medications to reduce stomach acid, or antacids at the same time; and don't wash down your iron tablet with tea. All can significantly decrease absorption.

Who's at risk for deficiency: Children; teenagers, especially teenage girls; premenopausal women; pregnant women; and vegetarians.

Good food sources: Lean beef, dark chicken meat, shellfish, and iron-fortified cereal products.

Cautions and possible side effects: It's best not to take supplements unless you are a woman with heavy menstrual bleeding or have been diagnosed with low iron status or anemia. May cause constipation. For people with hemochromatosis, taking iron supplements can be dangerous.

cles, that picks up and stores additional oxygen for use when muscles have to go at it long and hard. When you're low on iron, your capacity for exercise is reduced because your myoglobin can't transport enough oxygen to the muscles for the long haul.

The Energy Hand-Off

True, oxygen is needed for a cell's energy production, but iron plays another vital role in the energy-producing process as part of a cell's energy "assembly line."

In a cell's power plant, called the mitochondria, a set of proteins, some containing iron, are lined up in a bucket brigade called the electron transport chain. "These proteins transfer electrons from energy-yielding nutrients to oxygen, forming water and carbon dioxide, and in the process of respiration make a molecule called ATP, a cell's basic energy currency," says Paul Saltman, Ph.D., professor of biology at the University of California at San Diego. "Without enough iron, a cell's capacity to produce energy drops way off."

Iron also helps to oxidize compounds. It takes away electrons, a process that generates free-roaming, unstable molecules called free radicals that damage cells. In a way, this puts iron in head-to-head competition with vitamin E, which is well-known as an antioxidant that helps neutralize free radicals and prevent electron pilfering. "One is not necessarily better than the other," Dr. Saltman says. In fact, both processes are necessary for life, and they tend to balance each other out.

Iron is found in many enzymes so it plays a role in the enzyme activity that affects your cells. And this mineral is in the production line that leads to the making of amino acids, hormones, and neurotransmitters. It's on-site when beta-carotene is converted to the active form of vitamin A. It plays a walk-on part in the production of collagen, one of the body's major structural proteins. In the liver and intestines, iron also does essential emergency work, converting harmful toxins into safer compounds that can be more easily excreted.

Fighting Microbes, Helping Enzymes

Given iron's role in energy production and protein synthesis, it only makes sense that a shortage may decrease our resistance to infection. "We fight off infection by building up our armies of immunity—our white blood

Strange Cravings? Check Your Iron

It's not unusual to have a hankering for chocolate brownies, ripe watermelon, or a nice, juicy steak. But what if it's laundry starch, glue, or Styrofoam cups that you find yourself snacking on?

Doctors have a word for this bizarre disorder. It's called pica, a name that comes from the same Latin root as magpie, a bird known for its indiscriminate appetite. Over the years, doctors have reported cases of people with pica eating many unpalatable items including dirt, chalk, clay, library paste, paint chips, paper, cardboard, ice chips, and Styrofoam.

In one case, a 22-year-old woman showed up in the emergency room with undigested pieces of tube socks in her stomach. She had begun chewing socks to relieve the stress of moving away from her family. Unfortunately, instead of moving right along, the remains of the socks wadded up in her stomach, forming a painful, indigestible ball.

"Pica is a strange mix of the physical—usually an iron deficiency—influenced by psychological and even social settings," says William H. Crosby, M.D., a retired hematologist in Joplin, Missouri, who has a longstanding interest in pica. The condition tends to occur in pregnant women, who are often low in iron, and in some babies. The babies affected tend to be "milkaholics," meaning that they drink milk to the exclusion of other foods, thus lowering their intake of iron. No one knows why iron deficiency would cause such strange behavior, but often, when the deficiency is corrected with iron supplements, eating habits return to normal, Dr. Crosby says. Even the woman with a taste for socks got back to normal with iron supplementation.

Sometimes, people who are iron-deficient compulsively chew ice or gum or eat crunchy, salty, or sour foods such as potato chips, pickles, or unripe fruit, Dr. Crosby says. The name for this is food pica, which is the most common type in the United States.

Rather than put up with this behavior, see a doctor to be tested for iron deficiency and to get supplemental iron if necessary, Dr. Crosby says. A common problem in food pica is that people are ashamed about compulsively eating ice or other unusual items. "Don't let shame stop you from seeking a diagnosis," he says. "A good doctor will realize that this disorder can have an easily treated physical cause." People with pica are often amazed at how easily their compulsive behavior stops once they begin treatment, he says.

cells—and that takes lots of energy and protein," Dr. Saltman explains. Iron helps produce both.

Inside certain immune cells, iron plays an additional microbe-zapping role. Immune cells called macrophages, which can engulf and digest bacteria, rely on iron-containing enzymes. These enzymes are kept safely away from other parts of the cell inside special sacs. When they are released, they break down the bacteria that the macrophages engulf, Dr. Saltman says. "That whole system would be compromised in the case of iron deficiency."

Good for the Brain and Body

In addition to helping out macrophages, iron plays an important role in physical and mental functions. It is a crucial component of an enzyme, amine oxidase, that helps to produce three neurotransmitters, dopamine, serotonin, and norepinephrine. These brain chemicals are involved in dozens of different functions, including movement, intellectual performance, waking, sleeping, and emotional states like excitement, grief, happiness, and depression. No wonder iron deficiency has been strongly linked with changes in behavior and mood.

In adults, the symptoms are likely to be trouble concentrating, listlessness, and perhaps some irritability and trouble sleeping, Dr. Saltman says. Those problems get better when iron is restored.

Children who are iron-deficient may develop permanent problems. "There's growing evidence that children can have permanent brain damage if they are iron-deficient during critical times in brain development," Dr. Saltman says.

People with iron deficiency may have another problem as well—an impaired ability to maintain body temperature in a cold environment. In other words, they just can't get warm. "In this case, the lack of iron may be stopping the thyroid gland from functioning properly," Dr. Hunt says. It's because the thyroid controls the body's metabolism—its ability to burn calories for energy and for heat.

Your body must have iron on hand to be able to incorporate another essential nutrient, iodine, into molecules of thyroxine, the main thyroid hormone. Iodine activates thyroxine, letting it do its job of revving up your metabolism and letting you burn some calories as heat. No iron means no heat.

Coming Up Short?

Iron supplements used to be considered fairly safe for just about anyone, but now researchers have some reservations. High iron levels have been associated with a slightly increased risk of cancer and heart disease, probably because excess iron can cause cell damage. Plus, about 1 in every 300 people has an inherited disorder called hemochromatosis, which can cause a buildup of iron in your liver, spleen, heart, and other organs. This can be dangerous if you get lots of iron in your diet or from supplements, says James D. Cook. M.D., a hematologist and professor of medicine at the University of Kansas Medical Center in Kansas City. A blood test can reveal whether you have this condition.

Frequently, diets that are low in iron—like the diets of some vegetarians—are also low in copper, says Dr. Saltman. Be sure that there is some copper in your multivitamin/mineral supplement.

If you're a woman who is still menstruating, it's safe to take a daily supplement with up to 18 milligrams (the Daily Value) of iron, says Dr. Cook. If you think that you may be really short on iron, though, you should have your blood levels checked by a doctor. People who are consistently short on iron, as shown by blood tests, need to take much higher amounts initially to restore normal levels. After you reach a normal level, which is easily determined by a quick blood test, you may be able to slack off on supplementation after talking to your doctor. Anyone else—older women, men, children, and regular blood donors—should take supplemental iron only on a doctor's advice.

vitamin K

Consider blood. It has the remarkable ability to remain liquid even though it's loaded with all sorts of solid stuff—red and white blood cells, protein, vitamins, minerals, even gobs of fat from the last cheeseburger you ate. But blood can also become solid within seconds when a blood vessel breaks. That particular ability can spell the difference between life and death if you're seriously injured—and it requires vitamin K.

The vitamin got its name from the Danish researchers who discovered it. The "K" stands for "koagulation," the Danish version of "coagulation."

Your body needs it to make several blood proteins involved in clotting, including the most important, prothrombin. When bleeding starts, these proteins go through a quick series of changes that ends with a blood clot, says John Suttie, Ph.D., professor of biochemistry at the University of Wisconsin in Madison. If your body ran short of vitamin K, your blood would clot very slowly, and you might develop many symptoms that are a giveaway—easy bruising, frequent nosebleeds, or cuts that won't quit bleeding.

Potential Bone Builder

You need vitamin K to make two proteins found in bone. Without it, the bones produce an abnormal form of these proteins that can't bind to the minerals that normally form bone.

One Japanese study suggests that low vitamin K levels play a role in the breakdown of bone after menopause. Some researchers contend that postmenopausal women are at risk for a low-level vitamin K deficiency that the traditional blood-clotting test would not detect. "However," Dr. Suttie says, "much more needs to be learned about vitamin K's function in bone before we know for sure whether it plays a role in diseases such as osteoporosis."

Eat the Garnish

Most people get enough of this vitamin from their diets. The average intake is 80 micrograms or so a day, which is the Daily Value.

Good sources include leafy green vegetables such as parsley, spinach, watercress, turnip greens, kale, and broccoli. Vitamin K is also produced in the intestines by bacteria, but it's likely that these bugs in our guts don't produce all that much, Dr. Suttie says.

Vitamin K deficiency is not common, he says. People who are most likely to be deficient probably don't eat leafy green vegetables, or they have medical problems that interfere with fat absorption.

"People who are in the hospital for one reason or another are also at an increased risk for problems," Dr. Suttie says. That's because they may not have eaten anything for a while, and a deficiency can occur relatively fast—within a few days. There's an added risk of vitamin K–related complications for people who are taking anticoagulant (blood-thinning) drugs

SUPPLEMENT SNAPSHOT

▶ Vitamin K

May help: Bleeding problems associated with vitamin K deficiency.

Daily Value: 80 micrograms.

Special instructions: For best absorption, take a K-containing multivitamin with a meal that contains some fat. There is no need to take supplements unless prescribed by your doctor.

Who's at risk for deficiency: Newborns; people taking anticoagulants (blood thinners), long-term antibiotic therapy, or sulfa drugs; people who eat no green vegetables; and those who have problems with dietary fat absorption.

Good food sources: Broccoli, kale, parsley, spinach, turnip greens, and watercress.

Cautions and possible side effects: Don't assume that easy bruising or bleeding is being caused by a vitamin K deficiency; see a doctor if you have these symptoms. If you are taking the anticoagulant warfarin (Coumadin), do not take vitamin K without medical supervision.

such as warfarin (Coumadin), which block the action of vitamin K. Other causes of depletion are antibiotics or sulfa drugs that can wipe out bacteria in the intestines, making even this small supply unavailable.

Do You Need Special K?

Luckily, doctors check blood-clotting time in people who are taking anticoagulants or who appear to have bleeding problems. Any problems that might occur are easily corrected with an injection of vitamin K.

Doctors sometimes tell their patients who are taking anticoagulants not to eat anything that contains vitamin K, but that's not the best advice, Dr. Suttie says. "They should continue to eat the way they did before they started taking the drug and try to keep their intake pretty much the same from week to week," he says. This helps to stabilize the dose of anticoagulant.

Injections of the vitamin are routinely given to newborn infants, who tend to be low on it because it doesn't cross the placenta very well. Injections are also sometimes used for people who can't absorb nutrients well or who are on tube feedings.

Vitamin K is found in some multivitamins and in single supplements. If it's in a multivitamin, you'll find it listed on the label.

Large intakes of vitamin E—on the order of 2,200 international units (IU) a day—can reduce the absorption of vitamin K in the intestines, according to Dr. Suttie. "People who eat normal amounts of vitamin K–rich foods, however, can safely take 400 IU of vitamin E every day for long periods of time," he says.

kava kava

In the eighteenth century, when missionaries came ashore on the coral atolls and volcanic islands of the South Seas, they found native societies that had never learned to distill alcohol. The absence of demon rum must have seemed a blessing to the proselytizers of the Christian faith, but they soon found another evil abroad in the land—the drinking of kava kava, also known simply as kava.

The drink is made from the root of a native perennial shrub of the South Pacific that grows up to 18 feet tall when cultivated. Kava brought on euphoria and a sense of well-being and was considered sacred. It was used by the islanders to cure illness, welcome babies, send off the dead, celebrate marriages, and welcome important visitors.

The ritual of drinking kava goes back farther than the written history of the islands. The tradition was probably taken to the Eastern Pacific from the New Guinea–Indonesia area by the people who pioneered and settled the islands.

In religious ceremonies, the kava root was chewed by young men and women, who then spat the masticated mixture into a bowl and mixed it with coconut milk. This method of preparation appalled European sailors. Today, kava root is ground by mechanical means.

With true zeal, the missionaries tried to expunge kava from the rituals of island societies, and they very nearly succeeded. In fact, it wasn't until the 1940s that kava again became an important social and ceremonial drink in the South Seas.

In the meantime, scientists and Western herbalists had begun to study the plant. Before many years had passed, healers and practitioners began to use kava for medicinal purposes.

What they discovered was that kava seemed to be the perfect natural remedy for anxiety, depression, and insomnia. It was also used to treat muscle spasms, bladder spasms, and other ailments that called for antispasmodic medicine.

An Intoxicating Pepper

The milder, more medicinal effects of kava were overshadowed for some time, as English explorers who visited the South Seas described natives going into a stupor and falling asleep after drinking several cups of kava. Because of this, they gave the plant the botanical name *Piper methysticum*, or intoxicating pepper. The native word, *kava*, refers to its sharp, pungent taste.

In order to become so sedated on kava that you pass out, you would have to drink nearly toxic amounts, says Irene Catania, N.D., a naturopathic doctor and homeopathic practitioner in Ho-Ho-Kus, New Jersey. "The natives were literally overdosing on it," she says. "When you take kava medicinally, you use only a fraction of that amount, and it doesn't have an intoxicating effect."

In lower doses, kava helps to benefit the brain, relieve anxiety, and act as a mild sedative or tranquilizer. Unlike many pharmaceutical drugs used

SUPPLEMENTSNAPSHOT

▶Kava Kava

Botanical name: *Piper methysticum*; also known as kava.

May help: Anxiety, muscle spasms, tension, bladder infections, and insomnia.

Special instructions: For insomnia, take in the evening; for anxiety, take in the morning and afternoon.

Origin: Native to the South Sea islands.

Cautions and possible side effects: Kava is quite safe at medicinal dosages, but do not exceed the dose recommended on the label of the product you buy. Do not take with alcohol or barbiturates. Use caution when driving or operating equipment, as kava is a muscle relaxant and may cause drowsiness. Do not use if you are pregnant, trying to conceive, or breastfeeding. Do not use if you have liver disease. Note that kava has come under scrutiny for causing hepatotoxicity, or liver toxicity. Although there have been cases, the products that caused the problem were made from the root plus parts other than the root. Therefore, use only products that are made of 100 percent root.

for anxiety, such as diazepam (Valium) and alprazolam (Xanax), kava doesn't space you out or leave you with a kind of hangover, says Dr. Catania.

"That's one of the real benefits of kava. It's relaxing but not depressing. It doesn't deteriorate your mood," she says. "Most people feel more alert and have increased mental acuity."

Kava is good medicine any time there is anxiety from stress, mild depression, a phobia, premenstrual syndrome, or menopause. It also helps with insomnia when anxiety causes sleeplessness, says Dr. Catania. "The way it helps people get to sleep is by relaxing them and decreasing their anxiety level," she says.

For Nerves and Brain

Traditionally, only the main root of kava was used medicinally, but the lateral roots, sprouts, and peelings of the interior and exterior bark also contain active ingredients. What apparently brings on feelings of well-being is a group of chemicals known as kavalactones. They are especially abundant in the fat-soluble resin of the roots.

When researchers isolated kavalactones from the kava and gave study subjects only this one group of chemicals the tranquilizing effects were not as pronounced. People seemed to get more benefit when they took an extract that contained all of the ingredients. That may indicate that other chemicals are at work in addition to kavalactones, or it may be that kavalactones are more bioavailable—that is, more quickly taken up by the body—when taken in extract form.

Several European countries have approved kava extract to treat nervous anxiety. The extract is standardized to 70 percent kavalactones.

Exactly how kava works in the brain is still a bit of a mystery. What's clear is that it goes about its business differently than pharmaceutical drugs. Valium binds to certain receptor sites in the brain, which then change the chemical makeup of the brain itself.

Animal studies show that kava affects the limbic system, an ancient part of the brain and the principal seat of emotions. In other words, it may alter the way emotions are processed rather than having a tranquilizing, depressing action.

"Because it doesn't bind to the receptors, it also can be used a lot more safely than the anti-anxiety drugs," says Priscilla Evans, N.D., a naturopathic doctor at the Community Holistic Center in Chapel Hill, North Carolina. "Kava is nonaddictive, and you don't build up a tolerance to it as you do with drugs."

A Mellow Medicine

Kava's lack of side effects and its ability to relieve anxiety show up in several European studies. In one study, 58 patients who had anxiety were given either a very large dose of kava extract or an ineffective substitute that contained no kava (a placebo). The participants' anxiety levels were measured with standard psychological assessment tests. After just four weeks, the patients taking the kava showed a statistically significant reduction in feelings of nervousness. They also had fewer complaints related to anxiety, such as heart palpitations, chest pain, headaches, and dizziness. In addition, they reported no side effects from the kava extract.

In another study, German researchers tested kava extract with a group of 101 patients who had a range of anxiety and tension disorders. For 25 weeks, half of the group received a dried kava extract containing 70 percent kavalactones; the other half received a placebo. Once again, the group receiving kava showed significant mood improvement as compared to those given only a placebo.

A Body Balm

Kava's calming action occurs not only in the brain but also throughout the body. It has a pronounced antispasmodic or relaxing effect on skeletal muscles. Dr. Evans sometimes uses kava just to relieve muscle tension brought on by emotional stress or physical work. "It's effective for acute and chronic muscle spasms and tension," she says.

Dr. Catania has also successfully used kava to treat people who have gastrointestinal problems such as nausea or stomach pain that's caused by anxiety.

Kava is available in dried bulk form and as capsules and tinctures. Medicinal doses are generally no higher than 210 milligrams of kavalactones daily. In comparison, one cup of a typical kava drink as used traditionally in the South Pacific contains about 250 milligrams of kavalactones, and several cups are usually consumed at one sitting.

lecithin and choline

Imagine a supplement that could actually restore memory. Could we use it to reverse some of the memory loss that comes with aging? What if it could also enhance our ability to think?

The very thought is enough to make your head spin.

Unfortunately, we're not quite there yet, but research into the possibilities for lecithin has touched off some alluring expectations.

The supplement that's getting all this heady attention would seem, at first glance, to be a very unlikely candidate. Many of its effects have a lot more to do with digestion than with brain function. Yet there are components of lecithin that seem to play a critical role in nerve function—and our brains, of course, are nothing more or less than elaborate agglomerations of busy nerves making interesting connections with each other.

The Great Emulsifier

To see lecithin's action up close, put a chocolate bar in the freezer. When you take it out some time later, you'll notice that the whole bar is tinged with white.

You can chalk up that transformation to lecithin. Derived from soybeans and egg yolks, lecithin is often added to foods such as chocolate, cheese, margarine, and salad dressings. In these foods, it acts as an emulsifier, which simply means that it helps mix fats with water and keeps them from separating. When the chocolate bar is frozen, the lecithin-fat interaction falls apart. The fat rises to the surface, giving the candy that whitish tinge.

Lecithin forms naturally in all living cells of the body, and just as it does in food, it acts as an emulsifier. It helps keep fatty substances in bile, which is essentially a kind of juice produced by your liver. When lecithin is doing all it should, it also eases digestion and helps your body absorb valuable nutrients.

Lecithin also helps to maintain the structural integrity of cells, says

243

Steven Zeisel, M.D., Ph.D., professor and chair of the department of nutrition at the University of North Carolina in Chapel Hill. "Without lecithin, nothing would survive, because you wouldn't be able to separate the various compartments within cells, nor would you be able to separate cells from each other."

It also serves as a source of messengers used to help control blood pressure and regulate insulin, the all-important hormone that helps unlock cells so that blood sugar can be absorbed for energy. Without lecithin-derived messengers helping to coordinate these activities, many cells would be at a loss about what to do. "You wouldn't have the ability to send proper signals," notes Dr. Zeisel. "Everything would grind to a halt."

None of those admirable activities suggests a link between lecithin and brain power, however. For that, we have to look at one component of lecithin—a substance called choline.

The Choline Connection

Choline is a nutrient that's essential for helping to turn fat into energy within the liver. Although it's a component of lecithin, it's also sold separately as a supplement.

In addition to the way it helps the liver deal with fat, choline has another function: It helps transmit nerve impulses in the brain.

That transmission process isn't quite as straightforward as carrying cellular e-mail from one address to another. Instead, choline is a building

SUPPLEMENT SNAPSHOT

▶**Lecithin and Choline**

May help: Liver disorders, gallstones, heart disease, memory loss, depression, stress, and high cholesterol.

Good food sources: Soybeans, peanuts, and wheat germ; also available as an additive in chocolate, margarine, salad dressing, and cheese.

Cautions and possible side effects: Large doses of lecithin may cause upset stomach, sweating, salivation, and loss of appetite. Do not take doses of choline above 3.5 grams (equivalent to 23 grams of PC) without medical supervision. Regular supplementation with choline can cause a fishy body odor.

block of another chemical, acetylcholine, that actually carries messages between nerve cells. The brain uses acetylcholine for many purposes, including controlling memory, heart rate, and sweating, according to Dr. Zeisel.

Tantalized by the possibility that choline could help memory, researchers have been investigating the link. To date, they've found that acetylcholine is in short supply among some people who have neurological disorders, but that doesn't prove that more acetylcholine produces better brain function.

Related research has led to a more promising path. Researchers have run across another chemical in lecithin called phosphatidylserine (PS). The scientists have found that PS, a building block for brain cells, seems to have a particularly beneficial effect on the production and release of the chemicals that transmit messages, according to Parris Kidd, Ph.D., a biomedical consultant in Berkeley, California, and author of *Phosphatidylserine: The Nutrient Building Block That Accelerates All Brain Functions and Counters Alzheimer's.*

In fact, PS is the single best means for conserving memory and other higher brain functions as we age, says Dr. Kidd. In studies, PS has been shown to improve the quality of life for people with declining brain function. It improves function in people with mild to moderate Alzheimer's and counteracts some of the age-related memory loss among people who don't have Alzheimer's. According to Dr. Kidd, it also has some benefits that go beyond memory function: helping people cope with stress and, in some individuals, helping to alleviate depression.

"PS seems to have a global effect on brain functions," he says. "It helps memory, learning and concentration, mood, and daily rhythms. It seems to have a general revitalizing effect on the brain."

The type of PS that's been shown to work on memory is derived from bovine brain, says Alan Gaby, M.D., professor of nutrition at Bastyr University in Bothell, Washington. A soy-based PS is being tested, but the chemical structure is a little different, so we can't assume that its effects are the same, says Dr. Gaby. So far, it has not been shown to be effective, he says.

Lecithin in the Liver

Meanwhile, back in the digestive area, researchers can pinpoint many of lecithin's benefits when it comes to transporting valuable resources from place to place in our bodies.

We are constantly secreting lecithin into our bile, says Dr. Zeisel, and that helps enzymes mix with fat so that the fat is digested.

The liver exports fat. To do that, it must wrap the fat in an envelope containing lecithin and certain proteins. When lecithin is unavailable, no envelope can be made, and fat accumulates in the liver. Liver cells low in lecithin fill up with fat and then die.

"Humans who are fed intravenously with solutions that lack lecithin and choline start to have liver cell death," says Dr. Zeisel. "This can be reversed when you give them a lecithin or choline supplement."

One form of choline, phosphatidylcholine (PC), seems to be particularly beneficial to the liver. In clinical studies, PC helped with alcoholic liver damage, cirrhosis, viral liver damage, and drug-induced liver damage. Animal research showed that PC supplementation was superior to any other treatment for alcohol-induced liver damage and cirrhosis.

PC is found in small amounts in most lecithin supplements. Greater concentrations are available in supplements labeled PC or Leci-PC.

Closely related to the way lecithin benefits the liver is the way it helps to prevent gallstones. The lecithin has a blending effect on bile salts and bile components. Without lecithin, the proteins in bile would separate out and form gallstones, says Dr. Zeisel.

Should You Supplement?

The average adult diet in the United States provides 400 to 900 milligrams of choline a day. According to Dr. Zeisel, that's enough to meet your basic needs. If you take more, there's a chance that you might get some additional benefits, but that hasn't been definitely proven.

According to Dr. Kidd, lecithin offers safe nutritional support for energy and overall well-being. Supplements with additional PS benefit memory, and those with added PC benefit liver function and digestion, he says.

Lecithin is available in tablets or granules. Granular lecithin can be added to soups, casseroles, milkshakes, and other foods.

You can also get choline in tablet form, but there's a drawback to taking it this way. It can give you a bad case of B.O. if you take it on a regular basis, because choline breaks down into a fishy-smelling compound in the small intestine. Lecithin, on the other hand, doesn't cause an odor because it is absorbed before releasing choline.

magnesium

Magnesium doesn't get the kind of celebrity endorsements that calcium does, but it should. What other nutrient can claim chocolate as one of its better sources?

A real workhorse in the body, magnesium is essential for some 325-plus biochemical reactions, more than any other nutrient. Many of those tasks are basic and indispensable.

"Its function is so broad that it touches on almost all physiological systems, all the way from energy generation inside cells to the interaction of nerve impulses and muscles in the heart," says Henry Lukaski, Ph.D., research leader for mineral nutrient functions at the U.S. Department of Agriculture Human Nutrition Research Center in Grand Forks, North Dakota.

Getting enough magnesium has been hailed as an all-around protective measure. In research discussions, this mineral has been tentatively linked with protection from heart arrhythmia (irregular heartbeat), high blood pressure, migraine headaches, and heart attacks.

Energy Everywhere

Magnesium is needed so that the body can produce energy from any food we eat—carbohydrate, protein, or fat. It works in the energy-generating powerhouses inside cells, called mitochondria. There it plays an essential role in producing the body's basic energy currency. "Magnesium is needed for a cell to make ATP, the molecules that contain the energy, and then to break these molecules down to release the energy," explains Dr. Lukaski.

That's important, because our bodies produce a large number of ongoing chemical reactions, none of which can take place without ATP. We need ATP all the time to move nutrients and other substances in and out of cells to digest food; to break down molecules and rearrange them into new molecules, such as protein or hormones; and to make muscles and nerves work. Without magnesium helping to make ATP, that energetic activity would be reduced to zero.

In fact, Dr. Lukaski found that female volunteers who consumed 150 milligrams of magnesium a day—which is less than half the Daily Value

SUPPLEMENTSNAPSHOT

▶ Magnesium

Supplement forms: Magnesium lactate, orotate, glycinate, gluconate, oxide, and hydroxide.

May help: Heart arrhythmia, migraine headaches, angina, restless legs syndrome, Raynaud's disease, asthma, binge-eating disorder, osteoporosis, and pregnancy-induced high blood pressure; also used for chronic fatigue syndrome, intermittent claudication, celiac disease, menstrual cramps, PMS, tinnitus, mitral valve prolapse, kidney stones, diabetes, insomnia, endometriosis, leg cramps, and high blood pressure.

Daily Value: 400 milligrams.

Special instructions: Take a form of magnesium, such as magnesium lactate, orotate, glycinate, or gluconate, that is easily absorbed and least likely to cause diarrhea. Magnesium oxide and hydroxide are more likely to cause diarrhea at higher dosages. Do not take at the same time as calcium, which competes with magnesium for the same absorption sites.

Who's at risk for deficiency: People with uncontrolled diabetes, who lose magnesium through their urine; alcoholics; people taking "loop" or non-potassium-sparing diuretics; people who seldom eat magnesium-rich foods; and those under severe stress.

Good food sources: Wheat germ; unmilled grains such as whole wheat and brown rice; pumpkin, sunflower, and other seeds; cocoa; chocolate; unblanched almonds and filberts; rice bran; beans; lentils; tofu; spinach; Swiss chard; halibut; and mackerel.

Cautions and possible side effects: Do not take more than 350 milligrams a day as a supplement without medical supervision. Consult your doctor before taking if you have heart disease or arrhythmia, impaired kidney function, high blood pressure, or migraine headaches or if you are taking diuretics. May cause diarrhea.

but is the amount consumed by most women age 50 and older—soon began to slow down. After only two months on a low-magnesium diet, they were asked to ride a stationary bicycle at a moderate pace. On the low-magnesium regimen, volunteers used 15 percent more oxygen and had heart rates an average of 10 beats a minute faster than when they were getting higher doses of 350 milligrams a day.

"This means that people who are low in magnesium use more energy and have a greater strain on their hearts," Dr Lukaski says. "They can't exercise as long or as hard and they get tired faster. It may even limit their ability to work or to do daily activities."

There's more besides magnesium involved in energy production, but one thing's for sure: If magnesium is in short supply, your tail will soon be dragging.

Making Muscles Work

Together with calcium, magnesium is involved in making sure that muscles work properly. "It's the ratio of calcium to magnesium that's important," explains Burton M. Altura, Ph.D., professor of physiology and medicine at the State University of New York (SUNY) Health Science Center in Brooklyn.

Magnesium is important for muscles to be able to relax, while calcium helps them contract. Too little magnesium in relation to calcium (or low levels of both) can make muscles cramp more easily and may make some muscles, like the smooth muscles that wrap around big blood vessels, stay somewhat contracted, Dr. Altura explains. Magnesium deficiency can make muscles go into spasms easily. When you're short on magnesium, the waste products of metabolism, such as lactic acid, are harder to flush out, so you may get tired, burning, sore muscles.

Supplemental magnesium often helps people with migraine headaches or high blood pressure if they're low in magnesium, Dr. Altura says. Since magnesium can also relax muscles in airways in the lungs, it sometimes helps people with asthma breathe easier, he adds. Magnesium even helps some forms of angina—spasms of the coronary arteries that can cause chest pain.

Magnesium is also needed for the body to be able to construct its basic building materials, including protein, carbohydrates, fat, and nucleic acids, a cell's genetic material. In some cases, magnesium simply provides the energy needed for the body to link together the molecules of amino acids that make up a protein or the fatty acids that make up fat and cell membranes. At other times, it helps change the shapes of molecules so that they can bind together. In the case of genetic material, magnesium molecules bind to the "backbone" of the famous double-stranded DNA helix, helping to stabilize its structure and maintain order. This is important since each cell uses DNA as the blueprint for reproducing itself or parts of itself. Body maintenance and repair depend on accurate DNA blueprints.

Healthy Heartthrobs

Certain minerals play important roles in maintaining your heart's proper rhythm. These include potassium, magnesium, sodium, chloride, and calcium. Here again, a proper ratio is important.

When magnesium levels in the heart are low, people can develop certain types of heart arrhythmias, some of them potentially very dangerous, says Carla Sueta, M.D., Ph.D., assistant professor of medicine and cardiology at the University of North Carolina at Chapel Hill School of Medicine.

One type of potential arrhythmia problem affects the upper chamber, or atrium, of the heart. Another type, called ventricular arrhythmia, involves the lower heart chambers. In studies, intravenous magnesium reduced the incidence of death from several types of ventricular arrhythmia. "In fact, intravenous therapy with magnesium is now considered standard therapy for two types of ventricular arrhythmia," Dr. Sueta says.

Too little magnesium can also induce something called refractory potassium deficiency. Unfortunately, you can't correct a refractory deficiency simply by taking more potassium. But by getting more magnesium, you may ensure that this kind of deficiency never occurs in the first place.

Heart patients—and their doctors—need to pay heed to magnesium. Studies have shown that 65 to 75 percent of all people in intensive care units and 5 to 11 percent of people in general care sections of hospitals are deficient in magnesium. Also, magnesium deficiency can be caused by the very drugs meant to help heart problems. Some types of diuretics cause the body to excrete both magnesium and potassium, as does the heart-stimulating drug digitalis.

Overreactive Rodents

Years ago, German researchers dubbed magnesium a natural tranquilizer because it seemed to soothe jangled nerves. In people who are low in magnesium, it may do exactly that.

Magnesium is essential in the regulation of central nervous system functions, explains James Penland, Ph.D., head research psychologist at the USDA research center in North Dakota. Animals—and humans—low in magnesium have more "excitable" nervous systems that make them tend to overreact to stimulation. Rats, for instance, will jump in their cages at the sound of a closing door.

The human equivalent of the jumpy rat may experience symptoms of shakiness, insomnia, irritability, and anxiety, Dr. Penland says. He's found changes in brain waves in women who get a low dose of 115 milligrams a day of magnesium. "Even when they have their eyes closed, their brain waves indicate a state of enhanced vigilance, or hyperreactivity," he explains. In other words, their brains just can't relax completely.

Certainly, if you wake up several times during the night, if you're irritable or seem jumpy during the day, or if you are experiencing tremors or shakiness and you know you're not getting much magnesium, it's worth discussing with your doctor, Dr. Penland says. Taking 200 to 300 milligrams a day as a supplement is safe for most people. If you're severely deficient, though, you may need more than that amount, or injections. In that case, you need medical supervision.

Free-Radical Chaser

The less magnesium you consume, the greater your chances of developing atherosclerosis—clogged, inflamed arteries that cause heart disease and heart attacks. A magnesium deficiency promotes the generation of free radicals, the free-roaming, unstable molecules that can harm cells, including those lining arteries. When the arteries are roughed up by these renegades, it sets the stage for cholesterol deposits, explains Dr. Altura.

Magnesium deficiency also promotes heart disease by making it easier for harmful LDL cholesterol to be oxidized and for hearts to be overloaded with calcium. Both are steps in the development of heart disease, Dr. Altura says

Today, we get less magnesium in our diets than people were getting about a century ago. Back in 1910, the average was about 450 milligrams a day of magnesium, mostly provided by unprocessed foods and especially by whole grains. Nowadays, most people get less than 300 milligrams a day. Men average 185 to 250; women average 172 to 235. "This raises a real concern that people may be predisposed to chronic latent magnesium deficiencies that could have important health risks such as migraine headaches, heart disease, or high blood pressure," Dr. Altura says.

DV Delivery

If you're otherwise healthy but have reason to believe that you've been shortchanging yourself on magnesium, you can reach the Daily Value of 400 milligrams a day fairly easily by eating magnesium-rich foods. Alternatively, you can figure out about how much you normally get in your diet and then supplement to get yourself up into the 400-milligram range, Dr. Altura says.

If you're ill, however—if you have heart arrhythmia, kidney problems, high blood pressure, or migraine headaches—you should discuss magnesium supplementation with your doctor, Dr. Altura says. You may be so low in magnesium that you need quite a bit to get you back to normal. You may need extended treatment with oral supplements, and some people require injections.

To help determine true magnesium status, Dr. Altura and his wife, Bella T. Altura, Ph.D., research professor of physiology at the SUNY health center, developed a blood test that measures ionized magnesium, the active form of magnesium in the blood. Some specialists are now able to perform the test, according to Dr. Altura. If you're concerned about a possible magnesium deficiency, ask your doctor about this test.

melatonin

Astronauts orbiting the Earth see a new sunrise every 90 minutes. While that may be an awesome spectacle, it really does a number on their internal body clocks.

The human body clock relies on the complex interplay of certain chemicals, especially hormones, and your sensory organs, especially your eyes. In any 24-hour period, there's likely to be a time when your body says, "I'm sleepy, I need rest." That's when you should head for bed.

If that cycle is interrupted, however, you're likely to lose sleep. Orbiting astronauts, bothered by the frequent sunrises, are plagued by insomnia. They average only five to six hours of shuteye for every day in space. NASA is now studying whether the hormone melatonin is "the right stuff" to help them sleep.

Melatonin is produced by the pineal gland, a little cone-shaped structure in the brain that releases the hormone into the bloodstream. Darkness stimulates the pineal gland and causes it to produce more melatonin, which is why some call it the "hormone of darkness." Light puts the brakes on production.

During a normal night, production of melatonin peaks during the darkest hours—between 2:00 and 4:00 A.M. After that, production starts to decline, and it's essentially switched off when you wake up. The longer the night, the more melatonin will be secreted.

Under the Influence

Although we all have some melatonin in our systems, the amount doesn't remain constant during our lifetimes. Between the ages of 1 and 3, we have the highest levels. As we age, we produce and secrete less. When melatonin levels get too low, we may become sleep-deprived, which might be one reason that so many people over age 65 suffer from chronic insomnia.

Melatonin is also present in some plant and animal foods, although in very small amounts. Bananas have it, but you'd have to eat 40 at one sitting to get one milligram of melatonin. Supplements are the only source of significant concentrations.

When scientists isolated this hormone of darkness, they naturally began to wonder whether it could change sleep patterns. Today, melatonin is widely available as a supplement, and while some researchers think it may have many other properties, the most widely accepted use is for sleep-related problems.

When taken in proper doses at the appropriate time of day, this hormone can indeed increase sleepiness and help you fall asleep, says Irina Zhdanova, M.D., Ph.D., principal research scientist for the brain and cognitive sciences department at the Massachusetts Institute of Technology in Cambridge. Studies have shown that people who take melatonin may fall asleep faster, are less susceptible to awakening during the night, and feel that their sleep is more restful.

Supplementing with melatonin is not like taking a sleeping pill, however. Instead, it nudges you toward sleep by promoting general relaxation.

SUPPLEMENT SNAPSHOT

▶ Melatonin

May help: Insomnia; jet lag; seasonal affective disorder; depression and chronic fatigue syndrome associated with sleep problems; and delayed sleep phase syndrome, a type of insomnia.

Special instructions: As a sleep aid, take a half-hour before bedtime.

Cautions and possible side effects: Take no more than one milligram daily. Take only at bedtime and never before driving. Do not use if you have an autoimmune disease such as rheumatoid arthritis or lupus or a personal or family history of a hormone-dependent cancer such as breast, testicular, prostate, or endometrial cancer. Consult your doctor before using if you're on a prescription medication; rarely, interactions may occur. Do not take if you are pregnant or trying to conceive, and do not give to children. May cause headaches, morning dizziness, daytime sleepiness, depression, or upset stomach.

Changing the Clocks

Whether you're traveling east from San Francisco to Boston or west from L.A. to Singapore, you're probably going to lose some sleep. You are also likely to suffer other symptoms of jet lag, such as headache, irritability, and poor concentration.

Supplementing with melatonin appears to alleviate these symptoms. It fights jet lag in two ways, says Dr. Zhdanova. First, it helps you fall asleep. Second, it can reset your body clock, either forward or back, to help you adapt to a new time zone.

When you take melatonin in the afternoon, it tends to advance the body clock. In other words, if you take it at 3:00 or 4:00 P.M., you're likely to feel ready for bed earlier than you usually would. When you take it in the early morning—say, 3:00 or 4:00 A.M.—it delays the body clock so you're willing to stay awake longer than you normally would.

Because of these effects, melatonin has been studied as a sleep aid for shift workers, including those who rotate between day and night shifts. Most of us find it hard to stay alert at night, even if we sleep during the day. Night workers have an especially tough time and seldom adapt completely because they don't get the time cues they need from daylight.

The question of whether melatonin can help shift workers is not an easy one to answer, says Dr. Zhdanova. Individuals respond differently to melatonin. Even if they time it to help them adjust to new work schedules, it may actually make some workers more groggy and less alert as they move from a day shift to a night shift, then back again.

A Fountain of Youth?

Apart from its clock-adjusting effects, some researchers say that melatonin can help you "grow younger" and restore vitality to a tired sex life. There's little evidence to support either of these claims, says Richard L. Sprott, Ph.D., executive director of the Ellison Medical Foundation, an organization that funds research on the biology of aging, in Bethesda, Maryland.

How about claims that melatonin helps you live longer? Animal studies indicate that declining levels of melatonin may be associated with accelerated aging, but that decline could be a result, not a cause.

"The idea of living as long as possible is a very tempting idea," says Dr. Zhdanova, "but the few studies done with animals were inconclusive and left too many questions unanswered."

There is some evidence that melatonin may inhibit tumor growth, at least in animals. Research on the effects of melatonin on tumor growth in humans is conflicting, but most reports do show some kind of protective action. Studies continue, with the hope that some connection may be found that will guide future research, says Dr. Zhdanova.

A Little Melatonin Goes a Long Way

To many people who are feeling sleep-deprived, melatonin promises a shortcut to less insomnia and deeper rest, but some researchers urge caution.

"I would prefer that people wait until more research has been done on melatonin before they decide to supplement, but I'm realistic. I know that people are taking this supplement, sometimes with positive results. I urge them to be very careful," says Dr. Zhdanova.

Since low doses are the most effective, take no more than one milligram daily. "Increasing the dose does not increase effectiveness," Dr. Zhdanova says.

As a sleep aid, take melatonin a half-hour before bedtime. An ill-timed or larger dose could actually hamper sleep.

Available over the counter in health food stores and drugstores in the United States, melatonin is now regulated as a medication in Canada and in some European countries.

milk thistle

Poisons enter your body whenever you smoke cigarettes, drink alcohol, work with solvents and paints, take medications to combat pain, or walk down a city street breathing the exhaust of cars and buses. Even if you live in the country, hundreds of miles from an industrial hub, you probably breathe air laced with some of the 851 million pounds of toxic chemicals that are released into the environment each year.

What keeps these poisons from overwhelming your body is your liver. The liver breaks down toxins in the bloodstream and turns them into less harmful substances that are eventually flushed from your system. Your liver is the great detoxifier, and it has the capacity to serve you well for a lifetime.

When your liver becomes damaged by toxins, however, milk thistle, a plant with a long history as a liver tonic, may be helpful. This herb has been used to treat inflammation of the liver, hepatitis, mushroom and chemical poisoning, and liver damage from alcohol abuse or long-term use of certain medications.

"Milk thistle strengthens your liver and reduces the damage from environmental irritants like pesticides," says Jennifer Brett, N.D., a naturopathic doctor at the Wilton Naturopathic Center in Stratford, Connecticut.

The Liver's Bodyguard

Milk thistle is native to the Mediterranean but now grows wild in North America, especially California and the eastern United States. Although it was used for centuries in Europe as a liver tonic, by the beginning of the twentieth century, its value was nearly forgotten.

Some years ago, German scientists began investigating the chemical properties of the milk thistle fruit and discovered a concentrated group of flavonoid compounds called silymarin. Flavonoids in general are an important group of antioxidants that devour free radicals, the free-roaming, unstable molecules that rage through the body, harm healthy cells, and accelerate aging.

Silymarin is actually a group of flavonoids that functions as an antihepatoxic, meaning that it acts directly on the liver to protect it from poisons. It mounts the defenses on two fronts. First, it binds to the membranes of liver cells and creates a tough shield so that toxins have a more difficult time penetrating the cell walls. If toxins do make it into the cells and cause damage, silymarin stimulates the liver to speed up production of beneficial enzymes and proteins as part of a healing restoration.

"Silymarin is an antioxidant that acts very specifically on liver tissue. It also increases the activity of glutathione, the body's own antioxidant," says Alison Lee, M.D., a pain-management specialist and medical director of Barefoot Doctors, an alternative medicine practice in Ann Arbor, Michigan.

More Life for the Liver

The human liver has a remarkable natural capacity to regenerate itself after being damaged, and studies of people who have liver problems show that milk thistle can actually help a damaged liver grow new cells.

"Milk thistle enhances the liver's own healing process," says Dr. Lee. "It can be used both for short-term acute liver injury, like that resulting from exposure to a virus or mushroom poisoning, and for long-term, chronic problems such as cirrhosis as well."

SUPPLEMENT SNAPSHOT

▶ Milk Thistle

Botanical name: *Silybum marianum*.

May help: Hepatitis, cirrhosis, mushroom poisoning, liver inflammation, and liver damage caused by alcohol abuse, long-term use of medications, and chemical exposure; endometriosis; and Parkinson's disease.

Special instructions: For maximum absorption, take with food.

Origin: Native to the Mediterranean.

Cautions and possible side effects: Generally regarded as safe; may cause loose stools.

Swedish doctors have successfully used milk thistle as a kind of antidote for mushroom poisoning following accidental ingestion. But that doesn't mean that you can try to self-treat with milk thistle if you may have mushroom poisoning. See a doctor immediately.

The herb is commonly prescribed in Europe for a variety of liver conditions, including cirrhosis and hepatitis. It has sometimes been used as a digestive stimulant to encourage the release of bile, a fluid produced by the liver that plays an essential role in digestion. Mainly, however, it is employed as a liver tonic.

A Tonic for Toxicity

Who should take milk thistle, and how often? Most people would benefit from a daily supplement, according to Dr. Brett. She believes that Americans are routinely exposed to many toxins and that we should use it as a preventive. "It will not do you any harm and probably a lot of good, considering how toxic our society is," she says.

Milk thistle is most often sold in capsules or tablets. So far, Dr. Lee adds, there's no evidence to suggest any problems with taking the herb over the long term, which suggests that it's safe to take regularly as a preventive. Certainly, people who are regularly exposed to environmental hazards, such as painters, anyone who works around chemicals, folks who live in areas of heavy industrial pollution, and people recovering from alcohol abuse, are good candidates for milk thistle, she says. "That doesn't mean, though, that you can take milk thistle and just drink all you want. It doesn't work that way," she warns.

Dr. Lee often prescribes milk thistle to her new acupuncture patients, people who have been taking drugs for years to control inflammation or pain from chronic conditions. Many pain-relieving drugs—even common over-the-counter medications like acetaminophen—can be damaging to the liver with long-term use, she says. Milk thistle helps detoxify her patients' livers and helps while they are being weaned from medications, she says.

"If somebody is taking a lot of medications, their liver may not be as responsive as it might be," she adds. "I wouldn't recommend milk thistle for everyone. First, I do a simple blood test to determine liver function. If the test reveals a problem, I might recommend it."

nettle

When Roman soldiers invaded the dank climate of Great Britain, they kept warm by rubbing their chilled arms and legs with nettle, a common weed found along the trails. The hairy spines covering the plant released histamines and formic acid that caused their skin to burn and itch, but the soldiers from Mediterranean climes preferred the irritation to the chill.

As far back as biblical times, people throughout Europe practiced urtication, the practice of flogging or swatting themselves with nettle. They believed that by thus injecting irritating chemicals into their skin, they could ease rheumatism and arthritis pain.

Because the histamines in nettle limit the body's response to pollen and other irritating substances, nettle was also a favored treatment for asthma and allergies. The astringent or constricting quality of the roots and leaves led to its use to stop diarrhea, dysentery, and bleeding.

Old-time herbalists favored nettle for its diuretic action and prescribed it for many urinary tract conditions. Today, several companies in Europe manufacture a nettle extract to combat urine retention caused by an enlarged prostate.

"It was used for a long time as a detoxifying agent, helping to flush the body," says Debra Gibson, N.D., a naturopathic doctor in Woodbury, Connecticut. "A lot of folks drank nettle tea in the springtime when hay fever season came on. It was a spring tonic."

A Worldwide Weed

The common or stinging nettle is a perennial plant and common weed that grows in temperate climates throughout the world. It stands two to three feet high and has dark green, serrated leaves and small, inconspicuous flowers.

Young shoots of nettle are edible when cooked. They contain about the same amounts of beta-carotene and vitamin C as spinach and other greens. Other parts of the plant are used for healing.

In North America, nettle was a popular plant medicine with mainstream physicians throughout the nineteenth century and into the twentieth. A popular medical textbook published in 1928 mentions that people used it to reduce inflammation from sprains and arthritis. Since then, scientists have learned that nettle contains about 20 different chemicals, including lectins, phenols, sterols, lignans, and histamines.

Histamines, which occur naturally in the body, are the culprits behind allergic reactions, says Stanley W. Beyrle, N.D., a naturopathic doctor at the Kansas Clinic of Traditional Medicine in Wichita. When you are exposed to allergens—substances that cause allergic reactions—your body releases histamines, which in turn cause hives, constrict bronchial vessels, and inflame the skin.

The histamines in nettle attach to histamine receptor sites in your cells and keep your body's histamines from attaching to those cells during an allergic reaction. Nettle's action is very similar to that of pharmaceutical antihistamine drugs, says Dr. Beyrle.

"What's important here is that the plant histamines have a less sensitive trigger than the body's histamines. Although they attach to the receptor sites, they are so weak that they rarely cause any allergic reaction in the person," he says.

SUPPLEMENT SNAPSHOT

▶ Nettle

Botanical: *Urtica dioica*; also known as stinging nettle.

May help: Allergies, rhinitis, urinary problems, asthma, diarrhea, dysentery, hemorrhage, gout, hair loss, and prostate problems.

Special instructions: For maximum absorption, take with food.

Origin: Found in temperate zones throughout the world; cultivated in Europe.

Cautions and possible side effects: Rarely, may aggravate allergy symptoms; if you have allergies, take only one dose a day for the first few days. May cause stomach pain.

Allergic reactions to nettle itself are rare but not unheard of. Although it is a very benign herb, touching the plant may cause skin irritation similar to an allergic reaction, notes Dr. Gibson.

"People with extreme mold sensitivity should be cautious when using nettle teas, since the leaves may harbor molds that would be ingested," she says. "This is less likely to be a problem with capsules containing the freeze-dried herb or with tinctures." If you have allergies, take only one dose a day for the first few days to avoid aggravating symptoms.

Nettle may help people who have a tendency toward rhinitis, an inflammation of the mucous membranes in the nose that can be brought on by colds, dust, and allergies. Initially, nettle can prevent rhinitis by stifling allergic reactions, but its strong anti-inflammatory properties make it a kind of balm for red, swollen tissues.

In a study of 69 people in Portland, Oregon, researchers found that a freeze-dried extract of the herb was better than a similar but inactive substance (a placebo) at improving the symptoms associated with rhinitis. Some chemicals in the plant also seem to inhibit a destructive enzyme that's released into tissues during the inflammation.

Turning On the Flow

It's only been within the last 20 years—and mainly in Europe—that nettle root has been employed in the treatment of benign prostatic hyperplasia (BPH). BPH is a noncancerous enlargement of the prostate gland that constricts the urethra, the tube that leads from the bladder to the penis. Some men with this condition have problems with frequent urination, but they may also have trouble urinating when they have a strong urge. This can be particularly disruptive at night, when the urge to go is like a frustrating alarm clock.

No one is really certain how nettle helps. It's thought that the herb may limit the amount of testosterone, the male sex hormone, circulating in the blood, or it may inhibit an enzyme, aromatase, that leads to the formation of testosterone. BPH is caused mainly by an overabundance of testosterone, says Dr. Gibson.

Whatever the mechanism, German health authorities have concluded that nettle root extract is an effective treatment for urinary problems caused by BPH, but only when the prostate is slightly to moderately enlarged.

A French study found that men who had to get up several times a night to urinate found significant relief after taking an extract of nettle. Every eight hours, researchers gave a dilute extract of nettle root to 67 patients over 60 years of age. The men with the mildest problems found significant relief in just three to six weeks.

The results were less encouraging for men with more severe cases, as it took a few more weeks before any effect was noticed. Nevertheless, many of the subjects had fewer nighttime awakenings to urinate. The herb did not shrink the prostate but apparently reduced inflammation and swelling.

Commission E, a team of physicians, toxicologists, pharmacologists, and other specialists established by the German government to study herbal medicines, determined that nettle is also a good supportive therapy for inflammatory diseases of the lower urinary tract. All of these scientific conclusions fit with the traditional use of nettle as a diuretic, notes Dr. Beyrle. "This is really one of the great herbs for increasing the secretion of urine," he says. "I've also used it to treat chronic inflammation of the bladder."

Freeze-Dried Is Best

Nettle comes as a tincture, capsules, and dried root, from which you can brew a tea. "To get the full benefit of nettle, you really need a freeze-dried extract," says Dr. Beyrle. The freeze-dried preparation is made from nettle that is processed soon after harvesting, he says. Slow drying and processing remove many of the active ingredients.

niacin

Try to survive on a corn-based diet, and you run the risk of getting pellagra, a disease caused by niacin deficiency.

Corn lacks niacin. Years ago, people in the South who depended on corn grits as a diet staple suffered from this body-wide disease that leads to dermatitis, diarrhea, and depression. It can even lead to death, if deprivation continues long enough.

Today, nearly everyone gets sufficient niacin. Meat, poultry, and fish are rich in this B vitamin, and it's also added to flour and other cereal products to help ensure that our needs are met. Pellagra, for the most part, is a thing of the past.

Like most of the other B vitamins, niacin assists enzymes, the catalysts that help spark chemical reactions. An all-around booster shot for enzymes, it helps many of them do their jobs properly.

Niacin is also a major player in the process of breaking down food into a form of energy that the cells in our bodies can either use or store for future use. Niacin-dependent enzymes help "package" this energy and then release it in an orderly fashion as it's needed.

The niacin-dependent enzymes also play an important role in the body's handling of fat and cholesterol and the production of many biochemicals, including some hormones.

Confusingly, niacin has several different chemical structures, which also have different names. One of the forms prescribed by doctors is nicotinic acid. A second form is called niacinamide—also known as nicotinamide. And there's yet a third form—different from the other two—called inositol hexaniacinate.

Some forms are recommended for certain conditions but not for others. Niacinamide, for instance, is used to treat osteoarthritis and rheumatoid arthritis. Other forms may be selectively prescribed in large doses to treat high cholesterol and Raynaud's disease, a circulatory problem that causes cold hands and feet.

Clobbering Cholesterol

Large doses of nicotinic acid and inositol hexaniacinate do a good job of lowering cholesterol, possibly by affecting liver function.

Niacin also raises "good" HDL cholesterol. In fact, it does this better than any drug on the market. Several studies also show that regular doses of niacin can reduce the risk of death from heart disease. It is thus considered a good treatment choice when someone needs more than diet to control cholesterol, says Martin Milner, N.D., a naturopathic doctor who teaches at the National College of Naturopathic Medicine in Portland and Bastyr University in Bothell, Washington.

This is one treatment, however, for which knowledgeable medical su-

SUPPLEMENT SNAPSHOT

▶Niacin

Supplement forms: Nicotinic acid, niacinamide (nicotinamide), and inositol hexaniacinate; also known as vitamin B_3.

May help: Niacin and inositol hexaniacinate may help high cholesterol and Raynaud's disease; Niacinamide may help osteoarthritis, rheumatoid arthritis, and diabetes.

Daily Value: 20 milligrams.

Special instructions: Take with food to minimize side effects whenever you're taking high doses.

Who's at risk for deficiency: Alcoholics and people taking isoniazid (Laniazid) for long periods of time.

Good food sources: Meat, milk, eggs, fish, poultry, peanuts, and enriched breads and cereals. Coffee and tea also contain appreciable amounts.

Cautions and possible side effects: Do not take more than 35 milligrams a day of any form without medical supervision; do not take more than 35 milligrams daily if you have a history of gout, liver damage, peptic ulcers, gallbladder disease, or heart rhythm disturbances. Taking niacin in addition to certain cholesterol-lowering drugs ("statin" drugs) increases risk of liver damage. High doses can cause drops in blood pressure and can raise blood sugar in people with diabetes. May cause flushing and allergic reactions. Sustained release niacin can be hepatotoxic, so do not use if you have liver disease.

pervision is a top priority. In the large doses needed to lower cholesterol—1,500 to 3,000 milligrams a day—niacin can cause liver problems. In fact, problems can start with doses as low as 500 milligrams, although some effects might not show up for years.

Anyone who is taking high doses must have regular blood tests to measure three essential liver enzymes, says Dr. Milner. You may find timed-release forms of niacin on your drugstore shelf, but immediate-release niacin is less likely to cause liver damage.

Dr. Milner uses inositol hexaniacinate (Niacinol) because studies show that it is also less likely than the timed-release form to cause liver damage. There's also less chance of this form causing niacin flush, the characteristic reddening of the skin and itching that some people experience after taking niacin. Even though it's readily available from naturopathic doctors and at some health food stores, however, it's not something that you should try without regular monitoring, Dr. Milner says.

With inositol hexaniacinate, the doctor might start you on a dose of 1,500 milligrams. If you take regular niacin, your doctor will begin with a much lower dose and increase it gradually over a period of weeks to help minimize flushing, says Dr. Milner.

Helping Vessels and Joints

Niacin can help people with Raynaud's disease for reasons that are related to the way it causes blood vessels to expand. For someone with Raynaud's, the blood vessels in the hands essentially clamp down, cutting off a warming blood supply. When it's severe, the hands literally turn white with cold.

Because niacin helps blood vessels expand, it seems to be just what the doctor ordered for Raynaud's. Some doctors, usually naturopaths, do prescribe it for this condition. "Niacin's ability to dilate the superficial blood vessels of the skin, mostly around the chest and face but also in the hands, helps to stop bouts of Raynaud's," Dr. Milner says.

The rationale for using niacinamide for arthritis is based mostly on the work of William Kaufman, M.D., Ph.D., a doctor who pioneered nutritional therapy for people with the joint inflammation caused by this disease. Some naturopathic doctors recommend up to 500 milligrams twice a day. "This form acts differently in the body than niacin does," Dr. Milner says. "It's thought to improve certain functions in the cells. It does seem to be safe at these amounts, though."

pantothenic acid

Pantos is a Greek word that means "everywhere"—an appropriate prefix for the name of a vitamin that's found in most foods.

It's fortunate that this B vitamin is so plentiful, because it's very important to our bodies. "It is involved in many different metabolic pathways, including the conversion of food to energy, the synthesis of important hormones, and the body's utilization of body fat and cholesterol," says Won O. Song, R.D., Ph.D., professor of nutrition at Michigan State University in East Lansing.

This vitamin helps to convert carbohydrates and fats to energy and to break down and reassemble fats into new forms, some of which are used to make important hormones. It acts as a matchmaker between proteins and fatty acids, combining them into molecules called lipoproteins, which in turn make up the membranes that enclose our cells.

Pantothenic acid also plays an important role in making hemogloblin, the protein found in red blood cells that transports oxygen throughout our bodies. It helps our bodies detoxify a virtual Love Canal's–worth of nasty chemicals, and, at high doses, it could prove useful for chronic diseases such as rheumatoid arthritis.

Good—And Good for You

Pantothenic acid is an essential component of a substance called coenzyme A (coA). Enzymes are like spark plugs, helping to jump-start the chemical reactions that go on continuously in our bodies and allowing us to turn food into energy and produce the tissues that hold us together.

CoA plays an extremely broad role, especially in the production of energy. It helps to transport blood sugar, fatty acids, and even protein as these compounds are combined or converted to different forms. Our bodies also use it to detoxify many of the harmful manmade compounds found in herbicides, insecticides, and drugs, says Dr. Song.

Apart from its role in CoA production, pantothenic acid has some benefits on its own. Research suggests that it and pantethine, a form of the vitamin, may be therapeutic for some diseases.

Pantethine, in doses of 900 milligrams a day, has been shown in studies to significantly reduce cholesterol and triglycerides. This is important because high levels of either can lead to atherosclerosis (hardening of the arteries) and blockages in the blood vessels. Pantethine apparently inhibits the body's production of cholesterol while accelerating the use of fat as an energy source. Plain old pantothenic acid has no such effect, Dr. Song says.

Also in studies, pantothenic acid in the form of calcium pantothenate (50 to 2,000 milligrams a day) has been used to reduce the stiffness and pain of rheumatoid arthritis.

Acidic Action

Pantothenic acid is sometimes considered an anti-stress vitamin by doctors of alternative medicine because of its important role in the function of the adrenal glands, which produce hormones that help our bodies respond to stress. In studies in which people were made deficient in pantothenic acid by feeding them something that interfered with its use in the

SUPPLEMENT SNAPSHOT

▶ Pantothenic Acid

Supplement forms: Calcium pantothenate and pantethine; also known as vitamin B_5.

May help: Stress, rheumatoid arthritis, osteoarthritis, menopausal discomforts, and high cholesterol and triglycerides.

Daily Value: 10 milligrams.

Who's at risk for deficiency: Deficiency is thought to be rare, but people with serious drinking problems, older people on restricted diets, and people taking cholesterol-lowering drugs may be at risk.

Good food sources: Meat, fish, poultry, unprocessed whole grains, fortified cereals, legumes, peanuts, mushrooms, soy flour, and split peas.

Cautions and possible side effects: Generally regarded as safe.

body, symptoms of listlessness and fatigue developed after about nine weeks.

Deficiencies have been known to produce other problems as well. Possible symptoms include a burning sensation in the feet, depression, fatigue, insomnia, vomiting, and muscle cramping or weakness. Since pantothenic acid is so widely available in foods, such deficiencies are seldom seen, but some studies indicate that some people in the United States aren't getting enough. The Daily Value is 10 milligrams, and studies have shown that the average intake of most Americans is 5 to 10 milligrams a day.

Since up to 50 percent of the pantothenic acid in foods is lost in processing or cooking, the best sources are unprocessed whole grains, fortified cereals, and supplements. When sold as a supplement, pantothenic acid is sometimes labeled as vitamin B_5. Other forms include calcium pantothenate and pantethine.

pau d'arco

If you're a woodworker, you may be familiar with lapacho, a dense, extremely hard tropical wood. It makes beautiful, fine-grained furniture, but by woodworking standards, it's a challenge.

Lapacho resists sawing and bending. To put a nail in it, you have to pre-bore a hole. It doesn't take paint well and is impermeable to most wood preservatives. In the wild, lapacho is practically indestructible, yielding to neither termites nor decay.

The tree's resilience in the midst of the damp South American rain forest may have been what first attracted the attention of natives to its medicinal properties. Brazilian Indians used its inner bark to treat colitis, dysentery, snakebite, wounds, sore throats, ulcers, cancer, and a number of other ailments.

Pau d'arco, the phytomedicine made from the bark, is used today by herbalists to treat bacterial, fungal, viral, and parasitic infections. It's a common herb in health food stores and drugstores that carry herbal supplements.

Smothering the Bugs

You may hear the tree referred to interchangeably as pau d'arco and lapacho. In South America, the common name is trumpet tree. There are some 100 species native to tropical America.

The tree, which can grow 125 feet tall, has been well-studied by plant scientists because of its value as a hardwood. The wood is believed to contain between 2 and 7 percent of a compound called lapachol, which is considered by herbalists to be the most active ingredient. On microorganisms, lapachol acts as a respiratory poison, interfering with their oxygen and energy production.

When researchers purified an extract of the herb in an attempt to increase the amount of lapachol, however, the chemical was less effective.

This led them to believe that other ingredients, such as beta-lapachone and quercetin, were also active medicinally. One theory holds that beta-lapachone inhibits certain enzymes that viruses require to spread and grow. If that's the case, having more beta-lapachone in our bodies would be an effective way to block viruses, says Debra Gibson, N.D., a naturopathic doctor in Woodbury, Connecticut.

Fungus Fighter

Whatever its active ingredients, pau d'arco poses a death threat to a type of fungus called *Candida albicans*. Candida is always present to a small degree in our bodies, but it can reproduce uncontrollably under some circumstances. If your immune system is weak, you have diabetes, or you are pregnant, candida is more likely to take every opportunity to spread. You're also more open to candida if you are taking antibiotics or anti-inflammatory drugs.

"When you take antibiotics, you kill many of the bacteria in your body, including the good bacteria," says Dr. Gibson. "That leaves an opening for *Candida albicans*. It's an opportunistic organism. When there's no competition, it will grow."

Usually the fungus occurs on the skin or in the mouth, respiratory tract, or vagina. Many women know candida simply as a yeast infection.

Many people find relief by drinking a tea made with pau d'arco bark, says Kathleen Head, N.D., a naturopathic doctor in Sandpoint, Idaho, and senior editor of *Alternative Medicine Review*. A supplement will work as

SUPPLEMENT SNAPSHOT

▶ Pau d'Arco

Botanical name: *Tabebuia* species; also known as lapacho.

May help: Fungal infections, including candidiasis; viral, bacterial, and parasitic infections; and cancer.

Origin: Native to the West Indies and Central and South America; there are some 100 known species.

Cautions and possible side effects: Generally regarded as safe.

well, she adds. "If you're a woman who has recurring yeast infections, this would be a very good herb to try," she says.

Shrinking Tumors?

If you read up on pau d'arco, you're likely to come across references to its cancer-fighting properties. Although it's true that lapachol was studied by the National Cancer Institute and found to reduce tumors in rats, there's no evidence that it's effective against cancer in humans.

Some clinical trials used the compound lapachol on human cancers, but the trials were stopped after side effects, which included nausea, vomiting, anemia, and bleeding, were found to be too severe. Still, there are anecdotal reports of cancer patients who have had positive results after taking the herb, which doesn't cause the side effects associated with the isolated compound lapachol. Some herbalists and naturopaths still use pau d'arco as one of their cancer-fighting phytomedicines.

It's in the Bark

The active ingredients in pau d'arco seem to be most present in the bark, the part traditionally used by the South American Indians.

Pau d'arco is available as a tincture, in capsules, and as dried bark, from which you can make a tea. You can find lapachol in capsules and tincture. "It's really quite safe. It would be pretty hard to do yourself harm with it," Dr. Gibson says.

Although some animal studies of long-term, high-dose consumption of lapachol have shown that it may cause anemia—a reduction of red blood cells that can lead to extreme fatigue and other symptoms—Dr. Gibson says that anemia is very unlikely if you take typical medicinal doses.

phytonutrients

Despite the complicated sound of this word, there's no mystery to it. *Phyto-* simply means "plant," and phytonutrient supplements contain nutrients derived from plants.

Each of those nutrients is thought to have some sort of health benefit. Some can help reduce inflammation and aid digestion. Others may help protect your arteries from plaque, the sticky stuff that can clog up blood vessels and raise your risk of heart attack or stroke. Still others can help reduce cell damage.

Once isolated from the plant material, phytonutrients can be recombined in various ways. A phytonutrient such as isoflavone, for instance, may be isolated and concentrated from soybeans, then put into a pill. Add some lycopene from tomatoes, some beta-carotene from carrots, and a few anthocyanins from red cabbage, and you have a sort of vegetable soup in a pill that may, at least in theory, give you many of the health benefits of a real vegetable soup.

A Surfeit of Nutrients

Sometimes, there are so many nutrients included in a supplement that the soup is almost a stew. One well-known vitamin manufacturer, for example, makes a supplement called the MaxiLife Phytonutrient Protector. The greenish yellow, grassy-smelling capsules contain beta- and alpha-carotene, lutein, zeaxanthin, lycopene, citrus bioflavonoids, quercetin, bilberry extract, pine bark extract, red cabbage extract, red wine concentrate, grape skin extract, elderberry extract, green tea extract, soy isoflavone concentrate, citrus terpene extract, broccoli extract, garlic, rosemary extract, and turmeric extract.

Many of these food components have some potential value, at least when they are consumed as part of your diet. Rosemary, for instance, is a strong antioxidant that helps to protect cells from the kind of speeded-up aging and cell damage that can be caused by free-roaming, unstable molecules called free radicals. In fact, it works so well that rosemary oil extract is used as a food preservative.

Another phytonutrient source, turmeric, is a yellow spice that's often used in Indian cooking. It can help reduce inflammation and aid digestion.

But what if you are getting only a pill-size amount of the nutrient in a pill? "It is possible to isolate and then concentrate certain components from foods—such as isoflavones from soybeans—and come up with a pill that contains as many isoflavones as a serving of tofu," says Holly McCord, R.D., *Prevention* magazine's nutrition editor.

What the Labels Leave Out

It's hard to tell just by looking at the label of a supplement whether you're getting a substantial amount of a phytonutrient or just a smidgen. "Right now, it is very difficult to evaluate such products," says Ronald Prior, Ph.D., a research scientist at the Jean Mayer USDA Human Nutrition Research Center on Aging at Tufts University in Boston.

Since there's no standardization of such products, the only thing you can count on when shopping for phytonutrient supplements is a lot of in-

SUPPLEMENTSNAPSHOT

▶Phytonutrients

Individual names: Isoflavone, lycopene, carotenes, anthocyanins, lutein, and zeaxanthin, among others.

May help: Cancer, heart disease, stroke, restless legs syndrome, and macular degeneration.

Special instructions: Take with food.

Good food sources: Strawberries, blueberries, Concord grape juice, red wine, tea, oranges, grapefruit, lemons, limes, red onions, red cabbage, broccoli, carrots, kale, pumpkin, herbs, spices, garlic, and tomatoes.

Cautions and possible side effects: Don't take more than the recommended dosage. Never consider supplements as a substitute for food; the best variety and quantities of phytonutrients are found in a diet that's rich in fruits and vegetables.

consistency. Even though, based on their labels, products seem similar, the potency of each product is different.

"You can't knock all these products," concludes Dr. Prior. "Some are good and some not so good. Right now, though, there's no way for the consumer to really tell which ones are good just from reading the labels."

One product's daily dose offers 100 milligrams of soy isoflavone concentrate, which can help reduce the risk of breast and ovarian cancer. That's about the amount found in 1½ cups of tofu. It also has 25,000 international units of beta-carotene, which helps resist cell damage and reduces the risk of some kinds of cancer. You'd get only half that much in a nine-inch carrot. With the supplement providing an additional 100 milligrams of citrus bioflavonoid complex—another cell-protecting cancer fighter—you'll get about the same amount that you'd find in one or two Valencia oranges.

That same supplement product, however, contains only 5 milligrams of lycopene, the red pigment in tomatoes that's linked with a reduction in prostate cancer. By comparison, ½ cup of tomato sauce has 22 milligrams.

Even paying top dollar doesn't assure quality, Dr. Prior has found. "Some of the better products that we have evaluated are also the cheapest," he says.

Picking the Phytos

How can you make the best selection from the variety of phytonutrient products on the market?

You might think that the more, the better, but unfortunately, the quantity of phytonutrients doesn't determine the quality of the supplement. Three sources of flavonoids listed on a label, for instance, might seem impressive. But, notes Dr. Prior, that number is small compared to approximately 4,000 different flavonoids in all of the different fruits and vegetables.

The best policy is to select a major store brand or a product from a major manufacturer, who has more to lose if it's revealed that a product doesn't deliver what it promises, McCord suggests.

Avoid products that simply say "broccoli" or "parsley" in their list of ingredients. It means that you are getting only a costly, microscopic, freeze-dried serving of that vegetable. Instead, look for products whose labels say that they contain standardized extracts of a phytonutrient. It's no guarantee, but it at least suggests some initial quality control, Dr. Prior says.

Also, look for a mixture of those phytonutrients with the strongest evidence of health benefits. These include mixed carotenoids (just beta-carotene is not enough) including lycopene, suggests Andrew Weil, M.D., clinical professor of internal medicine and director of the program in integrative medicine at the University of Arizona College of Medicine in Tucson, and author of *Eight Weeks to Optimum Health*. Or look for a supplement that includes substantial amounts of a particular phytonutrient you want, he says.

If you're concerned about prostate cancer, for instance, look for lycopene. If you're worried about macular degeneration, a common cause of deteriorating vision in older people, look for capsules that contain lutein and zeaxanthin, the two phytonutrients that, in dietary studies, seem to be most strongly linked with reduced risk of this condition.

Whatever phytonutrients you take, it's important to keep in mind that they are not substitutes for real fruits and vegetables, says McCord. "I used to think it was just a philosophical thing, but there is more and more evidence that there does seem to be something beneficial about getting nutrients in the whole food package as opposed to just taking supplements." You still need to consume the natural sources of these health-conferring compounds.

potassium

If you have a family history of stroke or have had a stroke yourself, if you have high blood pressure or need to prevent it, and especially if you take diuretics to control high blood pressure, you'll want to learn all you can about potassium. It could save your life.

Potassium is one of those essential nutrients that's found pretty much everywhere in your body. It's especially concentrated inside cells. There, it helps maintain the proper balance of fluid and other electrolytes such as sodium and chloride, which allow a cell to act like a tiny battery with its own electrical charge. The ability to generate an electrical charge is what lets cells do their work—if they're in muscles, to contract and relax, if they're in nerves, to fire off signals, and if they're in glands, to secrete hormones.

The electrical charge also lets cells move things in and out through their membranes, activate enzymes involved in chemical reactions, and maintain proper pH (acid-base balance) within the cell walls. "Potassium plays a very basic and vital role in practically all aspects of cell activity," says Louis Tobian, M.D., professor of medicine at the University of Minnesota Medical School in Minneapolis.

Potassium does a balancing act with sodium, which is one reason that it's so vital in maintaining proper blood pressure, Dr. Tobian explains. It works with sodium but also helps to keep it in check. During nerve transmission and muscle contraction, potassium and sodium briefly trade places across the cell membrane. Then they swap again, returning to their original positions ready for action.

Proper Pressure

There's growing evidence that the more potassium you get in your diet, the less likely you are to develop high blood pressure. One reason for this probably has to do with potassium's interaction with sodium, says David B. Young, Ph.D., professor of physiology and biophysics at the University of Mississippi Medical Center in Jackson. "The more potassium you get in your diet, the greater your ability to excrete sodium in your urine," he says.

Think of sodium as a water magnet. "When you excrete sodium, you also excrete water," says Dr. Young. "Excreting water reduces your blood volume, which in turn reduces your blood pressure. Thus, potassium achieves the same goal as a diuretic."

Potassium also inhibits the release of a hormone called renin from the kidneys. Renin activates another hormone, called angiotensin, which throws the switch on a kind of internal suction pump. When angiotensin is activated, your blood vessels constrict and your kidneys start to retain sodium. Both of these actions bump up blood pressure. "Having low renin levels is good in terms of lowering blood pressure," Dr. Young says.

Some popular blood pressure medications such as captopril (Capoten)

SUPPLEMENT SNAPSHOT

▶ Potassium

May help: High blood pressure, stroke, leg cramps, and heart arrhythmia.

Daily Value: 3,500 milligrams.

Who's at risk for deficiency: People taking non-potassium-sparing diuretics such as furosemide (Lasix), digitalis, or steroids; those who don't eat fruits or vegetables, are heavy drinkers, have prolonged vomiting or diarrhea, overuse laxatives, or have eating disorders.

Good food sources: Baked potatoes, spinach (raw, microwaved, or steamed for highest potassium content), dried apricots, dried prunes, cantaloupes, honeydew melons, Adzuki beans, avocados, watermelon, acorn squash, and bananas.

Cautions and possible side effects: Appears to be safe at any amount in foods, even up to 11,000 milligrams a day, but do not get more than 5,000 milligrams a day from food and supplements without medical supervision. Large doses of supplements are available only by prescription; do not take without medical supervision. Excessive potassium can upset the balance of other minerals in the body and cause potentially fatal heart and kidney problems.

and enalapril maleate (Vasotec) work along similar lines by interfering directly with angiotensin. "Possibly, you could use potassium to get some of the same effects that these drugs provide," Dr. Young says. In fact, that's the approach that some doctors take.

Independent of its effect on blood pressure, high potassium intake also seems to have a protective effect on the kidneys, Dr. Young says. In animal studies, a high-potassium diet has been shown to help prevent thickening of the small arteries that feed blood to this pair of vital, blood-cleaning, urine-producing organs. Potassium also offers promise as a kidney-guarding mineral.

Keeping the Beat

A normal heartbeat may seem simple, but it's a highly coordinated event, directed by the sequential firing of nerves that signal each chamber of the heart. When all goes well, the lower chambers and the upper chambers work in sequence, pumping blood to the lungs and the rest of the body.

When things go awry, the nerve signals may be delayed, or the nerves may fire more often than necessary. The chambers may not pump in proper sequence. The end result is that the heart pumps blood less efficiently. In fact, instead of pumping, it may go into a kind of quivery state, or arrhythmia, called fibrillation, which can be fatal if it's not quickly corrected.

You need potassium for the muscles of the heart to stay strong, Dr. Young says. Even moderate potassium depletion weakens the heart muscle. Most people whose hearts are affected by low potassium already have some sort of heart damage, such as an enlarged heart or damage to the heart muscle from a heart attack. Then, if their potassium levels decrease, their risk for arrhythmia rises. That's why most heart doctors monitor their patients' blood levels of potassium.

Stop a Stroke

Because they can maintain low blood pressure and help your heart beat normally (which reduces your chances of developing blood clots), a potassium-rich diet and possibly even supplements have the potential to reduce your chance of having a stroke. In a study from the Harvard School of Public Health, doctors analyzed data from food questionnaires completed by nearly 44,000 healthy men ages 45 to 75. The conclusions of the study were based on two groups. Men in the high-potassium group consumed nine servings of fruits and vegetables a day. Men with diets that were lower in potassium ate only four servings of fruits and vegetables a day.

During the eight years of follow-up, doctors found that men in the first group had a 38 percent lower risk of stroke than men in the low-potassium group. Remarkably, the greatest benefit was seen among men who had a history of high blood pressure and were taking potassium supplements along with diuretics. Their risk was slashed by a whopping 64 percent.

Even if you can't seem to get your blood pressure down all that much, potassium still offers protection, Dr. Young says. In the arteries, for instance, it helps stop the buildup of cholesterol-laden plaque. "We believe it does this by interfering somehow with the action of certain immune cells, called macrophages, that attack LDL in the blood vessel wall," Dr. Young says.

Potassium also decreases the sensitivity of platelets—the parts of the blood that clot—to things that activate them and make them sticky. It also prevents the overgrowth of smooth muscle cells in blood vessels. This is important because thickened and stiffened blood vessels are more prone to blockage. "In several types of animals, we know that if we give extra potassium, we can prevent lesions in the arteries, and we can prevent blockages that occur after arteries have been reopened with a procedure such as balloon angioplasty," Dr. Young says.

Potato Chips versus Oranges

If you were to have a severe case of potassium deficiency, you might experience symptoms of muscle weakness, confusion, and heart irregularities. Most of us will never have that problem, however, because our bodies carefully regulate potassium levels.

"People don't develop severe potassium deficiencies unless they have some sort of endocrine or kidney problem, and then they are pretty sick for a number of reasons," Dr. Young says. While some diuretic drugs can seriously deplete the body of potassium, doctors monitor blood levels of potassium in people taking diuretics and supply extra potassium if necessary.

It's likely that a fair number of people in the United States are on the same kind of low-potassium, high-sodium diet that can cause high blood pressure and heart disease in animals, Dr. Tobian says. Many people just don't get their share of potassium-rich fruits and vegetables, and because of safety concerns, potassium isn't found in adequate amounts in multi-vitamin/mineral supplements.

While potassium from foods has not been associated with any ill effects, the same can't be said for potassium supplements. "You can kill yourself if you take too much potassium," Dr. Tobian says.

Prescription supplements do offer more potassium, but amounts need to be carefully monitored with blood tests, Dr. Tobian says. People might need prescription potassium supplements if they are taking diuretics that deplete potassium. For his patients with high blood pressure, those who have had strokes, or those who have family histories of stroke, Dr. Tobian combines a potassium-rich diet with supplements if necessary.

riboflavin

If you take a multivitamin that contains riboflavin, you may have noticed that your urine takes on a yellow-green glow soon after you pop the supplement. Whenever an excess of this B vitamin is excreted, you're likely to detect that mysterious glow.

Riboflavin does more than produce psychedelic urine, however. It is a key player in the body's production of energy from fat, carbohydrates, and protein. It also helps our bodies produce glutathione, which acts as an antioxidant by protecting us from the cellular damage that can lead to cancer and heart disease.

Riboflavin is also needed to help several other B vitamins go about their work. It changes vitamin B_6 into a form that the body can use, and it helps change the amino acid tryptophan into niacin, another essential B vitamin. "Even though we often focus on riboflavin's role in energy metabolism, it plays several other important roles throughout the body," says Donald McCormick, Ph.D., chairman of the department of biochemistry at Emory University in Atlanta.

Energy Relay

Like many of the other B vitamins, riboflavin helps us generate energy. Inside the mitochondria, a cell's tiny powerhouse, riboflavin acts as a kind of shuttle bus. It helps to move electrons derived from the foods we eat along a pathway called the electron transport chain. As the electrons are passed along, they release energy.

The energy is used to make a molecule called ATP that acts as the cell's basic energy currency. It is used extensively throughout our bodies any time energy is needed—to move muscles, make protein, and digest food. When it's in short supply, all body functions slow down, and we feel less energetic.

In addition, riboflavin seems to have the power to control migraines. While it's unlikely to rival aspirin as a headache stopper, researchers have noted that people with an inherited disorder that includes migraine headaches showed improvement with the supplement. "These people have fewer, less severe headaches when they get additional riboflavin," says Marc Lenaerts, M.D., a neurologist at the University of Oklahoma Health Sciences Center in Oklahoma City.

Given the results of these studies, "we decided to study the effects of additional riboflavin in people with 'normal' migraines," Dr. Lenaerts says. Their first study with migraine sufferers showed a 68 percent reduction in headache symptoms among people who took riboflavin. Another study four years later included a second group that was given an inactive substance (a placebo) instead of riboflavin; it was more carefully controlled to account for a possible placebo effect. It showed 37 percent fewer migraines, plus less nausea and vomiting, in people who took 400 milligrams of riboflavin a day as one daily dose.

"This improvement is similar to what can be achieved using conventional preventive migraine drugs," Dr. Lenaerts says. He's hoping to do

SUPPLEMENT SNAPSHOT

▶ Riboflavin

Supplement form: Riboflavin-5-phosphate; also known as vitamin B_2.

May help: Migraine headaches, cataracts, and sickle-cell disease.

Daily Value: 1.7 milligrams.

Special instructions: Since riboflavin is destroyed by light, buy milk in cardboard containers. A translucent plastic jug of milk sitting in a lighted dairy case for just one day can lose up to 70 percent of its riboflavin.

Who's at risk for deficiency: The elderly, who tend to eat fewer riboflavin-containing foods, people who are exercising and dieting; people who don't drink milk; alcoholics; those who are undergoing dialysis or taking diuretics, antibiotics, or barbiturates; and people with intestinal problems that interfere with absorption.

Good food sources: Eggs, lean meat, milk, broccoli, and enriched breads and cereals.

Cautions and possible side effects: May cause photosensitivity at high dosages (more than a few milligrams a day).

more studies to confirm this benefit of riboflavin for migraine sufferers and to determine if a lower dose might be just as helpful.

Free Radical Rounder-Upper

Riboflavin also helps our bodies make glutathione, a free radical scavenger that's produced by cells. Some people simply can't produce glutathione because of an inherited abnormality, and they have a marked increase in cell damage. Red blood cells break down more easily, while white blood cells and nerves are also affected. With more riboflavin to support the production of glutathione, it seems reasonable to assume that people would experience less cellular damage.

Animal research has led some scientists to believe that people who are deficient in riboflavin are more likely to develop cataracts, because glutathione helps to protect the eyes from damage by sunlight.

In one study on animal tissue, researchers found that riboflavin can help protect tissues from damage from oxygen that occurs when blood flow stops, then starts again. That stop-start pattern is exactly what develops when someone has a heart attack or stroke.

People with sickle-cell disease, in which misshapen cells occasionally clog blood vessels, may also benefit from additional riboflavin. In one study, people with sickle cell disease who were given five milligrams of supplemental riboflavin twice a day for eight weeks showed significant improvements in their health profiles.

Who Needs More?

The Daily Value for riboflavin is 1.7 milligrams, and most people get all that and more from the foods they eat, Dr. McCormick says.

The majority of people who seem to benefit from extra riboflavin, such as those with migraine headaches, may be relatively riboflavin-deficient because of the way their cells work, not because their food sources are letting them down, says Dr. Lenaerts.

Some people don't get enough riboflavin and other B vitamins simply because they don't eat well. These include alcoholics, elderly people who don't eat enough calories, and people who have sworn off dairy products, eggs, or meat. The lack of dairy foods is particularly telling, since most people get about half of their daily riboflavin from milk and milk products.

Vegans (strict vegetarians) can obtain ample riboflavin in their diets, especially if they include dark green vegetables. They can also get additional riboflavin from nutritional yeast, which is another good source.

People with intestinal problems that interfere with absorption and people undergoing dialysis may show symptoms of riboflavin deficiency.

Long-term use of some antibiotics can increase riboflavin excretion, and a class of psychiatric drugs called phenothiazines, which includes Thorazine, can interfere with the body's ability to use riboflavin, Dr. McCormick says. People who are taking these drugs may need supplementation.

Classic deficiency symptoms include cracks and redness at the corners of the mouth; a painful, smooth, purplish-red tongue; inflamed eyelids and sensitivity to light; and an unsightly skin rash called seborrheic dermatitis.

Shortages of other B vitamins can also cause these symptoms, and riboflavin deficiency can cause shortages of other B vitamins, notably B_6. If you suspect that you have a riboflavin deficiency, it's best to make sure that you're getting enough of all the B vitamins, Dr. McCormick says. If you do have a deficiency, your doctor may advise you to take supplements, he adds.

You need to be careful not to overdo it, however, since taking too much has the potential to cause photosensitivity. "If your body is saturated with riboflavin and you're sitting out in the sun, there is the possibility of injury to your skin or eyes," Dr. McCormick says.

royal jelly

Royal jelly is food fit for a queen—a queen bee, that is. This milky white substance, secreted from glands in a worker bee's head, is the life-sustaining food for all bee larvae for the first three days of life. After that, it's just for Her Majesty: Only the queen bee larvae get royal jelly for the rest of their larval lives.

This special diet is chiefly responsible for making the queen bee different from worker bees. Not only is she bigger than the other bees, she lives significantly longer. A hearty queen, raised on this high-powered jelly, lives for about six years, compared to only six weeks for worker bees.

Based on observations of the bee queen's royal lifestyle, many people think that royal jelly must have some specific nutritional advantages. Under laboratory analysis, this mystery food turns out to be mostly water, protein, sugars, and fatty acids. It also contains high levels of B vitamins as well as potassium and the trace minerals zinc, iron, copper, and manganese. Royal jelly also consists of 18 amino acids, 8 of which our bodies need but can't produce on their own, according to Steve Nenninger, N.D., a naturopathic doctor in New York City.

Many medicinal uses have been claimed for royal jelly. Some products are said to help rheumatoid arthritis, chronic fatigue, liver disease, kidney problems, pancreatitis, insomnia, stomach ulcers, and skin disorders. There have been no well-designed studies to support its use for humans, however.

A Royal Welcome

"Medically it's been used for two age groups—the very young and the very old," says Theodore Chebuliez, M.D., a physician in Scarsdale, New York, and president of the American Apitherapy Society, a nonprofit organization that advances the investigation of the healing use of products from the beehive. He believes that for infants, royal jelly has been successful in treating a condition known as failure-to-thrive syndrome.

"Failure to thrive is just that—newborns don't eat well and they don't grow well. Its origins may be allergic, emotional, or physical," he says. "But if you feed failure-to-thrive infants with royal jelly, many do improve and start resuming normal growth and eating habits."

Likewise, royal jelly helps restore poor appetite as well as lack of enthusiasm, or malaise, in the elderly, he says. "These indications are fairly well known but not well-studied. The evidence is anecdotal."

Dr. Chebuliez credits royal jelly with a third use, "priming the immune system," which he believes could prove helpful for people with rheumatoid arthritis, multiple sclerosis, scleroderma, lupus, and other autoimmune diseases. Again, the evidence is anecdotal. "I learned this from Chinese medicine. If you take royal jelly for several weeks, the immunological system will respond when it was not responding before," he says.

Bowls Full of Jelly

China is the number one supplier of royal jelly to the United States. To meet the demand, producers have special hives in which they create row upon row of queen cells with eggs, then wait for bees to fill the cells with royal jelly. When the eggs are swimming in the substance, workers suck the jelly out of each cell using a glass tube. Then the eggs are thrown away and replaced with fresh ones to continue the cycle.

Royal jelly has a slightly bitter, acidic taste. As a nutritional supplement, it's available in tablets, capsules, and liquid and is often combined with

SUPPLEMENT SNAPSHOT

▶ Royal Jelly

May help: Failure-to-thrive syndrome, malaise and poor appetite in the elderly, rheumatoid arthritis, multiple sclerosis, chronic fatigue syndrome, liver disease, kidney problems, pancreatitis, insomnia, stomach ulcers, and skin disorders.

Cautions and possible side effects: Do not take royal jelly if you have allergies or asthma. It has been linked to bronchial spasms, acute asthma, anaphylactic reactions, and even death. Those with a history of asthma or a predisposition to allergies are especially at risk.

Asian ginseng and other "energizing" substances. Liquid royal jelly should be stored in a tightly closed container and frozen until it's used, says Dr. Cherbuliez, who takes a gram a day by scraping it directly from the jar with a spoon.

Royal jelly can also be found in a variety of skin-care products, including creams, lotions, and soaps. Proponents believe that because of its high protein content, using royal jelly topically can slow aging. They also think that it provides the skin with the amino acids that form collagen.

St. John's wort

In an era centuries before scientific reasoning and modern chemical analysis, people observed herbs to understand their healing powers. They took clues from a plant's appearance and the places where it grew. The Chinese, for instance, thought of ginseng as a tonic for the whole body, in part because the root resembles a stick-figure human being.

When ancient peoples in Europe and the Mediterranean studied St. John's wort, or hypericum, they saw a plant with yellow blossoms that grew not in dark forests but in places with bright sunshine. So, based on the instant visual pharmacology of the time, they concluded that it must also shine favorably on the human spirit.

"It was yellow. It possessed the powers of sun and light. The flowers resembled shooting stars," explains Eran Ben-Arye, M.D., a researcher at the natural medicine research unit at Hadassah University Hospital in Jerusalem. For these reasons and more, it came to be revered as well as used.

For thousands of years, people considered St. John's wort a magic herb with supernatural powers, as implied by its Latin name, *Hypericum perforatum*, which means "over an apparition." Loaded with do-good potency, it was considered powerful medicine against evil spirits and protection against demonic possession. Herbalists called it the Devil's Scourge and prescribed it as a nerve tonic and to relieve depression.

Today, although the study of this herb is much more scientific, the conclusions reinforce those of yesteryear: For the despondent, discouraged, and depressed, hypericum holds promise of letting in the light.

A Rush to Hypericum

Chemical analyses, clinical trials, and a major study undertaken by the National Institutes of Health all support the benefits of St. John's wort. It appears to be an exciting new treatment for mild to moderate depression, says Andrew Weil, M.D., clinical professor of internal medicine and director of the program in integrative medicine at the University of Arizona College of Medicine in Tucson, and author of *Eight Weeks to Optimum Health*.

"Until recently, it was largely dismissed by our own medical community, but that's changing," says Dr. Weil. "It's been widely used in Europe for 15 years."

In any year, German physicians are likely to prescribe as many as 66 million doses of St. John's wort to treat depressive states, anxiety, nervous excitement, and other emotional or psychological disturbances. In Germany, for each single prescription written for the drug fluoxetine (Prozac), which is widely used as a pharmaceutical antidepressant, there are 25 prescriptions written for hypericum.

Interest in St. John's wort grew dramatically in 1996 after the *British Medical Journal* published a review of 23 scientific studies done on the herb in Europe. Looking at the results of the studies, the reviewers concluded that St. John's wort is significantly superior to a placebo (an inactive substance with no medicinal value) in treating patients with mild to moderate depression. Evidence is less conclusive that it works as well as standard pharmaceutical antidepressants.

Although the authors were cautiously optimistic about the herb's benefit, the news made big waves in the American medical community and the

SUPPLEMENTSNAPSHOT

▶St. John's Wort

Botanical name: *Hypericum perforatum*; also known as hypericum.

May help: Mild to moderate depression, binge-eating disorder, anxiety, nervous disorders, and viral infections.

Origin: Native to Europe and Asia; now grows well in parts of California and Oregon.

Cautions and possible side effects: If your doctor has prescribed MAO inhibitor antidepressants, or you are pregnant consult your doctor before taking. St. John's wort may cause photosensitivity. Although St. John's wort can be used in HIV treatment, it should be done under a physician's supervision. It has been demonstrated to lower the blood concentration of some HIV medications.

nutritional supplement industry. Currently, St. John's wort can be found in many drugstores, most health food stores, and some discount stores and supermarkets across the country.

With news spreading by word of mouth, through the Internet, and in media reports, the public has taken to St. John's wort, says Bernard Beitman, M.D., chairman of the department of psychiatry and neurology at the University of Missouri School of Medicine in Columbia.

"It's gotten very popular, partly because it's an herbal medicine. You don't need a doctor's prescription to get it," he says. "Plus, it fits with the whole new notion of 'Patient . . . heal thyself.' People are hearing about it and trying it on their own. I've had some women tell me that they are giving it to their husbands who are feeling depressed but won't go to the doctor," he says. "They tell me that their husbands are more fun, but the husbands don't notice anything different."

A Mild-Mannered Herb

Another reason that people are trying St. John's wort may be its apparent lack of side effects as compared to antidepressant drugs, says Dr. Ben-Arye. Dry mouth, headaches, nausea, digestive problems, insomnia, and loss of sexual desire are common problems with prescription medications. Users of St. John's wort only occasionally report some agitation and sleep loss. The most frequently mentioned problem is increased sensitivity to sunlight that causes a tendency toward sunburn, he says.

Although St. John's wort seems to be very safe compared to other antidepressants, that doesn't mean that people should self-medicate, especially if their depression is severe, warns Dr. Ben-Arye. It shouldn't be considered some sort of cure-all for depression, as it may not be strong enough to do the job. It's not recommended for treatment of severe depression or disorders that may include hallucinations and suicidal thoughts, he says.

"There are a lot of aspects to depression, and many treatments. You should be talking to a health professional about your problem, not just taking an herb or a drug," he suggests.

Magic and Myth

The folk use of St. John's wort goes back at least 2,000 years. Physicians and herbalists in Europe have used the plant to treat wounds and kidney and lung ailments as well as depression.

Native to Europe and Asia, the plant was first brought to the United States by European colonists. Although its main use has always been for psychological ailments and nervousness, St. John's wort has antiviral, anti-inflammatory, and diuretic properties.

An oil made from hypericum was used to heal bruises and sunburn. The herb's sedative effect helped reduce pain associated with nerve-related disorders like neuralgia and sciatica and rheumatic pain in the joints. It was sometimes given during menopause or menstrual periods to soothe irritability and mood swings.

Wort, another term for "plant," comes from Old English. The name St. John's wort may have come about because red or bloodlike spots appear on hypericum leaves in June, around the anniversary of the beheading of St. John the Baptist. During the Middle Ages, on the saint's anniversary, peasants slept with cuttings of the plant under their pillows. They hoped that St. John would appear in their dreams, bless them, and give them life for another year.

The primary medicinal part of the herb is the flower. In the United States, most medicinal supplies are grown in the eastern states and the Pacific Northwest. Western ranchers consider hypericum a noxious weed.

A Sum of Its Parts

The major known compounds in St. John's wort are hypericin and pseudohypericin, which are found in low concentrations in the leaves and in much higher amounts in the flowers. The plant also contains a broad spectrum of flavonoids. While these chemicals contribute to the herb's healing properties, there may be as many as 10 groups of chemicals that also have some effect.

It's likely that some of these chemical compounds work together, or synergistically, says Dr. Beitman. "You can compare it to a symphony orchestra giving a concert. We like what we hear, but we don't know who all the individual players are."

When the plant extract is used in studies, it usually includes a standard percentage of hypericin, the mostly widely known and studied active ingredient. Having standardized, measurable amounts of this ingredient in the plant extract ensures its quality, researchers believe.

Keeping the Good Stuff Flowing

Exactly how St. John's wort elevates mood isn't clear, but the mechanism is probably much like that of prescription antidepressant drugs, says Woodson Merrell, M.D., a specialist in alternative and complementary medicine and assistant clinical professor of medicine at the Columbia University College of Physicians and Surgeons in New York City.

Chemicals in the brain called neurotransmitters are used by nerve cells to communicate with one another. When the levels of some neurotransmitters fall, depression can set in. St. John's wort—like pharmaceutical antidepressants—helps to remedy the situation by normalizing the amounts of neurotransmitters. When that happens, you begin to feel better, says Dr. Merrell. "You get a better sense of well-being," he explains.

St. John's wort apparently binds more weakly to sites in the brain than its prescription counterparts. In other words, it seems to do its work more gently, says Dr. Merrell. That may be why the herb is more suited to mild or moderate depression for which the strength of prescription drugs isn't required. "Herbs, in general, tend to be gentler than prescription drugs, and that may make them safer, with fewer side effects," he says.

If you're already taking an antidepressant or other types of medications, however, there's reason to be cautious, says Dr. Beitman. Be sure to consult your doctor before taking this or any herb for a medical condition.

"Studies haven't been done on its interaction with other drugs," he says. "Just because it's been around for centuries and is thought to be safe doesn't mean that we know anything about its interaction with modern pharmaceutical drugs."

Turning On the Light

St. John's wort is widely available as a tincture and capsules. Look for a standardized extract that contains 0.3 percent hypericin, which approximates the standard used in Germany and in many of the medical studies. A typical dose of the extract is 300 milligrams three times a day.

Because of its mild action, St. John's wort takes more time to build up in your system than prescription antidepressants do, says Dr. Merrell. "It will take somewhere between four and six weeks before you'll start noticing any effect."

saw palmetto

If you've read anything about saw palmetto in the popular press, you probably know that it has come to be known as a guy herb. The guys most likely to want it are primarily middle-aged or older men who find that they're answering nature's call two or three times a night.

Typically, that call of nature ends up being an almost-false alarm: Even when it feels like a waterfall is about to pour forth, the result is more of a trickle. This problem is often a sign of benign prostatic hyperplasia (BPH), a noncancerous enlargement of the prostate gland that constricts the urethra, the tube that leads from the bladder to the penis. Picture what happens to your lawn sprinkler when you step on the garden hose, and you have a good idea of the problem.

Many men who take saw palmetto find that the herb shrinks the prostate and releases the squeeze so that urine flows normally, says Woodson Merrell, M.D., a specialist in alternative and complementary medicine and assistant clinical professor of medicine at the Columbia University College of Physicians and Surgeons in New York City.

How well saw palmetto works is still controversial because it may not be strong enough by itself to make a significant difference for some men, says Dr. Merrell. "It may be effective for moderate cases of BPH or when the prostate is just beginning to enlarge, however."

Purging the Pipes

Saw palmetto is a low, scrubby palm that grows in sandy soil in the southern United States, from South Carolina to Florida.

The Seminoles of the Everglades ate the berries for food, but it's not known if they valued the plant as a medicine. European settlers in the region used it as a diuretic to flush excess water from the body. In 1849, one herbal practitioner referred to the herb's "purgative property, often producing a copious evacuation."

Herbalists of that era also touted saw palmetto's anti-catarrhal properties, meaning that it seemed to relieve phlegm-producing conditions like colds and flu. The herb was used as an expectorant in some cough formulas.

Women took it to relieve painful periods and regulate the menstrual cycle. It has also been used for pelvic inflammatory disease and similar conditions.

Saw palmetto is known to stimulate the production of prolactin, a female hormone that, among other things, promotes breast enlargement and milk production in breastfeeding women, and prostate growth in men, says Tirun Gopal, M.D., an obstetrician and gynecologist who practices holistic and Ayurvedic medicine in Allentown, Pennsylvania. "There also are some claims that saw palmetto can be used for infertility when the problem is the absence of ovulation," he says.

Perhaps that is where the herb got a reputation as an aphrodisiac and a tonic to increase sexual energy and revive low libido in both sexes. Some research demonstrates that a compound in saw palmetto has aphrodisiac effects. Ironically, some herbalists have been known to use saw palmetto to treat honeymoon cystitis, bladder irritation that results from excessive sexual activity.

A Drug No More

Sexual matters aside, saw palmetto was widely and routinely used in the early decades of the twentieth century to treat urinary tract ailments, particularly chronic cystitis, an inflammation of the bladder. From 1906 to

SUPPLEMENT SNAPSHOT

▶Saw Palmetto

Botanical name: *Serenoa repens*.

May help: Prostate problems, bladder irritation, menstrual problems, and pelvic inflammatory disease.

Origin: Southern United States.

Cautions and possible side effects: If you have prostate problems, see your doctor for a diagnosis before using.

1950, it was officially listed as a drug in the United States, and it was prescribed both here and in Europe as a treatment for gonorrhea.

After World War II, it fell out of favor in the United States, but research continued in Europe. Scientists found that patients who consumed an extract of the berries had increased urine volume, a decrease in frequent urination, and more ease of urination.

As with many botanical medicines, it's difficult to identify exactly what active ingredients are working in saw palmetto. Scientists believe that it has steroidlike properties. In the case of BPH, it interrupts a critical chemical process, says William Page-Echols, D.O., an assistant clinical professor of family medicine who teaches alternative medicine at the Michigan State University College of Osteopathic Medicine in East Lansing.

BPH occurs when testosterone, the male sex hormone, is converted by an enzyme to a more potent hormone that causes cells and tissues to grow and proliferate. That growth is perfectly fine when the male sexual organs are developing, but later in life, when the organs are fully developed, the continued cell growth becomes a liability. Taken daily, saw palmetto inhibits the enzyme so the hormone conversion doesn't occur, says Dr. Page-Echols. Finasteride (Proscar), the prescription drug most often prescribed in the United States for BPH, has much the same action, he adds.

Several studies in Europe show that saw palmetto is an effective treatment for many men, especially those in the early stages of enlarged prostate. In Germany, it's sold over the counter as a treatment for BPH. One yearlong study of men with BPH found that an extract of saw palmetto reduced prostate size by 13 percent.

Gentle and Effective

Researchers have compared the effectiveness of saw palmetto with that of other drugs prescribed for BPH. Although results were somewhat mixed, tests showed that the herb produces fewer side effects than prescription drugs. Finasteride, for example, sometimes causes headaches, erection problems, loss of libido, and decreased ejaculation volume.

The German Federal Ministry of Health has determined that people experience few side effects from saw palmetto berries. In one three-year study, less than 2 percent of men taking an alcohol-based extract of the herb quit the study because of side effects. More than 80 percent of the men felt that the herb helped and improved their quality of life.

"When your medication is causing you to have decreased interest in sex and decreased capabilities, saw palmetto may be an important alternative to try," says Dr. Page-Echols. "A lot of men have come into my office asking about it. They've heard about it from friends."

Where to See Saw

When Dr. Page-Echols suggests saw palmetto, he usually advises using it in combination with zinc and plant-based medicines such as flower pollen. It's also available in capsule and tincture form.

Since saw palmetto isn't standardized for any active ingredient, your best bet is to look for a product made solely from the berries by a well-known company, says Dr. Merrell. Also, remember that like many herbs, saw palmetto has a fairly mild action. It may take weeks or months for it to work.

"Don't just start taking the herb without seeing your doctor," Dr. Merrell warns. "You shouldn't assume that your symptoms are due to BPH. Make sure that you have a benign condition first, then try the herb."

selenium

If you've heard anything about this essential trace mineral, it's probably been news that's related to cancer prevention. Studies from around the world suggest that where selenium intake is very low—usually because of selenium-poor soil—cancer rates tend to be higher than normal.

"Selenium has been associated with reduced cancer risk since the late 1960s, but findings were slow to be popularized because of exaggerated concerns about the potential for toxicity," says Larry Clark, Ph.D., associate professor of epidemiology at the Arizona Cancer Center in Tucson. "Selenium actually has one of the strongest bodies of literature supporting its role as an anti-cancer agent. The data are overwhelming."

A study done by Dr. Clark and his colleagues hints at selenium's potential. It was designed to look for a change in the rates of skin cancer and included more than 1,000 people (average age, 63) with a history of skin cancer.

The participants were divided into two groups and followed for six years. For about four years, one group received 200 micrograms daily of selenium from high-selenium yeast, which contains a special form of the mineral. The other group got inactive look-alike pills (placebos). When the study ended, the members of the group that had gotten the selenium had a 37 percent reduction in cancer risk. They also had a 50 percent reduction in cancer deaths.

Surprisingly, there was no reduction in the incidence of skin cancer. Instead, there were 63 percent fewer cases of prostate cancer, 58 percent fewer colon or rectal cancers, and 45 percent fewer lung cancers in the selenium group.

"It was a wonderful surprise," Dr. Clark says. "Not that we didn't expect selenium to reduce cancer rates, but we didn't expect it to have the power to produce such reductions in the short period of time of this trial."

Like vitamins C and E, selenium helps to prevent damage throughout the body from free-roaming, unstable molecules called free radicals. "Selenium's role in the body is complex, however, and not yet fully understood," says Orville Levander, Ph.D., a research leader at the U.S. Department of Agriculture Beltsville Human Nutrition Research Center in Maryland. "There are probably a dozen or so different selenium-containing proteins in the body," he says. "Some have antioxidant activity, and some apparently have other roles."

In addition to possibly helping to prevent cancer, selenium seems to inhibit certain viral infections. It also interacts with iodine to activate thyroxine, the thyroid gland's main hormone, and it promotes the infection-fighting ability of certain immune cells.

Kind to Your Heart and Cells

Selenium is an indispensable part of a free-radical–quenching enzyme called glutathione peroxidase, which, when teamed with another kind of selenium-containing enzyme, can help protect us from heart disease. We don't know exactly why selenium has this protective effect. Possibly, these enzymes offer protection by maintaining the essential fats that form a shield

SUPPLEMENTSNAPSHOT

▶Selenium

Supplement forms: Selenomethionine, sodium selenite, and high selenium yeast.

May help: Cancer, heart disease, angina, cataracts, hair loss, lupus, and HIV; may limit spread of chronic infections.

Daily Value: 70 micrograms.

Who's at risk for deficiency: People who get most of their food from selenium-poor soil. Deficiency is rare in countries where food is transported or imported and where diets include meat and shellfish.

Good food sources: Lobster, clams, crab, cooked oysters, and Brazil nuts.

Cautions and possible side effects: Don't take more than 200 micrograms in supplement form; higher amounts may cause fragile, thickened nails; stomach pain; diarrhea; loss of sensation in the hands and feet; fatigue; and irritability. Doses of about 800 micrograms have been known to cause tissue damage.

around cells in the artery walls, suggests Vladimir Badmaev, M.D., Ph.D., vice president of scientific and medical affairs for Sabinsa, a corporation in Piscataway, New Jersey, that makes selenium supplements. Without the selenium needed, Dr. Badmaev speculates, this shield could be damaged by free radicals, causing the arteries to collect plaque.

Some research indicates that selenium may prevent cancer by inhibiting tumor growth and inducing a kind of suicide in malignant cells, Dr. Clark says. "In tumor cells grown in the laboratory, selenium stimulates programmed cell death, which is a very late effect in the cancer process. This makes us think that it is never too late to start taking selenium, because it may have effects on actual tumors as well as on premalignant cells."

Other selenium-dependent enzymes can disarm a veritable toxic-waste dump's worth of harmful substances, including drugs, chemicals such as the herbicide paraquat, and toxic metals such as mercury, cadmium, and arsenic.

Virus Fighter

Researchers first became interested in selenium's role in viral infections when their attention was drawn to one area of China where the soil is low in selenium. People living in that low-selenium neighborhood were much more likely than normal to die of a form of heart disease called Keshan disease, which is characterized by cardiomyopathy, or weakening of the heart muscle. It is thought to be a result of a viral infection that occurs when a selenium deficiency causes a normally harmless virus to change into a deadly strain, Dr. Levander says.

Researchers know that in selenium-deficient animals, the harmless virus can mutate into a virulent form capable of causing heart damage and death. "In studies where the virus was removed from the selenium-deficient animals and injected into animals that were getting sufficient selenium, it remained in its deadly, mutated form," Dr. Levander says.

Several viruses are known to interact with selenium, according to Will Taylor, Ph.D., an AIDS researcher and associate professor at the College of Pharmacy at the University of Georgia in Athens. "The rate of progression from HIV to AIDS, for instance, has been strongly correlated with selenium status," he says.

In a study at the University of Miami, people with HIV who were deficient in selenium were 20 times more likely to die from AIDS within six months than people with normal selenium levels. Other viruses potentially linked with the mineral include hepatitis C and measles, Dr. Taylor says. No studies have been done on the effect of supplements, however.

Selenium apparently is used initially by viruses to help establish themselves in the body, so a viral infection can deplete the mineral. Later, however, during a long period when many chronic viral infections don't create symptoms, selenium appears to act as a kind of viral birth control. It seems to restrict rather than encourage the spread of the virus.

How Much Is Enough?

The Daily Value for selenium is 70 micrograms, and people in the United States get an average of a little more than 100 micrograms of selenium a day. If you're taking a selenium supplement, says Dr. Levander, you'll want to use one that doesn't put your total selenium for the day much above 350 micrograms (for a 154-pound person).

"We don't have good information on when selenium becomes toxic, but taking no more than 200 micrograms a day as a supplement seems to be within reason for most people if they choose to supplement," he says.

shark cartilage

Could the wide-mouthed creature that sometimes lunches on terrorized swimmers provide a dandy cancer treatment?

Some researchers and doctors think so, claiming that there's something in shark cartilage that can inhibit the growth of tumors in human beings.

Tumor growth involves a process known as angiogenesis, in which the body creates new blood vessels to feed a tumor with oxygen and nutrients as well as remove waste. If the blood supply is removed, the tumor dies. It's believed that shark cartilage does just that, stopping the development of new blood vessels and thereby starving the tumor.

"Sharks are unique in that they rarely get cancer," says I. William Lane, Ph.D., a biochemist and independent consultant at Cartilage Consultants, Inc. in Short Hills, New Jersey and author of *Sharks Don't Get Cancer* and *Sharks Still Don't Get Cancer*. "Only roughly one in a million has any signs of cancer, whereas fish get cancer at a rate of about three or four per hundred," he says.

Diving Deeper into Research

While promoters suggest that cancer can be cured with shark cartilage treatments, other doctors are frankly skeptical. "There are no cures. If there were, it would put me and every other cancer doctor out of work," says Charles Simone, M.D., founder of the Simone Protective Cancer Center in Lawrenceville, New Jersey, and author of several books, including *Cancer and Nutrition*.

Since 1994, Dr. Simone has been conducting one of the few shark cartilage studies approved by the Food and Drug Administration (FDA). The study combines shark cartilage with his own 10-point lifestyle plan that emphasizes proper nutrition, certain vitamin supplements, no smoking, no alcohol, exercise, stress reduction, and other lifestyle changes. The patients he treats are terminally ill, with cancer that has already spread to various parts of their bodies. All have failed to respond to chemotherapy or radiation therapy. In other words, their cancers are widespread and can't be cured with any conventional treatments.

Using shark cartilage and lifestyle modification, Dr. Simone has seen a response rate of about 15 percent in his patients, defined as a "reduction in tumor mass of at least 50 percent or more for at least four weeks." Not all types of cancers have responded, however. Cancers that occur in the upper part of the body—particularly those of the lungs, head, and neck—don't seem to be influenced by this treatment.

"We'll probably never see a lengthening of life span with any treatment," says Dr. Simone. "What we're looking for in this study is simply response: Can we shrink the tumor or not? The answer is yes, but in a limited number of patients."

Dr. Simone says that he can't be sure whether the shark cartilage, the 10-point lifestyle plan, or both have caused the reduction in tumors. "I wrote the study the way I did because I think it is unethical to withhold lifestyle changes from cancer patients," he notes.

Improving the quality of life for these terminally ill patients is an important component of Dr. Simone's study. He defines quality of life as whether the patient, not the doctor, indicates an improvement or not. By this definition, quality of life is enhanced in more than 75 percent of patients, he says. Dr. Simone emphasizes, however, that these are patients who are no longer getting chemotherapy or radiation treatments, so they aren't experiencing the painful or uncomfortable side effects of those treatments, either. That in itself could account for their temporary improvement in quality of life, he points out.

SUPPLEMENT SNAPSHOT

▶Shark Cartilage

May help: Inhibit tumor growth.

Cautions and possible side effects: Do not take if you are pregnant or have recently had a heart attack or surgery. Do not give to children. May cause gastrointestinal distress in doses of 10,000 milligrams or more.

Taking a Bite Out of Shark Claims

Robert Langer, Ph.D., professor of chemical and biomedical engineering at the Massachusetts Institute of Technology in Boston, who was one of the early trailblazers in the study of shark cartilage and tumor growth, has been involved in research to isolate the cause of biological activity in cartilage. The goal is to find the active component, purify it, clone it, and ultimately use it on cancer patients.

Oral supplements are created by grinding up shark cartilage. According to Dr. Langer, people who say that this ground-up cartilage can provide a cure for cancer are making some illogical leaps. "I make the following analogy: If somebody is diabetic, he gets pig insulin. Insulin is a large molecule that you can't swallow. You have to inject it. It took an enormous amount of work by a lot of people to purify that molecule. But just grinding up a pig and injecting it into a diabetic would do nothing." Similarly, chopping up shark cartilage and processing it into supplements that are taken orally isn't likely to produce results either, he says.

An Ocean of Uses

Dr. Lane has added fuel to the fire of controversy by claiming that cancer is not the only disease that may benefit from shark cartilage. "Cancer is the headline grabber, but shark cartilage will work on any growing mass, such as fibroids," he says.

A number of eye-damaging diseases, such as diabetic retinopathy, macular degeneration, and neurovascular glaucoma, may benefit from shark cartilage, says Dr. Lane, because, like tumors, their growth depends on the formation of new blood vessels.

Dr. Simone strongly disagrees. "There have been no studies, nor have there been any anecdotes to suggest that cartilage can benefit these medical disorders. It is not appropriate to make such speculation," he says.

Connecting with Arthritis

You may also see advertising claims linking shark cartilage to a treatment for rheumatoid arthritis and osteoarthritis. There's no solid evidence of animal or human studies published in medical journals to support this use, says Luke Bucci, Ph.D., vice president of research for Weider Nutrition International in Salt Lake City and author of several books on arthritis and nutrition, including *Healing Arthritis the Natural Way*. Besides, he adds, dosages are impractical and high, and the supplement itself is very costly. "I do not advocate shark cartilage supplements to anyone for anything," he explains. "We have so many better choices that we have good data on."

Similarly, bovine cartilage, another supplement used to treat arthritis, has been ineffective. Once researchers began to uncover the active components in cartilage, however, they came up with glucosamine and chondroitin sulfate, Dr. Bucci says. These components, both of which have been used effectively to treat osteoarthritis, are available as separate supplements.

"Thus, the components of shark or bovine cartilage, but not the actual cartilage powder itself, work on arthritis," says Dr. Bucci. "Cartilage powders are much cheaper than purified components. Some manufacturers use cartilage powders and claim that their products have chondroitin."

Land Sharks

You'll see shark cartilage powders and capsules in the natural foods aisle and in some mail-order catalogs. By Dr. Lane's estimation, as many as 95 percent of these supplements may be worthless because they have been denatured—that is, their molecular form has been altered during processing, making them largely ineffective against cancer and other illnesses.

"My best advice is to deal with clinical-quality, 100 percent shark cartilage brands from companies that specialize in the shark cartilage business," Dr. Lane says. This poses a dilemma for the average consumer. According to Dr. Lane, off-the-shelf products labeled "shark cartilage" may not be effective.

Meanwhile, research continues. To test the effectiveness of shark cartilage, Dr. Lane has initiated four FDA-approved research studies for a number of different kinds of cancer that have not responded to conventional medical treatments. To participate, patients must have failed to respond to at least two therapies, such as chemotherapy and radiation. The studies are designed to find out whether tumors respond to treatment with shark cartilage and also whether pain can be reduced, improving the patient's quality of life.

"The main thing we hope to achieve is tumor reduction and extension of life. If we can extend life in a quality manner by four or five years, that will be quite a victory," he says.

thiamin

To understand what thiamin does in your body, consider the word that describes thiamin deficiency: beriberi. This East Asian word means, literally, "I can't, I can't," and people with beriberi can't do a lot. They're tired, weak, and uninterested in things, especially food. They may have numb or burning feet, leg cramps, and sometimes mental confusion and an enlarged heart.

Recurrent canker sores may also be a tipoff to thiamin deficiency. A study by Israeli researchers found that 70 percent of people with that problem had low blood levels of thiamin, compared to only 4 percent of people who did not have canker sores.

Like the other B vitamins, thiamin is involved in energy metabolism. "That means it helps you to derive energy from the calories you get from food," explains Joanne Curran-Celentano, R.D., Ph.D., associate professor of nutrition and food sciences at the University of New Hampshire in Durham. "It helps to break down the molecules in foods and either re-arrange them into a form your body can use for energy or store them for later use as energy."

Thiamin interacts with several enzymes, the biochemical spark plugs that get chemical reactions going in your body. "Several of the enzymes involved in the process of breaking down carbohydrates for energy require thiamin," Dr. Curran-Celentano explains. The fatigue associated with thiamin deficiency is, figuratively, the equivalent of a clogged carburetor. You may have a full tank, but none of the gasoline is being burned to run the engine.

Brain Gain

Thiamin's ability to make energy available for the body has ramifications for the brain.

"If you dramatically reduce thiamin intake, you reduce the ability of the brain to use glucose (blood sugar). If you reduce that, you have impaired mental function," says Gary Gibson, Ph.D., professor of neuroscience at the

Burke Medical Research Institute of Weill Medical College of Cornell University in White Plains, New York. Unlike other body parts, which can switch to other fuels if they need to, the brain uses glucose pretty much exclusively, Dr. Gibson explains.

Thiamin is also very important in the synthesis of critical neurotransmitters in the brain, including one involved in memory and performance—acetylcholine. "We know that thiamin-deficient animals don't make much acetylcholine and that this lowers their ability to remember and respond," Dr. Gibson says. "So we believe that high levels of acetylcholine are important for proper brain function."

Just how much of a role thiamin plays in human mental performance has yet to be determined. In one study, though, young women with no signs of deficiency who took 50 milligrams of thiamin a day for two months reported feeling more clear-headed, composed, and energetic than those who weren't getting the supplements. Those taking the extra thiamin also had faster reaction times on tests than those without supplementation.

In other studies, thiamin deficiency has been found to cause mood changes, vague feelings of uneasiness, fear, disorderly thinking, and other signs of mental depression—symptoms that researchers say often affect memory, Dr. Gibson says.

SUPPLEMENT SNAPSHOT

▶ Thiamin

Also known as: Vitamin B₁.

May help: Beriberi, Wernicke-Korsakoff syndrome, and canker sores.

Daily Value: 1.5 milligrams.

Special instructions: For best absorption, don't take with alcohol, tea, or coffee.

Who's at risk for deficiency: Alcoholics, the elderly, strict dieters, and people who are critically ill.

Good food sources: Baker's and brewer's yeast, lean pork and ham, legumes, nuts, and whole-grain or enriched breads and cereals.

Cautions and possible side effects: No known problems from oral doses.

Thiamin deficiency clearly plays a role in the mental deterioration associated with alcoholism, since alcohol causes thiamin to be excreted faster, and many alcoholics don't get much of the vitamin because they eat poorly. Some alcoholics develop a condition called Wernicke-Korsakoff syndrome, which is characterized by the inability to form new memories, poorly organized retrieval of old memories, apathy, and emotional blandness.

Thiamin supplementation corrects this condition if it's caught before permanent nerve damage occurs.

An Alzheimer's Link?

In some ways, brain problems resulting from thiamin deficiency are similar to those seen with Alzheimer's disease, Dr. Gibson says. In both cases, he notes, there's degeneration of the nerves in some areas, and when this occurs, there's an accumulation of a protein that plays an important role in the development of Alzheimer's.

The only currently approved Alzheimer's drug, tacrine (Cognex), works in the cholinergic system, a body-wide system of nerve-cell receptors that are found in the brain, heart, and intestines and that respond to the body's release of acetylcholine. Thiamin is also needed to make the cholinergic system function.

Thiamin supplementation has been tried in patients with Alzheimer's, although without much success. Japanese researchers are continuing to study a fat-soluble form of thiamin—one that gets into the brain more easily than regular thiamin—in the treatment of Alzheimer's disease. "It's hard to draw any conclusions at this point, or to make recommendations," Dr. Gibson says. "We are simply trying to find out more about thiamin's basic functions in the brain."

In the United States, thiamin is one of the vitamins found in fortified flour and cereals, so deficiency is not common, Dr. Curran-Celantano says.

The Daily Value is 1.5 milligrams. Men typically get about 1.75 milligrams, and women get 1.05 milligrams. Deficiency is most likely to occur in people who abuse alcohol or who live mostly on empty calories, such as soda and sweets. Others who may develop deficiency-related health problems include older people in nursing homes and hospitals, people who are very ill, and strict dieters.

valerian

The old adage that if it tastes bad, it must be good for you is true for valerian, an herb that's been used through the centuries to calm nervous jitters and bring on sleep.

Modern herbalists call it the gym-sock herb because the medicinal parts of the plant—the dried roots or rhizomes—smell really rank. One eighteenth-century herbalist likened it to the urine of cats, so you can imagine that an herbal tea of valerian root is a less-than-exquisite sipping experience. Because of its strong smell, valerian is most commonly taken as pills or tincture.

Nevertheless, "valerian is a wonderful herb for relaxing the body, both the mind and the muscles," says Jill Stansbury, N.D., assistant professor of botanical medicine and chair of the botanical medicine department at the National College of Naturopathic Medicine in Portland, Oregon.

A Centuries-Old Cure

Valerian is a perennial plant that reaches a height of five feet and grows wild throughout Europe and parts of Asia. In many countries, it is cultivated for medicinal purposes. The plant's unmistakable odor emerges only during the drying process.

Herbalists in Europe have known about its calming properties for centuries. The ancient Greeks and Romans called it wild nard, but by the ninth century, it appeared in written records as valerian. It was recommended as a treatment for hysteria and emotional disorders. By the 1700s, physicians were recommending valerian for numerous complaints from living too luxuriously to having an ailment known as the vapors.

Valerian is classified as a mild tranquilizer. It's also considered an antispasmodic, meaning that it eases muscle spasms or cramps in the body, and it has been used to relieve menstrual cramps and premenstrual syndrome. In the 1800s, a physician wrote that it had a "remarkable effect in quieting the nervous agitation which prevents sleep in delicate and irritable females."

A Balm That Calms

A number of scientific studies have shown that valerian has a sedative effect on the brain and also relaxes muscles in the digestive tract that clench under stress. In herbal medicine today, it's primarily used for insomnia, mild anxiety, panic attacks, and tension in the body. The herb hastens sleep, improves sleep quality, and reduces nighttime awakenings. In England, dozens of over-the-counter sleep aids contain valerian. In the United States, you'll have no problem finding it in most drugstores and health food stores.

"It's a mild herbal relaxant. You take it when you're feeling stressed or when something is bothering you and keeping you awake," says Woodson Merrell, M.D., a specialist in alternative and complementary medicine and assistant clinical professor of medicine at the Columbia University College of Physicians and Surgeons in New York City. "It won't knock you out, but it can relax you enough so you can fall asleep."

Valerian isn't for long-term use, Dr. Merrell warns. If you have recurring insomnia, you should probably speak to a physician. If you're just a bit tense or restless at bedtime, however, it may be just the thing. "It tends to make you less nervous, and sometimes, that's all you need."

SUPPLEMENT SNAPSHOT

▶Valerian

Botanical name: *Valeriana officinalis*.

May help: Anxiety, insomnia, menstrual cramps, tension headaches, sleep problems associated with chronic fatigue syndrome, muscle cramps, and muscle spasms.

Origin: Europe and Asia.

Cautions and possible side effects: Do not use with prescription medications such as diazepam (Valium) or amitriptyline (Elavil). Don't use valerian if you experience heart palpitations or nervousness after taking it.

Mild and Nonaddictive

Its mild tranquilizing power has made valerian a popular treatment for anxiety; in Europe, it is often prescribed for that purpose. Unlike diazepam (Valium) and alprazolam (Xanax), the drugs often prescribed for anxiety in the United States, valerian has few side effects.

Some people confuse valerian and Valium, believing that their similar names imply that they are somehow related. They are not. Valium is a synthetic drug, a member of the benzodiazepine family, while valerian is derived from a plant.

There is a connection, however. The herb and the drug seem to affect the brain in a similar fashion, binding to the same receptors. The differences are that valerian appears to be nonaddictive, and its effects tend to be milder than those of Valium.

Unlike some pharmaceuticals, valerian doesn't interfere with the deepest part of the sleep cycle, called REM or dream sleep. There's no hangover or grogginess the next day and little chance of dependency, says William Page-Echols, D.O., an assistant clinical professor of family medicine who teaches alternative medicine at the Michigan State University College of Osteopathic Medicine in East Lansing.

"There's far less risk of building up a tolerance to valerian or becoming dependent on it," says Dr. Page-Echols. "In some cases of mild anxiety, people would do just as well taking a little valerian as opposed to a prescription drug."

If you're already taking sedatives or antidepressants, however, speak with your physician before taking valerian or trying to switch solely to the herb. Not everyone reacts to it in the same way, warns Dr. Merrell. "Valerian affects some people quite strongly. It really sedates them. For others, it's just the opposite: They actually become agitated after taking it. In general, though the herb has few side effects."

Still a Mystery

Although researchers have been studying valerian for many years to determine the effective ingredient, they have discovered that many chemicals contribute to its actions. The plant contains a volatile oil, which includes valeric acid and valerenal, and alkaloids known as valepotriates.

Scientists do know that valerian alkaloids seem to lower blood pressure, and there is some evidence from animal studies that valeric acid and valerenal may be most responsible for the herb's sedating qualities. That's why, in the drugstore or health food store, you're likely to see valerian supplements and tinctures standardized to a specific percentage of essential oils or valeric acid. That's only a best guess, however. It may be that several ingredients are involved or that the ingredients act synergistically, interacting with each other to create the herb's calming properties.

Many herbalists contend that herbs work best in their whole form and disagree with the notion that there is one best, most active compound in any plant. "Plants are wondrous and perfect combinations of numerous substances—some flashy active constituents and scores of enzymes, vitamins, minerals, and other compounds that all work in harmony with one another," Dr. Stansbury notes.

Knowing how valerian works from the Western scientific perspective may not be all that important right now, says Joe Selvester, an Ayurvedic herbalist in Gainesville, Florida. In Ayurveda, the herb has been used for thousands of years for vertigo, fainting, and hysteria as well as to calm muscle spasms and alleviate menstrual cramps. "In my opinion, this is one of the herbs that you should have in your medicine chest at home, just as you would aspirin," he says.

zinc

Scan a list of the health problems associated with poor zinc intake, and you'll get an immediate sense of this essential mineral's wide and varied roles in the body.

When children lack zinc in their diets, researchers have found, they tend to grow more slowly than normal, and their sexual maturity is delayed. Zinc deprivation has also been linked to poor appetite, decreased resistance to infection, slow wound healing, infertility, and low hormone levels, especially in men. Some people with zinc deficiency experience hair loss, skin and nail problems, taste and smell difficulties, night blindness, and ulcers on the surface of the eyes, among other ailments.

The deficiency doesn't have to be drastic for some of these problems to appear. "The body's immune system seems particularly sensitive to zinc status," says Philip Reeves, Ph.D., research chemist with the U.S. Department of Agriculture Human Nutrition Research Center in Grand Forks, North Dakota. "Even a mild deficiency can cause immunity problems, and a severe deficiency can have devastating effects."

Zinc is needed by more than 300 enzymes, the spark plugs that get chemical reactions going in our bodies. It's found in every organ and every tissue—anyplace there is protein—because it is needed for the process of making protein.

Producing Protein

Since protein is needed to make tissues such as skin and muscles, it's no surprise that a zinc shortage leads to slow wound healing, skin breakdown, or muscle loss. Additionally, it is used for immune cells that fight infection; hormones that regulate growth, appetite, and sex drive; neurotransmitters that allow our various body parts to communicate with one another; and even the pigments in the backs of our eyes that allow us to see.

Zinc's role in protein processing is varied. In some cases, proteins called zinc fingers reach out and grab specific parts of DNA so that it can begin the process of making other proteins. Zinc also helps to retrieve and copy the "recipe"—the amino acid sequence—for a particular protein from the cell's genetic material.

Zinc also participates when a cell needs to produce a copy of its genes as it prepares to divide. "Some enzymes that string together the bits that make up the long chains of DNA and RNA are zinc-dependent," Dr. Reeves says. "When these enzymes don't work correctly, a cell's genetic material isn't made." When there's a lack of genetic material, he points out, there's

SUPPLEMENT SNAPSHOT

▶Zinc

May help: Macular degeneration, cataracts, male infertility associated with low hormone levels, hair loss, wound healing, impotence, prostate problems, dermatitis, canker sores, bedsores, loss of appetite, low immunity, taste and smell problems, genital herpes, binge-eating disorder, osteoarthritis, HIV, and inflammatory conditions such as lupus and rheumatoid arthritis. Zinc throat lozenges may help treat colds.

Daily Value: 15 milligrams.

Special instructions: Take with food to reduce stomach irritation, but avoid taking with a lot of high-fiber foods, since fiber interferes with absorption. Calcium also interferes, so if your calcium intake from food and supplements is 1,200 milligrams daily, you should take 18 milligrams or more of zinc every day. Absorption can also be compromised by large amounts of iron; for best results, do not get more than 30 milligrams of iron daily from food and supplements. Since large amounts of zinc impair copper absorption, get 1 milligram of copper for every 10 milligrams of zinc.

Who's at risk for deficiency: Pregnant women, infants, elderly people who don't eat well, vegetarians, people with diabetes, and alcoholics.

Good food sources: Cooked oysters, clams, crab, red meat, poultry, fish, and beans.

Cautions and possible side effects: Do not take more than 20 milligrams a day of zinc (and no more than 2 milligrams a day of copper) unless directed by your physician.

a general slowdown in growth and tissue maintenance because new cells aren't being produced. There is a drop-off in the production of immune system cells and a breakdown in muscle and skin tissue.

Antioxidant Protection

Zinc is needed to make an important antioxidant enzyme called zinc-copper superoxide dismutase. Like vitamins E and C—other antioxidants that your body needs—this enzyme helps neutralize free radicals, the free-roaming, unstable molecules that can cause a chain reaction of damage throughout your body. "Superoxide dismutase is found in every cell in the body, but it's especially concentrated in the liver and kidneys, where it helps to neutralize toxins before they have a chance to cause problems," Dr. Reeves says.

Your lungs also get the support of this enzyme, which they need because they're constantly exposed to potentially damaging oxygen. Your eyes, too, get some protection from superoxide dismutase, as it helps shield them from the effects of ultraviolet light.

Zinc also helps to stabilize the structure of cell membranes, says Dr. Reeves. That's an important role because the membranes that surround cells act as a kind of security system. When they are intact and working right, they help to carefully regulate what goes in and out of a cell. Needed nutrients go in, and wastes go out.

"Zinc-dependent enzymes help to protect both proteins and fats in the membrane from being damaged by oxygen," Dr. Reeves observes.

If a cell's normally fluidlike membrane is damaged, though, it becomes rigid, interfering with the necessary flow of nutrients and wastes into and out of the cell. Specific receptor sites and transport systems—a cell's loading platforms—don't work. "The receptor sites for insulin, for instance, are one type that may be protected by zinc," Dr. Reeves says.

Are You Getting Enough?

Our bodies try to conserve zinc if we're not eating much, and we absorb more zinc from foods when it's available. "The absence of evidence of deficiency suggests that most people in the United States do get enough zinc, even if they're not always getting the Daily Value," says Janet Hunt, R.D., Ph.D., also with the USDA research center in North Dakota. In the United

States, people average about 10 milligrams a day of zinc, two-thirds of the Daily Value of 15 milligrams. Most of that comes from meat, fish, and poultry.

So who's most likely to be short on zinc? Vegetarians who aren't getting enough good nonmeat sources of zinc, such as beans; older people who simply aren't eating enough food; and people on diets that shortchange them on numerous nutrients. Severe zinc deficiency is also a well-known complication of alcohol abuse.

If you're taking a zinc supplement, you don't need to worry about the form of zinc in the tablet, Dr. Hunt says. Most commercial forms are readily absorbed and utilized.

Mingling Your Metals

Zinc can interfere with copper absorption at amounts as low as 20 milligrams a day, so you should get 1 milligram of copper for every 10 milligrams of zinc that you take in through diet or supplements. Most people don't need to take more than 15 milligrams of supplemental zinc and 1.5 milligrams of copper a day, Dr. Hunt says. These amounts of zinc and copper are available in many multivitamin/mineral supplements.

Large amounts of iron can interfere with your ability to absorb zinc, so if you are taking supplemental iron to correct iron-deficiency anemia, you should take it separately from any zinc supplements, Dr. Hunt says.

3

fighting disease
with
supplements

Alzheimer's disease and memory loss

Your brain is a vital organ, and like the other vital organs in your body, it can be damaged by poor diet, stress, exposure to toxins, and aging.

Just like your heart, your brain won't work as well if cholesterol deposits or high blood pressure damages the arteries that supply its blood. In fact, a study from the Netherlands found that the same high-saturated-fat diet raises your risk of having a heart attack or stroke also makes you more prone to developing dementia. That word doesn't mean demented, exactly. But dementia does include age-related memory impairment and Alzheimer's disease.

"What works for the heart, works for the brain, with some modifications," says Dharma Singh Khalsa, M.D., president and medical director of the Alzheimer's Prevention Foundation in Tucson and co-author of *Brain Longevity*. That's why many of the nutritional supplements recommended to shield your brain from age-related memory impairment also offer protection from heart disease.

"Memory loss used to be considered a somewhat normal occurrence with age, but it isn't," says Dr. Khalsa. "People don't have to inevitably decline."

Some researchers regard Alzheimer's disease as a kind of a subcategory of normal memory loss that's associated with aging, Dr. Khalsa says. "Experts now think that there is a continuum from age-associated memory loss into Alzheimer's disease, at least in some people."

Other researchers aren't so sure. When people have Alzheimer's disease, microscopic changes occur in the brain, and those changes are somewhat different from the changes seen in people who have declining memories as a result of the aging process, says Jay Lombard, M.D., assistant clinical professor of neurology at Weill Medical College of Cornell University in New York City and co-author of *The Brain Wellness Plan*. There's also a genetic component to Alzheimer's disease, so your risk may be higher if a parent or grandparent had it.

Some forgetfulness—and even some memory loss—doesn't mean that you're on the brink of Alzheimer's disease. In fact, there are a number of ways that you may be able to slow the progression, Dr. Khalsa says. "Reducing stress is really important because stress may be the main cause of memory problems in people under age 40," he says. The amount of sleep you get and the quality of your diet can also have a major impact on how fast your brain can compute.

Even exercise can protect your brain. One study showed that people who were least active from the ages of 20 to 59 were 2½ times more likely to have Alzheimer's disease than those who were most active.

Nutritional supplements or herbs can also help. Some can protect neurons in the brain from being damaged by free radicals. Unstable molecules can harm cells, and free radicals can sometimes prevent the breakdown of the important messenger chemicals called neurotransmitters, says Dr. Khalsa. Other supplements can actually stimulate the production of neurotransmitters. If you want to give your memory a boost, here's what is recommended.

Save Your Brain with Ginkgo

Ginkgo has long been used to improve mental function. In Europe, an extract of this herb is an approved treatment for dementia, including that caused by Alzheimer's disease. The first clinical study done in the United States found that 120 milligrams daily of ginkgo extract not only stabilized Alzheimer's disease but also led to significant improvements in mental function in 20 percent of the patients. The concentration used was standardized to 24 percent ginkgoflavoglycosides and 6 percent terpenelactones, which are believed to be the active agents. There were no side effects.

Ginkgo also acts as a potent antioxidant, says Dr. Lombard, so it can help to protect your brain from oxidative damage due to aging, heart disease, or toxins. It can also inhibit the breakdown of some kinds of neurotransmitters that are involved in mood and memory and enhance the release of others.

Ginkgo can be used to treat the early stages of Alzheimer's and to protect against further damage. Dr. Lombard recommends twice-daily doses of 120 milligrams of extract standardized to 24 percent ginkgoflavoglycosides. Don't expect immediate results, however. It may take up to six months of taking ginkgo consistently before the benefits begin to show.

Antioxidants Prevent "Brain Rust"

Our brains are prone to damage from free radicals just like the rest of our bodies. When they damage brain cells, we pay the price with memory loss. In addition, the immune system reacts to the damage with a process

Chinese Moss
May Help Restore Memory

D. Aug ??

A natural substance extracted from a rare moss found in the cold climates of China is being sold in the United States as a nutritional supplement that may alleviate symptoms of Alzheimer's disease.

Called Huperzine A, this substance can be extracted from the club moss *Huperzia serrata*, which has been used for centuries in China to treat fever and inflammation, says Alan Kozikowski, Ph.D., director of the drug discovery program at Georgetown Institute of Cognitive and Computational Sciences at Georgetown University Medical Center in Washington, D.C.

Huperzine A works by interfering with an enzyme that influences acetylcholine, an important brain neurotransmitter. An Alzheimer's drug on the market, donepezil hydrochloride (Aricept), works the same way. "Preventing the breakdown of acetylcholine allows the small amount that is present in the brain to exert its benefits so you can retrieve memories or form new ones," says Dr. Kozikowski. Several studies have shown that Huperzine A improves brain function in patients with dementia.

Huperzine A seems to have additional properties that may help it to slow the progression of Alzheimer's, Dr. Kozikowski says. One study showed that it can slow the formation of a harmful kind of plaque, a buildup of protein deposits in the brain. Other studies indicate that it can protect brain cells from glutamate, a neurotransmitter that becomes toxic when it is secreted in large amounts. Scientists suspect that the brain releases these super-high secretions when it's low on oxygen. Some research also indicates that Huperzine A helps to block the process of inflammation that occurs as Alzheimer's disease progresses, Dr. Kozikowski says.

The amount of Huperzine A used in the Chinese studies was four 50-microgram tablets a day. The dosage currently being recommended on the product sold in the United States is just half that amount—two 50-microgram tablets a day. More research on Huperzine A is currently under way in the United States, says Dr. Kozikowski.

that actually generates even more free radicals, so there's a cascade of free radical production. One study by Canadian researchers found evidence of significantly more free radicals than normal in samples of brain tissue from people with Alzheimer's disease.

There is good reason to believe that antioxidant nutrients, especially vitamin E, can help prevent damage to brain cells, Dr. Khalsa says. Vitamin E protects signal-sensitive neurons in the brain from free radical damage. Certain areas of the neurons, called neurotransmitter receptor sites, benefit from some fix-it work when vitamin E is present, he notes, "so vitamin E can not only prevent deterioration of the brain, it also actually reverses an important element of deterioration."

Vitamin E is fat-soluble, so it has a free pass around the brain, which contains a lot of fats. In its travels, vitamin E interacts with cell membranes, traps free radicals, and interrupts the rapid-fire chain reactions that produce even more free radicals. When scientists did animal studies using vitamin E, they found that this important antioxidant reduces the degeneration of cells in the hippocampus, which is precisely the part of the brain that's hit hardest by Alzheimer's. After blood flow was cut off for a time, vitamin E could help the cells recover, and it enhanced the recovery of motor function after spinal cord injury.

Some test-tube studies have also been done, and they suggest how vitamin E can do even more: It can help protect cells that have suffered from a lack of oxygen. It can also reduce cell death associated with a protein that causes damage in Alzheimer's disease.

A study that involved people with Alzheimer's showed some positive results when the participants took vitamin E. Recruited from 23 centers participating in the Alzheimer's Disease Cooperative Study, people with moderately severe disease received 2,000 international units (IU) a day of vitamin E for two years. According to researchers, those people survived an average of 230 days longer than those not getting supplements.

Both Dr. Lombard and Dr. Khalsa recommend taking antioxidant nutrients, including vitamin E. But they favor a mixture of antioxidants and less vitamin E than was used in the cooperative study. "If you are on an antioxidant program, you just don't need that much vitamin E," Dr. Khalsa says. "The antioxidants act synergistically, so 1 and 1 equals 11, not 2. A mixture of antioxidants is more effective than large amounts of just one."

Dr. Khalsa recommends 400 to 800 IU of vitamin E, 3,000 milligrams of vitamin C in divided doses, 10,000 to 25,000 IU of vitamin A, and 50 to 100 micrograms of selenium. In addition, he suggests that people take 100 to 200 milligrams a day of coenzyme Q_{10}, which acts as an antioxidant and helps energy production in cells throughout the body. With doses this high, however, it's important to have a doctor approve the supplement program.

Boost Your Brain with B Vitamins

Most of the B vitamins play a role in brain function. They help the breakdown of blood sugar, or glucose. Since the brain relies on a perpetual supply of glucose for energy, this is very important, Dr. Khalsa says.

Deficiencies of both vitamin B_{12} and folic acid have been associated with memory loss. When someone complains of problems with memory, a doctor usually begins an examination by checking for deficiencies of these vitamins, Dr. Khalsa says.

A study has helped establish the connection between these vitamins and Alzheimer's disease. Scientists at England's Oxford University and in Bergen, Norway, found that 76 Alzheimer's patients had lower blood levels of the two vitamins than 108 people of the same age with no signs of Alzheimer's symptoms. The researchers also found that the Alzheimer's patients had higher blood levels of homocysteine, an amino acid by-product that other studies have shown to be a factor in atherosclerosis (hardening of the arteries). This offers further support for supplementing with folic acid and B_{12}, since both are known to reduce homocysteine levels.

Diagnosing a deficiency of vitamin B_{12} can sometimes be difficult because a person can be low in the vitamin even if blood tests appear normal. Many doctors are now recommending a more sensitive screening to detect a B_{12} deficiency by measuring homocysteine levels. With some people who have Alzheimer's disease, homocysteine levels are abnormal, and Dr. Lombard has found that vitamin B_{12} treatment can be effective for them.

Since the B vitamins are generally beneficial, your best tactic may be to take a high-potency B-complex formula that includes 50 milligrams of most of the different kinds, Dr. Lombard says. Look for one that includes 1,000 micrograms of both vitamin B_{12} and folic acid along with the other ingredients.

A Memory Pill

Dr. Lombard suggests that people who have been diagnosed with Alzheimer's disease should also take 300 milligrams of a nutritional supplement called phosphatidylserine (PS) daily with meals. "Phosphatidylserine is an important component of cell membranes and helps cells in the brain to retain their fluidity—an important property for proper function," he says.

Several studies have shown PS to be helpful for age-related memory decline, Alzheimer's disease, or depression. In one six-month study, a group of people with moderate to severe senility were given three daily 100-

milligram doses of PS. In another group with similar symptoms, partici- pants received inactive pills (placebos). Researchers assessed both groups to measure their mental performance and behavior at the beginning and end of the study. Significant improvements were noted in the mental function and behavior of members of the group receiving PS.

The substance used in these studies was derived from cow brains. Since reports of mad cow disease began surfacing in the mid-1990s, cow brains are no longer considered a safe source, says Dr. Khalsa. The PS that is now on the market is derived from soybeans. "It appears to be pretty much the same and to have the same benefit, but there are no published studies to confirm that," he says.

Memory Aid from Acetyl-L-Carnitine *not as preventative*

Acetyl-l-carnitine, derived from the natural substance l-carnitine, is structurally similar to the memory neurotransmitter acetlylcholine and dis- plays similar actions in the brain, Dr. Lombard says.

Acetyl-l-carnitine protects nerve cell membranes from free radical at- tack. It also is essential for the production of energy in brain cells and helps transport fatty acids into the cells' tiny power plants, the mitochondria.

Several studies have shown that acetyl-l-carnitine is helpful for people with Alzheimer's disease, Dr. Lombard says. One multicenter study was done with 357 people age 55 or older who had Alzheimer's. It showed that the memories of those 65 or younger who received 3,000 milligrams of l-carnitine a day didn't decline as quickly as those of a comparative group of people who weren't given the supplement.

Dr. Lombard suggests 2,000 milligrams of acetyl-l-carnitine daily for treatment of people with mild to moderate memory loss. Take this supple- ment between meals, he advises.

As for using this supplement as a preventive, Dr. Khalsa advises against it. "It makes a lot of people feel overstimulated," he says.

anemia

If your blood doesn't contain enough red blood cells, you have anemia. You can also have anemia if you have enough red blood cells, but they just aren't doing their jobs. If they aren't carrying sufficient hemoglobin—the iron-rich red protein that transports oxygen—you'll have anemia just as surely as if you had a shortage.

The symptoms are noticeable, although at first you might not give them much attention. You'll probably look pale and feel pretty tired, but it's easy to write off these signs as the results of stress or of not getting enough sleep.

But maybe there's another reason for feeling drained: Perhaps your blood isn't delivering the oxygen needed to create energy. If you feel weak and short of breath, if your heart beats faster, and you find it hard to concentrate, it's time to ask your doctor to take a blood sample. It may take no more than a few minutes to find out whether your blood's falling down on the job.

The first thing your doctor needs to do is figure out why you are anemic. Anemia is often related to blood loss, says Michael DiPalma, N.D., a naturopathic doctor and director of natural medicine at the Village of Newtown Medical Center in Pennsylvania. For menstruating women, it may mean that they are losing more blood each month than their bodies are able to resupply.

Anemia could indicate blood loss from the intestinal tract, a bleeding ulcer, hemorrhoids, or even cancer. That's why it's important to get a proper diagnosis from your doctor. He will want to order a full laboratory evaluation appropriate for your specific symptoms. If internal bleeding is suspected, for example, he may check a stool sample for blood in addition to taking a blood sample for a complete blood count.

It's also possible that a nutritional deficiency is interfering with your body's ability to make new red blood cells, Dr. DiPalma says. "Iron deficiency is the most common, and it's possible to become iron-deficient if you're regularly losing blood or if you aren't getting much iron in your

Add to Your Iron with Yellow Dock

One problem with iron supplements is their tendency to cause constipation. That's why one popular herbal tonic for iron-deficiency anemia, Floradex, includes an herb called yellow dock. While the herb is a source of iron, it also produces a gentle laxative effect. Thus, while it's contributing to your body's stores of iron, it can also help counter supplemental iron's constipating tendencies, says Michael DiPalma, N.D., a naturopathic doctor and director of natural medicine at the Village at Newtown Medical Center in Pennsylvania.

"Yellow dock wouldn't be used alone to treat anemia, but it can be a helpful addition," says Dr. DiPalma. You shouldn't self-treat anemia without your doctor's approval, however.

diet." Other nutrients may play additional roles. Here are the things that you need to know.

Iron Out Anemia

Hemoglobin is so dependent on iron that your blood cells will look pale under a microscope if iron is lacking. And you must have healthy hemoglobin. It's the Federal Express of your blood cells, constantly picking up oxygen in the lungs and delivering it rapidly to be released in tissues where oxygen is low.

Your doctor can easily check your iron levels with blood tests, including a serum ferritin test, which can detect depleted iron stores before you actually become anemic, Dr. DiPalma says. Iron deficiency may be caused by increased iron requirements during pregnancy, an adolescent growth spurt, or heavy menstrual bleeding. It could also be a sign that you've severely decreased your dietary intake of iron—if you've gone on a diet, for instance, or switched to vegetarian meals without paying attention to the foods that provide iron.

Less commonly, the deficiency may be the result of absorption problems. You may even be donating blood more often than your body can handle. Often, the reason turns out to be a combination of factors, Dr. DiPalma says.

If your doctor determines that you are short on iron, you will need to take supplements until your anemia resolves, and then some. That is, you not only need to restore normal levels of iron, you also need to build up some excess in your system for future demands.

The amounts of iron used to correct anemia can vary widely. Some doctors initially prescribe large amounts—200 to 325 milligrams a day, usually in the form of ferrous sulfate, which is not easily absorbed and may lead to constipation. Others, such as Dr. DiPalma, use smaller amounts of a more absorbable form.

Dr. DiPalma often recommends that his patients take 30 milligrams of iron succinate or iron fumarate twice a day between meals. Or, if these supplements cause stomach upset, he may advise taking them with meals. He may also recommend an aqueous (liquid) liver extract because it provides heme iron, a natural food form that's also easily absorbed.

You should avoid using enteric-coated iron tablets or capsules containing slow-release granules, experts say. Both can interfere with the body's ability to absorb iron. Also, make sure that you continue your treatment for a sufficient period of time, under your doctor's supervision. Although your anemia will be corrected in 3 to 4 months, it takes an additional 6 to 12 months of therapy for iron stores to be replenished.

The B$_{12}$ Connection

A shortage of vitamin B$_{12}$ causes its own form of anemia, called pernicious anemia. Until 1934, this form was invariably fatal. That year, two Boston doctors demonstrated that a diet rich in barely cooked liver, which is rich in B$_{12}$, could ward off the deadly deficiency.

Since the symptoms of this type of anemia resemble those of other types, your doctor will need to do a blood test to figure out what's really going on, Dr. DiPalma says. If you do have a B$_{12}$ deficiency, your red blood cells suffer from what is called maturation arrest. They grow large, but they never mature into properly working cells. In fact, they may never make it out of the bone marrow, where red blood cells are normally created and released into your blood.

Doctors no longer recommend liver to correct a B$_{12}$ deficiency. Because liver is high in cholesterol, it can cause other health problems. Instead, you'll need supplemental B$_{12}$ to correct a deficiency. This deficiency is uncommon, however, except in people who are strict vegetarians (ve-

Liver without the Cholesterol

Calf's liver, and lots of it, used to be *the* remedy for anemia. Liver is loaded with an easily absorbed form of iron, plus it has lots of B vitamins and other minerals that stimulate the production of red blood cells. It also has some things that you don't want, however—it's high in cholesterol, and if you eat enough of it, you can exceed the recommended limits for fat-soluble vitamins A and D.

That's where aqueous extracts of liver come in. These liquid extracts are free of cholesterol and fat-soluble vitamins but are loaded with iron, vitamins B_6 and B_{12}, folate, riboflavin, copper, vitamin C, and protein, says Michael DiPalma, N.D., a naturopathic doctor and director of natural medicine at the Village of Newtown Medical Center in Pennsylvania. "These are all things that your body needs to rebuild blood."

Some doctors may think the use of liver therapy to treat anemia is a shotgun approach, but to others, "shotgun" is right on target. "It's really a whole-foods approach, which works better at resolving anemia than any single supplement," Dr. DiPalma says.

Concentrations vary, so follow the dosage directions on the liver extract label—and let your doctor know that you're taking it.

gans) or whose bodies have lost the ability to absorb vitamin B_{12}, Dr. DiPalma says. Absorption problems are most likely in older people with reduced stomach acid or those who have had stomach surgery. People who have Crohn's disease or other stomach or intestinal problems may also be susceptible.

Injections are one way to maintain adequate blood levels of B_{12}, Dr. DiPalma says, but some people without absorption problems can correct a deficiency by taking oral doses of 2,000 micrograms daily for at least one month. He advises taking methylcobalamin, the active form of B_{12}. After the first month, Dr. DiPalma has his patients take 1,000 micrograms daily. This form of B_{12} is taken sublingually—that is, under the tongue.

Other oral forms of B_{12} work well for some people, says Alan Gaby, M.D., professor of nutrition at Bastyr University in Bothell, Washington. You should follow this regimen under your doctor's supervision; he can determine whether you're absorbing as much B_{12} as you need.

The Folic Acid Factor

If you don't get enough folic acid, another B vitamin, your blood cells don't reach maturity. Instead, they become large, immature, egg-shaped cells that can't do their jobs well.

Folate (the naturally occurring form of folic acid) is found mostly in fruits and vegetables, so you're short-changing yourself if you're getting along on a very skimpy diet without those nutritional essentials. You might be short on folic acid during pregnancy, says Dr. DiPalma, and celiac disease or Crohn's disease can contribute to deficiency as well, he notes.

Unlike vitamin B_{12}, folic acid is not stored in large amounts in your liver. The liver's supply is used up within two to four months if none of the nutrient is incoming, so symptoms of this type of anemia can occur much more quickly than those of vitamin B_{12} deficiency. And it's not just anemia that shows up. A deficiency of folic acid can cause diarrhea; gingivitis; depression; cervical dysplasia; a swollen, red tongue; and elevated levels of homocysteine, an amino acid by-product that has been shown by research to be an independent risk factor for heart disease.

It takes only a blood test to determine if you are short on folic acid. "You may need large amounts of supplemental folic acid until blood levels are restored," Dr. DiPalma says. He recommends that his patients take 800 to 1,200 micrograms a day. High amounts of folic acid can affect the laboratory diagnosis of pernicious anemia, however, which means that some B_{12}-deficiency nerve damage could worsen even though the deficiency goes undetected. You should check with your doctor if you think you are deficient and want to take a supplement.

Add a Multi

In addition to iron, B_{12}, or folic acid, it's best to take a good multivitamin/mineral supplement when you're working to restore blood supplies, Dr. DiPalma says. For example, your body needs copper along with iron to make hemoglobin, and vitamin C helps many parts of the body function at their best, so look for a supplement that has these two nutrients. "People tend to get better faster when they are on a comprehensive program," Dr. DiPalma says.

angina

When you have angina, the pressurelike pain in your chest is more of a warning signal than a cry for help. It's usually a sign that something isn't right in the spaghetti-size arteries that deliver blood to your heart muscle.

That firm, relentless squeeze often means that the arteries have been narrowed by cholesterol-laden plaque. As plaque starts to clog those all-important pipelines, blood flow is reduced. When the arteries are starved of hearty red blood, with its supply of oxygen and nutrients, they are more likely to go into spasm, which reduces blood flow even more.

That squeezing in your chest is a tip-off that your heart muscle isn't getting enough oxygen-laden blood to meet its needs. Often, the attack hits when some other part of your body needs increased blood flow to feed your muscles or warm up your limbs. Maybe you've been exercising or are under a lot of stress. It can also occur in cold weather or after a big meal.

People with angina need to be on the same low-fat, high-fiber diet that lowers cholesterol, says Decker Weiss, N.M.D., a naturopathic doctor at the Arizona Heart Institute in Phoenix. He also recommends that his patients take a variety of supplements that may reduce the risk of heart disease.

Traditionally, physicians treat angina with medications such as nitroglycerin that improve blood flow to the heart. If the blockage is bad enough, a doctor might recommend an artery-opening procedure such as angioplasty or bypass surgery.

Certain nutrients and herbs, however, can also improve blood flow to the heart and enhance energy production in the muscle cells. With the aid of these nutrients, the heart muscle can work better even though blood supply is reduced, Dr. Weiss says.

If you have a history of angina, your doctor will want you to keep a medication such as nitroglycerin on hand, and, of course, you need to check with your doctor first about taking supplements. But many people are drawn to alternative treatments by the prospect of avoiding procedures such as angioplasty and bypass surgery. By taking helpful nutrients and pursuing other measures to ensure good heart health, you may be able to clear up the symptoms of angina and its causes as well, says Dr. Weiss.

Ease the Squeeze with Magnesium

At the top of Dr. Weiss's prescription list for angina is magnesium, a mineral that helps relax the muscles that wrap around blood vessels.

In several studies, intravenous magnesium was effective in stopping a type of angina characterized by spasms in the coronary arteries. In a British study that addressed another type of angina, intravenous magnesium again showed its power. People who received the magnesium had fewer angina episodes than those who didn't receive it.

"Magnesium dilates the coronary arteries, improving oxygen delivery to the heart," Dr. Weiss says. It also plays an important role in energy production in all cells, so magnesium is especially important to heart muscle cells, which are high energy producers, he says.

Magnesium deficiency can be induced by drugs meant to help heart problems, including diuretics, which help your body excrete excess fluid. You also have to watch out for deficiency caused by the commonly prescribed digitalis heart medications digitoxin (Crystodigin) and digoxin (Lanoxin). Signs of magnesium deficiency include muscle weakness, nausea, and irritability.

If you have angina, you probably have heart disease, so it's best to consult a doctor who's knowledgeable in nutrition before taking supplemental magnesium. Dr. Weiss recommends two forms—magnesium orotate and magnesium glycinate—but check with your doctor before you settle on a dosage of either.

Get Some 10, 6, and 3

Coenzyme Q_{10} is a vitamin-like substance that plays an essential role in producing energy. CoQ_{10}, as it's commonly called, actually increases oxygen delivery to heart muscle cells. For anyone with angina, it's a supplement to consider.

In one study, 12 people with one type of angina who took 150 milligrams of coQ_{10} daily for four weeks cut the frequency of angina attacks in half compared with a group taking inactive, look-alike pills (placebos).

If you're buying coQ$_{10}$ for the first time, you might wonder which kind to use—gel capsules or tablets. Since coQ$_{10}$ is fat-soluble, the gel capsules are more potent and more readily absorbed than the tablet form. If you opt for tablets, chew them with a fat-containing food such as peanut butter to maximize absorption.

Doctors also recommend two kinds of fatty acids—omega-3's and omega-6's—for people who have angina. These are found in fish oil, flaxseed oil, cold-pressed safflower or sunflower oil, and borage oil. "I recommend 1,000 to 3,000 milligrams a day of a mixture of these two essential fatty acids," Dr. Weiss says.

Experts also advise people with angina to cut back on saturated fats (those that are solid at room temperature), hydrogenated fats (margarine and shortening), and polyunsaturated fats (corn oil).

Get Help from Ginkgo and Amino Acids

"I absolutely recommend ginkgo for angina," says Dr. Weiss, noting that the herbal supplement can help stimulate blood flow around the damaged area of the heart.

Ginkgo also helps prevent platelets from sticking together, says Dr. Weiss. Platelets are components in blood that promote clotting, and they can also pile up at a site where an artery has been clogged by cholesterol. Dr. Weiss recommends 60 milligrams of ginkgo biloba extract (standardized to 24 percent ginkgoflavoglycosides) up to three times a day.

Another possible alternative for people who have angina is amino acids. These include carnitine, taurine, and arginine, Dr. Weiss says.

"Carnitine is vital, and I recommend it because many people with heart disease need extra carnitine to utilize the essential fatty acids that their hearts need," Dr. Weiss says. This amino acid helps transport fatty acids into the mitochondria, the tiny areas within cells where energy is produced. Supplemental carnitine may help the heart muscle better utilize its limited supply of oxygen, studies show.

The daily therapeutic dose for carnitine is 1,500 to 3,000 milligrams for an average person. Take three divided doses a day, advises Dr. Weiss.

Taurine is also important for the normal function of the heart and vascular system, says Dr. Weiss. It's the most abundant amino acid found in the heart. In Japan, taurine is widely used to treat various types of heart disease.

Arginine is involved in the production of nitric oxide, a compound formed by the cells that line the arteries. With increased nitric oxide, the arteries can relax and dilate, which helps augment blood flow to crucial heart muscle.

Your best bet for using these amino acids? Ask your doctor to recommend a formula that contains a balanced mixture. Recommended doses will vary depending on your current and past history of heart disease.

Hawthorn Helps Your Heart

Hawthorn is an herb with a long history of use for heart problems, with good reason. It improves the blood supply to the heart by dilating coronary arteries and aids the transformation of food into energy in your heart muscle cells. The herb can help eliminate some types of arrhythmia (irregular heartbeat), says Dr. Weiss.

"It is a wonderful herb for atherosclerosis," he says. Since atherosclerosis (hardening of the arteries) is a buildup of artery-blocking plaque, it leads to angina. "Taking hawthorn can lower the frequency, duration, and severity of angina."

Hawthorn takes two weeks to a month to work. It is available in several different forms, Dr. Weiss says. A typical tonic dose is ¼ teaspoon of liquid extract taken two or three times a day. Many people stir this syrupy extract of hawthorn berries into a glass of hot water. If you prefer a tincture, take 30 to 60 drops daily. For capsules, take 160 milligrams three times a day. If you have a heart condition, however, check with your doctor before taking hawthorn.

Nutrients That Ease Angina

Certain vital nutrients help prevent cholesterol buildup in arteries and protect the cells lining blood vessels from damage that makes blockage more likely. These protective nutrients include vitamins C and E and the trace mineral selenium. "I routinely suggest these nutrients to someone with angina," Dr. Weiss says.

In a study, supplements of vitamin E, along with vitamin C, vitamin A, and beta-carotene, reduced the incidence of angina. Vitamin E affects both cholesterol and platelets in a way that reduces the risk of heart disease, Dr. Weiss explains. He recommends 400 to 800 international units (IU) a day.

Vitamin C helps keep blood vessels open because it prevents the breakdown of nitric oxide, which helps promote blood flow, says Dr. Weiss.

Selenium, when teamed with vitamin E, can also offer some protection from angina. One study found that people with heart disease who took 200 IU of vitamin E and 1,000 micrograms (a very large dose) of selenium had a significant reduction in angina pain compared with people taking placebos. Doses of selenium over 200 micrograms must be taken with a doctor's supervision.

Doctors who recommend selenium supplements to their heart patients generally stick with no more than 50 to 200 micrograms a day. You'll also want to make sure that you're getting about 400 micrograms of folic acid, along with 1,000 micrograms of vitamin B_{12} and 50 to 100 milligrams of vitamin B_6, says Dr. Weiss. These B vitamins help your body process homocysteine, an amino acid by-product that can damage arteries by creating rough spots on artery walls that can pick up fatty deposits.

Bromelain and Curcumin: The Anti-Angina Duo

Dr. Weiss may also use a mixture of bromelain, a protein-dissolving enzyme found in pineapple, and curcumin, the yellow pigment in turmeric, for people with angina. Bromelain helps reduce the formation of fibrous tissue and clots in damaged arteries, and curcumin acts somewhat like aspirin, he says. It helps to reduce the tendency for blood to clot and also reduces inflammation.

For the best therapeutic effect, Dr. Weiss recommends divided doses. A standard dose of bromelain is 125 to 450 milligrams three times a day on an empty stomach, he says. Do not take bromelain with food, though, or it will simply act as a digestive enzyme.

Usual doses of curcumin are 400 to 600 milligrams a day, Dr. Weiss says. Ask your doctor what dosage is best for you.

asthma

Asthmatic lungs are oversensitive to triggers such as airborne allergens, exercise, cold air, emotional stress, and even certain foods. When an asthma attack hits, breathing passageways are narrowed, making precious oxygen scarce. Spasms in the bronchial tubes cause tightness in the chest and fits of coughing. And when inflammation lingers in the lungs, you'll start wheezing.

Chronic asthma is often treated with medications that are inhaled directly so the medicine reaches the air sacs in the lungs. If you have asthma, these drugs may help you breathe better. But they also offer their share of side effects.

If you use medication to control your asthma, supplements may help you gradually reduce the amount of medication you're taking. Giving these supplements a try may restore healthy breathing in a safe and natural way, but get your doctor's approval before taking supplements for asthma.

Try Magnesium for Immediate Relief

Quite a bit of research has linked magnesium with the improvement of asthma symptoms. One study at City Hospital in Nottingham, England, found that making an effort to take more magnesium can have a positive effect on asthma in a very short time.

Seventeen people took either 400 milligrams of magnesium or a look-alike supplement without magnesium (a placebo) for several three-week periods. Symptoms were significantly fewer when people in the study were getting the supplemental magnesium.

"Magnesium definitely has an antispasmodic effect on the smooth muscle of the upper respiratory tract," says Claudia Cooke, M.D., a holistic doctor in New York City. Since asthma is aggravated or worsened by spasms in the smooth muscles, which are involuntary muscles, magnesium's antispasmodic effects can be beneficial.

For an asthma attack, Dr. Cooke recommends taking 600 milligrams of magnesium along with any medications that have been prescribed by your doctor. If you get relief, she suggests, continue with a daily supplement of 600 milligrams, but don't take this much if you have any kidney problems or low blood pressure.

Keep Exercising—And Breathing— With Vitamin C

Asthma that's brought on by bouts of exercise can be particularly troubling for folks who are trying to stay fit. According to a study at Tel Aviv University in Israel, vitamin C may be able to prevent attacks among people who have exercise-induced asthma.

In the study, some people were given 2,000 milligrams of vitamin C one hour before they stepped on a treadmill for a workout. When researchers compared those who got the vitamin C to those who didn't, they discovered that those receiving the supplements showed less hyperreactivity in their airways. The results were probably due to vitamin C's ability to squelch certain inflammatory substances that are produced by overreactive lung cells.

It's smart to take vitamin C even if your asthma isn't exercise induced. People with asthma who get the lowest amounts of vitamin C have significantly more bronchial activity in general. For this reason, Dr. Cooke urges anyone with asthma to take vitamin C supplements. Take at least 2,000 milligrams a day in divided doses, suggests Dr. Cooke. If you start to get diarrhea from a dose this high, you should gradually reduce the dose until this side effect goes away.

Keep Inflammation Down with Omega-3 Oils

One of the newest pharmaceutical weapons against asthma is a class of drugs called leukotriene inhibitors. They work by halting the actions of compounds produced in the body that cause bronchial constriction and other allergic reactions.

In an emergency situation, drugs like these are probably the quickest route to relief, but supplements of omega-3 fatty acids work by a similar anti-inflammatory mechanism. Moreover, they can be nearly as effective for long-term asthma control, says Joseph E. Pizzorno Jr., N.D., president emeritus of Bastyr University in Bothell, Washington.

Omega-3 fatty acids are found in the oils of certain fish, particularly cold-water fish such as tuna, mackerel, and salmon, and in the oils of some plants, including flax. Although our bodies don't produce omega-3's, and we have to get them from one or more of these outside sources, we normally get enough from our diets to ensure that we maintain good health.

A supplement of omega-3's can improve the balance of fats, says Dr. Pizzorno. "Most of us eat way too many saturated fats and not enough of the omega-3 type. You do need both kinds, ultimately, but you need them in balance with each other."

Over time, supplementing with omega-3 fatty acids can dramatically reduce asthmatic wheezing. Some doctors recommend a daily dose of 1,000 to 3,000 milligrams of omega-3 fats or two teaspoons of cod-liver oil. If you want to use flaxseed oil, one tablespoon a day is reasonable, but it may not be as effective as fish oil, doctors say.

Breathe Easier with Bioflavonoids

The best food for helping asthma? Eat more fruits and vegetables, says Dr. Pizzorno. That's because of the special "ingredients" found only in those types of foods. All of them contain bioflavonoids.

There are almost as many different kinds of bioflavonoids as there are colors in nature. "Basically, they're the bright pigments that you see in produce," says Dr. Pizzorno. But they're more than pretty colors.

Bioflavonoids are growth regulators in plants. When you eat bioflavonoids in foods, you get the benefit of their potent anti-inflammatory and anti-allergic properties.

Some of the bioflavonoids available as supplements include quercetin, pycnogenol, grapeseed extract, and ginkgo extract. You can take any of these singly or as a blended combination: Many mixtures and concentrations are available in drugstores and health food stores. For dosages, just check the label and follow the instructions on the particular bottle you choose, says Dr. Pizzorno.

Using Pollen Prevention

According to Dr. Cooke, bee pollen is a valuable supplement to consider. But not always. Some people are actually allergic to this substance. If you are among them, your asthma may get worse rather than better. So check with your doctor before you try this therapy.

"It works through a process of oral tolerization," says Dr. Cooke. By taking bee pollen regularly, you can actually enhance immunity to the airborne irritants that stimulate some asthma attacks. It may sound complex, but Dr. Cooke says respiratory symptoms can really improve.

Take up to two tablespoons of pollen a day, she says. Start with a few grains and slowly work up to this dose over a few weeks. You can sprinkle pollen granules over cereal or yogurt. Or you can make your own supplements by buying empty gelatin capsules at a health food store and simply filling them with premeasured amounts of pollen.

bedsores

Bedsores are the bane of the bedridden. People who get these skin ulcers, caused by poor circulation and inactivity, are usually in poor health or are immobilized in traction.

Their conditions make treatment somewhat difficult but not impossible. The ulcers can open, close, and heal, but you can actually identify a trouble spot before it opens: The skin area of an unopened bedsore is dark pink, red, or blotchy.

Whether you have bedsores yourself or are caring for someone who has them, some basic procedures can help the healing go as quickly as possible.

A bedsore, or pressure ulcer, usually occurs over a bony prominence such as a hip or elbow. The sores are caused either by the weight of the body remaining in one position for a long time or by shearing action that exerts pressure on the tissues beneath the skin. Continually sliding down while in a wheelchair or in bed puts extra pressure on the skin and may set the stage for bedsores.

Cleanliness is essential to help prevent infection, says Kathy Foulser, N.D., a naturopathic doctor at the Ridgefield Center for Integrative Medicine in Connecticut, so change the bedclothes as often as possible. Because urine or feces contribute to the breakdown of the skin, it's essential to keep the area around the sore dry and clean. To help promote healing, suggests Dr. Foulser, apply a poultice with a saline solution, which is simply a cloth dampened with a low-concentration, sterile salt solution like those made by Bausch and Lomb.

If you're caring for someone who has bedsores, move the person every couple of hours so the pressure isn't always on the same part of the body. In a hospital, someone on the nursing staff may gently flex and extend the patient's legs and help her to sit up and lie down, says Dr. Foulser.

It helps to put some protective padding over any areas where the skin is thin and bony prominences press against the bed or chair. And keep all areas of the body clean and dry, Dr. Foulser says. "You can also gently massage the area to stimulate circulation. Anything that gets the blood moving can help," she suggests.

Get Your Vitamins

All of this requires a lot of attention from the caregiver. In addition, there are some supplements that may help, says Dr. Foulser.

Immediately after someone becomes bedridden, taking 500 milligrams of vitamin C four times a day is a good idea, she says. If a sore develops, she advises upping the doses to 3,000 to 4,000 milligrams four times a day. You'll need to be alert to possible reactions from amounts of vitamin C higher than 1,200 milligrams a day, however, since such high doses can cause diarrhea in some people.

Vitamin C is a good antioxidant and immune system booster. It also helps prevent the breakdown of body tissues. Despite the protective qualities of this important vitamin, however, elderly people often don't get enough of it. When there's a deficiency of vitamin C, the skin may become thinner, the underlying capillaries may become more fragile, and bedsores may be more likely to develop.

Another antioxidant, vitamin E, is important for wound healing. It may help avert the breakdown of skin and underlying connective tissues that occurs with bedsores. Dr. Foulser recommends taking between 1,000 and 3,000 international units (IU) of vitamin E daily as a possible preventive. Start with 100 to 400 IU and work up slowly, after discussing the dosages with your doctor.

Vitamin E oil or gel from the herb aloe vera also makes a good poultice as a topical treatment. Place a thin layer of the oil or gel on a sterile gauze pad and place it directly on the sore for a couple of hours, suggests Dr. Foulser.

Minimize Infection

If a bedsore opens, there's a high risk of infection. Dr. Foulser recommends taking 50 milligrams of zinc three times a day for a few weeks. This is a very important mineral for boosting the immune system and speeding the healing process. Consult your doctor before taking doses higher than 20 milligrams.

If someone is bedridden, her immune system probably isn't very strong to begin with. When circulation is impeded, as it's likely to be in someone who's not moving much, the protective, infection-fighting white blood cells have difficulty reaching the wound, notes Dr. Foulser.

Whenever you take a zinc supplement, you also need a bit more copper, because zinc and copper work in opposition to one another, says Dr. Foulser. Taking zinc alone can cause a copper deficiency. "Usually, it's enough that the patient is taking a multivitamin that contains about two milligrams of copper. That should keep everything in balance," she says.

Stimulate Skin Repair

Zinc also works well in combination with vitamin A in treating open, uninfected bedsores. Zinc is needed by the skin to produce new cells and grow new layers of skin, while vitamin A is critical in helping the body regenerate and heal tissue.

A multivitamin/mineral supplement that contains the recommended daily amounts of vitamin A and zinc is a good way to start. (If you're taking a daily supplement, just check the label to see whether it provides 100 percent of the Daily Value.) Frequently, though, those amounts aren't enough, especially for someone who has problems with absorption or has a poor diet, says Dr. Foulser. "I recommend 50 milligrams of zinc and no more than 12,000 IU of vitamin A," she says. Before taking more than 10,000 IU a day, though, you should talk to your doctor.

binge-eating disorder

It's a vicious cycle.

First, an irresistible urge compels you to eat large amounts of food in one sitting. Days later, you're at it again, wolfing down bagfuls of potato chips, cookies, or whatever else you can get your hands on. Extreme feelings of guilt and distress follow each episode, but even that doesn't stop you from repeating this uncontrollable eating pattern over and over again. More than likely, you hide your behavior from everyone, choosing to suffer in silence.

If this pattern sounds familiar, you might be among the one to two million Americans who have binge-eating disorder. The hardest part may be looking for help.

When you are get used to hiding a problem like this, it's extremely difficult to tell anyone about it—even your own doctor. Nevertheless, the first thing you should do is see your physician. You need to be diagnosed—and to find out what your treatment options are—before taking any nutritional supplement, says Nancy Dunne Boggs, N.D., a naturopathic doctor in Missoula, Montana.

Most of those who have binge-eating disorder are obese, and the condition is slightly more common in women, affecting three women for every two men. What's more, binge eating is the most prevalent eating disorder among African-American women, which may explain why they're twice as likely as white women over 30 to be obese.

Research shows that mild to moderate depression is the most common cause, says Dr. Boggs, so it's important to treat the depression with medication and counseling. Practitioners of alternative medicine say that one of the best ways to treat the depression associated with binge eating is to take a variety of nutritional supplements. Some vitamins, minerals, herbs, and other natural compounds can increase the levels of certain brain chemicals, or neurotransmitters, that lift your mood, suppress your appetite, and eliminate cravings.

Bring in the Bs

Because binge eaters tend to consume large quantities of high-fat foods that have little or no nutritional value, many are deficient in important B-complex vitamins and the minerals chromium, magnesium, and zinc, says Susan Kowalsky, N.D., a naturopathic doctor in Norwich, Vermont.

The B vitamins are needed to manufacture important brain chemicals, such as serotonin, that are responsible for regulating your moods, emotions, sleep patterns, and appetite. Vitamin B_6, in particular, helps convert tryptophan (an amino acid found in many foods) to serotonin in your brain, says Dr. Kowalsky. Serotonin is one of the chemical messengers that has been closely associated with many emotional states, including depression.

Vitamin B_{12} also facilitates brain cell communication so that other neurotransmitters can work together to help relieve depression. In addition, this vitamin helps your body make use of other mood-elevating brain chemicals such as dopamine and norepinephrine.

Dr. Kowalsky suggests taking a high-quality B-complex multivitamin daily. These may be labeled as B-50 or B-100 complex multivitamins, depending on whether they contain 50 or 100 milligrams of the B vitamins that are listed on the label. Many brands are available.

Mind the Minerals

Chromium and magnesium can help eliminate cravings and stabilize levels of blood sugar (glucose), which fluctuate wildly when a person binges on large amounts of food, says Dr. Kowalsky.

Take 200 micrograms of chromium and 500 to 700 milligrams of magnesium daily, says Dr. Kowalsky, but be sure to check with your doctor first if you have heart or kidney problems.

Another mineral, zinc, is also a player. Supplementing with zinc can help derail your appetite by activating a brain signal that tells you when you're hungry and when you're full. Dr. Kowalsky recommends taking 15 milligrams of zinc daily. If you take a multivitamin, you're probably getting all you need, since that's the amount found in most multis.

Boost Serotonin with 5-HTP

Binge eaters commonly produce low levels of serotonin, the chemical messenger that plays an important role in depression. As a result, their appetites become ravenous. They tend to crave high-fat carbohydrates and are less likely to receive a signal telling them that they're full.

That's where 5-hydroxytryptophan (5-HTP) can help. Shortly after you take 5-HTP in supplement form, the compound travels to your brain, where it is converted to serotonin. The boost in serotonin will suppress your appetite and activate the brain signal that tells you that you've eaten enough. You'll be in better spirits, your binge eating will be under control, and you'll eventually lose weight, says Dr. Boggs.

She suggests taking 50 milligrams of 5-HTP three times a day as a starting point. If you don't notice any decrease in your cravings and binge-eating episodes after six weeks, take 100 milligrams three times a day. If there is still no improvement after six weeks, increase to 200 milligrams three times a day, but don't exceed 900 milligrams daily. You can find this supplement in health food stores. Be sure you don't take it with other medications, especially antidepressants, however, unless you talk to your doctor.

Break the Cycle with St. John's Wort

St. John's wort is at the top of the list among herbalists for treating binge-eating disorder caused by mild to moderate depression, says Dr. Boggs. Like 5-HTP, this herb raises serotonin levels in the brain, but its action is different.

Researchers speculate that St. John's wort may inhibit the enzyme called monoamine oxidase (MAO), which breaks down serotonin molecules and other brain chemicals. Or perhaps it increases the action of serotonin at the nerve endings in the brain. (A number of pharmaceutical antidepressants work this way, too.) Attached to the receptor sites in your brain, the serotonin helps to boost your mood, stabilize your appetite, alert you when you're full, and prevent binge-eating episodes.

To get the benefits of St. John's wort, Dr. Boggs suggests taking 300 milligrams two or three times a day with meals. Look for a standardized extract containing 0.3 percent hypericin.

birth defects

Most people think that conception is the simple, no-planning-necessary part of having a baby. That's not quite right. Doctors say that if you want to ensure a healthy baby, you should start planning months before conception by eating a diet jam-packed with fruits and vegetables.

That little fertilized egg has a long way to go in nine months. It has to grow and divide. Its cells specialize to become bones, nerves, and other essential tissues. What helps make all of this happen without a hitch? Nutrients.

Sure, you can take other actions to protect a developing fetus. Avoid x-rays and environmental toxins, try to stay free of infections—especially German measles—and check with your doctor before taking any drugs. Apart from that, however, nutrients are your best insurance. They're the stuff that cells use to build your baby.

Both the contributors and the detractors deserve special attention in this baby-building process. On the plus side, you need folic acid. On the minus side, make sure that you don't get too much of potentially harmful nutrients such as vitamin A.

Plan Ahead

Around 1965, researchers began to suspect that a deficiency of folic acid, a B vitamin, during pregnancy could lead to central nervous system disorders called neural tube defects in the developing fetus. It seems that a high percentage of women who were taking anticonvulsant drugs (which interfere with the way your body incorporates folic acid) were giving birth to babies with these serious defects.

In a fetus, the neural tube is just a fold of tissue. When the baby is fully developed, that tissue becomes the spinal cord and brain. A baby whose neural tube doesn't close at the top is born with little or no brain and rarely lives more than a few days. A baby whose tube doesn't close at the bottom

Protecting the Unborn from Overdose

Making sure that you get the right amounts of nutrients is only half the battle when it comes to producing a healthy baby. The other 50 percent is avoiding the things that cause birth defects. One caution to be aware of concerns vitamin A—specifically, that you shouldn't take daily doses of supplemental vitamin A that exceed 5,000 international units or more. These levels, which are almost impossible to get from food alone, have been shown to cause various types of birth defects, says Aubrey Milunsky, M.D., professor of human genetics, pediatrics, and pathology and director of the center for human genetics at Boston University School of Medicine.

If you are currently supplementing with vitamin A, talk with your obstetrician about it to ensure that you're not taking an amount that's dangerous for your baby.

"I tell my patients not to take anything that they don't absolutely have to," says Priscilla Evans, N.D., a naturopathic doctor at the Community Wholistic Health Center in Chapel Hill, North Carolina. This includes herbs. It's a very complex matter, she says. Herbs that are safe to take during the second trimester, for instance, might not be safe during the first, when all of the baby's organs are being formed. "You should consult a qualified practitioner of herbal medicine before using herbs during pregnancy," she says.

is born with spina bifida, a condition that can cause paralysis of the lower body because the vertebrae don't join properly to protect the spinal cord.

Nearly 30 years after the first studies, neural tube defects still affected more than 4,000 babies born in the United States every year. We now know the cause, however, and have learned that many of these birth defects can be prevented. Studies have shown that getting adequate amounts of folic acid can protect infants.

"Folic acid is the most important supplement to take to avoid birth defects," says Aubrey Milunsky, M.D., professor of human genetics, pediatrics, and pathology and director of the center for human genetics at Boston University School of Medicine.

Studies have shown that women who take a multivitamin that contains folic acid while pregnant also have lower risks of delivering babies with cleft lip and palate—a split in the lip or in the roof of the mouth that occurs during fetal development. Multivitamins with folic acid also lower risk for a variety of heart defects, limb deficiencies, and urinary tract defects.

The catch is that folic acid is most important from the time of conception through the first six weeks—a time when many women don't yet realize that they're pregnant. If you are thinking about getting pregnant or are even of childbearing age, you should consider taking 400 micrograms of folic acid a day, says Dr. Milunsky.

Only about 25 percent of women of childbearing age get that daily amount of folic acid a day, according to the Council for Responsible Nutrition in Washington, D.C. Folic acid is essential for the DNA production that occurs during cell division.

Most prenatal vitamins contain enough folic acid, along with a host of other nutrients to support the mother and fetus, says Dr. Milunsky. Again, though, women often don't go to their doctors and start taking prenatal vitamins until after the crucial six-week period of organ formation has passed, he says.

Make Multivitamins a Must

"A good multivitamin is essential for pregnant women," says Willow Moore, D.C., N.D., a chiropractor and naturopathic doctor in Owings Mills, Maryland. "Probably, though, taking the full dose once a day isn't the best approach. I recommend that pregnant women take prenatal multivitamins that come in divided doses to be taken throughout the day." Your body is better able to absorb the nutrients if you take them in several smaller doses rather than in one large dose.

Researchers can't yet say exactly which vitamins within a multivitamin do the beneficial work. Apart from the effect of folic acid, there's some evidence to suggest that other B vitamins play vital roles. But we lack specific evidence. That's understandable, notes Dr. Moore, since researchers would never deprive pregnant women of nutrients that might prevent birth defects in order to study the effects of deficiency.

bladder infections

Having a frequent "urge to go," a burning sensation when you do, and achy lower abdominal pain are symptoms that many women recognize—and dread. They are symptoms of urinary tract infections (UTIs), which account for eight million doctor visits a year. Moreover, if a woman gets one UTI, there's a good chance that she'll have a flare-up later on.

Recommendations for preventing bladder infections include drinking plenty of water—and by "plenty," we mean two quarts or more a day. It also means urinating often, especially after intercourse. The idea is to make sure that urine doesn't stay in the bladder very long. All those fluids passing through help to wash away the bacteria that can flourish and fester there.

Bladder infections that are already raging are a little trickier. Doctors usually recommend antibiotics. Unfortunately, frequent antibiotic use may make the troublesome bacteria immune to the medication, leading to recurrent infections.

To combat a bladder infection, you need to take measures to improve your overall immunity, says Mark McClure, M.D., a urologist in Raleigh, North Carolina. You also need to target those bacteria and see if you can get rid of them as soon as they come back again. Supplements can help with both of these infection-prevention initiatives.

Add Some C to a Multi

Women with bladder infections would do well to address the cause of their problem, not simply the symptoms, says Dr. McClure. "Overall wellness issues and immunity should be the foundation from which you work to get well."

Stress, in particular, can predispose you to chronic or recurrent UTIs, he says, because it depletes the immune system and weakens your defenses against bacteria. "It affects the body in many negative ways, so I recommend yoga, breathing exercises, and meditation," he says.

Stress is caused by more than a hectic schedule or overly tense muscles, however. Poor nutrition is a form of stress that can affect immune performance, too, notes Dr. McClure. If you're not getting enough dietary fiber, you're loading up on sugar, and you have a lot of caffeine in your system, you reduce your body's defenses against infection, he explains. Eating better all the time should be your ultimate goal in order to prevent future infections.

Taking a good-quality, high-potency multivitamin daily is a step in the right direction, says Dr. McClure. If you're already doing that, add some extra vitamin C, he suggests. Taking 500 milligrams every two hours can help improve immune function by boosting white blood cell counts—a sign of better defenses. While this much C probably isn't needed on a daily basis, the body seems to require additional amounts of this nutrient in times of infection.

Prevention with Cranberry Extract

Long discussed and debated, the tart, red cranberry's bladder-friendly effects have finally been demonstrated. Cranberry really does help prevent the occurrence of UTIs.

A study conducted by cranberry researcher Edward Walker, Ph.D., professor of chemistry and director of the center for chemical technology at Weber State University in Ogden, Utah, showed that cranberry can help women with recurring UTIs.

In the study, 10 women were given capsules of solid cranberry concentrate for a period of three months. Then researchers switched them to a concentrate that looked like the same substance but didn't have any cranberry ingredients in it (a placebo). The results showed that when the women were taking real cranberry, they had half as many infections as when they were taking the placebos.

Cranberry has long been thought to work against UTIs by acidifying urine, making it into a less hospitable environment for bacteria. It's actually bacteria's ability to stick to the bladder or urinary tract walls, however, that causes infection to set in. Urine acidity doesn't seem to have much to do with it, researchers say. Besides, for cranberry to have an acidifying effect, you'd have to eat a veritable bushel of berries, according to Dr. Walker.

His research has found the active ingredient that gives cranberry its potent anti-adhesion properties, counteracting the sticky attack and making infection much less likely. When cranberry is present, the bacteria in the bladder or urinary tract can't hold on. Without firm footing, they are essentially rendered harmless.

"The bacteria will die on their own without a place to live," says Dr. Walker. Then the natural flow of urine gives the bad guys an easy ride out of town. "It's a lot gentler to just send them out of the body like this rather than use antibiotics," he says.

According to Dr. Walker's results, cranberry's strong suit is preventing—not curing—UTIs. "Our hypothesis was that cranberry would reduce the number of recurrent infections," he says—and that's exactly what happened. Other dark berries, such as blueberries, have similar anti-adhesion components.

For women plagued by regular infections, this news is as good as it gets. It means that you can use a cranberry supplement as a preventive measure. Take 400 milligrams of standardized cranberry extract twice a day, suggests Dr. Walker. The extract is available in health food stores.

An Herb to Squelch Infection

Uva-ursi, a strangely named shrub that grows in North America, can be a suitable stand-in for antibiotic infection fighters, says naturopathic doctor Tori Hudson, N.D., professor at the National College of Naturopathic Medicine in Portland, Oregon, and author of *Women's Encyclopedia of Natural Medicine.* "It's really the most important, most useful herb for treating bladder infections," she says.

While you can take uva-ursi as a tea, the dosage is more precise if you take supplements. If you find capsules that contain only powdered uva-ursi leaves, you'll need to take 500 to 1,000 milligrams three times a day, according to Dr. Hudson. A higher concentration is found in an extract of uva-ursi standardized to contain 20 percent arbutin, one of the active ingredients. If you take that concentration, you'll need only 125 to 250 milligrams three times daily, she says.

Stop taking uva-ursi when you feel well again. It could cause problems if taken over the long term. Also, it may be preferable to avoid taking cranberry extract at the same time, Dr. Hudson cautions, since arbutin works best in a nonacidic environment. You can take cranberry afterward to prevent recurring infections, she says. Pregnant women should avoid uva-ursi completely because it may bring on uterine contractions.

Uva-Ursi Knocks Out Bad Bacteria

For more than 1,000 years, people around the world have treated urinary troubles with the leaves of uva-ursi. Tannin and arbutin, the active ingredients, have important qualities that give this herb its impressive powers. Tannin is an astringent, which means that it causes tissue to contract in a way that can make an inhospitable environment for bacteria. In the urinary tract, arbutin becomes an antiseptic, which means that it directly battles the growth of bacteria and other organisms.

"Other plants do contain arbutin, but the highest amounts are found in uva-ursi," says naturopathic doctor Tori Hudson, N.D., professor at the National College of Naturopathic Medicine and director of A Woman's Time health clinic, both in Portland, Oregon.

While you can make a compress of uva-ursi and apply it directly to cuts and scrapes to help prevent infection, the herb is more often used to treat urinary problems than for minor first-aid. In addition to being sold in supplement form, uva-ursi is available in some specially blended teas.

Kava Root for Pain Relief

Painful urination is one of the earliest—and worst—symptoms of a bladder infection. The odd, uncomfortable spasms of pain can continue long after you've urinated.

The muscle-relaxing herb kava kava can be a boon to women who have substantial pain from a bladder infection, says Dr. McClure. Its active ingredients, called kavalactones, have a mild tranquilizing effect, and they also seem to create antiseptic and anti-inflammatory effects in the urinary tract. With that combination of benefits, kava is especially well-suited for treating UTIs.

Kava comes in tincture form as well as capsules. Follow the dosage directions on the label. With the tincture, for example, the instructions are often to dilute one to two milliliters in one cup of liquid and take it two to five times a day.

Using kava for up to three months appears to be very safe for most people, but it can cause drowsiness and interact with some medications. See page 240 for important information about kava.

Battle Bacteria with Goldenseal

Urinary tract infections are usually caused by one type of bacteria in particular—the awful organism known as *Escherichia coli*. Luckily, there's a natural weapon that has a special hatred for *E. coli*—its nemesis is the herb called goldenseal.

Goldenseal's antimicrobial and immune-stimulating properties make it a popular choice for treating infection in general, says Dr. Hudson. Berberine, the active ingredient, is what makes it specifically useful for UTIs, she says. Take 500 to 1,000 milligrams of goldenseal root extract daily, but don't take it for more than one week. Do not take this herb if you are pregnant, however.

breast cancer

There aren't many things worse than sitting in the chair across from your doctor and being told that you have breast cancer. In 1997, more than 180,000 American women found themselves in just that situation. Behind that dreadful scenario, however, there's a statistic that allows for more hope than ever before. Today, many experts think that at least 65 percent of all cancers—including breast cancer—can be prevented with the right lifestyle changes.

The catalog of cancer-preventing lifestyle changes is the same one that applies to all healthy living—exercise, eat right, and avoid cancer-causing agents. "Just four hours of exercise a week can reduce your risk of breast cancer by about 50 percent," says Jennifer Brett, N.D., a naturopathic doctor at the Wilton Naturopathic Center in Stratford, Connecticut.

On the dietary front, try to eat fewer dairy and animal products, she advises, and reduce the number of calories you get from fat. As for healthful additions to your diet, try to eat more fiber, fruits, vegetables, and soy products such as soy milk, tempeh, miso, tofu, and products made with soy flour. Avoiding alcohol use and pesticides on produce, both of which increase your risk of getting breast cancer, can also make a difference, she says.

Supplements can complement the primary strategy of eating right and exercising, says Dr. Brett. Also, as far as supplements go, there are a lot you can choose from, such as vitamins C and E and selenium. There are also herbs such as red clover and black cohosh.

There's one thing to keep in mind, however. Almost all of the studies on breast cancer–preventing agents have been done on foods, not supplements, says naturopathic doctor Tori Hudson, N.D., professor at the National College of Naturopathic Medicine in Portland, Oregon, and author of *Women's Encyclopedia of Natural Medicine*. Many times, the supplements that are recommended to prevent cancer are the key nutrients in the particular foods that have been shown to help, she says.

Fighting Free Radicals with Antioxidants

There are little scavengers in your body called free radicals. These molecules—natural products of the aging process—are each missing an electron, so they go around trying to steal electrons from molecules in healthy cells. When they succeed, the cell that was robbed is damaged or even dies. In some cells, the genetic material that tells them how to duplicate themselves is damaged. That's when cancerous changes begin.

Enter antioxidants. Antioxidants donate their own electrons to the free radicals and help prevent damage to cells.

Vitamins C and E, selenium, and carotene are all antioxidants, and studies have shown that they all help to prevent cancer. Initial studies of the supplement forms of these nutrients suggest, however, that vitamin E has the strongest cancer-preventing potential.

Researchers at Gazi University in Ankara, Turkey, compared vitamin E levels in the blood of 100 breast cancer patients and 70 healthy women. They found that the levels were much lower in women with breast cancer than in the healthy women.

To get the benefits of vitamin E, talk to your doctor about taking a dose of 400 international units (IU) a day, suggests Dr. Brett.

Vitamin E often gets top billing among antioxidants, but other supplements are effective, too. Numerous studies have shown that people who eat foods that are high in vitamin C can also reduce their risk of cancer.

In one review of studies that examined vitamin C intake in different populations, researchers concluded that women who get about 300 milligrams of vitamin C a day are 30 percent less likely to get breast cancer.

Dr. Brett is in favor of taking as much vitamin C as possible. The upper limit isn't the same for everyone, however, and the first sign that you're taking too much is a case of diarrhea. Dr. Brett suggests that you actually take enough vitamin C to give you diarrhea, then back off until you find a level that you can take without side effects. It might be best to take it in two or three divided doses so your body doesn't have to deal with a megadose all at once, she says.

As far as selenium goes, it's been shown in many studies that high levels of selenium are often associated with low levels of cancer, including breast cancer. For the best protection against breast cancer, take 200 micrograms of selenium daily, says Dr. Brett.

Carotene is also an effective cancer preventive, but not necessarily in the form of beta-carotene. Carotene capsules that contain natural carrot oil are much better for preventing cancer than synthetic beta-carotene, says Dr. Brett. "In fact, there's some evidence to suggest that taking synthetic beta-carotene could actually increase your risk of getting cancer," she says. "I typically recommend taking 25,000 IU a day of carotene, or about five carrots' worth."

Immunity Boosters

In order to successfully ward off disease of any kind, your body needs a sound immune system. Supplements that strengthen your immunity are a good idea if you're trying to prevent breast cancer, says David Perlmutter, M.D., a neurologist in Naples, Florida, and author of *Lifeguide*. In addition to the antioxidants mentioned earlier, two supplements that Dr. Perlmutter recommends for building immunity are zinc and Kyolic garlic, a brand that supplies standardized amounts of the herb. It's available in health food stores, drugstores, and many supermarkets.

Garlic has sometimes been called Russian penicillin because it figures in many Russian folk remedies to fight infection. The chemicals contained in its fragrant cloves help to activate the immune system. Garlic may also help your cells expel cancer-causing chemicals, and it can protect the genetic material of cells and improve the ability of certain enzymes to neutralize toxins. A typical dose of Kyolic garlic is two capsules three times a day.

Zinc helps by building new immune system cells and getting them ready to battle disease. "Adequate zinc stores get your body poised to fight at the first sign of cancer," says Dr. Brett. If you meet the Daily Value by getting 15 milligrams of zinc a day, you're probably getting enough, she says.

Estrogen-Lowering Herbs

"One of the biggest reasons that women get into trouble with breast cancer is that they have too much estrogen floating around in their bodies," says Dr. Brett.

One way to reduce free-floating estrogen is by following the dietary guidelines for breast cancer prevention mentioned earlier. In addition, Dr. Brett notes, there are some natural substances that will help to reduce estrogen levels. Your key allies are called phytoestrogens.

Phytoestrogens are simply the estrogens that occur naturally in plants. When you eat fruits and vegetables that contain those compounds, they act as a weak form of estrogen in your body. A woman's cells have specific receptor sites that are prepared to accept estrogen, and when the phytoestrogens come by, they move into those sites, taking the place of the body's estrogens. Because the phytoestrogens have taken the receptor spots, your body's much stronger estrogen has nowhere to go and is excreted as waste.

Researchers at the Royal Hospital for Women in New South Wales, Australia, reviewed all the studies conducted between 1980 and 1995 concerning the effect of phytoestrogens. They concluded that phytoestrogens were among the factors that protect vegetarians against breast cancer.

One of the most powerful phytoestrogens is soy. Women in Asian countries who consume a lot of soy products have much lower rates of breast cancer than women who eat a Western diet. Researchers have observed that rates of breast cancer among Asian women increase significantly when those women switch from an oriental to a Western diet.

Eating foods like tofu that are made with soy is a great idea, but if you're not fond of them, you can try taking genistein capsules, says Dr. Brett. Genistein is believed to be one of the active ingredients in soy, and as such, it can impart some of the same estrogen-reducing benefits.

However, there is debate regarding soy when breast cancer is present. Soy isoflavones may promote tumor growth through estrogen-dependant mechanisms, once a tumor has started. It is not recommended to take soy if a tumor is present without a physician's supervision.

If you decide to try genistein, you can find it as a supplement in health food stores. A typical dose is 45 milligrams a day.

Red clover and black cohosh are two herbs that are also phytoestrogens that work to reduce potentially dangerous levels of estrogen.

"Red clover is an old, old cancer remedy," says Matthew Wood, a professional member of the American Herbalists Guild in Minnetrista, Minnesota, and author of *The Book of Herbal Wisdom*. "It works to break down tumors and keep cancer from spreading. Like soy, red clover contains genistein."

If you are taking a number of different supplements to help prevent cancer, follow the directions on the labels of the products you buy, says

The Power of Red Clover

Red clover not only contains vitamins and minerals, it may also have some power to balance the female hormone estrogen. "I think we're going to be hearing a lot about red clover in the coming years," says Jennifer Brett, N.D., a naturopathic doctor at the Wilton Naturopathic Center in Stratford, Connecticut.

Among the important vitamins and minerals that red clover offers are vitamins B and C, calcium, magnesium, and potassium. Because it can help balance estrogen, this herb is widely recommended for treating menstrual and menopausal problems. This capability also makes it a prime choice for women who are looking to prevent breast cancer, Dr. Brett says. It should never be taken during pregnancy, however.

Herbalists have found many other uses for red clover. It's one of the best alternative remedies for eczema and psoriasis in children, they say. Because it can help relax nerves, it's a good treatment for bronchitis, asthma, and whooping cough—conditions that can be relieved to an extent by relaxing the breathing muscles.

The use of red clover dates back centuries. The Chinese used the sap to help treat colds and influenza. It was a popular remedy in England and Germany and came with the American colonists when they immigrated from those countries.

On the American continent, it was taken up by many Native American tribes, including the Iroquois and Cherokee, who began using it to ease the discomforts of menopause. At the beginning of the twentieth century, it was often brewed into a tea to relieve spasmodic coughing and had a reputation as a "blood purifier." In Mennonite communities today, red clover is still widely used to relieve croup and whooping cough.

Dr. Brett. A typical dose for black cohosh, for instance, is 40 milligrams twice a day.

With red clover, Wood sometimes recommends large doses as part of a cancer treatment program. For very large doses of this herb, you'll need the advice of an herbal practitioner or a naturopathic doctor, he says. Even when clover shows results, he cautions that it is important to continue with medical supervision.

Flaxseed Packs a One-Two Punch

Taking flaxseed will add two powerful anti-cancer weapons to your arsenal: lignans and alpha-linolenic acid (ALA).

In 1990, when the National Cancer Institute decided to single out certain plant chemicals for extensive study, flaxseed was the first item on the list. Early results suggested the existence of powerful anti-cancer compounds.

The plant compounds called lignans are believed to be part of the reason that flaxseed exerts such powerful effects. Like soy phytoestrogens, lignans tend to take up space on estrogen receptor sites. With fewer sites that it can call home, your body's estrogen tends to be excreted rather than affecting breast tissue.

Lignans have another benefit as well, as they increase production of a compound that helps with the excretion of excess estrogen. Research has shown that breast cancer rates are lower in women who excrete higher amounts of lignans in their urine.

The other beneficial compound in flaxseed is ALA. When researchers examined the levels of ALA in the breast tissue of 121 women with breast cancer, they found that the ALA seemed to be producing some distinct benefits. Among women who had low levels of ALA, the cancer was much more likely to have spread from the breast to the lymph nodes in the armpit and to other areas as well. After considering all other factors, the researchers concluded that low levels of ALA were the most significant predictor of whether a woman's breast cancer was likely to spread.

cancer

If your body had a slogan, it would probably be something like "Divide and copy." That's because every day, cells split and replicate, over and over again. But we all make mistakes—even at the cellular level.

Once in a million or so divisions, something goes wrong, and the mistake produces an abnormal cell. Normally, the immune system corrects these mistakes. When abnormal cells go unnoticed and uncorrected, cancer becomes a possibility.

Just like normal cells, damaged cells will copy themselves, reproducing the mistake in every generation. As more and more cancerous cells pile up, a tumor begins to grow.

Preventing mistakes in the first place can help stop cancer from occurring. To do that, oxidative damage—the prelude to cell mutation—must be kept to a minimum. That's where antioxidant vitamins and minerals come in.

Even when cancerous cells do appear, our bodies almost always dispatch them without a hitch. Certain nutritional supplements can help support your ability to squelch cancer before it grows out of control or even to inhibit early tumor growth.

Get an Edge with Antioxidant Vitamins

Researchers speculate that up to 30 percent of cancers are affected simply by what we eat. One study, for example, indicates that people who eat meat nearly every day have more than double the risk of colon cancer of those who eat meat about once a week. Plus, researchers have noted that people who favor vegetables, grains, and fruits have less risk of cancer than those who eat fewer of these plant foods.

Why is there such a strong connection between certain foods and reduced risk of cancer? For one thing, a steady diet of red meat and fatty foods brings an excess of free radicals into the body. These free-roaming,

The Goodness of Green Tea

Some people think that green tea—a favorite of the Japanese—is an acquired taste. If so, there's a good reason to acquire it.

The traditional pale-green brew that accompanies Japanese food appears to have potent anti-cancer properties, according to Jerzy Jankun, M.D., a cancer researcher and associate professor in the department of urology at the Medical College of Ohio in Toledo.

Green tea contains a substance called epigallocathechin-3 gallate (EGCG). Dr. Jankun's research shows that EGCG inhibits urokinase, the enzyme that allows tumors to grow and spread. "By inhibiting urokinase, those processes *could* be stopped," says Dr. Jankun. "EGCG has been known to possess other anti-cancer activity, but inhibition of urokinase seems to be the most important factor."

How much green tea should you sip? You can follow the lead from the East: Asian tea lovers commonly drink up to 10 cups a day. While this may seem like a lot, research suggests that consuming such a large quantity may be necessary to reap green tea's anti-cancer benefits.

Regular green tea contains caffeine. Although it has only about one-third as much as the same amount of black tea, regular consumption might give you more caffeine than you want. Fortunately, you can find decaffeinated varieties in some supermarkets and health food stores—and the decaf kinds have equivalent amounts of EGCG.

If you prefer your protection in capsules rather than cups, green tea extract is available in supplement form, says Dr. Jankun. Sometimes an equivalent in cups will be noted on the label, or the label will give the concentration of green tea in milligrams. Since potencies are different, follow the directions on the label. Most brands advise taking one or two capsules two or three times a day.

Just don't go overboard when supplementing with green tea capsules. The potential dangers of taking excessive amounts of green tea in a purified form are still unknown, according to Dr. Jankun.

unstable molecules can damage cells and make them more susceptible to cancer.

Eating plenty of vegetables and fruits actually supplies the body with an armory of antioxidants—protective substances that can help destroy free radicals and protect fragile structures inside your cells from the damage that may lead to cancer.

Getting the requisite five or more servings a day of fruits and vegetables is the first step in defending yourself against cancer. While prevention may start on your plate, though, you can go even farther with specific antioxidant supplements known for their anti-cancer actions, says Keith Berndtson, M.D., medical director of the American Wholehealth Centers of Integrative Medicine in Chicago. In addition to a healthy diet, he says, "I'd stick to a high-potency multiple vitamin with additional antioxidants for cancer prevention."

Two of the most important antioxidants are also the most well known—vitamin E and vitamin C. These two are favorites when it comes to improving overall health, and for cancer prevention, they seem to be all-stars.

Oily vitamin E is hard to get in abundance from dietary sources alone. Supplemental amounts from 400 to 800 international units (IU) a day are recommended by W. John Diamond, M.D., medical director of the Triad Medical Center in Reno, Nevada, and co-author of *An Alternative Medicine Definitive Guide to Cancer*.

Water-soluble vitamin C is relatively easy to find in foods. Even though the Daily Value (DV) for C is only 60 milligrams, Dr. Diamond suggests much more for the prevention and treatment of cancer. He recommends between 1,000 and 8,000 milligrams in divided doses throughout the day.

Stop Cancers with Selenium

The essential trace mineral selenium has been connected with protection against cancer since the late 1960s. While we still aren't sure how selenium works in the body, researchers continue to gather evidence that it seems to have anti-cancer effects.

Initially, researchers thought that selenium might help reduce the incidence of skin cancer. In a trial done by the Nutritional Prevention of Cancer Study Group at the Arizona Cancer Center in Tucson, researchers tried to determine whether the mineral helped prevent basal and squamous cell carcinoma, commonly known as skin cancer. The results were disappointing, but only when researchers focused on skin cancer. To their surprise, they learned that people getting selenium had significantly fewer

Toxins and Your Body

The very word *toxins* seems to reek. Think of bootleg liquor and bad, cheap wine. Imagine jumbles of jumbo helpings of junk food, deep-fried in week-old oil. Picture bad clams slurping up wastewater from Pollution Bay. Or how about ominous-looking barrels of lead, cadmium, and mercury?

Yes, these are all carriers of toxins. There's another carrier, however, that you're less likely to guess—you.

Even in its best moments, your body is a toxin factory. You produce various chemicals that are considered toxins when you digest food, process hormones, or send a message via your nervous system. Moreover, the constant stream of toxins produced as a matter of course inside your body vastly outranks the number of toxins that enter it from the outside.

Luckily, our bodies are usually able to handle the big job of getting rid of accumulated waste. "Contrary to what most people think, though, detoxification is not as simple as pooping and peeing," says Sidney M. Baker, M.D., a physician in Weston, Connecticut, and author of *Detoxification and Healing*.

It's easier to understand the process of detoxification if you compare your body to a small city and think of detoxification as the city's sanitation efforts, says Dr. Baker. In this city, a full 80 percent of the budget goes toward supporting sanitation by buying new garbage trucks. And these aren't just any old garbage trucks—each one is specialized to pick up a certain kind of trash.

In your body, that means that more than three-quarters of your daily energy expenditure goes toward creating specialized molecules (the garbage trucks) to usher various toxic molecules (trash) out of your body. In reality, detoxification is a process of building things rather than breaking them

prostate, colorectal, and lung cancers than people who weren't getting the supplement.

Selenium supplements appear to encourage the death of potentially cancerous cells grown in laboratory dishes as well as inhibiting tumor growth. This leads researchers to predict that taking supplemental selenium may deliver cancer protection soon after you start taking it.

Selenium comes from the soil, and fruits and vegetables that come from selenium-rich soil are more likely to contain the mineral. Of course, there's

down. It's more a process of synthesis than of trash-hauling, Dr. Baker points out. "It's just like growing or healing."

In the body, transporting toxins follows fairly standard procedures. Some toxic molecules are safely moved to the intestines, liver, kidneys, or sweat glands for disposal. Others, like some metals, are sent to the hair or nails for long-term storage. After those toxins arrive, however, various things can happen—and some aren't so good.

If the toxin was made inside the body—such as a molecule of hormone—the "garbage truck" simply drops off the toxin and returns to circulation, seeking more toxins to dispatch. Trouble arises when an externally produced toxin—like a molecule of pesticide or heavy metal—is taken to the dump. The garbage truck founders at the dumpsite and gets stuck there, unable to return to service. After all, our trucks were designed before the days of strange toxins like petrochemicals. Our living systems don't know quite what to do with them, Dr. Baker suspects. Cleaning up external toxins uses up more of the body's resources.

That's why it's smart to do your best to limit your exposure to external toxins. "Fresh, organically grown, unadulterated food is where we would all start from, ideally," says Dr. Baker. He stresses, though, that a body that is fed even the purest diet still produces internal toxins that need to be cleaned up.

Good nutrition is the most important support for your body's detox abilities, says Dr. Baker. Be sure to get the Daily Value of all of the essential nutrients, he advises. That means eating a healthy diet as well as taking vitamin and mineral supplements. If you think you need extra help, turn to naturally detoxifying herbs like ginseng, garlic, or milk thistle, he says.

no way to know exactly whether you're getting adequate selenium from the produce you buy in the supermarket. Supplements are the surest way to make sure that you get enough.

In the Tucson study, the people who showed increased resistance to cancer were taking more than 200 micrograms of selenium a day. According to Dr. Berndtson, this is a safe and effective amount to include in your anticancer supplement program. You should take amounts of selenium over 200 micrograms only under your doctor's supervision.

Can Isoflavones Protect You?

You can find supplements of isoflavones, the plant estrogens found in soy and red clover, on the shelves of health food stores and even national drug-store chains. The isoflavone most likely to be in these supplements is genistein, and doctors are hopeful that this isolated substance, or other isoflavones from soy, will produce the same benefits that people get from soy-based diets, such as reducing the risk of breast and prostate cancer, heart disease, and osteoporosis.

Genistein and other isoflavones appear to be promising substances, and "this is a very active area of research right now," says Stephen Barnes, Ph.D., professor of pharmacology and toxicology at the University of Alabama at Birmingham.

Some researchers, however, are doubtful that isoflavones such as genistein have the protective potential of soy proteins. Most studies have looked at soy proteins contained in foods such as tofu and tempeh rather than studying the benefits of isoflavones taken as supplements. There's not enough evidence to confirm that isoflavones alone provide the same benefits as soy-based foods, according to some researchers.

Most evidence of the potential benefits of isoflavones comes from Japanese populations that eat a traditional diet, including many soy-based foods. In these populations, the incidence of cancer, heart disease, and osteoporosis is lower than in the United States.

Fight Harder with Folic Acid

Many doctors recommend folic acid for women who are pregnant because it's been shown that this B vitamin will reduce the risk of birth defects.

In food, folic acid comes in a form known as folate. This nutrient is essential. If it is in short supply, the body may produce abnormal cells, known as dysplasia, that can add up to cancer.

Among some other beneficial effects, folic acid seems to help prevent colon cancer. Studies indicate that men who don't get enough have a greater risk of this type of cancer than men who do.

The Nurses' Health Study at Harvard Medical School found that folic acid is good for women, too. In fact, the amount of folic acid found in many

The positive effects of soy, such as lowering cholesterol levels, seem to come from a combination of soy protein and isoflavones, Dr. Barnes says, and a supplement may not provide the same benefits. Isoflavones alone, however, do seem to improve artery elasticity, another component of circulatory health, he says.

With regard to cancer, the focus has turned to genistein. Studies with laboratory animals suggest that this isoflavone may be useful in both protecting against and treating prostate cancer.

Population studies focusing on cancer seem to be reassuring, since people who eat lots of soy foods are less likely to get cancer than people who eat a meat-based diet, Dr. Barnes says. Again, though, the same results might not occur with isoflavones.

"It's true that there are clinical questions that will take some time to answer," Dr. Barnes says. In the meantime, if you want soy's protective effects, you can eat 50 to 60 milligrams of isoflavones a day, he says. The amount of isoflavones in soy foods varies. A half-cup of tofu offers 35 milligrams, one cup of soy milk has 20 to 30 milligrams, and ¼ cup of dry soy protein granules provides 60 milligrams.

If you do opt to take isoflavone supplements, it's still prudent to stay within the 50- to 60-milligram range, Dr. Barnes suggests. "We think that's safe because people have been getting that amount from foods," he says.

multivitamins was enough to cut women's colon cancer rates by more than 75 percent.

In the study, researchers examined data for more than 120,000 female nurses who were selected in 1976 and reported their health status every two years thereafter. The longer the women took the vitamin containing folic acid, the smaller their risk of cancer became. "After 15 years of use, their risk was markedly lower," says Edward Giovannucci, M.D., Sc.D., lead researcher in the study and assistant professor of medicine at Harvard Medical School and Brigham and Women's Hospital in Boston.

The nurses with the lowest incidence of colon cancer were getting at least the DV for folic acid—400 micrograms, an amount found in many multivitamins. There's evidence, however, that we get the best anti-cancer benefits if we take more than the DV.

Taking a multivitamin that contains folic acid is a good policy, says Dr. Giovannucci. You can also enhance your daily diet with folate-rich foods. Among the best are broccoli, pinto and navy beans, chickpeas, spinach, sunflower seeds, and fortified breakfast cereals.

Include the Carotenoid Crew

Research has connected a group of substances called carotenoids with a reduced risk of cancer. In most of the studies, however, researchers studied the effects of carotenoid-rich foods rather than supplements.

Sometimes called carotenes, carotenoids are named for the vegetable that is one of the richest food sources—the lowly carrot. That's not the only vegetable that contains this valuable nutrient, though. The giveaway is vivid color. Red vegetables like tomatoes, deep orange ones like squash, and dark leafy greens like kale also contain ample amounts of various types of carotenoids.

Of all the carotenoids that have been studied, however, beta-carotene is the most prominent. In initial studies, researchers found that the group of people who got the largest amount of this nutrient from foods also had substantially fewer cancers. Beta-carotene was hailed as the newest antioxidant vitamin, able to protect both the insides and outsides of cells against free radical damage.

When researchers started studying supplements of beta-carotene, however, they observed that the benefits didn't apply to everyone who upped their consumption. For smokers, beta-carotene may have a negative effect. Two studies showed that smokers who got high doses in supplement form were actually more likely to develop lung cancer than smokers who took no beta-carotene.

These results have led experts to be wary of recommending supplemental beta-carotene to everyone. True, a nutrient that poses a risk to smokers may be beneficial rather than harmful to nonsmokers. Smokers are already at high risk for cancer, and perhaps because of that, they react differently to beta-carotene than nonsmokers. Researchers are wondering, though, whether it might be harmful to take beta-carotene in isolation from the rest of carotenoids, and with that question still hanging, a beta-carotene supplement can't be recommended as an across-the-board preventive. The moderate doses of carotenoids that come from foods, however, continue to show substantial anti-cancer promise.

If you want to add to that diet, you might try a supplement called mixed carotenoids, says Dr. Berndtson. Look for one that supplies beta-carotene, gamma-carotene, lycopene, lutein, and zeaxanthin, he advises.

Addressing the Calcium Question

Not too long ago, calcium seemed poised to become a big anti-cancer supplement. Studies suggested that taking ample amounts of this bone-boon mineral could do more than keep your skeleton solid. In particular, precancerous polyps that can lead to colon cancer seemed to appear much less often in people who took more than the DV of calcium.

Then along came a study from Harvard Medical School, and some experts began to question whether high-dose calcium was really all that helpful in preventing cancer. Researchers examined the eating habits of nearly 48,000 men who were taking part in a six-year survey called the Health Professionals Follow-Up Study. They found that rates of prostate cancer went up when the men had more calcium in their diets. The increased cancer rates were especially prevalent among those who got more than 2,000 milligrams a day, according to Dr. Giovannucci, who was co-author of the study.

What causes the contradictory effects of calcium? It could be that another nutrient plays an opposing role, according to Robert E. C. Wildman, Ph.D., assistant professor of human nutrition at the University of Delaware in Newark. "It seems that greatly increased calcium intake may depress the active form of vitamin D," he says. According to Dr. Giovannucci's study, vitamin D may play a role in preventing the uncontrolled cell growth that can lead to prostate cancer.

So how do you safely resolve the calcium quandary? Premenopausal women and all men under 65 need a daily 1,000-milligram supplement. Women who are past menopause and not taking hormone replacement therapy and men who are over 65 need 1,500 milligrams daily. Don't exceed these amounts unless your doctor deems it medically necessary, Dr. Wildman says.

The DV for vitamin D is 400 IU a day for everyone. Stay on the safe side, recommends Dr. Wildman, by being sure to get your share of this important nutrient. Look for a multivitamin supplement that supplies the DV, or take it as a separate supplement.

canker sores

Canker sores may be out of sight, but they're not out of mind. They lie on the inner lining of your lips and cheeks or on the base of your tongue, the floor of your mouth, or your soft palate. Eat anything hot or spicy, and they'll burn like fire.

These painful critters, also called recurrent aphthous ulcers, are yellowish gray or white with red borders. They're tiny, round, and appear individually or in bunches.

Fortunately, they're not contagious and normally heal within 7 to 14 days. But that's faint praise. When they do make their cameo appearances, they can turn the simple pleasures of eating, talking, and even brushing your teeth into harrowing experiences.

It's a good thing that help is just around the corner. There are some dietary and other natural measures that you can take to keep these little buggers out of your mouth.

Start by eliminating the top canker sore triggers from your diet, such as chocolate, nuts, tomatoes, green peppers, strawberries, and oranges and other citrus fruits. Try to avoid eating sharp-edged corn chips and pretzels, because they can irritate and injure the lining of your mouth and produce an ulcer.

After you've eliminated the troublemakers, you can reintroduce each of these foods into your diet one at a time every two to three days to determine which is the source of the trouble.

Canker sores can also be caused by food sensitivities to wheat products. See your doctor to determine whether food allergies are causing your problem.

Once you've taken these steps, if you still suffer from an occasional canker sore or two, a certain type of licorice supplement will relieve the pain and shorten the duration of the ulcer. You can also take a high-quality multivitamin/mineral supplement daily to prevent them altogether.

Zap Canker Sores with Licorice

The kind of licorice that stops canker sores is a far cry from the black, stringy stuff that kids love to gnaw on. What you want is deglycyrrhizinated licorice, or DGL.

"DGL has anti-inflammatory properties. It speeds the healing process and soothes the discomfort of canker sores," says Michael Traub, N.D., a naturopathic doctor and director of the integrated residency program at North Hawaii Community Hospital in Kamuela.

In one study, 20 people with recurrent canker sores used a DGL mouthwash. Fifteen people experienced at least a 50 percent improvement within one day and were completely healed by the third day.

Among those who recovered was one patient who had had recurrent canker sores for over 10 years. He had several sores on his tongue and lips, inside his cheek, on his soft palate, and in the back of his throat. By the seventh day after he started using the DGL solution, he was completely free of sores.

To begin the healing process, take two 200-milligram tablets 20 minutes before meals, says Dr. Traub, or chew one or two tablets two or three times a day. While chewing, use your tongue to position the tablet residue on the sore to promote even speedier healing. You should use DGL, which is available at health food stores, until the sore heals, he adds.

In addition, you can empty the powder from a capsule into ½ cup of lukewarm water, dissolve the DGL, and swish the solution around in your mouth, says Dr. Traub. Repeat this at least two or three times a day until the sore has healed.

A High-Potency Multivitamin to Cover Your Bases

Deficiencies of B vitamins, including B_{12} and folic acid; zinc; and iron appear to be prevalent among people with canker sores. When the deficiencies are corrected, the sores often show improvement or complete remission. "Evidence of a vitamin deficiency often shows up inside your mouth and throat because of the rapid cell turnover rate that's characteristic of the mucous membranes," says Jennifer Brett, N.D., a naturopathic doctor at the Wilton Naturopathic Center in Stratford, Connecticut.

"Low levels of some B vitamins can cause swelling of the tongue and canker sores. If you're not getting enough zinc, you won't heal as quickly from small injuries like biting the inside of your mouth. And without enough folic acid and iron, you won't maintain the necessary rapid cell division that you need to keep the lining of your mouth healthy," says Dr. Brett.

A high-potency multivitamin purchased at a health food store should give you the nutrients that are necessary to prevent recurrent canker sores, says Dr. Brett. Take 500 to 1,000 micrograms of vitamin B_{12}, 10 milligrams of iron (if a man or postmenopausal woman, consult a doctor first), 800 micrograms of folic acid, and 15 to 20 milligrams of zinc, she says. If your multivitamin doesn't include all you need, simply add separate supplements to make up the difference.

C and Thiamin: More Sore Solutions

If your canker sores are a result of food allergies, take 1,000 to 1,200 milligrams of buffered vitamin C daily to help reduce the level of histamines in your body, says Dr. Brett. Histamines are the immune system chemicals that are released by white blood cells and cause inflammation and irritation. To enhance the effectiveness of the vitamin C, take 1,000 milligrams of quercetin or 100 milligrams of grapeseed extract daily as a preventive, she says. These are both bioflavonoids, compounds that inhibit histamine release, reduce inflammation, and speed healing.

Other research shows that a deficiency of thiamin can lead to recurrent mouth ulcers. In a study, researchers determined levels of a thiamin-dependent enzyme in 120 people. Forty-nine of the 70 participants with recurrent canker sores had low levels of the enzyme, compared to only 2 among the 50 in the group without ulcers. Dr. Brett recommends taking 100 milligrams of thiamin daily as a preventive.

carpal tunnel syndrome

What makes your foot go numb when you sit too long with your legs crossed? Bad circulation, right? That's why it helps to stand up and stomp the pins and needles out. It gets the blood moving again.

What's really going on doesn't have anything to do with blood flow, though. The numbness occurs when a nerve, not a blood vessel, is compressed. That's the same thing that happens—in a different part of the body, of course—when someone has carpal tunnel syndrome (CTS).

Instead of being compressed by a weight, the median nerve that runs to your thumb and first two fingers is constricted when your body's tendons and tissues swell and press against it. The nerve and the nine tendons that move your fingers are encased in a sheath called the synovium, making a sausagelike bundle that passes through the bony, hourglass-shaped passageway on the underside of the wrist that's known as the carpal tunnel.

When you're doing things like typing or bowling, the repetitive motions of your hand and wrist can cause the tendons and synovium to become inflamed and swollen. Even slight swelling in the wrist area can press the nerve enough to short-circuit the signal.

Women, especially pregnant women, are more prone to CTS than men. Regardless of your sex, however, you're at greater risk for CTS if you're overweight and if you don't exercise very much. Women's risk is also increased by taking oral contraceptives and during menopause.

The first symptoms of CTS aren't that far removed from the sensation you get in your foot when it "falls asleep." You may experience tingling, numbness, or pain in the hand and fingers, especially in the thumb and first two fingers. The more you use your hand, the more it will hurt. As the condition progresses, your hand can become so weak that you can't even grip a glass. For severe cases like this, a doctor may recommend surgery to relieve pressure on the entrapped nerve.

Naturopathic doctors recommend that you first take steps to avoid surgery by working on the mechanical problem of CTS as well as taking supplements. You may be able to get relief and reduce inflammation right away with simple measures like splinting your wrist in a neutral position and altering your activity. You can also use heat and cold to help relieve your symptoms.

In addition you'll probably want to try some of the supplements that can help. Here are some vitamins and herbs to soothe and heal the irritated nerve.

Vitamin B$_6$ Gets a Boost

Vitamin B$_6$ seems to help relieve the symptoms of CTS, says Jill Stansbury, N.D., assistant professor of botanical medicine and chair of the botanical medicine department at the National College of Naturopathic Medicine in Portland, Oregon.

While doctors aren't sure why this supplementation works, some speculate that CTS is actually caused by a deficiency. Although you can get B$_6$ pretty readily from everyday foods like potatoes, brown rice, bananas, green vegetables, and chicken breast, the average diet doesn't usually provide the Daily Value of two milligrams.

Also, the content of your diet doesn't really tell the whole story when it comes to CTS. Low levels can be caused by other factors, says Dr. Stansbury. "Some people may just need more of this vitamin because they use more up," she says. "Stress is one factor that can increase your need for B$_6$ as well as other B vitamins."

Researchers hit on the link between low levels of this vitamin and CTS in the late 1970s. One early study found that 22 of 23 people who took between 50 and 300 milligrams of B$_6$ for 12 weeks got complete relief from pain and tingling in their hands. How this happens is still a bit of a mystery, says Dr. Stansbury.

The problem is that B$_6$ has so many roles in the body that doctors have had difficulty pinpointing any one key action that could have a direct effect on the carpal tunnel area. Like other B vitamins, B$_6$ works with enzymes, the chemicals that spark reactions in your body. It is an essential part of many chemical reactions involved in the body's production of energy, protein, and fats. "It gets around," says Dr. Stansbury. While that emphasizes the fact that we really need this vitamin, however, it doesn't say anything about the direct role that it plays in helping to relieve CTS.

Vitamin B_6 seems to work best on mild to moderate cases of CTS, says Thomas Kruzel, N.D., a naturopathic doctor in Portland, Oregon. To end the tingling, take 50 milligrams of B_6 each day, he suggests, and give it time to work. It usually takes 12 weeks to get the full benefit.

You can boost the healing power of B_6 by taking at least 10 milligrams of riboflavin along with it, says Dr. Kruzel. The riboflavin seems to improve the effect by converting B_6 to a more active form that is essential to more than 60 chemical reactions in your body.

An Herb with Nerve

Widely known for its ability to treat depression, St. John's wort also helps nerves recover when they are damaged, inflamed, or strained, says Dr. Stansbury. Thousands of years before doctors coined the term *carpal tunnel syndrome*, the relaxing herb was used to heal nerve pain and tingling, she says.

For the squeezed median nerve, St. John's wort helps in two ways. Its sedative effect helps to reduce pain, while its anti-inflammatory activity can help shrink swollen nerve tissue. Don't expect the kind of quick pain relief that comes from popping a pharmaceutical like aspirin or ibuprofen, though; St. John's wort typically takes a few weeks to start working.

Start out with 150 to 250 milligrams of extract standardized to 0.3 percent hypericin three times a day, says Dr. Stansbury. You should start to see some improvement in about two weeks. If you don't, take a little more, she says—300 to 400 milligrams three times a day.

While St. John's wort is generally very safe, pregnant women should not take it without a doctor's okay.

Some Wrist Action for Pineapple

When it comes to inflammation, sometimes your body just doesn't know when to stop. With CTS, you need to reduce the inflammation in the swollen tendons and synovium in order to relieve the pain. Pharmaceutical anti-inflammatories like aspirin or ibuprofen might be all you need, but some people find that they experience side effects from these drugs, particularly upset stomach and ringing in the ears.

For relief with fewer side effects, you have the option of trying some supplements that can be very effective. One of these is bromelain, an enzyme found in pineapple that is nature's anti-inflammatory medicine. This hungry enzyme can take a bite out of pain and swelling and help you heal faster, says Dr. Kruzel. Just be sure you don't blunt its effect by taking it with meals. If you do, all of its enzymatic energy is just digested. If you take it between meals, however, it goes to work digesting the products of inflammation.

When the tingling pain of CTS strikes, take two 500-milligram tablets or capsules of bromelain between meals two or three times a day, says Dr. Kruzel. Bromelain is measured in milk-clotting units (mcu) or gelatin-dissolving units (gdu). The higher the number, the greater its potency. Look for a supplement with a strength between 1,800 and 2,400 mcu or 1,080 and 1,440 gdu in each capsule.

Pouring On the Flaxseed Oil

You can also soothe the inflamed nerve and tissues with flaxseed oil, a supplement rich in omega-3 essential fatty acids, says Ellen Potthoff, D.C., N.D., a chiropractor and naturopathic doctor in Pleasant Hill, California. Any type of inflammation responds well to essential fatty acids because no matter where it hurts, they interrupt the process of inflammation early.

You should feel better in two to four weeks if you start taking one tablespoon of flaxseed oil every day, says Dr. Potthoff. Taste is one way to tell if you're getting good-quality flaxseed oil. "It should have a really nice, nutty flavor and a dark amber color," she says.

The Power of Turmeric

Turmeric is an herb that contains a powerful anti-inflammatory chemical called curcumin. The herb has traditionally been used in India's Ayurvedic medicine to treat pain and inflammation.

The effect of turmeric has been compared to that of cortisone, the pharmaceutical sometimes used to treat CTS symptoms. Although turmeric's pain-fighting power is not as strong as cortisone's, the herb is a lot easier on your system, says Dr. Kruzel.

Turmeric's action is similar to that of bromelain. For some relief, opt for capsules of the standardized extract. Unlike the turmeric on your spice shelf, the capsules contain 95 percent pure curcumin.

Dr. Kruzel gives people with CTS 250 to 500 milligrams of curcumin a day. Keep taking this dose until the inflammation has been reduced, he advises, then take half that dose for one to two weeks until your symptoms are gone.

If the symptoms return, repeat with the high dose and return to the lower dose again after they improve. Do not use turmeric supplements without talking to your doctor, especially if you are pregnant.

You might also consider adding bioflavonoids to your supplement arsenal, suggests Dr. Potthoff. Rich in powerful antioxidants, bioflavonoids are used to treat injuries because they relieve pain and promote healing, she says. She recommends taking 1,000 milligrams of a broad-range bioflavonoid supplement that contains citrus bioflavonoids and quercetin three times a day.

cataracts

If your doctor tells you that you're developing a cataract, it means that the lens in one of your eyes is becoming less transparent. As this normally crystal-clear disk begins to cloud over, you might have trouble seeing into the distance, words on a page may appear blurry, or you could find yourself wishing that your eyeglasses were stronger.

Oddly enough, cataracts may actually cause strange improvements in vision when they first occur. If you suddenly notice that you no longer need your reading glasses to scan the newspaper, suspect a cataract.

Cataracts ultimately interfere with clear vision, but if they are treated properly, they generally aren't blinding or life-threatening. "Ninety-nine percent of the time, cataracts are not an emergency," says Robert Abel Jr., M.D., clinical professor of ophthalmology at Thomas Jefferson University in Philadelphia and author of *The Eyecare Revolution*. You should go to an eye doctor for a thorough examination at least once every two years. Your doctor will be able to tell you if you have cataracts, and if so, what stage they've reached.

The progression of cataracts can be slowed or even reversed with the right vitamins, says Dr. Abel, but he advises that you check with your doctor before taking supplements. "The perfect people to try supplements as treatment are those with early or intermediate cataracts—the kind they may not even be aware of yet," he says. By taking some supplements for as little as six months, some people can get out of what Dr. Abel calls the cataract surgery zone.

Antioxidants Keep Things Clear

Most of the evidence for supplements' effect on cataracts points to vitamins C and E and selenium.

The lens of the eye has the second highest concentration of vitamin C of any organ in the body, says Mark Lamden, N.D., a naturopathic doctor and adjunct faculty member at Bastyr University in Bothell, Washington. Any vitamin C that you get—from food or supplements—can help your lenses in a big way.

There's another reason to take vitamin C, however. It's an antioxidant, and you need its power because the eyes are prime sites of what are called oxidative processes. Any time we burn energy, it's a metabolic process that involves oxygen molecules. The eyes, says Dr. Abel, are the most metabolically active parts of the body. "For the eyes, it's constant oxidation," he says, "and even though oxidation is a normal life process, it exerts a lot of wear and tear."

Research suggests that when it comes to vitamin C and cataract prevention, commitment is the key. A study of 247 nurses at Tufts University in Boston showed that women who took vitamin C supplements for 10 years or more were much less likely to have signs of cataracts than those who never took the vitamin.

If you have cataracts, you should take 3,000 to 5,000 milligrams of vitamin C in divided doses throughout the day, recommends Dr. Lamden.

Scavengers for Better Vision

Vitamin E and selenium are other antioxidants that have been associated with reduced risk of cataracts. Like vitamin C, they scavenge free radicals, the free-roaming, unstable molecules that wreak a lot of damage on cells. Because of their free radical–scavenging abilities, vitamin E and selenium help prevent or clear up cloudiness in the lens. Research has shown that people with cataracts often have low levels of selenium in their blood and in the aqueous humor—the fluid within the eyeball—compared to people without cataracts.

Although vitamin E and selenium are present in some foods such as whole grains and vegetable oils, you would have a hard time getting significant amounts of either nutrient from food. "There's no way you could eat enough of the right foods to get the high doses necessary for real nutrition therapy," says Dr. Lamden. Fortunately, that's where supplements come into the picture.

For people already diagnosed with cataracts, Dr. Lamden recommends 800 to 1,200 international units (IU) of natural vitamin E and 400 micrograms of selenium a day. To help keep cataracts from forming in the first place, a lower daily dose of 400 to 800 IU of Vitamin E is ample. Since these are high doses of both supplements, however, you should talk to your doctor first.

The mineral zinc is another nutrient that can help halt hazy sight, says Dr. Lamden. In studies, it has been noted that the lenses of people with cataracts tend to be lacking in zinc. If you have cataracts, Dr. Lamden recommends 30 to 60 milligrams of zinc every day. These doses also require medical supervision.

A good dose of riboflavin—which boosts glutathione levels in the body—may also help prevent cataracts. A study at the State University of New York at Stony Brook found that people who received the most riboflavin were much less likely to have cataracts than those who received smaller amounts. The connection, once again, appears to be antioxidants. The body uses riboflavin to manufacture glutathione, a powerful compound that battles free radicals. When you don't get enough riboflavin, glutathione levels fall, and that gives free radicals more time to damage the eyes.

celiac disease

Some folks who have celiac disease find themselves in an ironic situation. They eat a balanced diet of meat, dairy, fruits, vegetables, and whole-grain foods, yet their guts growl constantly with gas, diarrhea, and stomach cramps, alternating with constipation. It's as if their insides were rebelling against what, for most people, would be a healthy and nutritious diet.

If you have celiac disease, you're intolerant of gluten, the protein in wheat, rye, barley, and oats that makes dough sticky and gooey. Unless the condition is treated, your system can't absorb enough nutrients from food to carry on body functions, a condition known as malabsorption. If you lose weight, become listless, and appear malnourished, you may have celiac disease.

"If left untreated, it can become life-threatening. People can waste away," says Kristin Stiles, N.D., a naturopathic doctor at the Complementary Medicine and Healing Arts Center in Vestal, New York. That's why it's important to get a proper diagnosis from your doctor if you experience these symptoms.

Get the Gluten Out

Fortunately, the treatment is fairly simple once you know the cause. The disease, which often runs in families, was initially identified in the first century A.D. It wasn't until World War II, however, that a Dutch pediatrician discovered that his patients improved because there was no bread available. It seems that some people lack an enzyme that breaks down and helps digest gluten. When this enzyme is absent, a toxic substance builds up and damages the mucous membrane lining the small intestine. Frequently, the damaged area becomes inflamed.

When injured, the intestinal lining has difficulty soaking up the nutrients in food. That's why people with celiac disease may also develop anemia. Anemia often results from a lack of iron in the blood, and that's one of the nutrients that is blocked when the intestinal lining can't do its job. Other deficiencies may show up, too, such as shortages of folic acid and other B vitamins and vitamins A, D, E, K, and beta-carotene.

The first and most effective treatment is to eliminate gluten from your diet. This isn't quite as easy as it sounds because so many processed foods use wheat, which contains gluten, for filler and flavoring. If you're aware of risky food products and avoid them, a gluten-free diet can restore small intestine function within a few days to a few months. Once the mucous membrane is no longer inflamed, the absorption problem usually disappears.

Replace Lost Nutrients

In the meantime, until the healing process does its work, it's a good idea to take vitamin and mineral supplements to prevent deficiencies and malnutrition, says Pamela Taylor, N.D., a naturopathic doctor in Moline, Illinois.

At the very least, you'll want to take a multivitamin/mineral supplement that includes calcium and magnesium, says Dr. Taylor. Magnesium deficiency often occurs in malabsorption syndromes and may contribute to osteoporosis, the rapid bone loss that can lead to hip fractures and other skeletal problems. This mineral is also important for proper tissue healing, so you need to get enough to help your body heal itself. To make sure that you get magnesium, be sure that your diet consists of moderate amounts of protein and plenty of steamed leafy green vegetables like kale, collard greens, and mustard greens. These greens are also good sources of calcium, she adds.

In addition to a multivitamin each day, Dr. Stiles tells her patients to take a high-potency B-complex supplement. This type of supplement contains 50 milligrams or the equivalent of B vitamins like niacin, thiamin, and riboflavin, as well as 400 to 800 micrograms of folic acid. Typically, one or two tablets daily with food are sufficient, she says. Your doctor can determine through blood tests how much you should take, she adds. If you take more than 35 milligrams of niacin, though, be sure to let your doctor know.

"You definitely want to supplement B vitamins, because those are not well-absorbed when the intestines are aggravated," says Dr. Stiles. "Also always take the supplement with food. If you take it on an empty stomach, you won't absorb it."

Even after your intestinal inflammation has subsided and you're absorbing nutrients the way you should, you probably should continue taking a multivitamin, says Dr. Taylor. "A good multivitamin/mineral tablet can catch and fill in the deficiencies and make sure you're getting what you need each day."

Speed the Healing

The inflammation in the intestine won't go away until you eliminate gluten, but you may be able to speed healing by taking an herbal combination of echinacea and goldenseal, says Dr. Stiles. These two immune system boosters are often packaged together in capsule form. Take one capsule three or four times a day, she suggests. If you use tincture, take 10 to 15 drops of each herb in water or juice three or four times a day, with or without food.

You may also find echinacea and goldenseal in combination with slippery elm, marshmallow, geranium, and other herbs. If you can't find this combination at a drugstore, check at a health food store. This supplement goes by the generic name of Robert's Formula, which is made by a number of different supplement makers. It is a naturopathic mixture that treats the digestive tract by creating a slimy goo that is healing to gut tissues.

Echinacea and goldenseal are important healers because they have anti-inflammatory and antibacterial properties. One cautionary note, however: Don't take these herbs continuously. Dr. Stiles recommends two weeks on and two weeks off for a period of one to two months. "You quickly build up a tolerance to echinacea, and it's no longer effective," she says.

Vitamins can also speed healing. Dr. Taylor often recommends that her patients take a combination supplement of vitamins A, E, and C, along with a chelated form of zinc supplement. She suggests that you follow the dosage directions on the bottle. A typical dose, for example, is 5,000 to 10,000 international units (IU) of vitamin A in the form of fish oil, 200 to 500 milligrams of vitamin C, 100 to 400 IU of vitamin E, and 15 to 30 milligrams of chelated zinc. You'll need to check with your doctor before taking more than 20 milligrams of zinc, however.

Dr. Taylor recommends taking the supplements with food. You may need to continue supplementation for two to four months, she says.

chronic fatigue syndrome

Sure, we're all tired, at least some of the time. But people with chronic fatigue syndrome (CFS), have more than that occasional pooped-out feeling.

CFS, in fact, has an official definition that's used for diagnosis in the medical community. It's defined as debilitating fatigue that lasts for at least six months, accompanied by a number of other symptoms such as sleep disturbances, tender lymph nodes, sore throat, trouble with short-term memory, and various aches and pains.

Needless to say, if you have such continuous fatigue, the first thing you need to do is see if you and your doctor can find a cause, since many health problems can cause a similar range of problems. If no other cause can be found, it's possible that you have CFS.

Although CFS is still something of a medical mystery, doctors and researchers are continually learning more about it. "Many experts now think that chronic fatigue syndrome may be an example of the hypothalamus failing to properly regulate the brain's influence on the immune system," says Jay Lombard, M.D., assistant clinical professor of neurology at Weill Medical College of Cornell University in New York City and co-author of *The Brain Wellness Plan*.

The hypothalamus is a regulatory gland in the brain. It normally stimulates the production of an important hormone called corticotropin. Corticotropin in turn is needed to stimulate the adrenal glands, which are located on top of the kidneys. When the hypothalamus isn't doing its job and you don't get enough corticotropin, your adrenal glands don't produce enough cortisol, the body's main stress hormone. "Clearly, chronic fatigue syndrome involves faulty communication among the nervous system, the immune system, and the endocrine system," Dr. Lombard says.

Lots of people with CFS also have low blood pressure, and a few studies suggest that some may also have difficulty producing and utilizing energy inside cells, Dr. Lombard says. Plus, some people have digestive problems that can cause improper digestion and absorption of critical nutrients, says Jeanne Hubbuch, M.D., a doctor in Newton Highland, Massachusetts.

One problem, called leaky gut, occurs when portions of improperly digested food elements seep through the lining of the intestine. Some experts speculate that this leakage sets off an immune response that can ultimately lead to attacks on the body's own cells.

Nutritional supplementation for CFS really depends on your particular symptoms, says Dr. Hubbuch. Doctors may use a wide array of supplements, each geared toward dealing with a particular symptom. Even doctors who consider themselves quite familiar with CFS, though, admit that it's not easy to treat.

"Treatments may sound great in theory, but in practice it is a very difficult matter," Dr. Lombard says. "Chronic fatigue syndrome is a difficult disease to treat, medically and nutritionally. Often, there are psychological issues that may not be causing the disease but that certainly play a role."

With that in mind, here are the nutritional and herbal treatments.

The Gut Connection

Practitioners of natural medicine advise that people with CSF have a comprehensive digestive stool analysis. This analysis will show whether they're having problems with bacterial or yeast overgrowth in the intestines or with the incomplete breakdown of foods, Dr. Hubbuch says.

A wide variety of nutritional supplements might be used to treat digestive problems, says Dr. Hubbuch. These include foods such as garlic or grapefruit seed extract, which can help kill bacteria or yeast.

Some people try introducing "friendly" bacteria such as *Lactobacillus acidophilus* and *Bifidobacterium bifidum* to restore a healthy balance of beneficial bacteria in the intestines and help crowd out the bad bugs. Others with CFS can benefit from enzymes that help the body break down food into digestible particles, she says. You may also want to take fiber formulas derived from plants, such as those made from psyllium seed, kelp, agar, pectin, and oat bran, to help elimination. It's best to talk to your doctor about how much of each one to take.

Garlic is most effective if it's fresh and raw, and it's good to use at least one clove a day, says Dr. Hubbuch. If you are taking garlic supplements, you need a daily dose of at least 10 milligrams of allicin, the active ingredient in garlic that helps fight fungal infections. As for *L. acidophilus* and *B. bifidum*, you should get 1 to 10 billion viable organisms a day, so check the dosage on the product you use.

Follow the directions on the label or your doctor's directions if you're taking digestive enzymes. Dr. Hubbuch says that she normally suggests taking 5,000 units of lipase, 20,000 units of amylase, and 20,000 units of trypsin. You can also take 3 to 5 grams or more of soluble fiber each day at meals, she says.

Improving Immunity

Because so many people with chronic fatigue syndrome also have weakened immune systems, Dr. Lombard recommends several nutrients that have been shown to strengthen immunity. A high-potency multivitamin/mineral supplement may provide what you need. Look for these amounts in the supplement you choose: 30 milligrams of zinc, 25,000 international units (IU) of vitamin A (part can be from beta-carotene), 50 milligrams of B-complex vitamins such as pantothenic acid and riboflavin, 200 micrograms of selenium, 2 milligrams each of copper and manganese, and 400 IU of vitamin E. Dr. Lombard also recommends 4,000 milligrams of vitamin C a day in divided doses. For such a high amount, you'll need a separate vitamin C supplement.

Herbs can stimulate your immune system, notes Dr. Lombard. He suggests 500 milligrams of a standardized extract of astragalus daily for long-term use. "Astragalus enhances antibody response, increases helper T lymphocytes and natural killer cell activity, and aids in immune system self-regulation," he says. "You should take this especially during periods of stress, such as during cold and flu season."

Along with astragalus, Dr. Lombard recommends 250 milligrams of a standardized extract of echinacea daily for 7 to 10 days with three-week rest intervals between dosage periods. "Echinacea stimulates macrophages, enhances the action of white blood cells, and stimulates the production of immune system–regulating biochemicals," he says. You need to take some time off between dosage periods, however, because echinacea loses its effectiveness after you take it for a while and your body builds a tolerance to it.

Dr. Hubbuch also recommends echinacea, often in combination with another immune-enhancing herb, goldenseal. "These are really good if you have a lot of viral symptoms, such as a sore throat, swollen glands, low-grade fever, or herpes," she says.

If you have only occasional flare-ups, you can use the herbs when symptoms start, as long as you consult your doctor. For flare-ups, you can take a 250-milligram capsule two or three times a day (a total of 500 to 750 milligrams) of a combination of echinacea and goldenseal, says Dr. Hubbuch. To suppress symptoms or as a maintenance dose, you can use two capsules twice a day, she adds.

You can also take echinacea and goldenseal as a tincture, using 15 to 20 drops—about a dropperful—three times a day if you have active symptoms. For maintenance, when the symptoms quiet down, you can take the tincture twice a day.

Aiding Sleep

Tired as they may be, people with CFS often have trouble sleeping, To help improve sleep, Dr. Hubbuch recommends 5-hydroxytryptophan (5-HTP) and melatonin.

In your body, 5-HTP increases levels of serotonin, a chemical that helps regulate sleep patterns. Studies show that 5-HTP can shorten the time it takes to fall asleep and make you less likely to waken during the night. When Dr. Hubbuch prescribes this supplement, she instructs people to take 50 milligrams one hour before bedtime.

You can increase the dosage up to 150 milligrams at night if necessary, but don't go any higher than 200 milligrams, advises Dr. Lombard, since higher doses can cause disturbing dreams.

You should not take 5-HTP if you are currently taking antidepressant medication or have taken it recently, as the combined effects could cause a possibly fatal condition called serotonin syndrome. Otherwise, you can use 5-HTP safely for long periods of time, Dr. Hubbuch says. Decrease the dose if you are sleeping well, she advises. Along with the 5-HTP, she suggests taking 50 milligrams of vitamin B_6.

In addition to 5-HTP, some people may need to take melatonin, which can also be a sleep aid, Dr. Hubbuch says. She recommends two milligrams of timed-release melatonin at bedtime. For those who need still more help falling asleep, she suggests valerian, a calming herb that can help hasten sleep, improve the quality of sleep, and reduce nighttime awakenings.

In his book *The Green Pharmacy*, James A. Duke, Ph.D., a botanical consultant and former ethnobotanist with the U.S. Department of Agriculture who specializes in medicinal plants, says that some naturopaths whom he respects suggest drinking valerian root tea about 30 minutes before retiring. Others suggest taking 150 to 300 milligrams of a standardized extract (0.8 percent valeric acid). Do not use valerian with sleep-enhancing or mood-regulating medications such as diazepam (Valium) or amitriptyline (Elavil), however. If stimulant actions such as nervousness or heart palpitations occur, discontinue use.

Try one of these sleep remedies at a time and see if it works for you, Dr. Hubbuch says. If you don't notice results after one to two weeks of using one product, try another. "Sometimes, you do use all of them," she says. "It depends on how bad your sleep problem is." It is safe to use all three, according to Dr. Hubbuch.

Enhancing Energy

People with CFS may also have impaired energy metabolism within the mitochondria, the energy producing areas of the muscle cells, Dr. Lombard says. The cells just don't make or use energy as well as they should, for unknown reasons.

To improve this situation, he recommends coenzyme Q_{10} (coQ_{10}). This substance helps charge up the mitochondria. Both he and Dr. Hubbuch recommend taking 200 milligrams a day.

Dr. Hubbuch suggests taking a type of coQ_{10} that is placed under the tongue (sublingual), where it dissolves and is absorbed through the mucous membranes, rather than the kind you swallow. "It is helpful in quite a few people," she says. "It's better absorbed and seems to work better."

If you start taking coQ_{10} and it helps, the results usually show up in about a month, says Dr. Hubbuch. "Try it for a month and see if it is worth it for you. If it's not doing anything, then just stop." You can take it at any time of day, she says.

Many of the B vitamins as well as the amino acid l-carnitine are also essential for energy production. They're important because they all appear to work together to boost muscle energy levels. You can make sure that you're getting all of the B vitamins by taking a high-potency B-complex supplement, Dr. Lombard says. Look for one that includes about 50 milligrams of most of the B's.

Since you should get more folic acid and vitamin B$_{12}$ than what's provided by a B-complex supplement, you'll probably need to take additional supplements, says Dr. Lombardo. He recommends a total of 1,000 micrograms of folic acid and 1,000 micrograms of B$_{12}$ a day. In addition, he suggests supplementing with 500 milligrams of l-carnitine daily. But don't take extra B-complex vitamins if you are already taking them to boost immunity, he cautions.

Have Some Magnesium

An essential mineral, magnesium, is also necessary for energy metabolism. Doctors have found that many people with CFS have low levels of magnesium in their red blood cells, and several studies have shown some improvement in energy levels with magnesium supplementation.

Typically, magnesium comes as magnesium oxide or carbonate, but other forms may be better absorbed orally and utilized in the body. These include magnesium lactate, orotate, glycinate, and gluconate.

Helping Your Hormones

People with CFS may need to reduce the amount of stress on their adrenal glands. That means limiting sugar and caffeine and taking vitamins, minerals, and herbs that help the glands function properly, Dr. Lombard says.

"The adrenal glands contain the highest concentration of vitamin C in the body," he says. Vitamin C helps influence neurotransmitters, the essential messenger chemicals that carry signals from one part of the body to another. Dr. Lombard recommends 4,000 milligrams of vitamin C a day, taken in divided doses. If you are already taking this amount to boost immunity, however, you don't need to take more.

He also suggests 50 milligrams of pantothenic acid, 30 milligrams of zinc, and 600 milligrams of magnesium in divided doses. "These nutrients all play necessary roles in the manufacture of hormones by the adrenal glands," Dr. Lombard says. If you are already taking these nutrients for other reasons, though, there's no need to add more.

Siberian and Asian ginseng can also help support the adrenal glands, increase resistance to stress, and exert a number of beneficial effects on immune functions that may be useful in the treatment of CFS, Dr. Lombard says. In one study, people who took 10 milliliters a day of a liquid extract of Siberian ginseng had a significant increase in T-helper cells and in natural killer cell activity, both of which are of value in treating CFS. Dr. Lombard recommends 500 milligrams a day of standardized extract of Siberian or Asian ginseng.

Licorice for Low Blood Pressure

Licorice is also helpful in supporting the adrenal glands and increasing the production of cortisol, an important hormone, by this gland, Dr. Hubbuch says. Low amounts of cortisol or other adrenal hormones in the body can lower blood pressure. "Some people with CFS have problems with low blood pressure. As a result, they may feel dizzy and light-headed, especially when they are changing positions," she says. If you notice that you become dizzy when you stand up suddenly, low blood pressure may be the reason. Licorice can help relieve this symptom.

How much licorice you need to take depends on your symptoms and the type you use. A standard dose is 1,000 to 2,000 milligrams of powdered root or two to four milliliters (roughly ⅓ to ⅔ teaspoon) of liquid extract. Alternatively, you can take 250 to 500 milligrams of dry, powdered extract.

Be careful not to overdo it, though. You should talk to a doctor if you're taking these amounts, since high daily doses for more than four to six weeks can cause symptoms such as headache and lethargy and may even lead to impaired heart or kidney function. Also high blood pressure is the most common side effect.

Help from DHEA

Dr. Hubbuch will also sometimes recommend dehydroepiandrosterone (DHEA), an adrenal hormone that the body can convert to various other hormones, including testosterone. People with CFS may produce inadequate amounts of it. She recommends that you have your doctor check your level of DHEA with a simple blood or saliva test before you supplement with it.

"I would try it only if other treatments aren't helping enough and if DHEA levels are low," she says. In men, low DHEA levels are often associated with low sex drive. In women, often the only symptom is fatigue, Dr. Hubbuch says.

DHEA is available over the counter. If you have a prescription from your doctor, a compounding pharmacist can make up a specific dose, says Philip Mease, M.D., a rheumatologist at Minor and James Medical Center and clinical associate professor of medicine at the University of Washington Medical School, both in Seattle. DHEA has not been studied in chronic fatigue patients, but Dr. Mease says, "I have heard reports from patients that this hormone supplement can be helpful for reducing pain and fatigue."

The dose of DHEA varies depending on the strength of the product you are taking. If you can get the tincture from a pharmacist, the instructions are usually to take drops under the tongue twice a day, according to Dr. Mease. "My experience has been that the DHEA made by pharmacists is more effective than the capsules you'd get at a health food store," he says. Whatever you do, it's wise to work with your doctor if you want to take DHEA, Dr. Mease advises.

colds and flu

With more than 200 cold viruses floating around and a new strain of flu just waiting to claim its next victim each year, it seems almost impossible *not* to get sick.

When a cold or flu hits, you may want to go stock up on to the drugstore and over-the-counter remedies. Before you buy those cough suppressants, decongestants, and antihistamines, though, you should consider nutritional supplements to speed your recovery.

You can try a combination of nature's most powerful herbs, such as echinacea, goldenseal, and astragalus, to shift your immune system into overdrive so that your body can fight off the infection naturally. To back up this herbal defense team, you can use an array of infection-fighting vitamins and a mineral that can shorten the duration of your cold or flu, lessen the severity of symptoms, or continue to build your immunity until you start feeling like yourself again.

If these and other remedies don't have an effect, however, you may have to be on guard for other kinds of infection. Be sure to see your doctor if your cold does not improve within 14 days or if you have green or yellow phlegm. And check with your doctor if you have trouble breathing, or if your temperature tops 102°F.

Powerful Herbs to the Rescue

Echinacea and goldenseal, taken in combination, are top cold and flu fighters among medicinal herbal supplements, says Kristy Fassler, N.D., a naturopathic doctor in Portsmouth, New Hampshire.

Echinacea, also known as purple coneflower, Kansas snakeroot, and black Sampson, is a potent herb that forcefully stimulates the production of natural killer cells. The aptly named killer cell is a type of white blood cell that fights off viral infections.

While boosting the population of killer cells, echinacea also increases levels of immune system chemicals such as interferon and properdin that kill bacteria and viruses. It speeds up destruction of bacteria and viruses by enhancing the activity of cells called phagocytes.

Similar to echinacea, goldenseal stimulates white blood cell activity and contains antiviral and antibacterial compounds, chiefly berberine. It works well with echinacea because it has properties that enable it to reduce inflammation and mucus production. When you take goldenseal, it helps break up nasal and chest congestion and also reduces the swelling of mucous membranes, says Dr. Fassler.

When symptoms strike, take 300 milligrams of each of these herbs every two to four hours for the first two to three days, says Dr. Fassler. Continue with the same dosage of each three times a day until symptoms disappear.

A Root from the Orient

For thousands of years in China, the herb that has been used to enhance immunity is astragalus root. This potent herb is considered by herbal practitioners to be a tonic that strengthens the body's resistance to disease. Astragalus can stimulate practically all of the processes of your immune system. It increases the number of stem cells in bone marrow and speeds their growth into active immune cells.

Astragalus also may help boost levels of interferon, one of your body's potent fighters against viruses, says Chris Meletis, N.D., professor of natural pharmacology at the National College of Naturopathic Medicine in Portland, Oregon. A heightened level of interferon can help prevent or shorten the duration of colds and flu. Astragalus even boosts production of white blood cells called macrophages, whose mission is to destroy invading viruses and bacteria.

To stamp out a cold or flu in its earliest stages, take one 500-milligram capsule of astragalus four times a day until symptoms disappear, says Dr. Meletis. Then take one capsule twice a day for seven days to prevent a relapse.

Tap into a Trio of Infection Fighters

It's a good idea to stock your medicine cabinet with vitamin C, vitamin A, and beta-carotene supplements, say Dr. Fassler and Dr. Meletis. These nutrients help you fight back fast, before the virus takes up residence and multiplies in your body.

Studies show that vitamin C can shorten the duration of common colds and flu and even prevent them. Taken in large enough doses, vitamin C can rev up your immune system by pumping enough fuel into white blood cells to destroy invading viruses and bacteria, says Dr. Meletis.

Vitamin C increases interferon levels and has interferon-like properties itself. It acts as a natural antihistamine that helps dry up watery eyes and reduce nasal and chest congestion, according to Dr. Meletis. It is also a powerful antioxidant that can help prevent the damage that your body endures when viruses or bacteria attack your immune system, he says.

At the first sign of cold or flu symptoms, take 500 milligrams of vitamin C with bioflavonoids or rose hips four to six times a day, says Dr. Meletis. "The bioflavonoids and rose hips strengthen the vitamin C's infection-fighting power by 35 percent," he says.

Vitamin A is known as the anti-infection vitamin. It battles viruses and bacteria in two ways. By keeping the cells healthy all along your respiratory tract, it provides a barrier that resists microorganisms. If some invading microorganisms manage to breach the barrier, you want to have antibodies and lymphocytes ready to destroy them. Vitamin A helps your body provide those reinforcements.

As soon as you notice cold or flu symptoms, take 100,000 international units (IU) of vitamin A daily for three days, says Dr. Fassler, then reduce the dosage to 25,000 IU for one week or until symptoms disappear. She cautions, however, that these are very high doses, and you need to check with your doctor before taking this much.

Vitamin A's precursor beta-carotene is brimming with antioxidant power and antiviral properties. It bolsters immunity and protects the thymus gland, the main headquarters where a certain type of white blood cell matures and learns to recognize foreign invaders, says Dr. Meletis.

"Beta-carotene also protects you from viruses by enhancing mucous membrane secretions. By producing the secretions, the beta-carotene prevents the virus from setting up housekeeping in your body," says Thomas Kruzel, N.D., a naturopathic doctor.

If you feel a cold or flu coming on, take 100,000 IU of beta-carotene for 10 to 14 days, says Dr. Kruzel, then cut the dosage to 50,000 IU a day to prevent future respiratory infections.

A Zinc Prescription

Of all the trace minerals found in multivitamins, zinc is probably the most important for keeping your immunity strong. It stimulates the immune system by generating new white blood cells and whipping them into shape to battle viruses. If you have too little zinc, your production of white blood cells may drop, and that can increase your risk of catching a cold, flu, or other upper respiratory infection.

In one study, children who got 10 milligrams of zinc daily for 60 days were much less likely to get respiratory infections than children getting less. In fact, the children who got enough zinc were 70 percent less likely to have fevers, 48 percent less likely to have coughs, and 28 percent less likely to have mucus buildup.

While it's best to get zinc from foods, you can get what you need from supplements. Be careful not to take too much, though—more is not necessarily better. In fact, doctors recommend taking no more than 15 milligrams a day. If you check with your physician, you can take 30 milligrams a day with food for 7 to 10 days, but don't take more unless you have your doctor's consent.

Zinc gluconate in lozenge form has been found to shorten the duration of cold symptoms. In a study, participants who sucked on one zinc gluconate lozenge (containing about 13 milligrams of zinc) every two hours while awake got rid of their coughs, nasal congestion, sore throat, and headaches three to four days sooner than those who didn't get any supplementation. After checking with your doctor, you can take the lozenges to help shake off these symptoms. Don't take them for longer than one week, cautions Dr. Meletis, because they can weaken your immune system.

lick

cold sores

A tingling sensation outside your mouth or above your lips is usually the telltale sign. Within two to three days, a painful, fluid-filled blister appears. It swells, ruptures, and oozes fluid that forms a yellow crust. Eventually, it peels off and reveals new skin underneath. The blister usually lasts 7 to 10 days, but while it's in full view, you may be tempted to go into hiding or cover your mouth with your hands until the unsightly sore disappears.

What causes cold sores, commonly called fever blisters, is herpes simplex virus type 1 (HSV-1). About 90 percent of all people are infected with this virus, and if you get a sore once, you can be pretty sure that you'll get one again. If you change your diet and take some other natural measures against these sores, however, you might be able to shorten the time that they stay on your mouth and lips.

To prevent cold sores, some naturopathic doctors advise that you eat more foods that are high in the amino acid lysine, such as yogurt, chicken, fish, and vegetables. At the same time, they say, you should cut back on foods that are high in arginine, another amino acid. The foods to avoid include chocolate, nuts, seeds, and gelatin.

As for supplements, lysine is near the top of the list. Also, certain vitamins and minerals stimulate your immune system so that your body can fight off the virus more effectively. They can shorten the time it takes for cold sores to heal, inhibit the growth and spread of the virus, and reduce pain and swelling. You should also know about some herbal supplements that are chock-full of antiviral compounds that can destroy the virus. They, too, can help build up your immune system.

Heal Them with Lysine

Lysine is an amino acid that inhibits the replication of herpes simplex. Research suggests that a diet high in lysine and low in arginine can prevent the virus from multiplying. Although it relies on arginine to thrive, the virus can't distinguish between lysine and arginine, so it's easily tricked into attaching itself to the lysine. But unlike arginine, lysine blocks the steps the virus must take to replicate.

To keep lysine levels high, take 500 to 1,500 milligrams daily at the first sign of symptoms, says Jennifer Brett, N.D., a naturopathic doctor at the Wilton Naturopathic Center in Stratford, Connecticut. Continue with that dosage until symptoms disappear.

If you're having an outbreak, take 3,000 milligrams of lysine daily until the lesions go away.

Zap 'Em with Vitamin C and Bioflavonoids

Vitamin C with bioflavonoids should be your next line of defense. These supplements will boost your immune system by stimulating production of white blood cells, the infection fighters in your body. The blisters will heal faster as a result, says Dr. Brett.

Bioflavonoids, chemical compounds related to vitamin C, can help reduce the inflammation and pain that's associated with cold sores, says Dr. Brett. You can buy a formula that includes both bioflavonoids and C or take each as a separate supplement.

In one study, 20 people with cold sores took 600 milligrams of vitamin C and 600 milligrams of bioflavonoids three times a day for three days. Another 20 took 1,000 milligrams of C and 1,000 milligrams of bioflavonoids five times a day for the same amount of time. Ten participants received look-alike pills that didn't contain either of the active ingredients (placebos).

At the end of the study, researchers found that the vitamin C and bioflavonoids stopped the cold sores from blossoming into unsightly blisters. They also concluded that the therapy achieved the best results when people took the supplements at the first sign of symptoms.

This research also showed that taking the two together inhibits the progression of the virus. Those who were treated with 1,000-milligram doses had cold sores for a little more than 4 days. Those treated with placebos had sores for more than twice as long—at least 10 days.

To prevent cold sores, take 1,000 milligrams of vitamin C with bioflavonoids daily, Dr. Brett advises. To speed the healing of existing sores, she recommends taking 3,000 milligrams of vitamin C daily in divided doses and 1,000 milligrams daily of quercetin, a commonly used bioflavonoid.

Zinc 'Em, Too

Upping your intake of zinc can also reduce the frequency, duration, and severity of cold sore outbreaks. This mineral has been shown in test-tube studies to block the reproduction of the virus. It produces T lymphocyte cells, which are important body defenses against viral infections.

During a cold sore outbreak, take 50 milligrams a day of zinc in divided doses with food, says Michael Traub, N.D., a naturopathic doctor and director of the integrated residency program at North Hawaii Community Hospital in Kamuela. As a preventive, take 20 milligrams a day. Also, since zinc supplementation can lead to copper deficiency, you should take 1 to 2 milligrams of copper for every 25 milligrams of zinc you take, says Dr. Traub. Don't exceed 2 milligrams of copper daily, however.

A Pair of Antiviral Herbs

Medicinal herbs such as echinacea and St. John's wort can also speed healing, lessen the severity, and shorten the duration of cold sores, says Dr. Traub.

Echinacea strengthens the immune system. It also increases the levels of a chemical called properdin, which activates the part of the immune system responsible for shoring up defense mechanisms against viruses and bacteria.

Dr. Traub recommends taking one 300-milligram capsule of echinacea four times a day during a cold sore outbreak. For prevention, take one 300-milligram capsule daily during times of stress or as soon as you feel a cold sore coming on, he says.

St. John's wort has strong antiviral properties that may help to prevent the herpesvirus from replicating. In fact, this herb's antiviral activity is so significant that high concentrations of it have decreased HIV (the virus that causes AIDS) in a laboratory setting. The active ingredients that possess these antiviral properties are hypericin and pseudohypericin.

During a cold sore outbreak, take one 300-milligram capsule of St. John's wort daily, says Dr. Traub. Buy the standardized extract that contains 0.3 percent hypericin.

constipation

Constipation is defined as difficult or infrequent bowel movements.

Difficult? We know what that is. But what does infrequent mean? Surely, each person's routine is different.

Even if the definition isn't crystal clear, most of us know when we're constipated. We might not know what's causing the problem, however.

"A lot of constipation just comes down to diet, water, and exercise," says Melissa Metcalfe, N.D., a naturopathic doctor in Los Angeles. See a doctor, though, if you are constipated frequently and every attempt at a bowel movement involves a lot of pain. There may be a blockage, and you may need a doctor's immediate attention to have it removed.

If that's not the problem, and you just have occasional, ordinary, run-of-the-mill constipation, it might be a long-term and fairly constant struggle. There are many possible causes. You may be suffering from stress, dehydration, hemorrhoids, or anal fissures. A colon with weak muscle tone can also cause constipation.

"If there aren't serious underlying causes, the cure is pretty simple," says Dr. Metcalfe. That's where some diet and lifestyle changes, and possibly supplements, can help set things in motion and spare you the strain.

Drink Up

Your first self-treatment is an all-natural combination of two hydrogen molecules and one oxygen molecule joined together in a glass.

That's right—H_2O. Water adds soft bulk to stools. It's also required by the cells of the colon to lubricate the stool's passage, says Dr. Metcalfe.

At the very least, you should drink 8 full eight-ounce glasses of water a day, says Dr. Metcalfe. If you're physically active or drink coffee and other caffeinated beverages that make you urinate often, you should drink 12 glasses a day, she says.

"You need to compensate for that dehydration," says Dr. Metcalfe. "I tell patients to put two liters of water in the fridge and make sure it is gone at the end of the day."

She believes that most people probably don't drink enough water because they don't like the taste of water that comes from the tap. In that case, buy bottled water or some type of filtering system, she suggests. "If dehydration is your only problem, you can be having a normal bowel movement in less than 24 hours," Dr. Metcalfe says.

Fill Up with Fiber

Dietary fiber absorbs water and makes stools fuller and easier to pass. The result is faster transit time through the intestines.

Both soluble and insoluble fiber absorb water. Soluble fiber essentially turns into a kind of gel in your intestine. Good food sources include prunes, apples, kidney beans and other legumes, and oats.

For insoluble fiber—the kind that doesn't turn jellylike but helps to "sweep" your system clean—you'll need to turn to different sources. You can get it from bran, wheat, and vegetables like celery, carrots, and spinach. Fiber is so important to digestion and regularity that experts hold to the recommendation that you should get 25 grams a day.

"Fiber works wonders pretty quickly. Within a few days of getting your daily fiber, you'll notice a difference," says Dr. Metcalfe.

Although it's best to get your fiber from food sources, you can also take a supplement when your meals aren't supplying enough. Dr. Metcalfe recommends taking two tablespoons daily of a fiber/nutritional supplement that contains psyllium. You can also add two tablespoons of flaxseed to yogurt or make a "smoothie" with blended yogurt, fruit, and flaxseed. "At the same time, though, you should be working to get more fiber in your diet," she says.

Move to Have Movement

If you think sitting on your bottom all day can give you constipation, you're not far wrong. To get things moving down below, you have to get off your duff, says Pamela Taylor, N.D., a naturopathic doctor in Moline, Illinois.

Two layers of muscles around the small intestine work together in a process called peristalsis, the wavelike contraction that moves digested food and waste products through the gastrointestinal system. People who are sedentary, particularly if they're older, often lack muscle tone in the abdominal area.

"Exercise can tone abdominal muscles, massage the abdominal organs, and increase blood flow to the area. All of that can help restore good bowel function," says Dr. Taylor.

See about Senna

Sometimes, if diet and lifestyle changes don't do the trick, as a last resort you can try senna, a strong-acting herb that stimulates peristalsis, says Dr. Metcalfe. Its active ingredient, a chemical called anthraquinone, is responsible for this effect.

You might want to use senna as a one-time option, suggests Kristin Stiles, N.D., a naturopathic doctor at the Complementary Medicine and Healing Arts Center in Vestal, New York. It's not safe to use for long-term, chronic constipation. If you take senna repeatedly, your bowel may lose the ability to function on its own.

Dr. Metcalfe recommends that you purchase senna tea bags at a health food store and start off with no more than one cup of senna tea each morning. "Senna is probably going to cause some cramping at first. It really increases peristalsis quickly, so you want to start off slowly with it," she cautions.

Senna works well in combination with psyllium. In a short-term study at the University of Wisconsin-Madison, 42 people who had been having less than three bowel movements a week were given psyllium or psyllium with senna. Although both laxatives increased the frequency of bowel movements, people who took the combination had more moisture in their stools and experienced more relief.

Because senna is a powerful herb that has some risks, you should seek the advice of a naturopathic physician before taking it. Women who are pregnant or breastfeeding should not take senna.

depression

The ups and downs of everyday life can often leave you feeling blue. When your low spirits turn into a never-ending state of sadness, however, you may have depression. While you may not be able to tell the difference between feeling blue and being depressed, a doctor usually can.

In fact, a diagnosis of depression needs to be made by a doctor. There are many possible signs, ranging from sleeplessness and irritability to feelings of guilt or thoughts of suicide. Whether or not you have these symptoms, though, you should seek professional help if you have a blue mood that lasts more than two weeks.

Many doctors prescribe medication for depression, and if you're already taking medication, you shouldn't take supplements without talking to your doctor. Often, dietary and lifestyle changes can help lift your mood, says C. Norman Shealy, M.D., Ph.D., founder of the American Holistic Medical Association and director of the Shealy Institute, a holistic and alternative medicine clinic in Springfield, Missouri. In fact, just 20 minutes of aerobic exercise five days a week can put that pep back in your step, says Dr. Shealy.

Studies show that any kind of exercise prompts the release of mood-enhancing brain chemicals called endorphins that help restore your sense of well-being. Also if you avoid caffeine, alcohol, sugar, and refined carbohydrates (found in cakes and white bread, for instance), you'll prevent brain chemical imbalances that are known to cause depression.

Some natural antidepressant supplements might also be helpful. Certain vitamins can cheer you up by helping to create and stabilize a variety of brain chemicals responsible for mental and emotional health.

Pump Up Some Essential Vitamins

The most common deficiencies in people who are depressed are the B-complex vitamins and vitamin C, says Dr. Shealy.

The B vitamins help energize brain cells and manufacture important chemicals to keep your moods high. Vitamin B_6, for example, plays a starring role in the making of serotonin, a brain chemical that has a direct impact on your moods, emotions, appetite, and sleep patterns. Too little serotonin, and you'll walk around feeling down in the dumps.

What's more, B-complex vitamins enhance communication between brain cells so that other important brain chemicals can work in concert to keep things running smoothly, says Ray Sahelian, M.D., a physician in Marina del Rey, California, and author of *The New Memory Boosters: Natural Supplements That Enhance Your Mind, Memory, and Mood.*

Another B vitamin that has been linked to depression is folate, the naturally occurring form of folic acid. In fact, depression is considered the most common symptom of a folate deficiency.

Harvard Medical School researchers reviewed the literature on depression and found that as many as 38 percent of adults diagnosed with depression had low levels of folate in their blood. Other research shows that low vitamin B_{12} levels are common in elderly people with depression and that folic acid and B_{12} work together to boost low spirits, says Dr. Shealy. Vitamin B_{12} also helps metabolize other mood-elevating brain chemicals and keep nerve tissue healthy.

Another vitamin that's just as important in maintaining high spirits is vitamin C. Low levels can leave you feeling gloomy, says Dr. Sahelian. Vitamin C helps manufacture serotonin and two other essential brain-related chemicals, dopamine and norepinephrine, which lift your mood, keep you alert, and sustain your sex drive.

For mild to moderate depression, you may want to take a high-potency multivitamin/mineral supplement daily after talking to your doctor, says Dr. Shealy. He also suggests 100 milligrams each of thiamin, riboflavin, niacin, and B_6, along with 400 micrograms of folic acid, 100 micrograms of B_{12}, and 2,000 milligrams of vitamin C in divided doses daily.

Help from St. John

If you haven't heard by now, St. John's wort is the quintessential herb of choice for mild to moderate depression. In fact, it is one of the most researched natural antidepressants around. The herb's active ingredients include hypericin, flavonoids, and other compounds that work in unison to raise serotonin levels in the brain, says Jennifer Brett, N.D., a naturopathic doctor at the Wilton Naturopathic Center in Stratford, Connecticut.

Studies show that St. John's wort is just as effective for mild to moderate depression as the widely prescribed antidepressant drugs imipramine (Tofranil), fluoxetine (Prozac), sertraline (Zoloft), and paroxetine (Paxil), says Dr. Shealy.

While it's not understood exactly how the herb increases serotonin levels, researchers speculate that the underlying mechanism is probably similar to that of the prescription drugs, says Dr. Brett. St. John's wort may inhibit an enzyme that breaks down serotonin molecules and other brain chemicals, or it may increase the action of serotonin at the nerve endings in the brain. The serotonin is available so that your brain can further utilize it to regulate your moods and emotions more effectively, she says.

The advantage of St. John's wort over the prescription antidepressants is that it's associated with very few side effects. Some people do get mild stomach irritation, and others have reported sun sensitivity and insomnia. If you are pregnant, check with your doctor before taking this or any other supplement. If you are already taking antidepressant medication, you should also talk to your doctor before taking St. John's wort.

Dr. Shealy suggests taking one 300-milligram tablet or capsule three times a day with meals if you have mild to moderate depression. For maximum effectiveness, buy a standardized extract containing 0.3 percent hypericin, he says. If you don't feel better after four to six weeks, it's unlikely to help, he adds.

Some Good from Ginkgo

Although it's not as strong as St. John's wort, ginkgo can be used as a mild antidepressant. Ginkgo greatly improves blood flow, mental alertness, and memory, and—as a by-product—relieves depression, says Dr. Sahelian. "Poor blood circulation to the brain can cause the brain to malfunction, which can lead to imbalances in serotonin levels and other neurotransmitters that regulate moods and emotional stability."

In one study, 40 patients, ages 51 to 78, were given either 80 milligrams of ginkgo extract or an inactive pill (placebo) three times a day in addition to their antidepressant medication. After eight weeks, researchers found that those who took the ginkgo showed more improvement than those who took the placebo.

If you're over age 50 and have mild to moderate depression, take one 40-milligram capsule of ginkgo three times a day, says Dr. Shealy. Choose capsules or tablets that contain 24 percent ginkgoflavoglycosides for maximum strength.

Brain Chemicals in a Pill

Another natural supplement that might have the edge over antidepressant prescription drugs is 5-HTP. This is a natural compound produced by the body from tryptophan, an amino acid found in many foods. It's also a precursor of serotonin, which means that more serotonin is produced when 5-HTP is present.

When you take 5-HTP in supplement form, it's absorbed in your gastrointestinal tract and then journeys to your brain, where it's converted into serotonin, says Dr. Sahelian.

If you've been diagnosed with depression and you have a doctor's approval, you can take 50 milligrams of 5-HTP late in the evening, says Dr. Sahelian. But he doesn't advise taking larger amounts. Any dosage over 50 milligrams can cause vivid dreams, nightmares, and nausea, Dr. Sahelian points out.

dermatitis

Dermatitis is a general term for an inflammation of the skin. The symptoms are usually itching, crustiness, blistering, and a watery discharge from pustules. In other words, just about any annoyance on the surface of your skin—ranging from the mildly itchy to the downright distressing—is dermatitis. One of the most common forms is eczema, an itchy kind of skin rash.

As for the causes, they're numerous. In some people, stress alone can lead to dermatitis. Others have allergic reactions to any number of things, from poison ivy and poison oak to certain metals. In other cases, a general infection displays itself in dermatitis as well as other symptoms.

If you get standard medical treatment, your doctor might prescribe creams, lotions, or ointments that contain cortisone, or you might buy an over-the-counter hydrocortisone cream that helps soothe itching or quell the inflammation. There are alternatives, however.

Rev Up the Immune Response

When dermatitis strikes, you want to kick your immune system into high gear so that it can combat the irritation and inflammation, says Michael Gazsi, N.D., a naturopathic doctor in Ridgefield, Connecticut.

Your best immune booster is the old herbal standby echinacea, according to Dr. Gazsi. This herb increases the number of white blood cells, or killer cells, that are responsible for beating up foreign invaders. Echinacea speeds up the process of phagocytosis, which means that the killer cells hunt down and destroy the causes of infection.

"Echinacea enhances the ability of your immune system to get rid of the poison," Dr. Gazsi says. "That can be very helpful when the dermatitis has been caused by a foreign substance like poison ivy. I'd use it for a week or two. It's most effective during the initial stages of inflammation," he says. He recommends taking two or three 300-milligram capsules a day.

Interrupt Inflammation

For most skin conditions, you can benefit by taking either evening primrose oil or flaxseed oil supplements, says Dr. Gazsi. Flaxseed oil is a rich source of omega-3 fatty acids, beneficial fats that are important for skin health. Evening primrose oil is a great source of gamma-linolenic acid (GLA), which the body transforms into several hormonelike substances, including prostaglandins, which have anti-inflammatory effects. Both oils are particularly effective at treating eczema, the mild, itchy kind of dermatitis that can flare up over and over again.

Some people lack GLA due to reduced enzyme activity, says Irene Catania, N.D., a naturopathic doctor and homeopathic practitioner in Ho-Ho-Kus, New Jersey. "When you get more GLA into your system, your body may be able to bring down inflammation on its own," she says. "I've found that evening primrose oil and flaxseed oil are especially effective with eczema." Fish oil is also highly recommended.

You can find evening primrose oil in liquid or in soft gel cap form. Dr. Gazsi recommends taking 500 to 1,000 milligrams every day for 12 weeks.

Omega-3 fatty acids also nurture the immune system and help the body get protection from the bad substances that might be causing a skin outbreak, says Dr. Gazsi. "I tell people to take two tablespoons a day of flaxseed oil," he says. "You can simply drink the oil or put it on foods such as salads."

Don't expect immediate results, warns Dr. Gazsi. "If your condition has been chronic, I'd wait six weeks to a few months to judge how well it is working. The skin responds pretty slowly."

Combine Vitamin A and Zinc

People who have chronic skin problems may be deficient in vitamin A or zinc, says Dr. Gazsi, and some people lack both. These deficiencies show up in people with liver disease, vegetarians who don't eat healthy meat substitutes like beans or wheat germ, and people who are eating nutritionally poor diets or following faddish weight-loss diets. Alcoholism can also cause these deficiencies.

You need vitamin A for your body to properly regenerate outer layers of skin. If this critical vitamin is absent, your skin may develop a sandpaper-like texture. Zinc, too, is necessary for the skin to produce new cells and maintain new layers of skin.

"Vitamin A and zinc really work together, which is why I usually recommend them in combination," says Dr. Gazsi.

You can begin by taking a multivitamin/mineral supplement that contains the recommended daily amounts of vitamin A and zinc. Frequently, though, those amounts aren't enough if there are some problems with a person's vitamin absorption or diet, says Dr. Gazsi. Your doctor can perform a test to determine whether you have absorption problems.

"If you're looking to clear up dermatitis, I'd recommend 50 milligrams of zinc and no more than 12,000 international units of vitamin A," he says. You should definitely talk to your doctor before taking vitamin A and zinc at these doses.

Attack the Rash Topically

Since dermatitis involves the skin, topical treatments are helpful in combating itching and any resulting rash, says Kathy Foulser, N.D., a naturopathic doctor at the Ridgefield Center for Integrative Medicine in Connecticut.

If your dermatitis is caused by an allergic reaction—to a poison plant, for example—you can get some relief by taking an oatmeal bath. Simply pour a cup of regular or colloidal oatmeal (such as Aveeno) into lukewarm water and soak for 15 minutes, recommends Dr. Foulser.

Aloe is another topical standby. At most health food stores, you can buy aloe in gel, cream, and liquid forms. Just rub the aloe into the itchy, damaged skin, says Dr. Fousler.

"Aloe makes a really nice, gooey mix that sits on the skin," she says. "It's really soothing for most skin problems."

diabetes

If there's one good thing that can be said about type 2 (non-insulin-dependent) diabetes, it's that this disorder usually responds very nicely to diet and lifestyle changes. The nutritional and herbal supplements that are recommended here are no substitute for the fundamental lifestyle changes that can help you control this kind of diabetes. You have to eat right, control your weight, and get regular exercise, says Rebecca Wynsome, N.D., a naturopathic doctor in Seattle.

"There's absolutely no doubt that dietary changes and weight loss can have a major impact on this disease," she says. If you lose just 10 pounds, for instance, you may be able to decrease insulin resistance. That's a significant breakthrough because insulin ushers blood sugar, or glucose, into your cells. In order for your cells to get the life-giving energy they need, they must accept rather than resist insulin.

Once you've embarked on the dietary changes that you need to make, though, nutritional supplements and herbs can complement your efforts. Supplements may help reverse deficiencies that have developed as a result of diabetes, protect your body from diabetes-related damage, improve your metabolism so you have more energy, and help to stabilize blood sugar, says Dr. Wynsome.

It's best—and safest—to work with a doctor who can develop the right program for you and then help you maintain it, Dr. Wynsome says. "Many of these nutrients and herbs have a profound effect on drug doses and regulation and often work in combination," she says. "There is often a period of transition and adjustment as your body adapts to its new regimen, and having medical supervision during this time is critical." Here's what she recommends.

Fiber Puts the Brakes on Absorption

The more slowly and evenly you absorb the carbohydrates you eat, the better control you'll have over your blood sugar levels, Dr. Wynsome says.

The Herb That Blocks Sugar Cravings

Several herbs are known to be very helpful for controlling diabetes or helping to prevent its complications. One of the cornerstones of herbal treatment is *Gymnema sylvestre*, an Indian herb, says Rebecca Wynsome, N.D., a naturopathic doctor in Seattle. "This herb is a tonifer, or regulator, and it is fairly safe," she says. "I always recommend it to people with diabetes in addition to the nutritional supplements they may need."

When drops of gymnema extract are put on the tongue, components in the herb block the sensation of sweetness. "People say that taking the herb this way is helpful for stopping sugar cravings," says Dr. Wynsome.

The extract also boosts production of insulin in people with diabetes, an action that may reduce blood sugar levels and the need for supplemental insulin, Dr. Wynsome says. In one study, 22 people with type 2 diabetes were given gymnema extract along with their regular medications. All had improved blood sugar control, and 21 were able to considerably reduce their dosages of medications. In fact, 5 of the people were able to discontinue their medications and maintain blood sugar control with the herb alone.

Animal studies suggest that gymnema might actually regenerate insulin-producing cells in the pancreas, but human studies have not been done to confirm that it actually works this way, Dr. Wynsome says.

For both type 1 and type 2 diabetes, the dose for gymnema extract is 400 milligrams a day, taken in three or four divided doses. The herb has no apparent side effects. It does not cause low blood sugar and does not affect people whose blood sugar is normal, Dr. Wynsome says.

If you are on insulin or other blood sugar–lowering drugs, you shouldn't take gymnema unless your doctor okays it.

Fiber, especially soluble fiber, slows absorption in the intestines. If there is plenty of soluble fiber in a meal, you absorb small amounts of carbohydrates over a longer period of time. This helps to prevent a rapid rise in blood sugar, which in turn prevents excessive secretion of insulin. When less insulin is secreted, your liver and tissues become more sensitive to insulin, improving their uptake of blood sugar.

Get as much soluble fiber in your diet as you can by eating foods that are rich sources, such as beans, oat bran, and most fruits and vegetables. "I ask my patients with diabetes to get 25 grams a day of fiber, which isn't that easy to do," Dr. Wynsome says. That's the equivalent of two ½-cup servings of the highest-fiber bran cereal you can buy.

In addition to a high-fiber diet, she recommends a fiber supplement that contains pectin, pea fiber, or psyllium. Amounts of fiber vary in different supplements, so read the labels for the right dose and check with your doctor if you have any questions.

If you find that you're taking a fiber supplement that causes gas or cramping, try one that does not contain psyllium or oat bran, Dr. Wynsome suggests. "Some people have a sensitivity reaction to these ingredients," she says.

Chromium Helps Insulin Work Better

Studies of people with diabetes have shown that supplementing the diet with a trace mineral, chromium, can lower fasting blood sugar levels, improve glucose tolerance, and reduce insulin levels.

"Chromium helps insulin work better and bind better to cell receptors so that the cells can take in glucose," Dr. Wynsome explains. "Many people with type 2 diabetes have enough insulin, but it doesn't work right. Their cells have resistance to insulin." Chromium helps overcome this.

A large study clearly documented the benefit of chromium for people with type 2 diabetes. In the study, 180 people were divided into three groups. The first group received inactive pills (placebos), the second group received 100 micrograms of chromium picolinate twice a day, and the third group received 500 micrograms of chromium picolinate twice a day. All of the participants continued their regular medications.

In both groups taking chromium, there was a significant decrease in glycosylated hemoglobin, which is a measure of long-term blood sugar control. There was also a significant reduction in fasting insulin levels and insulin levels when tested two hours after meals. Blood cholesterol levels were also lower in the people taking chromium.

Dr. Wynsome recommends chromium to all of her patients with diabetes. The form that she recommends—one of the forms that's well-absorbed—is chromium picolinate. For patients who need it and are under close medical supervision, the initial dose may be as high as 1,000 micrograms a day of this supplement, she says.

If you're taking chromium on your own, Dr. Wynsome recommends only 200 to 400 micrograms. "Since chromium does make the insulin that you have work better, you need to be careful when you take it," she says. "It can cause low blood sugar until your insulin levels out, so your doctor should monitor your blood sugar levels while you're taking it."

The amount and form of chromium do appear to be important, says chromium researcher Richard Anderson, Ph.D., lead scientist in the nutrient requirements and functions laboratory at the U.S. Department of Agriculture Beltsville Human Nutrition Research Center in Maryland. In most of the studies where chromium proved beneficial, people were taking the type recommended by Dr. Wynsome, chromium picolinate, in doses of at least 200 micrograms a day. Since most multivitamin/mineral supplements contain chromium chloride, a less absorbable form, you probably can't count on a standard multivitamin to help you get the dose you need.

Vanadium Ups Insulin Action

Another trace mineral, vanadium, seems to enhance insulin action in people with diabetes, according to several studies. In one study, people with type 2 diabetes who took 50 milligrams of vanadium twice a day for four weeks had a 20 percent decrease in fasting blood sugar levels. The form they took was vanadyl sulfate.

"Vanadium also has an insulin-like effect, and it decreases blood sugar levels," Dr. Wynsome says. "If people take supplemental vanadium, they may need less chromium." She might start someone on five micrograms of vanadyl sulfate three times a day with meals, then cut back to five micrograms once a day as blood sugar levels move into a normal range. The dosage needs to be regulated by your doctor, however, so don't take vanadium without medical supervision.

Not everyone does well on this mineral, Dr. Wynsome says. "Some people say they feel more clear-headed, their blood sugar is stabilized, and they feel great. Others feel just the opposite, however—light-headed, spacy, and shaky." If you experience these reactions, you should stop taking vanadium, she advises. The safety of long-term use has not been demonstrated, and results of some animal studies suggest concern about long-term toxicity.

There's also the possibility of stomach upset. In one study, six of eight people reported diarrhea, abdominal cramps, gas, and nausea the first week they took vanadium. After that, though, their symptoms stopped.

Antioxidants Provide All-Around Aid

Two of the antioxidant nutrients, vitamins C and E, provide important protection for people with diabetes, studies confirm. Both can help prevent the major long-term complications of diabetes, such as blindness, kidney disease, and nerve damage due to high sugar levels. Here's how they work.

Both vitamins help to prevent a process called glycosylation, a reaction between sugar and protein that alters the protein's structure so that it can't be used, says John Cunningham, Ph.D., professor of nutrition at the University of Massachusetts in Amherst. Glycosylated proteins are thought to contribute to many of the long-term complications of diabetes, he says.

Vitamin E improves insulin action as well, Dr. Cunningham says. "Because vitamin E helps to protect cell membranes, some speculate that it might help insulin receptor sites on the surfaces of cells to remain functional."

Vitamin C protects cells in another way. It prevents sugar inside cells from being converted to sorbitol, a sugar alcohol that cells can neither expel nor burn for energy. "Sorbitol buildup has been implicated in diabetes-related eye, nerve, and kidney damage," Dr. Cunningham says.

In a study by researchers at the University of Massachusetts, the levels of sorbitol in red blood cells responded within one month to doses of vitamin C. In people with type 1 (insulin-dependent) diabetes, blood sorbitol levels dropped from double the normal amount to normal after they took 100 or 600 milligrams of vitamin C a day for 30 days.

Another study, from Finland, supports these findings. Researchers showed that supplemental vitamin C improved blood sugar control and reduced blood cholesterol levels in people with type 2 diabetes.

Studies have shown benefits with 100 to 1,000 international units (IU) a day of vitamin E and with 100 to 1,000 milligrams a day of vitamin C, Dr. Cunningham says.

Dr. Wynsome recommends 100 to 500 milligrams a day of vitamin C and 400 to 800 IU of vitamin E. She suggests that you work with your doctor to determine the right amount of both of these vitamins, because vitamin E carries a small risk of raising blood pressure, and vitamin C can cause diarrhea. If you have late-stage diabetes, your doctor will probably advise against either of these supplements because there is a risk of kidney failure. In this situation, all supplements are potentially dangerous because you can't excrete the excess.

Why You Need the Bs

B-complex vitamins are essential for your body to convert sugar and starches to energy, a chemical process called carbohydrate metabolism. A shortage of any one of them can cause problems. Vitamin B_6 deficiency has been linked to glucose intolerance, which is an abnormally high rise in blood sugar after eating.

Shortages of B vitamins can also lead to nerve damage in the hands and feet. Some studies indicate that people with diabetes develop less of the numbness and tingling associated with diabetes-related nerve damage if they take supplemental B vitamins, Dr. Wynsome says.

People with diabetes tend to use up their B vitamins. Also, poorly controlled diabetes causes these nutrients to be excreted in the urine, Dr. Wynsome says. She recommends a supplement that includes 50 to 100 milligrams of most of the B vitamins. Look for a type called B-50, she advises.

Some people may need additional amounts of biotin and B_{12}, some B vitamins as well, Dr. Wynsome notes. She may give 3,000 to 6,000 micrograms a day of biotin if tests of metabolic function show that someone isn't utilizing this vitamin properly or has symptoms of dermatitis, high cholesterol, nausea, and muscle pain.

Dr. Wynsome gives vitamin B_{12} by injection if tests suggest that someone is having trouble absorbing this vitamin properly. She recommends injections if people have symptoms of tingling, numbness, or poor nerve conduction or if they have slowed reflexes related to their diabetes.

Keep an Eye on Niacinamide

One B vitamin in particular, a form of niacin known as niacinamide, may actually help keep type 1 diabetes from developing in high-risk people, Dr. Cunningham says.

Type 1 diabetes is distinctly different from type 2, the more common type. People with type 1 develop antibodies that attack and destroy the cells in the pancreas that produce insulin.

Bitter Melon Tames Ups and Downs

It's a green, cucumber-shaped fruit with gourdlike bumps all over it. Called *Momordica charantia* or bitter melon, it's common in Asia but harder to find in the West, and it has long been used as a way to reduce blood sugar levels.

The blood sugar–lowering action of fresh juice or an extract of bitter melon have been clearly established in several studies. "Bitter melon has several compounds with confirmed antidiabetic properties," says Rebecca Wynsome, N.D., a naturopathic doctor in Seattle.

"If someone is going through a transition period or any kind of destabilization of blood sugar control, I am likely to recommend 50 milligrams of an extract of this herb for two to three months, then evaluate the effect," Dr. Wynsome says. "Bitter melon has strong glucose-regulating effects." Just be sure to talk to your physician or a well-informed practitioner before taking it.

"Niacinamide seems to help protect insulin-producing cells from attack," Dr. Cunningham says. Having enough on hand also helps your body produce more energy and facilitate chemical reactions.

Niacinamide is crucial in making a molecule that is central to the energy-production process, he says. In large doses, niacinamide can also inhibit the formation of certain types of free radicals, the free-roaming, unstable molecules that set off destructive chain reactions in your cells.

Researchers from New Zealand did a two-year study using high doses of niacinamide. Among children with early signs of reduced insulin production, only 20 percent of those who took high doses of niacinamide progressed to type 1 diabetes. In contrast, 80 percent of a group of children with the same early signs of type 1 who did not take niacinamide did develop insulin dependence.

In a similar study with adults, only 15 percent of those taking niacinamide developed type 1 diabetes, compared with 40 percent of the adults in a group that didn't take the vitamin.

It's extremely important not to take more than 500 milligrams of niacinamide without medical supervision, says Dr. Wynsome. In large amounts, this vitamin can cause liver damage. She advises that you consult your doctor to determine the safe effective dose.

Mind Your Magnesium

Like the B vitamins, the mineral magnesium is involved in several aspects of carbohydrate metabolism, Dr. Wynsome says. Magnesium also helps vitamin B_6 get inside cells, where both the mineral and the vitamin play central roles in energy production. Some people with diabetes have low levels of magnesium, and there's some evidence that getting enough may help prevent complications such as damage to the retina of the eye and heart disease.

"I tell people to eat more magnesium-rich foods such as beans, whole grains, leafy greens, tofu, nuts, and seeds, because they will get magnesium and lots of other good nutrients," says Dr. Wynsome. She recommends 500 milligrams a day from supplemental sources that are easy for your body to absorb, such as magnesium gluconate or citrate.

People who are very low in magnesium may need to start out by taking even higher amounts, but they should do so only under medical supervision, she says.

Other minerals are probably just as important for people with diabetes, so it's a good idea to take a multivitamin/mineral that covers all your bases, Dr. Wynsome says. Manganese and zinc, in particular, are also involved in blood sugar control.

The Fats You Need

Too often, we think of fat as bad, especially when we've been told that we need to lose weight.

Everyone needs some fat, however, and certain types actually help diabetes, Dr. Wynsome says.

The most needed fats are the two essential fatty acids—omega-6, or GLA, which is shorthand for gamma-linolenic acid, and omega-3's, which have eicosapentaenoic acid (EPA) and docosahexaenoic acid (DHA). Omega-6 fatty acids protect against the development of diabetic neuropathy, the nerve dysfunction that can result from diabetes. Omega-3's help prevent damage to blood vessels and enhance insulin secretion.

In one study, researchers worked with people who had mild neuropathy: All showed some nerve damage. The group took 480 milligrams a day of GLA for one year. Nerve health was assessed with tests that measured how fast their nerves conducted signals, their muscle strength, and other factors. At the end of the year, all of the functions had improved in the people taking GLA, and most showed significant change for the better.

You can get omega-6 fatty acids with GLA in borage oil, evening primrose oil, or black currant oil. Omega-3's are provided by fatty fish such as mackerel or salmon; you can also take fish-oil capsules or supplements of flaxseed oil, which also provide omega-3's.

"I usually recommend 1,000 to 3,000 milligrams a day of omega-6's or the same amount of a mixture of omega-3's and -6's," Dr. Wynsome says.

If you're a woman nearing menopause, says Dr. Wynsome, the better choice might be flaxseed or evening primrose oil. These supplements help contend with hormone fluctuations. A man with heart disease, on the other hand, might be better off with fish oil, which has less influence on hormones but more benefit for people at risk for heart disease.

In some studies, however, large amounts of omega-3 fatty acids impaired blood sugar control. Dr. Wynsome suggests that a safe dose for most people is no more than 900 milligrams a day of purified EPA. To further ensure the safety of these doses, she recommends that her patients take antioxidants such as vitamin E and vitamin C. She usually prescribes 600 IU of vitamin E and 100 to 200 milligrams of vitamin C a day.

Bilberry Spares Eyes

People with diabetes run a high risk of eye problems, including a degeneration of the retina called retinopathy. The retina is a sheet of light-sensitive cells that act as "film" at the back of the eye, capturing the images that enter through the lens at the front of the eye.

In people with diabetes, blood vessels may leak, swell, and cause scar tissue that can permanently blur vision. Much of the damage to the retina is oxidative, related to free radicals generated in the eye as a result of high blood sugar or high insulin levels, Dr. Wynsome says. Thus, antioxidant nutrients such as vitamins E and C are vital to protect the retina.

An herb called bilberry or European blueberry can provide valuable antioxidant protection directly to the eyes. Bilberry contains flavonoids, or anthocyanins, that have a special affinity for the blood vessels of the eyes and retina. They're especially helpful in the macula, the area of the retina responsible for fine vision.

Bilberry extracts have been prescribed for diabetic retinopathy in France since 1945. The standard dose for an extract is based on its anthocyanidin content, which is usually standardized to 25 percent. Research studies have used 80 to 160 milligrams three times a day, but some doctors have found that 60 to 120 milligrams three times a day is effective.

Head-to-Toe Help from Ginkgo

People with diabetes frequently develop circulatory problems, especially in their legs. If these problems aren't resolved, the toes, feet, and legs can be damaged by impaired circulation. In worst cases, the damage can lead to amputation. One of the most common reasons for toe, foot, or leg amputations, in fact, is impaired circulation from uncontrolled diabetes, Dr. Wynsome says.

Ginkgo is an herb that helps to improve circulation, especially in the smaller arteries that feed blood to our legs, hands, nerves, and brains, Dr. Wynsome says. Among its many benefits, it helps stabilize cell membranes, acts as a powerful antioxidant, and enhances use of oxygen and blood sugar.

"I recommend ginkgo to everyone with diabetes, to be taken along with other nutritional supplements," Dr. Wynsome says. Look for a standardized extract that contains 24 percent ginkgoflavoglycosides. She recommends 40 milligrams three times a day.

diarrhea

For most people, diarrhea is not a serious problem but rather an awkward, embarrassing dilemma for a day or two. Usually, it goes away on its own, unless it is a symptom of a more serious problem such as food poisoning, Crohn's disease, ulcerative colitis, or an adverse drug reaction.

If you try some remedies and use the supplements that doctors recommend, they should start to work in 24 to 48 hours. If your diarrhea lasts for more than three to four days, however, if there is blood in the stool, or you feel dehydrated and very weak, see a doctor.

One thing you have to be concerned about is the loss of fluids. You may not feel like drinking when your stomach is doing somersaults, but it's necessary. You should always try to sip water to avoid dehydration, says Kristin Stiles, N.D., a naturopathic doctor at the Complementary Medicine and Healing Arts Center in Vestal, New York.

Whenever you lose fluids and don't replace them, you also lose calcium and electrolytes, including sodium, magnesium, and potassium. These minerals regulate many of the body's essential processes, such as blood pressure, heart rate, and muscle movements.

If an infant or elderly adult has diarrhea that lasts more than 12 to 24 hours, the nutrient loss can be severe, so they should get medical attention as soon as possible. In an otherwise healthy adult, the most important task is to make up for lost fluids and electrolytes.

Sports drinks may be intended for athletes, but they're perfect for anyone with diarrhea, too. These drinks contain a hearty dose of electrolytes—sodium and potassium along with simple sugar. Sip at least four ounces every hour for as long as the diarrhea lasts, says Dr. Stiles.

Help Out with Herbals

If your diarrhea is due to bacteria or some type of food poisoning, goldenseal and garlic can help your body do away with the bad bugs. Both have antibacterial properties. Take 100 to 250 milligrams of goldenseal or 200 to 400 milligrams of garlic three times a day until your diarrhea subsides, recommends Dr. Stiles.

When your digestive system is trying to get rid of the contents of your stomach and intestines, there's a lot of inner activity called peristaltic movement, which sometimes causes cramping. Plus, you may get gas because the material in your intestines is starting to ferment, says Pam Taylor, N.D., a naturopathic doctor in Moline, Illinois. To help alleviate spasms in the gastrointestinal tract, try taking a capsule or two of ginger, Dr. Taylor recommends—a dosage of 200 to 400 milligrams.

Ginger helps prevent the stomach spasms and stimulates the release of gastric juices, pancreatic juices, and the enzymes that enhance digestion. "Ginger normalizes peristaltic movements and has pain-relieving properties, and it's a good tonic for the stomach," Dr. Taylor says.

Another herb that's good for relieving intestinal spasms is valerian. "Most people think of valerian only as a sleep tonic, but it also relieves stomach cramping and reduces the formation of gas," says Dr. Stiles. She recommends taking a 100- to 300-milligram capsule of valerian twice a day.

Glutamine for GI Health

With severe diarrhea or a bout that lasts a few days, the intestines may remain inflamed, says Dr. Stiles.

Try glutamine, an amino acid supplement frequently used by naturopathic doctors for gastrointestinal diseases, she says. Glutamine encourages the quick turnover or production of cells along the wall of the stomach and the small intestine, she says. It makes the body heal a bit faster.

"While you're healing, I would recommend 500 milligrams of glutamine three times a day," suggests Dr. Stiles. Continue this dosage for about two weeks or until you have no more discomfort, she adds.

With these remedies, you can expect diarrhea to clear up within 24 to 72 hours. But don't hesitate to call the doctor if you have bloody diarrhea, localized pain, fever, or dehydration. Signs of dehydration include decreased urine output, dry mucous membranes, or sunken eyeballs.

diverticulitis

It's a series of intestinal developments just waiting for trouble to happen.

Maybe you've been straining a lot during bowel movements, or maybe the walls of your colon have weakened a bit. Little pouches and sacs called diverticula have formed in the lining of your colon.

In these little dead end streets, seeds, bacteria, or other debris may become trapped. When those troublemakers aren't flushed out of your system, they ferment, decay, and inflame tissues—and you have diverticulitis.

People who develop diverticulitis often have had previous symptoms of constipation and difficult bowel movements with hard stools, according to Kristin Stiles, N.D., a naturopathic doctor at the Complementary Medicine and Healing Arts Center in Vestal, New York.

The problem announces itself with a wide range of symptoms. Even your doctor may be puzzled about the exact cause. Among the signs are alternating diarrhea and constipation, gas, bloating, and chronic cramping and pain in the intestines. Since these mimic many of the symptoms of irritable bowel syndrome (IBS), it takes some medical sleuthing to determine what you have. Your doctor will make the initial diagnosis through information that you give him and observation in his office. After treatment to help reduce the inflammation, he will probably want to do a follow-up colon examination to find out whether diverticulitis is really the problem.

Once you know that you have diverticulitis, your doctor may help you find ways to improve your diet. Some supplements can help you recover more quickly. Here's what experts suggest.

Prevent It with Fiber

"When I see this problem, it's usually because the person is eating a high-fat, high-sugar, low-fiber diet—basically a junk diet," says Dr. Stiles. "I immediately get him onto a high-fiber diet."

You should consume between 25 and 30 grams of soluble and insoluble fiber each day, advises Dr. Stiles, and she advocates getting most of that through diet. Fiber is found in fruits and vegetables, legumes, and grains like whole wheat, oats, and rye.

All the same, getting this much fiber from food may be a challenge. "I wouldn't recommend that you eat foods with any seeds, like sesame or sunflower. You don't want a lot of hard stuff in the stool passing through this really irritated area," says Melissa Metcalfe, N.D., a naturopathic doctor in Los Angeles. When your colon is very irritated, she adds, it may be best to start out with a fiber supplement rather than eating a lot of rough fiber like bran.

If you're not getting the recommended amount of fiber from food, Dr. Stiles recommends taking two tablespoons daily of a fiber supplement that contains psyllium.

Since fiber absorbs large amounts of water, make sure that you drink plenty, whether you're increasing your food fiber or taking supplemental fiber. Dr. Stiles suggests that you drink 8 to 10 eight-ounce glasses of water daily. The water adds bulk to the stool and helps soften them for easier transit through the colon.

Healing Your Irritation

When you're in the throes of diverticulitis, your immediate problems are inflammation, infection, and irritation of the colon. Several herbs, called demulcents, have the ability to soothe and coat mucous membranes. By direct contact, they help heal irritated and inflamed tissues, says Pamela Taylor, N.D., a naturopathic doctor in Moline, Illinois.

These herbs form a coating that bathes the walls of the large intestine and helps heal the lining.

Some health food stores carry a naturopathic herbal combination known as Robert's Formula that is very good for gastrointestinal irritation, she says. The combination includes herbs such as slippery elm, marshmallow root, and geranium. It may also contain echinacea and goldenseal, two botanical ingredients that help boost your immune system.

Robert's Formula is produced by a number of different companies with varying combinations of ingredients. It is generally available in capsules or as a tincture. If you choose to try it, simply follow the directions on the label, recommends Dr. Taylor. A usual dose is two "00" capsules three times a day. Capsules are best taken with food so the herbs will be carried to the large intestine.

A Soothing Spice for a Grumpy Gut

If you need an excuse to go out and eat some hot Indian food tonight, here's one: It's good for you.

Turmeric, the main ingredient in curry powder, is a powerful anti-inflammatory that can help reduce the puffiness and soreness of irritated tissue. It's also an antioxidant, so it helps defuse the free-roaming, unstable molecules called free radicals that can seriously damage your cells. Plus, it's a digestive aid. For all of these reasons, naturopathic doctors sometimes recommend it as a treatment for diverticulitis.

The spice was used as a healing herb in China. In the tradition of Ayurvedic medicine practiced by doctors in India, it has been used as a medicine for thousands of years. Today, Indian doctors use it for many inflammatory conditions, from rheumatoid arthritis to sprains. They sometimes make poultices of turmeric that are applied directly to sore muscles and painful joints.

Ayurvedic practitioners believe that the herb has a number of benefits for the gastrointestinal system. In animal studies, it has been shown to reduce the amount of gas that's produced in the intestine and increase the secretion of gastric juices. It protects the stomach, possibly helping to prevent ulcers. Given in combination with other herbs, it has also been used to help treat liver disorders.

Although turmeric has several active ingredients, curcumin seems to be the most important for medicinal purposes. In fact, because it comes in a highly concentrated form, curcumin alone can be more effective than turmeric. It is available in capsules at health food stores.

You can also take some of the herbs separately. Slippery elm alone is a powerful demulcent. Usually you'll find it in 100-milligram capsules. Take three a day, recommends Dr. Metcalfe.

Turmeric also works well as an anti-inflammatory, she says; try taking a 200- to 400-milligram capsule twice a day.

Chamomile is another good anti-inflammatory that's also soothing to gastrointestinal tissues. Dr. Metcalfe suggests taking two 400- to 500-milligram capsules three times a day.

You can continue to take any of these supplements as long as you have problems with diverticulitis, she says.

Killing the Infection

Infection is always a concern with diverticulitis. If it is not controlled, doctors sometimes recommend surgery to remove affected portions of the intestine. You can help your body fight any infection in the colon by taking a combination of echinacea and goldenseal, says Dr. Stiles.

Both herbs have anti-inflammatory and antibacterial properties. Goldenseal is also astringent to the mucous membranes in the intestine, says Dr. Stiles—that is, it helps to tighten the tissues, which can help provide some relief.

"You don't want to take either of these herbs for too long, however. I'd recommend two weeks on and two weeks off until the infection subsides," says Dr. Stiles. "You can quickly build up a tolerance to echinacea, so it becomes less effective."

A typical dose is one 200- to 250-milligram capsule of echinacea and one 50- to 60-mlligram capsule of goldenseal three or four times a day, she suggests. Health food stores and some drugstores also carry combination capsules. Alternatively, you can take 10 to 15 drops of an extract of each herb in water or juice three or four times a day, with or without food.

Vitamins for Healing

To heal the damaged mucous membranes, Dr. Taylor sometimes recommends that her patients take vitamins A, E, and C and a chelated form of zinc. Many companies market these nutrients in a single supplement, says Dr. Taylor. She uses the following daily amounts, based on a body weight of 150 pounds: 5,000 to 10,000 international units (IU) of vitamin A in the form of fish oil, 200 to 500 milligrams of vitamin C, 100 to 400 IU of vitamin E, and 15 to 30 milligrams of chelated zinc. You'll need to check with a naturopathic doctor to determine the dosages appropriate for your weight and follow his advice on when to take the supplement.

As you recover from diverticulitis, the inflammation will heal, but you still need to pay attention to the factors that may have contributed to the problem in the first place. Be sure to maintain a low-fat, high-fiber diet, exercise regularly, and drink adequate amounts of water, says Dr. Stiles.

"If you keep things moving and improve the muscle tone of the bowel, the outpouchings won't be such a problem," she says.

emphysema

Somewhere in your grade-school education, you probably yawned your way through a science class in which your teacher compared your lungs to inflatable party balloons. Like balloons, our lungs hold air and are very elastic, expanding and contracting easily. But what would happen if you let the air out of a balloon and it *didn't* deflate? As weird as it sounds, that's basically what happens when you have emphysema.

This smoking-related disease causes your lungs to lose the resilience they need to fully collapse every time you exhale. Since you're not pushing out all of the "waste" of breathing—the carbon dioxide—that toxic gas begins to build up in the semi-deflated lungs. Breathing becomes difficult and not very efficient. You may have a constant sensation of breathlessness. Often, you have a cough along with the other symptoms.

If you're a smoker with emphysema, the doctor will certainly tell you to stop smoking. She'll also urge you to stay away from environmental air pollution.

Currently, there's no cure for emphysema, but people in advanced stages of the disease who need to use supplemental oxygen may find that nutritional supplements will protect their lungs from further damage.

Emphysema can be prevented, however. The most obvious step, if you're still smoking, is to quit. But taking supplements can also help.

An Antioxidant Twosome

For severe emphysema, some people take supplemental oxygen to help them breathe more easily. There's something you should know about O_2, however. While it's true that humans can't live without it, oxygen in its purest form isn't purely beneficial.

"Oxygen itself is what we call an oxidizing agent," explains James Scala, Ph.D., a nutritionist in Lafayette, California, and author of *Prescription for Longevity*. Oxidation is what happens to bananas when they brown, iron fences when they rust, and people when they age. The process involves unstable molecules called free radicals that circulate in the body. In order to regain its electrical balance, a free radical must swipe an electron from another molecule, and this starts a chain reaction of cellular damage.

Some free radicals are produced in our bodies when we're breathing in normal amounts of oxygen, but many more of these troublesome molecules are generated by outside forces like the sun's rays, alcohol, cigarette smoke, and other forms of air pollution. Supplemental oxygen also generates an oversupply, according to Dr. Scala.

Antioxidant supplements can help prevent emphysema from worsening. Plus, says Dr. Scala, if your lungs are already in the pink, antioxidants can help keep them that way.

Two antioxidants in particular are especially important to respiratory health. "A person who takes vitamin E and vitamin C supplements is less likely to develop emphysema than a person who doesn't, all other things being equal," says Dr. Scala.

Vitamin E, an oily antioxidant found in blood fats and cell membranes, is important for proper lung function. "Studies show that if you put athletes on a treadmill and get them burning rubber while you monitor their breath, the ones who took vitamin E will have less oxidation by-products coming from their lungs," says Dr. Scala.

Take a multivitamin and a separate supplement containing 200 to 800 international units (IU) of vitamin E to give your precious lungs an edge over emphysema, he says. If you are considering taking amounts above 400 IU, though, discuss it with your doctor first.

Vitamin C is a water-soluble antioxidant that's found in every body fluid. Besides protecting the rest of the body from cancer, heart disease, and cataracts, it also shields the respiratory system. According to Dr. Scala, studies of elite athletes show that those who take vitamin C are less likely to get the kinds of lung problems that often crop up in marathon runners. Even if you're not a top-speed runner, though, vitamin C is a good bet for your twin airbags. "Most people could use at least 500 milligrams a day," says Dr. Scala.

endometriosis

What a mysterious process! For some reason, the tissue that normally lines a woman's uterus begins to migrate and grow in other areas within the abdomen while still behaving like uterine tissue. That means that other internal organs may have an island of tissue that swells and sheds blood every month. Since that foreign tissue is not supposed to be there, and your organs don't know how to handle its strange behavior, you may begin to feel a lot of pain.

This is what doctors call endometriosis. It affects an estimated 10 to 15 percent of all premenopausal women.

Hormone therapies and surgery are the favored treatments in conventional medicine. If you have endometriosis, you should work with a doctor to help manage it. There aren't any known cures. There are, however, a number of ways to help relieve the pain and influence the hormonal balance that plays an important part in the condition, according to naturopathic doctors.

Getting your diet in order can be a big step. First, cut down on foods that might be increasing your estrogen levels, says Barbara Silbert, D.C., N.D., a chiropractor and naturopathic doctor in Newburyport, Massachusetts, and president of the Massachusetts Society of Naturopathic Physicians. Commercially raised animals are often given hormones for more robust growth and milk production, so if you eat meat or dairy products, you might be absorbing extra estrogen. Another possible concern with meat is that foods that are high in saturated fat have a tendency to make estrogen more available to the body.

Phase out meat and dairy products in favor of soy foods (tofu, tempeh, miso, and soy milk) and fiber-rich foods, says Dr. Silbert. Soy contains phytoestrogens, compounds that help regulate estrogen levels. Fiber makes stools firm and easy to pass, which is especially important if endometrial tissue is encroaching on the bowel area.

She also recommends regular exercise—at least 30 minutes three times a week—to help relieve the pain and cramping associated with endometriosis. With exercise, you step up production of endorphins, your body's natural pain blockers.

Then there are supplements. "Because endometriosis is a complex thing to deal with," says Dr. Silbert, "I always use a combination of herbs, vitamins, and minerals." It may take a few months for supplements to work, but there are many to try. She cautions, however, that you need to get a proper diagnosis and then work with your doctor to see if supplements are right for you.

Some supplements can lower estrogen levels by helping you excrete it. Others can help your liver and kidneys flush out as much as possible, which may help you control endometriosis. Still others can help relieve the pain. Here's what experts recommennd.

Three Estrogen Reducers

"In order to get endometriosis under control, you have to reduce the amount of estrogen in your body," says Jennifer Brett, N.D., a naturopathic doctor at the Wilton Naturopathic Center in Stratford, Connecticut. The herbs red clover and black cohosh and genistein, a supplement derived from soybeans, can help your body excrete estrogen.

These three supplements are phytoestrogens, or plant forms of estrogen. They bind with estrogen receptor sites, which are like dedicated landing sites on your cells. These sites would normally be occupied by your body's much stronger estrogen, but when plant estrogens start to hog the sites, your estrogen has no place to go and ends up being excreted, says Dr. Brett. "That's exactly what you want to happen with endometriosis."

If you reduce the amount of estrogen circulating in your body, you'll probably also reduce the pain of endometriosis, says Dr. Brett.

When taking red clover or black cohosh, follow the directions on the package. Label directions on one brand of red clover supplements call for two 430-milligram capsules three times a day. A typical black cohosh brand recommends one 540-milligram capsule three times a day. Black cohosh is particularly effective at relieving cramps, notes Dr. Brett.

You can get genistein by taking a supplement of mixed soy isoflavones according to the directions on the label. A typical dose is one 540-milligram capsule a day.

Flush Out Toxins

The other strategy to take with endometriosis is to get your body working to flush out as much estrogen as it can, says Dr. Brett. In the case of endometriosis, estrogen could be considered a toxin. Your body has too much of it and it's causing harm.

Having a body full of toxins is like having a full vacuum cleaner bag, observes Dr. Silbert. To empty the bag, you need to help the liver and kidneys function at peak capacity, since they're the organs that do most of the cleaning up and cleaning out. Supplements can help keep them working at their best. "Your body works a whole lot better when there aren't so many toxins clogging up the works," she says.

Magnesium is an all-purpose toxin flusher. One of its jobs is to transmit fluids to and from cells, your bloodstream and lymphatic system (whose primary job is immunity), and your tissues. The Daily Value for magnesium is 400 milligrams. In supplement form, 350 milligrams should be effective when taken in combination with other supplements that also help to flush out estrogen and toxins, says Dr. Silbert.

B_6 and Milk Thistle

You may also want to consider taking vitamin B_6 and the herb milk thistle. Both will help the liver break down and dispose of excess estrogen, says Dr. Brett. Studies have shown that when you supplement with B vitamins, you also help relieve other ailments associated with having too much estrogen, such as premenstrual syndrome (PMS).

Try taking 50 milligrams of vitamin B_6 twice a day, says Dr. Silbert. Because some women's bodies have trouble metabolizing this vitamin in its standard form, she recommends taking pyridoxal-5-phosphate (P5P). This is the activated form of vitamin B_6 that everyone's body can handle. If you take 50 milligrams of P5P twice a day, you'll get the equivalent of the same dose of vitamin B_6.

When you're taking milk thistle, follow the dosage directions on the package, typically one or two 150-milligram capsules three times daily.

Yarrow Restores Hormone Balance

Throughout history, yarrow has been used to stop bleeding, get rid of urinary tract infections, relieve digestive troubles, and ease the symptoms of female ailments. According to Greek mythology, Achilles packed yarrow into the wounds of soldiers 3,000 years ago in the Trojan War, using the only herbal on hand to stanch the bleeding of his fallen men.

Yarrow contains more than 120 compounds. One of these, azulene, is an effective anti-inflammatory and fever reducer.

Yarrow is also used to stimulate the liver so it does a better job of flushing out body wastes, and this is the function that's helpful if you have endometriosis and need to flush excess estrogen, says Jennifer Brett, N.D., a naturopathic doctor at the Wilton Naturopathic Center in Stratford, Connecticut. Because yarrow also helps to balance hormones, it's often prescribed by herbalists to treat heavy menstrual bleeding, fibroid tumors, and menopausal hot flashes.

Yarrow has antispasmodic properties that help relax muscles that cramp or contract, so it can ease your uterine and abdominal muscles.

Yarrow capsules are available in drugstores and health food stores. It's not recommended if you're pregnant, however.

Other Factors

Lipotropic factors are another supplement that will help your liver excrete toxins, says Dr. Silbert. The lipotropic factors choline (a component of lecithin), inositol, and methionine enhance liver function and chemical reactions that promote detoxification. In general, they work to unclog the liver so it can do its job better, she says.

Look in health food stores for a product labeled lipotropic factors. Select a product with a one-to-one ratio of two of the nutrients (choline and inositol are widely found together), and take an additional supplement of the third nutrient in the same amount. Check the label for directions.

To make sure that your kidneys are doing their share of the work, drink plenty of water—at least eight full eight-ounce glasses every day, advises Dr. Brett. And she recommends the herb yarrow. Not only will it help get your kidneys in prime working order, it may also ease the painful cramps that can accompany endometriosis. Dr. Brett advises following directions on the package. A typical dose is two or three capsules of between 250 and 350 milligrams taken twice a day.

Feel Better with Evening Primrose Oil

A natural anti-inflammatory, evening primrose oil can help reduce the pain of endometriosis, and is especially helpful with cramping, says Dr. Brett.

Traditionally, evening primrose oil has been used by herbalists and naturopathic doctors to help relieve symptoms of a wide range of women's ailments. Often recommended by naturopaths to relieve PMS and deal with menopausal discomforts, it can also work well if you're troubled by endometriosis.

fibromyalgia

Fibromyalgia is one of those mysterious ailments with no identifiable cause, vague symptoms, and no standard treatment. Some medical textbooks and dictionaries don't even list it as a disease or condition.

Nevertheless, people who have fibromyalgia clearly have common complaints of muscle pain, fatigue, and increased sensitivity to pain. The condition appears to have both physical and psychological roots, which include stress, lack of sleep, poor diet and digestion, a suppressed immune system, and perhaps a deficiency of some important vitamins and minerals.

"Fibromyalgia tends to manifest itself like chronic fatigue syndrome, but the pain is the predominant factor. Also, people who have fibromyalgia tend to be malnourished," says Hope Fay, N.D., a naturopathic doctor in Seattle. "There are lots of different theories, treatments, and supplements out there. Some work for some people, others don't. It is one of those conditions that you try to treat very broadly."

If you suspect that you have fibromyalgia, see your doctor. Although there is no specific test for it, your doctor may be able to rule out other causes with testing, says Dr. Fay.

Support Your Immune System

For chronic conditions like fibromyalgia, many natural healers believe that the first step is to help the body help itself. That begins with nurturing and strengthening the immune system, says Elizabeth Wotton, N.D., a naturopathic doctor at Compass Family Health Center in Plymouth, Massachusetts.

"People with this condition often just get laid out by colds and flu. They're up, then they're down. They just don't have very good resistance," she says. Recovering from fibromyalgia can be a lengthy process, so Dr. Wotton likes to prescribe the herb astragalus, a long-term immune booster.

Astragalus provides what is known as deep immune support. Studies show that it helps guard your body by increasing the activity of protective cells and raising the level of antibodies in your system. The exact mechanism isn't clear, but the herb seems to work within the bone marrow itself, where immune cells are manufactured. That's quite different from the action of echinacea, another popular immune-boosting herb, which rallies or speeds infection-fighting white blood cells to the site of an infection.

Dr. Wotton recommends taking one teaspoon of astragalus liquid extract three times a day. You can also take astragalus capsules. If the supplements are 500 milligrams, a typical dose would be one or two capsules three times a day with meals.

"Astragalus begins to build up the immune system to provide support on a long-term basis. It's really good for this type of chronic condition because it gives you some stability," she says. "You should take it for at least four to six months."

Get a Lift with Ginseng

Deep weariness is one of fibromyalgia's most nagging symptoms. It's a weariness brought on by pain, stress, and lack of energy. To give her patients a lift, Dr. Wotton recommends ginseng. "It's a tonic herb that makes you feel less run-down," she says.

Although ginseng has a reputation as an energy booster, it's not actually a stimulant but rather an adaptogenic herb. It can help your body adapt to different conditions. In the case of stress and fatigue, the adrenal glands may be functioning erratically. If they are working too hard—pumping out too many hormones—ginseng will reduce this action. If they aren't functioning well and aren't releasing enough hormones, ginseng can stimulate them to produce more.

"By supporting the adrenal glands, ginseng increases endurance and strengthens a person's ability to withstand stress," says Dr. Wotton. "In that way, it can boost energy and bolster the immune system, even though it doesn't have a direct effect on the immune system itself. People with fibromyalgia sometimes get in their situation because they don't let up and either can't or won't give themselves and their bodies a break. Finally, their bodies just get worn down."

She recommends one to two teaspoons of the liquid extract twice a day or one 200-milligram capsule twice a day. But don't take ginseng after

2:00 P.M., she cautions, because it can keep you awake at night. It may also cause irritability if taken with caffeine or other stimulants.

Magnesium for Your Muscles

Many fibromyalgia patients seem to have low levels of magnesium, which may be a significant cause of their muscle pain, says Dr. Wotton.

Calcium and magnesium work together to tense and relax muscles, with magnesium acting as the primary relaxation mineral. When it's lacking, the muscles remain tense and inflammation can build up. This may be one source of muscle pain, says Dr. Wotton.

It isn't really known why some people lack magnesium. Perhaps they don't absorb it well or aren't getting enough in their diets. Whatever the reason for the shortage, the solution is to take a magnesium supplement. That usually relaxes the muscles, allows blood to flow into the constricted areas, and flushes out the waste products of inflammation, says Dr. Wotton. Your doctor can do a white blood cell magnesium test to determine if you are lacking this mineral, she says.

Another theory suggests that the muscle pain and soreness stem from a lack of adenosine triphosphate (ATP), the basic fuel source for muscle cells. A combination of magnesium and a substance called malic acid will increase the production of ATP. "This theory says that the muscles aren't getting enough energy to do their job, so they feel sore and tired all the time," says Dr. Wotton.

By adding magnesium to your diet, you spur the production of ATP, which could help relieve that sore, tired feeling. Look for a magnesium supplement that contains malic acid in health food stores, she says. Take 200 milligrams three times a day for four to six months.

Put Fat on the Fire

Reducing any kind of inflammation usually brings about some improvement, says Dr. Fay. In fibromyalgia, there is clearly inflammation in the muscles and probably in the intestinal tract as well.

You may be able to lessen inflammation throughout your body by reducing your consumption of meat and taking essential fatty acid supplements that do not contribute to inflammation, Dr. Fay says.

Saturated fats from meat contain arachidonic acid, which is used by the body to make inflammatory chemicals called leukotrienes. Evening primrose oil, however, contains gamma-linolenic acid (GLA), a substance that won't produce those chemicals.

"GLA has a different pathway that leads away from inflammation," says Dr. Fay. "Giving your body more GLA can make a significant difference. When you reduce inflammation, you also reduce pain and fatigue."

She suggests a 1,000-milligram capsule of evening primrose oil three or four times a day. Some people do better if they start with small amounts and increase with time, says Dr. Fay. You can take this preparation at this dosage for three to six months and then gradually begin to cut back, she advises.

Increase Your Vitamins and Minerals

Malnourishment seems to be part of the problem for many fibromyalgia patients. Either their diets are quite poor, food allergies are involved, or the people just aren't extracting enough energy and nutrients from food, says Dr. Fay.

She tells her patients to cut out coffee, sugar, and refined foods and start on healthier diets that include more fresh fruits and vegetables, more whole grains, and less red meat. Also, she suggests that they take multivitamin/mineral supplements that provide nutrients in amounts higher than the Daily Values.

Boost Enzymes and Stomach Acid

Sometimes, deficiencies are due to poor absorption of minerals and vitamins in the digestive tract. People with fibromyalgia often have low levels of stomach acid, which leads to an incomplete breakdown of food, says Dr. Fay.

To increase stomach acid, she suggests taking a 650-milligram capsule of betaine hydrochloride with each meal. The supplement is available in health food stores. But before taking betaine hydrochloride, you should check with your doctor to determine if you indeed have a problem with low stomach acid.

"If you get any type of burning sensation, just take a capsule with one or two meals instead of three," she says. "I'd keep it up for several months, minimum. Eventually, your body should start producing more hydrochloric acid on its own." But you need to do other things as well—eat a low-fat, high-fiber diet, regular exercise, and make other healthy lifestyle choices, says Dr. Fay.

The other important players in breaking down food are digestive enzymes. Dr. Fay prescribes plant-based enzyme supplements that contain amylase, lipase, and protease enzymes. Enzyme Process, a supplement manufacturer, markets an appropriate product called Enzyme Process Digeszyme-V. The standard dose is three capsules a day with meals.

"Whatever supplement you get, look for a product that contains a broad mixture of enzymes," she says. "If you have had your gallbladder out, you'll need one that contains bile salts and acids to help digest fats."

Plant the Good Bugs

Occasionally, digestion and absorption problems may be caused by an overgrowth of yeast (candida) in the gut, says Dr. Fay. Yeast is naturally present in the body in small numbers, but a poor diet, mercury dental fillings, or a course of antibiotic drugs can cause it to grow out of control, she explains. She suggests working with a naturopathic doctor or doctor of oriental medicine to determine the exact nature of your condition.

Yeast can crowd out the good bugs such as acidophilus in your system and increase inflammation, aggravate food allergies, and interfere with the assimilation of minerals and vitamins, says Dr. Fay.

Garlic and pau d'arco are two effective herbal treatments for killing yeast. Dr. Fay suggests taking two 250-milligram capsules of garlic three times a day with meals. Alternatively, you can take an extract of pau d'arco bark. Nature's Plus, for example, makes several pau d'arco products that are available at health food stores. Supplements are available in 100-milligram tablets, and the typical dose is three a day.

While you're killing the candida, you can recolonize your gut with *Lactobacillus acidophilus*, the good bacteria that help maintain intestinal health, says Dr. Fay. She recommends taking one acidophilus tablet in the morning and another at night. "With my patients, I do the recolonizing for at least three to four months," she says.

fingernail problems

Take a look at your hands, specifically your fingernails. What do you think they say about your health?

A lot, actually. To someone with a practiced eye, fingernails are like little signposts that reveal whether you're deficient in vitamins and minerals and whether you're digesting your food well. Some experts say that fingernails can even reveal whether you have a condition like heart disease or diabetes.

"Usually, fingernail symptoms are a sign of something else happening in the body," says Leon Hecht, N.D., a naturopathic doctor at North Coast Family Health in Portsmouth, New Hampshire.

Soft nails that look scooped out—called spooned nails—may indicate anemia or an iron deficiency. Nails with white spots may be a result of a zinc deficiency. If your nails are brittle and break easily, you may need more vitamin B_{12}. Discolored nails could mean trouble with your blood sugar. Nails that separate from the nail bed may caused by a fungal infection or a thyroid problem.

"When you have nail problems, it's always important to have your thyroid checked first," says Michael Gazsi, N.D., a naturopathic doctor in Ridgefield, Connecticut. "If your thyroid is okay, you could try some self-treatment with supplements."

Dose Up

If a doctor has determined that you don't have a thyroid problem or some other serious condition that requires immediate treatment, there are some supplements that will help you have generally healthier nails.

Your first action should be to take a high-potency multivitamin/mineral supplement, says Dr. Gazsi. "I often recommend vitamins that exceed the daily allowances."

If white flecks on your nails concern you and the multivitamin doesn't

435

help, you might consider a daily supplement of zinc, somewhere between 30 and 50 milligrams, in addition to your multi, says Dr. Gazsi. Your total daily intake of zinc should be between 30 and 50 milligrams.

Pack In More Protein

Nails and hair are made of protein. "When the body isn't doing a good job of assimilating protein, it may show up in the nails," says Dr. Hecht. The signs could be weak, peeling, or brittle nails.

This can happen with alcoholics who have damaged stomach cells, or it may be caused by some autoimmune diseases. Often, however, it is simply the result of aging. As we grow older, our bodies produce less hydrochloric acid and pepsin, an important digestive enzyme secreted in the stomach.

"Hydrochloric acid and pepsin are really important for breaking down proteins and absorbing minerals," says Dr. Hecht. "If you have a hydrochloric acid deficiency, you don't extract all the nutrients from your food. You can aid your digestion and absorption of vitamins and minerals by taking two to six 500-milligram capsules of a hydrochloric acid supplement (betaine hydrochloride) with each full-size meal." Take the capsules after the first few bites of food.

Some people experience digestive side effects such as heartburn, gastric reflux, and a burning feeling in the chest or stomach from hydrochloric acid. Check with your doctor before taking this supplement, and be sure to follow the recommendations given on page 498. "I recommend taking hydrochloric acid for a couple of months and watching what effect it has on your nails," says Dr. Hecht. "It will take time to work."

Eventually, you may be able to stop the treatment, he says, but that's not always the case. "For some people, it's necessary to take low doses of hydrochloric acid (typically, two 500-milligram capsules with each meal) for the rest of their lives," says Dr. Hecht.

Fatty Acids Are Essential

To have healthy nails and skin, you also need essential fatty acids, Dr. Gazsi points out. Some people who have poor, unbalanced diets often don't get enough of these.

Essential fatty acids are easily obtained from eggs, nuts, vegetables, butter, and whole milk. You can also get them from a supplement like flaxseed oil or evening primrose oil.

Flaxseed oil can be used in place of olive oil on a salad, or you can take it straight by the spoonful, says Dr. Gazsi. He recommends two tablespoons daily. For evening primrose oil, he recommends a 500-milligram capsule a day. "Don't expect anything to happen overnight, though," he says. "It might take several months."

Go for the Bs

In a few cases, fingernail problems may be related to a B-vitamin deficiency. Dr. Gazsi recommends taking a B-complex or B-50 supplement—one in the morning and one in the evening. If you have a supplement that provides 100-milligram strengths of the B vitamins, take just one capsule daily, preferably with a meal. "There are a lot of good B formulas out there in the health food stores," he says.

If you're feeling run-down and fatigued, you can take a supplement of B_{12}, which has been shown in some studies to boost low energy. Dr. Gazsi suggests 1,000 micrograms twice a day for up to four months.

gallstones

Whenever you eat a high-fat meal, your body has to secrete bile to help you digest the fat. Bile is manufactured in the liver and stored in the gall-bladder. From there, it's dumped into the small intestine, where it goes to work, helping to break down the fat that comes from foods like steaks, ice cream, and potato chips.

As you might conclude from this scenario, if you're regularly eating high-fat items, your gallbladder is working overtime.

Just because it takes a lot of gall to break down fat doesn't necessarily mean that you're going to have a lot of gallstones. Gallstones form from excess cholesterol, the same notorious fat that has a reputation for clogging arteries, and some people are just more prone to them than others. Doctors have found that women are more likely to get gallstones than men, particularly if they're pregnant. Both sexes are at higher risk if they're overweight.

If you've had gallstones, you're definitely at risk of getting them again, so it makes sense to take preventive steps. When gallstones are inside the gallbladder, they sometimes cause intestinal discomfort or nausea, but only a doctor, with the help of x-rays, can tell you whether those symptoms are being caused by stones.

Once the stones start to move into the bile ducts—the exit ramps from the gallbladder and the liver—pain is not far behind. They can be dangerous, too, causing jaundice or serious infection from blocked ducts.

If you have had gallstones and you recognize some familiar symptoms returning, see the doctor. You might need to have the gallstones dissolved or have the stones or your gallbladder surgically removed.

The Food Factor

"I believe that your first defense against gallstones is to change what you're eating," says Kristin Stiles, N.D., a naturopathic doctor at the Complementary Medicine and Healing Arts Center in Vestal, New York. "You have to cut back on the fat and get more fiber in your diet."

Some specific foods are said to help. "I've had people get really effective relief from gallbladder pain with beet greens," says William Warnock, N.D., a naturopathic doctor in Shelburne, Vermont. When steamed, beet greens are unusually high in minerals, vitamin A, and a substance called betaine. According to Dr. Warnock, betaine stimulates the production of bile and simultaneously thins it out. Also, betaine causes the muscles surrounding the gallbladder and bile ducts to contract and move things along.

Filling with Fiber, Not Fat

Getting more fiber into your diet is a simple way to decrease excess fat. Dietary fiber binds with bile salts, which are a primary part of bile, and cholesterol in the intestines and prevents both from being absorbed by the body. You can up your fiber intake by eating as many fruits and vegetables as possible, along with brans and whole grains like wheat, oats, and rye, says Dr. Stiles.

Fiber absorbs large amounts of water, and water-soaked fiber bulks up and softens the stool. A well-hydrated stool absorbs lots of wastes and by-products of digestion, such as fat. With less fat around, the process of gallstone formation may be interrupted.

The recommended daily amount of fiber is 25 to 30 grams, says Dr. Stiles. If you find that you can't eat enough high-fiber foods to achieve that level, an alternative is to try one of the fiber/nutritional supplements found in drugstores and health food stores. Dr. Stiles recommends a supplement that contains psyllium. She suggests stirring two tablespoons of the supplement into a glass of water and drinking it at breakfast time each day.

Turning to Lecithin

According to naturopathic doctors, one nutritional substance that might help prevent gallstones is lecithin. Also called phosphatidylcholine, lecithin is a major ingredient in cell membranes. It's found in animal tissues, especially the nerves, liver, and semen.

Lecithin is important because it helps water and fat mix together more easily. Usually, fat stays separate from water, but lecithin is an emulsifier, a kind of go-between that reconciles these opposites and allows the two substances to combine.

In the body, lecithin can help make cholesterol (a fat) mix with water. Because lecithin is such a good emulsifier, naturopaths believe that cholesterol is transported more easily when there's plenty of lecithin around.

Indeed, some naturopathic doctors say that low levels of lecithin in the body have been linked to the formation of gallstones. If you supplement with lecithin, gallstones are less likely to occur. You can also get lecithin from foods such as soybeans, wheat germ, and peanuts.

Lecithin can't dissolve stones that are already in your gallbladder, says Dr. Stiles, but it might help prevent new ones. The typical dose of lecithin is 500 to 1,000 milligrams a day, she says. You should supplement for several months at the same time that you're working to improve your diet.

Making Bile Flow

If you can just "keep the juices flowing," you may help prevent gallstone problems, herbalists believe. You can get some aid from herbs that have what are called choleretic properties, meaning the ability to increase the amount of bile the liver produces and also boost the flow of bile from the gallbladder. At the same time, herbalists believe that herbs with choleretic properties stimulate gallbladder contraction.

Milk thistle is one herb with these properties. "It gets things moving and helps flush out the small stones," says Dr. Stiles. It is also believed to help improve the digestion of fats, she adds.

Although some supplement formulas are made up of a number of choleretic herbs, Dr. Warnock favors milk thistle taken by itself. "What usually happens when you put a lot of herbs into one capsule is that you don't end up with high concentrations of any of them," he says.

For the most effective concentration, you need a standardized extract of milk thistle that contains 80 percent silymarin, the herb's primary active ingredient, says Dr. Warnock. The typical dose is 70 to 210 milligrams three times a day. A naturopathic doctor can recommend a specific amount.

"It may take three to six months before it has a beneficial effect," says Dr. Warnock. You should never take it during a gallstone attack, however. If you already have gallstones that begin to cause persistent pain or a fever, you should see a doctor immediately, not wait months to find out whether the herb is effective.

genital herpes

The herpes simplex virus is a sneaky little devil. Most of the time, it lies dormant in the nerve cells near your spine. The moment it notices that your immune defenses are down, it comes to life and makes a beeline for the skin's surface surrounding your genitals. There, the virus forms clusters of painful, fluid-filled blisters that can hang around for two weeks or more.

Each year, at least 500,000 people in the United States contract genital herpes. Once herpes moves in, it becomes a permanent guest. While a lucky 40 percent of people infected with this sexually transmitted disease (STD) never have another outbreak after their initial episodes, the not-so-lucky majority may have five or more recurrences a year.

Fortunately, you can keep this annoying virus in check by making a few significant adjustments to your lifestyle and diet. Daily exercise such as brisk walking, cycling, jogging, and stretching can melt away stress and fatigue, two of the most common triggers of recurrent outbreaks. Moreover, doctors say that if you eat more foods high in the amino acid lysine, such as chicken, fish, and vegetables, you can help keep the virus at arm's length. They also say you should try to avoid fare such as chocolate, nuts, seeds, and gelatin, foods that are high in another amino acid, arginine.

In addition, a variety of nutritional supplements can give you extra protection. Certain herbs can relieve stress and strengthen your immune system. Some vitamins and minerals can alleviate the painful warning signs of an imminent outbreak, and others can reduce the number of recurrent infections, shorten the duration of the episodes, and speed the healing of lesions. Supplementing with lysine also can help keep the virus at bay.

Chill Out with Siberian Ginseng

One of the most common triggers of recurrent herpes outbreaks is physical and emotional stress. Too much stress weakens your immune system,

441

A Gland's Best Friend

If you are plagued by recurrent genital herpes infections, chances are your thymus gland isn't performing up to par. This gland is your immune system's main headquarters, where virus-fighting white blood cells are activated.

To improve the health of your thymus gland, you might consider taking supplements that contain a bovine thymus gland extract, says Thomas Kruzel, N.D., a naturopathic doctor in Portland, Oregon. Available in most health food stores, these extracts are believed by naturopathic doctors to boost immunity and prevent the number and severity of recurrent herpes outbreaks.

"There's some evidence that taking glandular material from a certain animal will strengthen the corresponding human gland and the immune system's response to the herpesvirus," says Dr. Kruzel.

"Your body will absorb the glandular molecules from the extract in a useful form, and they will be used as food for your own thymus gland," says Susan Kowalsky, N.D., a naturopathic doctor in Norwich, Vermont.

Age, oxidation, and poor nutrition all contribute to the poor health of the thymus gland, she adds. Keeping this gland healthy will better equip your immune system to keep herpes outbreaks away.

making you more susceptible to repeated infections. The less stressed you are, the fewer outbreaks you'll experience, says Susan Kowalsky, N.D., a naturopathic doctor in Norwich, Vermont.

Enter Siberian ginseng. This medicinal herb is most noted for its ability to protect your body from the negative effects of stress. Siberian ginseng is often referred to as a tonic for your adrenal glands—the glands that produce stress hormones—because it maintains their overall health. It's an herb that can relieve stress and improve stamina without adverse side effects.

Dr. Kowalsky suggests taking 2,000 to 4,000 milligrams of Siberian ginseng three times a day. Everyone's response to ginseng is different, so start off with the lower dosage and increase it over time. If you find that you're experiencing irritability, nervousness, or insomnia at higher doses, cut back by at least half until you don't experience any side effects, then gradually work back up over a few weeks, she says.

An Herbal Medicine Chest

Two other medicinal herbs that can inhibit outbreaks of the herpesvirus are echinacea and licorice.

Echinacea is a potent antiviral and antibacterial herb that strengthens your immune system by stimulating white blood cell production. It increases levels of a chemical in your body called properdin, which activates a certain part of your immune system that destroys viruses.

Moreover, echinacea raises levels of interferon, another immune system chemical that blocks the replication of herpesvirus proteins, says Dr. Kowalsky. So your outbreaks should be few and far between.

Take 500 milligrams of echinacea twice a day at the first sign of symptoms to help prevent an outbreak or to speed the healing of lesions if you're already having a recurrence, says Thomas Kruzel, N.D., a naturopathic doctor in Portland, Oregon. Continue taking this dose until symptoms and lesions disappear, he says. If you need to take it for more than eight weeks, however, talk to your doctor.

Similar to echinacea, licorice turbocharges your immune system and builds your resistance to the herpesvirus, says Dr. Kowalsky. Glycyrrhizin, one of the herb's eight antiviral compounds, inhibits a number of processes involved in viral replication, such as the ability to penetrate healthy cells and reproduce their genetic material. What's more, certain compounds in licorice boost interferon levels and make it especially hard for the herpesvirus to survive, she says.

Take 1,000 to 2,000 milligrams of powdered licorice root in capsule form three times a day during an outbreak or when symptoms arise, says Dr. Kowalsky, but be sure to talk to your doctor if you're taking these doses and especially if you are pregnant.

Boost Immunity with Vitamin C

Since the herpesvirus tends to resurface whenever your immunity is low, a vitamin that supports your immune system is a real ally in your battle with herpes. Vitamin C is such a vitamin. It can recharge your immune system by strengthening white blood cells that will fight off the virus. Vitamin C can also help speed healing—and the faster you heal, the less pain and discomfort you'll experience from the lesions. According to Dr. Kowalsky, this vitamin can also prevent damage to healthy cells and boost interferon levels.

"It's known that viruses deplete vitamin C residing in white blood cells, so we know that if you want your immune system to stay strong, you need to take extra vitamin C," says Dr. Kowalsky. To prevent herpes outbreaks, she recommends 1,000 to 3,000 milligrams daily in divided doses. She also suggests taking it with food to avoid stomach irritation.

If you're having an outbreak, you'll need to take even more. Dr. Kowalsky recommends 3,000 to 12,000 milligrams of vitamin C. Along with that, she recommends taking 1,000 to 3,000 milligrams of citrus bio-flavonoids, compounds that may help fight inflammation, halt viruses, and control the oxidation process that can lead to premature aging of cells. Citrus bioflavonoids boost the absorption of vitamin C and shorten the duration of herpes outbreaks, according to Dr. Kowalsky.

Think Zinc for Relief

Like vitamin C, the mineral zinc can help rev up your immune system. Zinc helps boost production of T-lymphocyte cells, which are important body defenses against viral infections. "Zinc also disrupts the replication of the herpesvirus by blocking it from going into its reproductive cycle," says Dr. Kruzel. He recommends taking 15 to 30 milligrams of zinc daily to prevent outbreaks.

If you're having a recurrence, take 30 to 45 milligrams daily until the lesions clear up, says Dr. Kowalsky. Don't exceed 20 milligrams of zinc a day without first discussing it with your doctor.

A Trio of Infection-Fighting Nutrients

Vitamin A, beta-carotene, and vitamin E all qualify as strong contenders in the fight against recurrent herpes infections.

Vitamin A arms your immune system with the ammunition it needs to battle the virus. It can alleviate symptoms of an impending outbreak and reduce the number of recurrences. Since doses of vitamin A above 10,000 international units (IU) are not usually recommended, a safer alternative is to take beta-carotene, according to Dr. Kowalsky. Beta-carotene is the antioxidant that increases antibody production and white blood cell activity, and it converts to vitamin A in the body.

"Beta-carotene encourages new cell growth and strengthens your cells' outer layers so that the virus can't penetrate, duplicate itself, and spread like wildfire," says Dr. Kruzel.

When symptoms of a possible outbreak occur, take 100,000 IU of beta-carotene daily in divided doses to jump-start your immune system, says Dr. Kowalsky. Although you should also check with your doctor before taking this high daily dose, beta-carotene doesn't pose the same risks as vitamin A.

Vitamin E also protects your white blood cells from invading viruses and strengthens other aspects of your immune system. It can help speed the healing of the lesions as well, says Dr. Kowalsky. She recommends taking 400 IU a day during an outbreak and continuing after the symptoms are alleviated.

The Lysine-Arginine Connection

Research shows that a diet high in lysine and low in arginine can prevent the herpesvirus from surfacing.

In one study, people with genital herpes took 1,000 milligrams of lysine daily for six months while eliminating arginine-rich foods from their diets. At the end of the study, lysine was rated effective or very effective at preventing herpes outbreaks in 74 percent of those who took it.

To keep lysine levels high, take 500 to 1,500 milligrams daily at the first sign of symptoms and continue until symptoms disappear, says Dr. Kruzel. If you're having an outbreak, take 9,000 milligrams daily until the lesions go away and for four to five days afterward. Doctors caution, however, that you shouldn't take this dosage for more than two weeks.

gingivitis

When you're savoring a meal or munching on a snack, it's pretty distasteful to visualize the soft, sticky film of bacteria that's getting a grip on your teeth. Nevertheless, it's always there, poised and ready to form a layer called plaque all around your teeth, between them, and even under your gum line. If you don't brush or floss the film away, it will harden into a substance called tartar, which will eventually irritate your gums and cause them to turn red, swell, and even bleed.

These are warning signs of early gum disease, or gingivitis. Plaque is the number one cause of gingivitis, which is responsible for at least 80 percent of dental problems in adults. In fact, nearly 85 percent of the population has some form of gingivitis.

In the early stages, gingivitis is reversible as long as you conscientiously clean your teeth at home and visit your dentist a couple of times a year for professional cleanings. Untreated, gingivitis can lead to periodontitis, an advanced stage of gum disease that causes receding gums, pockets forming between the teeth and gums, infection, loss of bone, and, finally, tooth loss.

Your best weapons against gum disease are a soft-bristle toothbrush, fluoride toothpaste, and dental floss. To prevent plaque buildup, brush your teeth after every meal and floss at least once a day. Follow that with regular visits to your dentist, and you should be fine, says Meena Shah, D.D.S., a dentist in Lake Grove, New York.

If you're already practicing good dental hygiene, but your gums are still a little inflamed and bleed periodically, visit your dentist. Meanwhile, you can make some choices about your diet that can reduce the progression of gingivitis.

Eat lots of high-fiber foods, such as fruits and vegetables, and less sugar-laden fare, says Dr. Shah. Dietary fiber acts as a cleaning agent for your teeth. Sugary foods such as cookies, cake, and candy and sticky foods like raisins increase plaque buildup on your teeth and breed bacteria, she says.

446

Supplements can help, too. Taking extra vitamin C, folic acid, and other nutrients can rev up your immune system to battle the infection, reduce inflammation, and stop the bleeding. Certain medicinal herbs such as echinacea can also boost immunity as well as heal and strengthen damaged gum tissue. Here's how the supplement lineup can help keep your gums and teeth in tip-top shape.

Combine Vitamin C with Bioflavonoids

One important nutrient that can help heal red, swollen gums is vitamin C. This antioxidant boosts your immune system, brings down inflammation, and speeds up wound healing. In fact, a deficiency of vitamin C can lead to gingivitis, which may cause teeth to become loose and even fall out.

Vitamin C has proven to be vital for the production of collagen, the basic protein building block for the fibrous framework of all tissues, including gums. The vitamin strengthens gum tissue and helps the gum lining resist bacteria.

Vitamin C can repair and rebuild connective tissue. "Moreover, it will boost your immune system so that you can fight off the infection," says Liz Collins, N.D., a naturopathic doctor and co-owner of the Natural Childbirth and Family Clinic in Portland, Oregon.

Dr. Collins recommends taking 3,000 to 4,000 milligrams of vitamin C daily in divided doses. As part of your daily vitamin C regimen, Dr. Collins also recommends taking bioflavonoids. Naturopathic doctors believe that these nutrients are very effective at reducing inflammation and repairing and healing gum tissue. They're strong antioxidants that can prevent damage from free radicals, the free-roaming, unstable molecules that harm cells. Bioflavonoids are also known to boost the effectiveness of vitamin C.

"You should always take bioflavonoids with vitamin C," says Dr. Collins. You can buy a vitamin C and bioflavonoid combination formula or take the bioflavonoids separately.

Two of the most effective bioflavonoids are quercetin and grapeseed extract. Take 1,000 to 2,000 milligrams of quercetin or 100 to 200 milligrams of grapeseed extract daily, says Jennifer Brett, N.D., a naturopathic doctor at the Wilton Naturopathic Center in Stratford, Connecticut.

Folic Acid Treatment

Several studies have shown that folic acid can reduce inflammation, bleeding, and plaque buildup on the teeth when taken in pill form or used as a mouthwash. Research has also shown that it can help treat periodontitis, the advanced stage of gum disease.

"Folic acid is a B vitamin that keeps the cells in your mouth healthy. Your mouth contains some of the fastest-dividing cells in the body, and any cell that divides quickly needs folic acid to replicate properly," says Dr. Collins.

Take 400 to 800 micrograms of folic acid daily to treat gingivitis, she says. You can also make a mouthwash, which some studies say is more effective. Twice a day, empty a folic acid capsule into four ounces of lukewarm water and stir. Swish the solution in your mouth for a couple of minutes, then swallow it, says Dr. Collins. Repeat until you've finished the liquid.

Coenzyme Q_{10} for Healthy Gums

Coenzyme Q_{10}, or coQ_{10}, is a vitamin-like compound found in human tissue that stimulates the immune system. It's chemically similar to vitamin E and is a powerful antioxidant that helps treat gingivitis and maintain healthy gums and other tissues by increasing the flow of oxygen to cells. Food sources include salmon, sardines, beef, peanuts, and spinach. In Japan, coQ_{10} is widely used to treat gum disease.

When researchers reviewed seven studies that used coQ_{10}, they found that 70 percent of the 332 people with periodontal disease who took supplements of the substance showed signs of improvement. In one of these studies, the group taking coQ_{10} showed a reduction in inflammation, receding gums, and tooth mobility.

Dr. Brett recommends taking 150 to 200 milligrams daily if your gums are inflamed and bleeding. As soon as the bleeding stops and the inflammation goes down, you can stop taking it.

Herbal Remedies

Medicinal herbs such as echinacea, burdock root, and Siberian ginseng can help battle a gingivitis infection, says Ellen Evert Hopman, a professional member of the American Herbalists Guild, a lay homeopath in

Amherst, Massachusetts, and author of *Tree Medicine, Tree Magic*. She recommends taking these herbs in capsule form.

Dosages vary, so follow the directions on the label. If the echinacea supplements are 380 milligrams, a typical dose would be one to three capsules three times daily with water at mealtimes. For 425-milligram capsules of burdock root, a common recommendation is to start with one capsule twice a day and build up to two capsules three times daily over a three-week period. For Siberian ginseng, if the supplements are 410 milligrams, a usual dose would be two capsules three times daily. Take these supplements with water, and be sure to drink plenty of water throughout the day.

Echinacea stimulates the immune system by galvanizing white blood cell production, Hopman says. It increases levels of a chemical in the body called properdin, which activates the part of the immune system responsible for shoring up defense mechanisms against bacteria and viruses.

Burdock root is a blood purifier that can strengthen immunity to help get rid of the infection and reduce inflammation, says Hopman. Its roots and seeds contain a variety of chemicals and nutrients.

Siberian ginseng, which is mainly used to restore vitality, boost energy, and protect the body from the negative effects of stress, can stimulate the immune system and repair inflamed, tender gum tissue, says Hopman.

gout

There was a time when people were reassured by the swelling and red-hot pain of a gouty foot. Since the pain zeroed in on a distant extremity, the big toe, it seemed to signify that all the nerves in the far reaches of the body were working well. Therefore, people surmised, maybe all was perfectly well with everything in between.

Gout is no all-clear signal, however. "That pain in the joint is the end result of a long breakdown process," says Luc Maes, D.C., N.D., a chiropractor and naturopathic doctor in Santa Barbara, California. It means that the kidneys are not doing a good job.

Your blood transports the chief troublemaker, uric acid. Like a traveler toting a heavy suitcase through an airport, blood that has a burden of excess uric acid begins looking for a dump site, says Dr. Maes. Down around the big toe, circulation is sluggish, and it's easy for the blood to drop its load. The uric acid deposited in the joint forms needle-shaped crystals that can trigger an inflammation so severe that even the weight of a bedsheet causes pain.

Purine-rich foods just make matters worse. Purines are chemicals found in foods such as alcohol, seafood, and organ meats. Normally, they don't do any damage, but if you're prone to gout, these foods can cause crystal formation.

It helps to drink as much water as possible to help flush purines and uric acid from your system—and by all means, eliminate purine-rich foods from your diet. It also helps to limit your intake of animal fats and refined carbohydrates, which increase the production of uric acid.

Along with those measures, nutritional and herbal supplements are good allies, say alternative medicine experts. Many can help improve the kidney, the liver, and the blood, according to Dr. Maes. Others can help fight inflammation. But he emphasizes that supplements can't make amends for a diet that includes lots of animal fats and refined carbohydrates. "If you eat a poor diet for a long time, your body gets too much of certain nutrients and not enough of others," he says.

Fight the Flame with EPA

When you eat saturated fats—the kind that come from meat and dairy foods—you're inviting the overproduction of inflammatory chemical. "Gout is a state of inflammation," says Dr. Maes. "Things are on fire."

Studies have shown that you can help reverse this pattern and correct the nutritional imbalance by taking fish oil or flaxseed oil. Fish-oil supplements are particularly rich in an omega-3 fatty acid called eicosapentaenoic acid (EPA), which discourages inflammation, says Priscilla Evans, N.D., a naturopathic doctor at the Community Wholistic Health Center in Chapel Hill, North Carolina. EPA is only available from fish.

Like throwing a track switch to reroute a train, EPA reroutes the chemicals in your body early in the inflammation process. With the flick of that switch, the chemicals start to fight inflammation.

Supplements can't do the whole job, Dr. Evans emphasizes. "It's very important to cut back on oils and saturated fats that promote inflammation. Just adding fish oil is not enough if you're still eating a lot of red meat and fat."

Dr. Maes advises people with gout to take 1,500 milligrams of fish oil a day, but not all at once. Divide the doses and take the supplements with meals.

You should also take 400 to 1,200 international units of vitamin E a day with the fish oil, she says. It works along with the EPA to act as an anti-inflammatory and also serves as an antioxidant.

If you're a vegetarian or don't like fish, you may be able to get similar benefits by taking one to two tablespoons of flaxseed oil every day, says Dr. Maes. This oil contains alpha-linolenic acid, however, not the more valuable EPA, and only a portion of it is converted to EPA by the body.

The Bromelain Benefit

An enzyme with an appetite, bromelain, which comes from pineapple, is nature's anti-inflammatory medicine. Because it's an enzyme and enzymes help with digestion, you can take it with meals. You can also take it between meals. When you do, it works as an anti-inflammatory agent. "Bromelain inhibits those proteins that are promoting inflammation in the body. It kind of digests the products of inflammation," says Dr. Evans.

Celery Seed Extract: A Natural Diuretic, and More

Medieval magicians put celery seed in their shoes in order to fly, but you're more likely to use this spice-cupboard staple to add some flavor to soup. These tiny, flavorful seeds are natural diuretics and anti-inflammatories that have been used since ancient times for treating gout and arthritis as well as colds and flu.

The healing properties of celery seed are in the volatile oil, which acts as an antiseptic. In the urinary system, the oil helps clean out the organs that carry urine.

Celery has been used for centuries in Asia as a folk remedy for high blood pressure. Today, some herbalists also use celery seed for its sedative and tranquilizing effect and prescribe the extract for treating insomnia and anxiety. "It's a clearing kind of herb," says Betzy Bancroft, a professional member of the American Herbalists Guild in Washington, New Jersey.

To test it, researchers at the University of Chicago injected animals with a small amount of a chemical compound that is found in celery and celery seed. Within a week, the animals' blood pressures dropped an average of 12 to 14 percent. The chemical injection relaxed the muscles lining the arteries that regulate blood pressure and also reduced the amount of stress hormones in the blood. With reduced stress hormones, there was less constriction of blood vessels.

Celery seed is so tiny that one ounce contains about 72,000 seeds, but it's also rich in calories, with more than 100 calories an ounce. Each seed contains the nutrients calcium, phosphorus, magnesium, potassium, iron, and zinc.

You can buy the extract in capsules or tablets that are standardized by the percentage of volatile oil they contain.

Dr. Evans recommends 500 milligrams of bromelain three times a day between meals to help reduce the inflammation during acute gout attacks. For milder cases of gout, you'll probably want to start out with a smaller dose, since bromelain sometimes causes a burning feeling in the gut.

Although an attack of gout can last as long as a few weeks, you should take high doses of bromelain for only four to five days. After that, if the gout lingers, take 125 to 250 milligrams three times a day to control in-flammation, advises Dr. Evans.

Folic Acid at Work

Folic acid also has a dampening effect on uric acid production, studies show. This B vitamin gets in the way of the enzyme responsible for pro-ducing uric acid, and when that enzyme is blocked, uric acid production takes a nosedive. Folic acid won't resolve an acute attack, but in high doses, it may help ward off future attacks.

For gout, the recommended dosage is 10,000 to 50,000 micrograms of folic acid daily. That's 25 to 100 times the Daily Value of 400 micrograms, Since that's far more than you should take without a prescription, you need to contact your physician if you would like to try folic acid as a preventive. Also, research has shown that you need to take some vitamin C along with the folic acid in order for it to work.

Boon from Berries

Help in another form comes from bioflavonoid molecules, which are found in cherries, blueberries, and other fruits. In the 1950s, researchers dis-covered that cherries could decrease uric acid levels and prevent a gout at-tack. You'd have to eat a lot of cherries—a half-pound a day—or the equivalent amount of unsweetened juice to make a dent in gout. Blueber-ries work as well.

For the same results, you can take a bioflavonoid supplement or 2,000 milligrams of berry extract a day, says Dr. Maes. The best are those that have a combination of all the bioflavonoids or the extracts of several dif-ferent berries, he says.

Bioflavonoids affect other body processes as well as uric acid produc-tion. Researchers have found that they help in tissue building and can pre-vent the release of some compounds that promote inflammation.

Soothing with Celery

When doctors prescribe a drug for gout relief, it's often allopurinal (Zy-loprim), which controls the levels of uric acid. A natural alternative is celery seed extract, a supplement that acts as a diuretic, helping to flush fluids out of the system.

The pharmaceutical and the natural supplement were tested and compared by James A. Duke, Ph.D., botanical consultant, former ethnobotanist with the U.S. Department of Agriculture who specializes in medicinal plants, and author of *The Green Pharmacy*. After taking allopurinal prescribed by his doctor for acute gout, Dr. Duke learned that celery seed extract might help just as much, so he decided to try it. The extract was supposed to help his body eliminate uric acid and prevent it from reaching the critical levels that induce an attack of gout.

Dr. Duke took two to four tablets of celery seed extract every day instead of allopurinol, and his attacks of gout disappeared. "I've now found an herbal alternative in celery seed extract, which I expect to continue taking as long as the threat of gout hangs over me," he says.

Settle on Nettle

Nettle, a natural antihistamine that has long been used by old-time herbalists to treat inflammation of the joints, also works as a diuretic to help to lower uric acid levels. "Nettle works as a blood cleanser and detoxifying agent," says Dr. Maes.

To get the full benefit, take 300 to 600 milligrams of a freeze-dried extract daily, he advises. Nettle may be used long-term, but Dr. Maes recommends not using it for more than two to three months at a time. Avoid tinctures of nettle. They contain alcohol and may aggravate gout.

hair loss

If you're looking for a cure for male pattern baldness, you won't find it here. Hair loss is a trait inherited through the maternal side of the family.

If your mom's dad or her brothers are bald, the cards are stacked against you. Unless you're willing to spend hundreds of dollars a year on hair-raising new drugs that may or may not produce results, you'll just have to resign yourself to a future of diminishing strands.

Not all hair loss is inevitable, however, nor is the decline entirely controlled by genes. Stress, hormone changes, and vitamin or mineral deficiencies can lead to fast fallout. Moreover, you're likely to lose hair faster if your hair follicles become inflamed or if you get skin disorders that affect your scalp.

Even women aren't immune to some of the fallout from these problems. "I've had women patients who have lost all their hair due to major stresses in their lives," says Hope Fay, N.D., a naturopathic doctor in Seattle. "When you're under stress from illness or work, sometimes the circulation in the scalp is so constricted that the hair follicles lose blood supply, which causes them to die and fall out." Dr. Fay is quick to add, however, that if women lose their hair, it often grows right back in when they're no longer under extreme stress.

To help the hair return when the loss isn't a matter of inherited baldness, you can try a number of tactics. The solution usually lies with improving your diet and making lifestyle changes to relieve stress, says Dr. Fay. In addition, you can supplement your diet with nutrients that aid in hair growth, she says.

In other words, you've got to feed your head.

Mine Minerals, Pluck Nettle

When a mineral or vitamin deficiency is at the root of your hair loss, you simply need to correct the deficiency. Maybe it's the result of improper digestion, or perhaps you're not absorbing the necessary vitamins and minerals as well as you need to, notes Elizabeth Wotton, N.D., a naturopathic doctor at Compass Family Health Center in Plymouth, Massachusetts.

Deficiencies of selenium and zinc generally lead to hair loss, researchers have observed. These minerals aid in immune function and in the utilization of protein that your body needs to help produce hair.

Selenium and zinc are known as trace minerals because the body does not need large amounts of them. Normally, plants get these minerals from the soil, animals get them from plants, and humans acquire their needed amounts of trace minerals with breakfast, lunch, and dinner.

It doesn't always work that way, however, says Dr. Wotton. "Unfortunately, in some areas of the United States, some trace minerals just aren't in the soil in high enough quantities," she observes. "So they aren't being taken up by food crops. You could be eating what you think is a good diet but still be lacking."

If that's your problem, there's a quick fix. Simply go down to the local health food store or drugstore and pick up a trace mineral supplement. It should include a wide variety of trace minerals, including amounts such as 200 micrograms of selenium and 20 milligrams of zinc.

"I would just follow the dosage directions on the bottle and try it for several weeks." says Dr. Wotton. "It will be a while before you know if it's working."

You can also try taking 30 milligrams of zinc daily and see if you stop losing hair or even start to grow it back, says Dr. Wotton. If your hair loss is due to a zinc deficiency, you could see regrowth in as little as a week. You should talk to a doctor before taking this amount of zinc, however.

While you're at the store, you might also look at some herbs that could help. One is nettle. "It's really high in mineral content and can make your hair much healthier," Dr. Fay says.

Nettle can be found as capsules. Simply follow the dosage directions on the bottle. For 480-milligram capsules, for example, the typical dose is one capsule twice a day. The tincture form does not contain minerals. You have to eat plant material to get minerals. Extraction in vinegar pulls some minerals out, but eating the plant is best.

Regulating Hormones

In the first few months after their children are born, some women are distressed to find that their hair begins to fall out. The problem is usually due to hormonal changes. The body's hormone ratios are radically revised during pregnancy. After delivery, the body has to establish a new balance.

Hormone upsets aren't limited to new mothers, however. Stress, menopause, and illness can also bring on changes.

To ease hormonal transitions, Dr. Wotton suggests giving your body the nutritional building blocks it needs to manufacture and regulate hormones. You can begin by eating more foods containing phytoestrogens, plant compounds that mimic the biological activities of female hormones. These foods include legumes and soy products, such as tofu.

Dr. Wotton also suggests supplementing your diet with a few important minerals and vitamins. She recommends 150 milligrams of magnesium twice a day, 400 to 800 international units (IU) of vitamin E daily, and a daily vitamin B-complex supplement that contains 100 milligrams of B_6 and 50 micrograms of biotin.

"With these supplements, you're giving your body all the right raw materials," Dr. Wotton says. "If hormones are your problem, your body should eventually right itself."

In addition, you might consider supplementing with essential fatty acids from flaxseed oil or evening primrose oil, says Dr. Fay. These kinds of fats form the biological backbone of many hormone molecules. The oils are rich sources of omega-3 and omega-6 fatty acids, good fats that are important for healthy skin and hair.

Dr. Fay suggests taking 1,000 milligrams of evening primrose oil three times a day or one teaspoon of flaxseed oil once or twice a day. You can take the flaxseed oil by the spoonful or put it on salads and other foods.

headache

If you are prone to headaches, chances are you were born with a slightly different brain chemistry than people who get don't get them. You might have imbalances in the chemical serotonin, which is a messenger that helps regulate the diameter of blood vessels.

Medical researchers now believe that in the majority of headaches, certain factors trigger fluctuations in serotonin levels. Once the serotonin is out of balance, the blood vessels in your brain become inflamed and you end up with a head that's throbbing with pain.

More than 90 percent of all headaches are classified as tension headaches, which occur when the muscles in the back of your neck and scalp tighten. When you have a tension headache, you'll probably feel a generalized dull head pain. That's a signal that the nerves running through the muscles have become inflamed and irritated.

Migraines are another kind of animal. The pulsating throb of a migraine headache is less common but more likely to send you to the doctor in quest of relief. Migraines occur more often in women than in men and can last from a few minutes to a few days.

A third type, the cluster headache, is even more acute but also much more rare.

Whichever type of headache you're prone to, chances are that the underlying cause is your genetic makeup. "We are clearly dealing with a biological disorder, not a psychological one," says Fred Sheftell, M.D., a psychiatrist, headache specialist, and co-founder of the New England Center for Headache in Stamford, Connecticut.

Pay Attention to Triggers

Just because you were born with a predisposition for headaches doesn't mean that you have to get them, according to Dr. Sheftell. If you can avoid the pain triggers, you might be able to avoid the headaches.

Heading up Dr. Sheftell's Top Ten list of triggers are sensitivities to foods such as chocolate, certain food components such as alcohol and caffeine, and the food additive MSG. Other possible triggers are hormone fluctuations during the menstrual cycle, changes in the weather or season, sleeping late or not enough, bright lights, and odors. Last but certainly not least is that old bugbear, stress.

Traditional over-the-counter medications may get rid of the pain once it hits, but they won't help you have fewer headaches. With nutritional measures, you can take a preventive approach, says Dr. Sheftell.

Which supplement you try will depend on which type of headaches you get and what's causing them. Each supplement acts in a different way. You can take supplements in combination without any problems, but your best approach, says Dr. Sheftell, is to try one or two at a time until you find the custom formula that works for you.

Try Riboflavin for Migraines

Riboflavin is a benign B vitamin. In super-high doses, it can help ward off a migraine attack by helping the brain cells utilize energy, says Dr. Sheftell.

In a Belgian study of 49 people who frequently got migraines, researchers got good results with daily doses of 400 milligrams of riboflavin. At that dose, about half of the people in the study became migraine-free. Among the others, the intensity of pain was reduced by about 70 percent.

How does riboflavin work? Researchers have found that some people who get migraines may not have enough energy stored in their brain cells. Riboflavin helps the enzymes in the body tap into the energy stored in those cells.

Researchers speculate that flooding the system with riboflavin stirs up more energy in the cells. Helping to regenerate the lethargic cellular energy system defuses the migraine, says Seymour Solomon, M.D., professor of neurology at the Albert Einstein College of Medicine of Yeshiva University in the Bronx.

Riboflavin is found in milk. Four glasses will give you the Daily Value of 1.7 milligrams. The doses needed to help prevent migraine are many times higher, however. In fact, since you would need to drink about 62 gallons of milk a day to get the 400-milligram dose that was used in the Belgian study, supplementing is essential.

A Mineral for Facial Pain

It's not hard to recognize a headache when it's happening, but what if you're having pain in your face rather than your head?

Frequently, the source of facial pain—sometimes called trifacial neuralgia—is the trigeminal nerve. Known as the great sensory nerve of the head, it comes out of the cranium right above the jaw. The extensions of that nerve form a web across much of your face. If you have inflammation or infection or if the nerve is injured, you might feel the pain signals all around your face.

Many people have this kind of facial pain as the result of temporomandibular disorder (TMD), a problem with the temporomandibular joint in the jaw. If your jaw doesn't line up correctly, it may grind or click whenever you're chewing and talking. TMD can lead to muscle spasms, pain, and eventually inflammation, which in turn leads to more pain, says Anne McClenon, N.D., a naturopathic doctor at the Compass Family Health Center in Plymouth, Massachusetts.

If you have facial pain caused by TMD, try some kind of physical bodywork, suggests Dr. McClenon. Chiropractic, craniosacral therapy, or massage therapy can relax the muscles and allow the joint to line up properly. If this doesn't help, you may need to see a dentist who specializes in TMD, she says.

For TMD, Dr. McClenon also recommends magnesium, which is an effective headache cure. Magnesium is the critical mineral in getting muscles to relax. Take 300 to 350 milligrams a day, suggests Dr. McClenon. "Usually, people take it in the evening so that muscle relaxation hits about bedtime," she says. "That way, they can get a good night's sleep."

"Almost as a matter of routine, all of our patients are put on riboflavin. We start them on 200 milligrams for a week and then bring them up to 400 milligrams," Dr. Sheftell says.

According to Dr. Sheftell, some people experience nausea when they take as much as 400 milligrams. If that happens, you can just return to the 200-milligram dose. It may take some time to get relief, so stick with the supplements for two to three months before you decide whether they have any benefit, says Dr. Sheftell.

Adding Some Magnesium

Another promising migraine fighter is magnesium. This mineral plays a key role in regulating both blood vessel size and the rate at which cells burn energy. Researchers estimate that 50 percent of migraine sufferers are magnesium deficient, says Burton M. Altura, M.D., professor of physiology and medicine at the State University of New York Health Science Center in Brooklyn. At the center, studies on more than 1,000 migraine sufferers have shown that an intravenous dose of 1,000 milligrams of magnesium sulfate can relieve some acute headache attacks.

Does this mean that you can pop a few magnesium tablets to get rid of a headache? Not quite, but the supplement may be useful in preventing them.

"We believe that everyone should be taking 500 to 600 milligrams of magnesium a day in a combination of diet and supplements," says Dr. Altura. "If people would bring up their total consumption of magnesium, they could reduce the frequency of recurring migraine headaches."

The trouble is, that dose of magnesium has to be absorbed if it's going to do its job, and absorption can be a challenge. Magnesium supplements often cause diarrhea, says Jacqueline Jacques, N.D., a naturopathic doctor and specialist in pain management in Portland, Oregon. This all-too-common side effect is a sign that the supplement is not being absorbed.

If you want to get the most from a magnesium supplement and minimize the chance of diarrhea, Dr. Jacques advises taking magnesium glycinate instead of magnesium oxide or magnesium chloride. Magnesium glycinate is a form that is readily absorbed, which means two things. First, it can go right to work and do what it is supposed to do—prevent constriction of the blood vessels in your brain and scalp. Second, since it is easily absorbed, it spends less time in the gut and is less likely to cause loose stools.

Feed on Feverfew

Don't wait until you're hurting to take feverfew, says Dr. Sheftell. A cousin of dandelion and marigold, feverfew has long been used to prevent headaches of all kinds, but medical doctors took little notice of this folk remedy until 1985. That was the year that a British survey of 270 migraine sufferers found that 70 percent had fewer headaches and less pain when they ate feverfew leaves daily.

"It's important to understand that when you use a remedy preventively, it takes a fair amount of time to evaluate its effectiveness," says Dr. Sheftell. "You need to take 125 milligrams of feverfew every day for about six to eight weeks."

Pain Relief from Fatty Acids

If you're not getting the relief you need from other pharmaceuticals and supplements, you might try adding omega-3 essential fatty acids to your diet. Found in high amounts in fish oil and flaxseed oil, these key fats provide eicosapentaenoic acid (EPA). This nearly unpronounceable substance changes your body chemistry so that your body produces fewer chemicals that increase sensitivity to pain and cause constriction of the blood vessels. Thus, you conquer the pain and also counteract the cause. In addition, EPA reduces serotonin activity.

In studies, EPA seems to be effective in people who have migraines. Several studies in the 1980s suggested that in some people, migraines can be prevented by taking high doses of fish oil. In one, at the University of Cincinnati College of Medicine, eight people with severe migraines took 15 grams of fish oil daily. At the end of a six-week period, it was found that they had about half their usual number of migraines when they were taking the supplement.

There's also a good chance that you'll get fewer migraines, and less intense ones, if you take one to two tablespoons of flaxseed oil every day, says Brent Mathieu, N.D., a naturopathic doctor in Boise, Idaho. Although you could see an improvement in as little as a few days, four to eight weeks is more typical.

Flaxseed oil contains a substance that the body converts to EPA, so it is an indirect source of the important omega-3 fatty acid. "Fresh, cold-pressed flaxseed oil is the best natural source of omega-3 fatty acids," says David Perlmutter, M.D., a neurologist in Naples, Florida, and author of *Lifeguide*. For some people, however, fish oil may work better because it is a ready-made source of EPA.

If you take fish oil, take 1,000 to 2,000 milligrams a day in divided doses with meals, says Dr. Mathieu. The capsules sometimes cause unpleasant, fishy-tasting burping unless you take them with food.

An Herbal Massage

When your head is in the viselike grip of a tension headache, take small doses of an herbal supplement that includes a mixture of valerian, passionflower, and skullcap, says Priscilla Evans, N.D., a naturopathic doctor at the Community Wholistic Health Center in Chapel Hill, North Carolina. This trio of herbs can help relax muscles in your shoulders, neck, and scalp. "Valerian is great for relaxing the nervous system, relieving tension, and providing general pain relief. Passionflower and skullcap help to calm stress," she says.

While antidepressants are often prescribed for people who frequently get tension headaches, herbs can offer benefits as well. The natural supplements are useful tools for stress management, says Dr. Evans.

If you anticipate a stressful period that could trigger a tension headache, these soothing herbs can help minimize the impact. Stick with the manufacturer's recommendations if you choose a ready-mixed supplement. Typical instructions are to take 225 milligrams with meals or water twice a day. If you're using a tincture that combines the three herbs, take 10 drops three or four times a day, says Dr. Evans.

Better Than Aspirin

For pain relief from tension headache, use a supplement of white willow bark. This is the same salicylate-containing herb that led to the development of aspirin, says Dr. Mathieu. For effective relief, take one or two 400-milligram doses of dried bark capsules every two to four hours as needed.

If willow bark and aspirin both have the same components—salicylates—why not just take an aspirin? "Willow bark is naturally buffered and acts gently, so it generally does not upset and irritate the stomach," Dr. Mathieu says.

The herb also contains small amounts of vitamin C and quercetin and other bioflavonoids, which combine with the salicylate to relieve both pain and inflammation. The trade-off is that it's hard to regulate the dosage with herbs. "There's a wide variation in the quality of the plant and how it was prepared, so you never know exactly how much of the active substance you're getting," says Dr. Mathieu.

Although its active ingredients are less concentrated than the drugstore product, you shouldn't take willow bark if you are allergic to aspirin, says Dr. Mathieu.

heart arrhythmia

A heartbeat is a highly coordinated event. Nerves need to fire in precisely the right sequence to stimulate muscles that contract the chambers of the heart. When a heartbeat goes perfectly, blood flows through your heart and out to your lungs and the rest of your body.

When this process goes awry, it results in heart arrhythmia. If nerves fire out of sequence, the chambers of the heart don't contract properly.

Usually, arrhythmia is the result of damage to the heart muscle. The cause could be coronary artery disease or even a viral infection, says Decker Weiss, N.M.D., a naturopathic doctor at the Arizona Heart Institute in Phoenix. "Anything that affects the heart adversely can affect the nerve conduction system of the heart, which is what controls the heartbeat."

Sometimes, and often in conjunction with heart disease, mineral imbalances can interfere with the heart's normal nerve function. These imbalances may be brought on by drugs that have been prescribed to treat high blood pressure or congestive heart failure.

You need to be under a doctor's care if you have arrhythmia, but there are some mineral and herb treatments that can go hand in hand with medications to help keep the nerves firing smoothly. Just make sure your doctor knows what supplements you're taking.

Two minerals, potassium and magnesium, play an especially important role in helping your heart beat properly.

Potassium Powers the Pump

If you're a heart patient, your doctor will monitor your blood levels of potassium. Low potassium can cause heart arrhythmia, and certain types of diuretics, such as thiazide (Hydrodiuril), can leach this mineral from your body, says Carla Sueta, M.D., Ph.D., assistant professor of medicine and cardiology at the University of North Carolina at Chapel

464

Hill School of Medicine. Digitalis, a common heart medication, can also lower potassium.

Potassium deficiency affects more than your heart. It can also weaken your muscles and lead to mental confusion.

The amount of this mineral that you need depends on your blood levels. The Daily Value for potassium is 3,500 milligrams, but food gives most people what they need. Potassium supplements in amounts higher than 99 milligrams per tablet are available only by prescription. Too much potassium is as bad as too little, so it is essential that you work with your doctor if you need supplemental potassium to control your heartbeat, Dr. Sueta says.

Magnesium Keeps the Beat

When magnesium levels in the heart are low, people can develop certain types of heart arrhythmia. Some of them are potentially dangerous, Dr. Sueta says. The effects of magnesium are so well proven that doctors sometimes give it intravenously to prevent certain kinds of arrhythmia. Studies have shown, for instance, that intravenous magnesium reduces the incidence of death from ventricular arrhythmia, which involves the lower chambers of the heart. "In fact, intravenous therapy with magnesium now is considered standard for two types of ventricular arrhythmia," Dr. Sueta says.

Just as diuretics and digitalis can cause potassium deficiency, these medications can also induce a shortage of magnesium. Moreover, magnesium is often at the bottom of what's called refractory potassium deficiency, says Michael A. Brodsky, M.D., professor of medicine at the University of California, Irvine, and director of the cardiac electrophysiology/arrhythmia service at the university's medical school.

"The amount of magnesium in the body determines the amount of a particular enzyme that determines the amount of potassium," says Dr. Brodsky. "If you are magnesium deficient, you may in turn be potassium deficient, and no amount of potassium is going to correct this unless you are also getting enough magnesium."

It's best if your doctor monitors your blood levels of magnesium, because how much you need depends on the amount that's in your blood. A test that measures ionized magnesium—the active form of magnesium in the blood—can detect a deficiency before it reaches a critical level, Dr. Sueta says.

Smoother Beating with CoQ$_{10}$

Along with magnesium, Dr. Weiss may recommend coenzyme Q$_{10}$ (coQ$_{10}$) for heart arrhythmia.

This vitamin-like substance is made in the body, particularly in the cells of the heart muscle, where it is used to produce the energy that the muscle needs. Additional coQ$_{10}$ seems to provide more energy to the muscle cells, an action that can be of great benefit for heart disease, Dr. Weiss says.

CoQ$_{10}$ also seems to help reduce stiffening of the heart muscle. This stiffening can produce abnormalities called diastolic dysfunction, says Peter Langsjoen, M.D., a cardiologist in Tyler, Texas. Dr. Langsjoen has been using coQ$_{10}$ in his practice to treat heart disease since 1985.

The diastolic, or filling, phase of the cardiac cycle actually requires more energy than the systolic, or contraction, phase, Dr. Langsjoen says. "Relaxation of the muscle actually requires energy," he points out. "This stiffening of the heart muscle returns to normal with supplemental coQ$_{10}$, and people have less fatigue." In his observation, coQ$_{10}$ not only improves irregular heart rhythm but also reduces chest pain. "It's as dramatic as watering a dried-up houseplant."

The need for additional coQ$_{10}$ depends on your symptoms. Dr. Weiss starts with a minimum dose of 120 milligrams a day divided into four 30-milligram doses. To aid absorption, he suggests taking it between meals with omega-3 and omega-6 fatty acids. If you're taking the blood thinner warfarin (Coumadin) for heart disease, though, be sure to talk to your doctor, since taking coQ$_{10}$ can cause a slight decrease in its effectiveness.

Dr. Langsjoen starts people on twice that much, 240 milligrams a day, and may raise the level as high as 360 milligrams, divided into three daily doses, if symptoms are severe.

Some people respond quickly to coQ$_{10}$, while others show little or no response for weeks or months, says Dr. Weiss.

This supplement is expensive, so you'll want to stay with the lowest dose that relieves your symptoms. Studies show that there are no side effects or toxicity.

CoQ$_{10}$ is fat-soluble, which means that your body will absorb more of the active ingredient if it's in a gel cap rather than a powder or tablet. If you do use tablets, you'll get the most from them by taking them with a meal that contains some fat or with a fat-containing food such as peanut butter.

Fats That Help Your Heart

Dr. Weiss recommends cutting back the fats that can harm your heart, including the saturated fats that come from animal sources and hydrogenated fats found in many high-fat food products. Instead, he urges getting more of two essential fatty acids that help to protect your heart.

The sought-after ingredients are the omega-3 fatty acids found in fish oils and omega-3's and omega-6's from flaxseed oil and borage oil respectively, among other sources. Dr. Weiss recommends that people with heart arrhythmia get 1,000 to 3,000 milligrams a day of a mixture of these two fats. They are available as gel caps or, in the case of flaxseed or borage oil, in liquid form.

Strengthen with Hawthorn

When someone's heart is additionally weakened by cardiovascular disease or congestive heart failure, Dr. Weiss may add hawthorn, an herb known for its heart-strengthening effects. Hawthorn contains bioflavonoids, compounds that act as heart-protective antioxidants.

"Hawthorn's bioflavonoids are considered to be very specific for blood vessels," Dr. Weiss says. German researchers report that it gently increases the strength of the heartbeat. Typically, it also helps the heart muscle beat at a normal rhythm and simultaneously increases blood supply to the heart.

Hawthorn is used while the current problem exists, explains Dr. Weiss. If a patient's heart function is improving due to diet and lifestyle changes such as exercise and weight reduction, Dr. Weiss will wean him off hawthorn.

Although Dr. Weiss says that he has monitored patients on hawthorn for many years without seeing any problems with the supplement, he still advises that you get your doctor's advice before you use it, especially if you are taking other heart drugs. You may require lower doses of other medications, such as blood pressure drugs, since hawthorn has been shown to lower blood pressure.

As for dosage requirements, the amount of hawthorn you should take depends on your symptoms and the type of hawthorn you're using. A typical tonic dose is ¼ teaspoon of standardized extract taken two or three times daily.

heartburn

It's high time that heartburn had another name. Since it has nothing whatever to do with the heart and a lot to do with a little door in the digestive tract, it would be much more appropriate to call it stomach burn.

Whether or not that new name is accepted in the lexicon of common complaints, the uncomfortable sensation will remain the same. It's a burning, painful feeling that occurs behind your breastbone whenever stomach acid flows back up from your stomach into the main entryway, the esophagus.

Many of us are familiar with the over-the-counter antacid medications that are designed to relieve the symptoms, but these products will not cure heartburn. While commercial antacids will provide relief, many natural healers believe that we should try to do more than just reduce the acid. For one thing, it helps to improve your diet and digestion so the acid stays where it belongs—in the stomach. It also helps to use herbal and nutritional supplements that can heal the irritation and burning caused by any acid backup, says William Warnock, N.D., a naturopathic doctor in Shelburne, Vermont.

"Normally, stomach acid is confined to the stomach by a valve between the stomach and the esophagus," says Dr. Warnock. "When that valve malfunctions and the acid is able to pass from the stomach into the esophagus, it can cause irritation there, so the first thing you want to do is prevent the irritation from continuing."

If you're plagued with the symptoms of heartburn, you may want to consider changing your eating habits. Fatty, fried, or high-protein foods, alcohol, and coffee are often the culprits behind heartburn, says Pamela Taylor, N.D., a naturopathic doctor in Moline, Illinois.

People who eat quickly and gulp their food often get heartburn, says Dr. Warnock. He advises people to eat regular meals and above all, chew food slowly, savoring the smell and taste.

Also, pay attention to the final meal of the day, suggests Dr. Taylor. "I tell patients not to eat within four hours of their bedtimes and that their last meal of the day should be oriented toward foods such as steamed vegetables, baked or broiled fish, and nonwheat grains such as rice or quinoa," she says.

Coat, Soothe, and Heal

Even if you're a deliberate eater, you may have chronic heartburn. There are many possible causes, including stress, age, and poor digestion. You may have chronic heartburn because you've been infected with *Helicobacter pylori*, the same bacteria that contribute to stomach ulcers.

People are more prone to heartburn if they take medications that affect the muscles of the esophagus. And they're more likely to get it if they have a hiatal hernia (a hernia of the diaphragm).

Whatever the source of the problem, the mucous membranes of your esophagus are probably inflamed and irritated, says Melissa Metcalfe, N.D., a naturopathic doctor in Los Angeles. That's one area where supplements might be able to lend a helping hand.

An excellent herb to soothe those tissues is deglycyrrhizinated licorice, or DGL, according to Dr. Metcalfe. For one thing, DGL has antispasmodic action, which means that it helps to control various muscle actions that can affect your digestive tract. The herb also helps reduce acid reflux by calming a cramping stomach, she says.

The primary medicinal benefit of DGL, however, is its ability to increase and build up the protective substances that line the digestive tract. By stimulating the body's natural defense mechanisms, licorice helps prevent the formation of ulcers and lesions due to the irritating acid, says Dr. Metcalfe. It's also a powerful, localized anti-inflammatory.

"It's the first thing I recommend to people—it's a great initial treatment," says Dr. Metcalfe. The typical dose is two 250-milligram capsules taken 20 minutes before mealtime.

Rather than swallowing the DGL with water, Dr. Metcalfe suggests that you suck on the capsules and let them dissolve slowly in your mouth. You can also get DGL in chewable tablets, which dissolve as you chew them. "You want the licorice to coat the inside of your throat and esophagus to cover those inflamed and irritated tissues," she says.

Use it for four weeks and then assess if it's working, she suggests. If it is, your throat should feel less irritated. If not, see your health-care practitioner.

Link Up with Licorice

If you've known licorice only as a gummy, stringy candy—a general-store forebear of Gummi Bears—it may be time to bone up on its history.

Derived from the root of a perennial shrub, licorice was first used in Chinese medicine thousands of years ago. It also became a flavoring agent for candy and sweet-smelling pipe tobacco.

Licorice root has been used to treat female disorders, peptic ulcers, stress, colds, and several types of bacterial infections. It's a well-studied herb, and some of these traditional uses have been verified scientifically.

Licorice is especially useful for relieving symptoms of premenstrual syndrome and menopause, according to herbalists. It has phytoestrogenic action, which means that its plant compounds have an effect in a woman's body much like that of the female hormone estrogen.

Despite this benefit, there are some safety factors to consider if you use large amounts of licorice regularly for more than four to six weeks. One of the active ingredients, called glycyrrhizin, can cause high blood pressure and loss of potassium. It can also contribute to retention of fluids and sodium. Because of these effects, you should use licorice cautiously if you have high blood pressure or heart problems.

To sidestep these side effects, licorice is also sold in a form from which 97 percent of the glycyrrhizin has been removed. The extract of deglycyrrhizinated licorice is known as DGL. In animal studies, it has been shown that flavonoids, the active ingredients in DGL, are especially effective in protecting gastrointestinal tissues from ulcer formation. DGL appears to promote the release of compounds in saliva that may stimulate the growth and regeneration of stomach and intestinal cells.

If you are pregnant or nursing or have diabetes, however, you should avoid medicinal amounts of any form of licorice.

Get at the Inflammation

Another healing substance for damaged mucous membranes is glutamine, an amino acid that's available as a nutritional supplement. Dr. Metcalfe frequently recommends it for gastrointestinal disorders whenever inflammation is a problem.

Glutamine encourages the turnover or disposal of damaged cells, and it increases the production of new cells along the gastrointestinal walls, says Dr. Metcalfe. It's also a potent antioxidant, helping to protect cells from the damage caused by free-roaming, unstable molecules called free radicals. All of these actions equate with faster healing, she says.

"I tell people to take one 500-milligram capsule four times a day until they are feeling better," says Dr. Metcalfe. "Usually, that's about a month."

Kill the Bacteria

If bad bacteria—usually *H. pylori*—are the source of your problem, you could consider taking goldenseal, says Dr. Metcalfe. First, though, get a proper diagnosis from your doctor.

For best results, Dr. Metcalfe recommends that you combine a goldenseal supplement with colloidal bismuth, which is the active ingredient in many over-the-counter stomach medications like Extra-Strength Pepto-Bismol. Besides coating the stomach, the bismuth helps the herb adhere to the mucous membranes of the stomach.

Take two or three 400-milligrams capsules of goldenseal daily along with one tablespoon of Extra-Strength Pepto-Bismol four times daily, Dr. Metcalfe suggests. "When you take bismuth, be aware that your stools will turn black. It's nothing to worry about." Don't use goldenseal if you are pregnant, however.

Relief on the Run

You don't need to go to the health food store for relief. In fact, you don't have to look any farther than the spice rack.

"When people are traveling and have heartburn, I tell them to stop at a supermarket and buy some ginger," says Dr. Taylor. You can get either fresh ginger in the produce section or the powdered spice.

Ginger relaxes the smooth muscle along the walls of the esophagus, says Dr. Taylor. "If your digestion is working better, you're less likely to get that reflux, or backwash, of stomach acid," she says. "Ginger is an excellent tonic for the whole gastrointestinal tract."

If you're using ginger to prevent heartburn, take it 20 minutes before a meal. You can take it as a capsule, make a tea from the fresh root or the powder, or eat candied or pickled ginger as it comes from the jar. Ginger tincture is also available.

To use it in capsule form, take one or two "00" capsules and wait for a half-hour. If your symptoms don't improve in that time, you may repeat the dose. You can also empty the contents of the capsules into hot water, let it steep, and drink it as a tea, Dr. Taylor says.

Candied ginger has a long history as a digestive aid. Use a small amount, about the size of the tip of your little finger. Chew it slowly and well, incorporating a fair amount of saliva before swallowing, Dr. Taylor says. You can repeat this dose in 10 minutes or so if your symptoms have not lessened.

For tincture, she recommends a dose between 15 and 60 drops. "Always use the smaller amount, in a little water if possible. Repeat the 15-drop dose every 15 minutes, up to a total of 60 drops, if necessary."

Because ginger is considered a "hot bitter," people with very sensitive stomachs may find it too strong. If symptoms do not resolve with the above recommendations, consult your health-care practitioner.

high blood pressure

If you have high blood pressure (consistently higher than 140/90) and see a conventional doctor, chances are pretty good that the doctor will tell you that you'll have to take drugs, probably for the rest of your life.

If you're willing to try some changes in your diet and lifestyle, though, there's a good chance that you can bring your blood pressure into normal range—or at least reduce it somewhat. Losing just a little weight can work wonders. So can a modest cutback in salt. In one study, dropping about eight pounds and reducing sodium intake by 25 percent allowed half of the participants to lower their blood pressures enough to stop taking medication. Eating less saturated fat and more fiber can also reduce pressure, studies have shown.

There's more. Doctors and practitioners who use alternative medicine have an arsenal of nutritional supplements—including herbs—that go hand in hand with dietary measures and weight loss. Some of these supplements help regulate blood volume and relax blood vessel muscles so that arteries can dilate, which reduces blood pressure. Others reduce your risk of developing atherosclerosis (hardening of the arteries), which eventually also causes high blood pressure. Still others, such as coenzyme Q_{10} (coQ_{10}), help your heart pump more efficiently, which also reduces blood pressure, especially in people with damaged hearts. If you have high blood pressure, though, always check with your doctor before you take any supplements.

A Trio of Helpful Minerals

The people who are most susceptible to salt's blood pressure–elevating effects may be low in other minerals, such as potassium, magnesium, and perhaps calcium, says David McCarron, M.D., professor of medicine and head of the division of nephrology, hypertension, and clinical pharmacology at Oregon Health Sciences University in Portland.

Potassium, magnesium, and calcium have a direct effect on blood volume or influence the ability of blood vessels to relax. Increasing blood volume is like opening up a faucet, and it increases blood pressure. If blood vessels are constricted, pressure also rises. When the vessels relax, blood pressure tends to go down.

"Each of these minerals has some effect separately, but all three interact and may have a better combined effect," Dr. McCarron says.

Potassium Power

Potassium affects blood volume because it helps you excrete sodium, says David B. Young, Ph.D., professor of physiology and biophysics at the University of Mississippi Medical Center in Jackson. When you excrete sodium, you also excrete water, which reduces blood volume and in turn reduces blood pressure.

How much should you get? The Daily Value (DV) is 3,500 milligrams, an amount provided by eight to nine servings of fruit and vegetables, and that much will help to reduce blood pressure. "More potassium will reduce it even more, however," says Dr. Young. "I'd like people to aim for twice that amount, 7,000 milligrams or more a day."

The safest way to get potassium is from foods, he says. In supplement form, a prescription is needed for dosages higher than 99 milligrams per tablet. If you are taking a non-potassium-sparing diuretic for high blood pressure, though, you may need supplemental potassium, Dr. Young says. In this case, your doctor will monitor your blood levels.

More Magnesium?

Magnesium helps to relax the smooth muscles in blood vessels, which allows them to dilate, says Decker Weiss, N.M.D., a naturopathic doctor at the Arizona Heart Institute in Phoenix. Supplemental magnesium has been effective in people who have high blood pressure due to kidney damage, pregnancy-induced high blood pressure, and the type of high blood pressure that's caused by diuretics.

If you're taking non-potassium-sparing diuretics such as thiazides to treat high blood pressure, they will begin to deplete your body of magnesium and potassium, the very minerals that you need to help regulate your pressure, notes Dr. Weiss. If your doctor has prescribed a diuretic for blood pressure control, it may stop working after six months or so because magnesium has been drained from your system. "Supplemental magnesium sometimes makes the diuretic more effective again," he says.

It's safe for most people to use up to 350 milligrams a day of supplemental magnesium, Dr. Weiss says. The preferred forms are magnesium orotate and magnesium glycinate.

Calcium sometimes also helps to reduce blood pressure, although it has less effect than potassium or magnesium. It seems to work best in women who develop high blood pressure during pregnancy and in children who are calcium-deficient, says Matthew Gillman, M.D., assistant professor of ambulatory care and prevention at Boston University Medical School. In one study, pregnant women who took 2,000 milligrams a day of calcium reduced the incidence of high blood pressure by 54 percent.

The DV for calcium is 1,000 milligrams, an amount that many of us fail to consume in our daily diets. Even if you're not getting the DV, though, if you already have high blood pressure, you should check with your doctor before taking supplemental calcium, Dr. Weiss says. "I don't normally recommend it for high blood pressure unless I'm seeing an older woman who also has osteoporosis, because too much calcium can interfere with magnesium's muscle-relaxing ability."

Herbs That Take the Pressure Off

Herbs can provide additional help in controlling blood pressure, Dr. Weiss says. Many different herbs are used for this purpose. With most you need medical supervision.

Among the safer and more popular herbs is dandelion leaf, which acts as a natural potassium-sparing diuretic. "I will prescribe a leaf tincture of dandelion for up to a few months if someone has excess fluid that needs to be reduced," Dr. Weiss says. How much you need to take depends on your blood pressure. If you have gallbladder disease, however, you should not use dandelion preparations without the approval of your doctor.

Fiber Fills the Bill

Dr. Weiss routinely prescribes a high-fiber diet for people concerned about heart disease, and there's some evidence that fiber can also help reduce high blood pressure. In a large study of more than 40,000 nurses whose lifestyles and diet patterns were followed for four years, researchers discovered that those who got the highest amounts of fiber were least likely to develop high blood pressure. In another study, with animals whose blood pressures had been elevated by a high-fat diet, switching to a low-fat diet and fiber supplements reduced pressure by 10 to 15 points.

Of the two kinds of fiber—soluble and insoluble—it's the soluble type that's more important for lowering blood pressure, Dr. Weiss says. This fiber is found in fruits, beans, and oats. If you want additional fiber, look for a supplement that contains mixed soluble fibers such as psyllium, gums, and pectin, he says.

Fish Oil and Flaxseed Oil Smooth the Way

Doctors recommend that you do some serious fat-swapping if you have high blood pressure. Cut back on saturated fats, they say, including animal fat, butter, and the kind of fat that's in many baked goods. As much as possible, avoid hydrogenated fats, the kind found in margarine and shortening, and polyunsaturated fats, such as corn oil.

Instead of these "unhealthy" fats, Dr. Weiss suggests that you get more of two essential fatty acids, omega-3's and omega-6's. Omega-3's are found in fish oil and flaxseed oil. Borage oil supplies omega-6's.

"I recommend 1,000 to 3,000 milligrams a day of a mixture of these two essential fatty acids," he says. The fatty acids change your body chemistry so that you produce fewer harmful prostaglandins, hormonelike substances that can jack up blood pressure.

Vitamins to the Rescue

High blood pressure can also develop over time from atherosclerosis, as arteries clogged with fatty deposits become narrow and hardened, like a pipe clogged with mineral deposits. Not everyone with high blood pressure has atherosclerosis, but if you have high cholesterol and high blood pressure, Dr. Weiss recommends adding nutrients that help prevent atherosclerosis. These include vitamins C and E, which help reduce the formation of fatty deposits and clots inside blood vessels.

Vitamin C may have additional blood pressure–lowering effects, Italian researchers report. They found that it helped blood vessels dilate normally. In some people with high blood pressure, the vitamin stopped the breakdown of nitric oxide, a blood vessel–dilating chemical that is secreted from the walls of the blood vessels.

"I routinely prescribe these to anyone who wants to prevent heart disease and related problems," Dr. Weiss says. He recommends 400 to 800 international units of vitamin E and suggests using the type labeled "mixed tocopherols." "And I recommend 1,000 to 2,000 milligrams a day of vitamin C in divided doses," he says.

You'll also want to make sure that you get about 400 micrograms of folic acid, 1,000 micrograms of vitamin B_{12}, and 100 to 250 milligrams of vitamin B_6, Dr. Weiss says. Doses of vitamin B_6 above 100 milligrams a day must be taken under medical supervision.

These three B vitamins are important because they help your body chew up homocysteine, a substance that you can easily do without. Homocysteine is an amino acid by-product that can damage arteries, says Dr. Weiss. It creates rough spots on artery walls, and those roughened areas can pick up fatty deposits that harden into artery-clogging plaque. Taking these B vitamins can help preserve smooth-walled arteries.

Coenzyme Q_{10} Helps Your Heart Help You

This substance is made naturally in the body, but perhaps it's in short supply. If high blood pressure is accompanied by heart damage or weakness, you might need coQ_{10}, Dr. Weiss says. It improves energy supplies to the heart muscle cells, so it helps your heart to pump more efficiently, with less effort. That in turn helps to lower blood pressure.

In one study of 109 people with high blood pressure, more than half were able to stop or reduce their medication after four months of treatment with coQ_{10}. Dr. Weiss recommends 30 milligrams three times a day. To improve absorption, he says, it's best to take it at the same time you take fish oil or flaxseed oil.

high cholesterol

High cholesterol isn't a disease, it's more like an alarm signal. The state of your cholesterol levels tells you something about your risk of developing the United States' number one killer, heart disease, or coronary artery disease.

The higher your blood levels of "bad" low-density lipoprotein (LDL) cholesterol, the greater your risk of developing coronary artery disease, the life-threatening condition that occurs when the arteries to your heart become clogged with cholesterol. One form of LDL cholesterol, called lipoprotein (a), or Lp(a), has been found to be even more damaging than ordinary LDL. In fact, the risk of heart disease for people with high levels of Lp(a) is 10 times higher than that of people who simply have elevated levels of LDL cholesterol. That's because Lp(a) sticks to artery walls much more easily than LDL does.

When doctors look at cholesterol levels for a profile of your risks, they also consider other kinds of fats, or lipids, that affect arterial health. Two of those factors, one bad and one good, are triglycerides and high-density lioprotein (HDL) cholesterol. Triglycerides are simply partners in crime with LDL, and when your blood profile shows high triglycerides, there's reason for concern. HDL, on the other hand, is a fat that campaigns for free-flowing blood, and it never sticks around to cause trouble in the arteries. For this reason, it's easiest to think of HDL as the good cholesterol; the higher your HDL levels, the lower your risk of heart disease.

Eating a diet low in fat, especially saturated fat, and high in fiber is always a primary strategy for lowering the bad cholesterol and raising the good. You need to pursue that diet even if your cholesterol is so high that your doctor has prescribed cholesterol-lowering drugs, says Decker Weiss, N.M.D., a naturopathic doctor at the Arizona Heart Institute in Phoenix.

If you know that your LDL cholesterol is high and you're already on cholesterol-lowering drugs, some vitamin or herbal supplements might come in handy for reducing the side effects of those drugs. Other supplements directly lower cholesterol levels or reduce your risk for atherosclerosis, the notorious hardening of the arteries that results from a buildup of blood-slowing plaque along the arterial walls. Supplements can reinforce your cholesterol-control efforts on a number of different fronts. Here's how they stack up.

Antioxidants Help Disarm Cholesterol

"Cholesterol doesn't hurt you when it's just floating around in your blood," Dr. Weiss says. As soon as the fatty substance clings to your artery walls, however, it becomes a threat, and a serious one at that.

Harmful LDL cholesterol doesn't go looking for trouble when it's traveling along in its free-floating form. Before it can stick to your artery walls, it has to be oxidized. To prevent the chain of events that leads to oxidation of cholesterol, you need a good dose of the antioxidant nutrients that can disarm free radicals, the free-roaming, unstable molecules that do the damage. Many antioxidants are found in foods. Others are most available from supplements, particularly when you want vitamin E or large amounts of vitamin C.

Dr. Weiss recommends taking 400 to 800 international units (IU) of vitamin E every day. "While it doesn't actually affect cholesterol levels, vitamin E does help to lessen the potential harmful effects of high cholesterol levels," he says.

In your body, vitamin E helps prevent LDL cholesterol from being oxidized. A study showed that at least 400 IU is needed to significantly reduce LDL oxidation.

C: What It Does

Vitamin C apparently can have a more direct effect on cholesterol levels. Dozens of studies have shown that higher blood levels of vitamin C correspond to lower total cholesterol and triglyceride levels and higher HDL levels. In a study at the Jean Mayer USDA Human Nutrition Research Center on Aging at Tufts University in Boston, researchers found that people with low blood levels of ascorbic acid (vitamin C) who took 1,000 milligrams a day for eight months had an average 7 percent increase in HDL. Researchers say that eating five servings of fruits and vegetables a day would bring your vitamin C levels into the normal range.

Dr. Weiss recommends taking 1,000 to 3,000 milligrams of vitamin C daily in divided doses.

More on the Antioxidant Front

Additionally, Dr. Weiss recommends lipoic acid, an antioxidant that plays a role in energy production. This antioxidant has a unique property: It is effective against both fat-soluble and water-soluble free radicals. It has been found to raise blood levels of vitamin C and of glutathione, another powerful antioxidant that is made in the body. You can get lipoic acid in either capsules or tablets. A standard dose is 20 to 50 milligrams a day.

Dr. Weiss also recommends bioflavonoids, or proanthocyanidins. These powerful antioxidant compounds are found in many plants and in red wine. The proanthocyanidins used in supplements come from grape seeds and pine bark.

Laboratory studies indicate that, in theory, "proanthocyanidins can trap a variety of free radicals and inhibit the damaging effects of several enzymes, including enzymes that degrade collagen, the body's main connective tissue," says Dr. Weiss. If you're using proanthocyanidins to prevent heart disease, a daily dose of 50 milligrams is enough. If you already have heart disease, you should raise the dose to 150 to 400 milligrams a day, he says. Of course, be sure to tell your doctor which supplements you are taking.

Lipotropic Compounds Aid Your Liver

Believe it or not, most of the cholesterol floating around in your bloodstream is made in your liver. In order to make that cholesterol, the liver relies on the fats you eat for raw material. That's why it deserves attention if you have high cholesterol, Dr. Weiss says.

He recommends a combination supplement of lipotropic compounds that have multiple benefits for the liver. The mixture may include choline, betaine, methionine, vitamin B_6, folic acid, vitamin B_{12}, milk thistle, and dandelion. The combination helps to promote the flow of bile to and from the liver, in effect decongesting it. It helps to promote improved liver function and improve the way your body burns fat.

Take enough lipotropic compounds to get a daily dose of 1,000 milligrams of choline and 1,000 milligrams of either methionine and/or cysteine, recommends Michael Murray, N.D., a naturopathic doctor and co-author of *The Encyclopedia of Natural Medicine.*

Double Up on Fiber

Along with a lipotropic compound, Dr. Weiss recommends a high-fiber diet. Fiber, especially the soluble kind, can bind up the bile that's secreted by your liver into the small intestine. Bile is laden with cholesterol. When fiber binds with the bile and escorts it from your body, it means that the fats won't be reabsorbed, "so the combination of fiber and a lipotropic compound is often an effective way to lower cholesterol," Dr. Weiss says.

You need to get somewhere between 15 and 30 grams of fiber a day in order to see an impact on your cholesterol levels, according to Dr. Weiss. The average intake in the United States is about 12 grams, so he says that you should aim for about twice that amount. Beans, berries, whole grains, and bran, such as oat or wheat bran, can provide good amounts of fiber.

If you need to get more, use a supplement of mixed soluble and insoluble fibers, including pectin, gums, psyllium, and oat bran, Dr. Weiss recommends.

Helping the Heart

Our bodies use both blood sugar (glucose) and fat as fuel. The energy that the heart muscle relies on, however, is supplied mostly by fatty acids. Dr. Weiss recommends cutting back on the fats that can harm and going for the ones that can heal. The harmful kinds are saturated and hydrogenated fats, found in red meat, hydrogenated oils, and many processed foods.

The two essential fatty acids that help to protect your heart are omega-3 and omega-6 fatty acids, found in various proportions in fish oil, flaxseed oil, and borage oil. Moreover, fish oil has additional benefits. Studies show that substituting it for saturated fats or other unsaturated fats can significantly reduce triglycerides.

Dr. Weiss recommends that people with high cholesterol get 1,000 to 3,000 milligrams daily of a combination of fish oil and flaxseed or borage oil. This mixture is available in gel caps, or you can get flaxseed oil separately as a liquid.

Niacin Nixes the Bad Stuff

In large doses, niacin, a B vitamin, is sometimes used to lower LDL cholesterol. Niacin also raises HDL and lowers levels of Lp(a) and triglycerides. It also lowers fibrinogen, a blood protein that causes clot formation. Dr. Weiss cautions, however, that niacin is not universally effective, since there are some inherited forms of high cholesterol that it won't improve.

Also, niacin is not a supplement that you can automatically substitute for a cholesterol-lowering drug. Some people are better off with one of the "statin" drugs, such as simvastatin (Zocor), says Dr. Weiss. "Either niacin or a statin drug may be an appropriate choice for a particular patient, depending on the patient's lipid profile."

If triglyceride levels are high, you might get better results from niacin, Dr. Weiss notes. Statin drugs, on the other hand, are more likely to be your doctor's first choice if you've just had a heart attack and have very high LDL levels that need to be reduced quickly.

Even though niacin is available at health food stores, you need to talk to a doctor before you take the high doses—1,000 to 3,000 milligrams a day—that are needed to lower cholesterol. At high doses, niacin can cause liver damage, especially timed release niacin.

Your doctor will want to monitor your liver enzymes while you are taking niacin. If you are taking a cholesterol-lowering drug, never add large amounts of niacin without your doctor's approval. Such a combination can also cause serious liver damage.

Added Protection: Coenzyme Q_{10}

If you're taking a statin drug, Dr. Weiss recommends taking coenzyme Q_{10} (coQ_{10}), a vitamin-like compound that's made in your body. It acts as an antioxidant and is also essential for the production of energy. "Statin drugs deplete your blood of coQ_{10}, so I have my patients use supplements while they're taking a statin drug," says Dr. Weiss.

CoQ_{10} may help your liver cells withstand the toxicity of the statin drugs and reduces side effects such as liver problems and muscle aches. As for how much to take, Dr. Weiss suggests a dose ranging from 30 to 50 milligrams a day.

An Ayurvedic Approach: Gugulipid

Doctors will sometimes use a compound from an herb from India to lower cholesterol. The compound, called gugulipid, is derived from the resin or sap of the mukul, or myrrh tree. (Myrrh, a treasured spice in ancient times, was one of the three gifts offered by the Wise Men.)

"I might use gugulipid to lower cholesterol if someone has liver damage, is intolerant of niacin or has diabetes along with high cholesterol, since niacin sometimes makes blood sugar levels harder to control," says Decker Weiss, N.M.D., a naturopathic doctor at the Arizona Heart Institute in Phoenix.

Gugulipid has a long history of medical use in India, especially for lipid disorders and obesity. Studies show that it can indeed lower cholesterol and triglyceride levels, raise HDL levels, and promote weight loss. Like niacin, it acts in the liver, stimulating liver cells to increase the amount of LDL cholesterol they gather from the blood. In 1986, gugulipid was approved in India for marketing as a lipid-lowering drug.

There's no standard dose, and how much you need to take depends on a number of factors, says Michael Murray, N.D., a naturopathic doctor and co-author of the *Encyclopedia of Natural Medicine*. In studies, people were able to lower their cholesterol if they had doses of 25 milligrams of gugulsterone—the active ingredient—three times a day.

To get that amount of the active ingredient in an extract that's labeled as 5 percent gugulsterone, you'd need to take a dose of 500 milligrams three times a day. Gugulipid has an excellent safety record and does not affect liver function, blood sugar control, or kidney function, according to Dr. Murray.

Garlic Gobbles Up Cholesterol

If you're a garlic fan, go ahead and eat your fill. Having plenty of fresh raw or lightly cooked garlic may be all you need to do to lower your cholesterol, Dr. Weiss says.

The benefits of whole garlic are well-known, and Dr. Weiss has found that the experience of his patients supports the good press about garlic. "I had one lady whose cholesterol and blood pressure were really out of whack, and the only thing she did was to eat 10 to 15 steamed cloves of garlic a day—she loved it. Everything normalized in three weeks."

For many people, however, consistently eating five or more cloves a day to lower cholesterol is just a bit more than they can relish. If you're among the lukewarm fans of whole garlic, the pills are worth a try before you consider cholesterol-lowering drugs, Dr. Weiss says.

Look for dried garlic powder preparations in enteric-coated tablets or capsules. These are designed to pass through the stomach and then degrade in the alkaline environment of the intestine, where the beneficial conversion of one compound, alliin, into the active ingredient, allicin, takes place.

In studies, it's been found that people can lower total cholesterol by 10 to 12 percent and LDL and triglycerides by about 15 percent with supplements. HDL levels usually increased by about 10 percent. For these kinds of results, you'll need a preparation that provides a daily dose of at least 10 milligrams of alliin or a total allicin potential of 4,000 micrograms. You'll probably need to allow one to three months before you begin seeing a change in your cholesterol levels.

HIV and AIDS

For some people living with HIV or AIDS, the breakthroughs in research and treatment have literally written a new lease on life. Having life-saving drugs is only part of that new lease, however. People also need to make the most of a drug's healing properties and enhance their quality of life. It's here that supplements can be most useful.

AIDS is caused by the human immunodeficiency virus (HIV), which is found in infected blood, semen, or vaginal fluids. The most common way that people contract HIV is by engaging in unprotected sex—that is, having sex with an infected partner without using a condom to block transmission of the virus. People who use intravenous drugs can be exposed by sharing HIV-infected needles. It can also be spread through transfusions of contaminated blood, platelets, or plasma.

Once HIV enters the body, it attacks the immune system and sets out to destroy white blood cells called T cells, which help battle infection. The virus uses the genetic material of the T cells to reproduce itself, and as these cells die off, new HIV particles are released into the bloodstream to infect other white blood cells. The end result is a severely weakened immune system that can't fight off opportunistic illnesses such as skin and fungal infections, pneumonia, and some cancers.

Today, there are several antiviral drugs and nutritional supplements that you can take in combination to slow the progression of the disease. The antiviral drugs include AZT, DDC, and DDI. These, as well as drugs called protease inhibitors, can reduce the amount of virus in your body and prevent opportunistic illnesses. Anyone taking these drugs, however, will attest that they can cause many unpleasant side effects.

Supplementing your drug regimen with antioxidants such as vitamin E, lipoic acid, and selenium and some herbs can inhibit replication of the virus while meeting your body's basic nutritional needs. Herbs such as licorice, turmeric, and St. John's wort have antiviral properties that can help suppress the virus. And the amino acid carnitine can bolster immunity, help the antioxidants do a better job, and prevent drug toxicity. Of course, you shouldn't start using any of these supplements without your doctor's advice.

Antioxidants to the Rescue

Several studies have shown that people who have HIV and AIDS are deficient in many antioxidant vitamins and minerals. To understand why these shortages occur, you have to look at the way the antiviral drugs work and also consider the behavior of virus itself, says Brad Lichtenstein, N.D., a naturopathic doctor and clinic supervisor of the HIV immune clinic at Bastyr University in Bothell, Washington. He recommends a number of nutritional supplements to hinder the progression of HIV to AIDS.

Vitamin E. Of all the antioxidants that may help stop the virus in its tracks, research shows that vitamin E has the most consistent and best results. In one study, HIV-positive men with the highest levels of vitamin E in their blood were 34 percent less likely to develop AIDS than men who had the lowest levels of the vitamin.

Vitamin E's antioxidant power prevents cell damage caused by HIV, so it inhibits the replication of the virus, says Susan Kowalsky, N.D., a naturopathic doctor in Norwich, Vermont. What's more, vitamin E can help stimulate production of red blood cells in bone marrow, which comes to a screeching halt if you're taking the drug AZT. Dr. Lichtenstein suggests taking 400 to 1,000 international units (IU) of vitamin E daily. Make sure you take d-alpha tocopherol, the natural form of vitamin E, he says.

Vitamin A and beta-carotene. Low levels of vitamin A and beta-carotene are associated with a decrease in T cells, says Dr. Lichtenstein, and supplementation will aid in the growth and reproduction of these immune cells.

Research shows that when vitamin A levels are low, T-cell counts also take a beating. People who are HIV-positive but also have normal levels of vitamin A will be more likely to have a higher count of T cells. Despite this, though, people with HIV should not automatically load up on vitamin A. The problem is that when vitamin A is taken in very high doses, it may speed the replication of the virus rather than slow it down. Alternative practitioners pay close attention to the amount that's given. Vitamin A has been shown to slow the progression of HIV to AIDS when taken in moderate doses of 10,000 to 20,000 IU daily.

To get around the risk of accelerating virus replication, practitioners often prefer to recommend beta-carotene rather than vitamin A, says Dr. Lichtenstein. Beta-carotene converts to vitamin A in the body, so you'll get the same benefit. In one study, researchers gave 30 milligrams (50,000 IU) of beta-carotene to participants twice daily for four weeks, followed by six weeks without treatment. The total counts of several essential blood factors were measured at the beginning of the study, at the end of four weeks, and finally, six weeks later. Researchers found that one of the significant blood factors—the immunity-boosting lymphocytes—increased by 66 percent as long as people continued to take the beta-carotene supplements.

Dr. Kowalsky recommends taking 50,000 to 200,000 IU of beta-carotene.

Selenium. Levels of this antioxidant usually dip dangerously low in people with HIV and AIDS. But we all need it, because selenium helps maintain a strong immune system. It's very effective at protecting the body from free radicals, the free-roaming, unstable molecules that can damage cells, weaken immunity, and lead to various infections and diseases.

What's more, selenium works closely with vitamin E to produce the antibodies that fight infection. It also raises levels of glutathione, a vital and powerful antioxidant produced in the liver that detoxifies bacteria and other harmful substances. Glutathione helps maintain red blood cells and protects white blood cells from harmful viral attacks; it has been shown to help slow the progression of HIV into full-blown AIDS.

Consult a physician to determine your nutritional deficiencies and find out how much selenium you should take.

Vitamin C. Like selenium, vitamin C can boost glutathione levels when taken in moderate doses, says Dr. Kowalsky. Research has shown that it inhibits replication of HIV in test tubes. Although there's not much evidence to indicate that vitamin C can do the same in humans, it's still considered a powerful antioxidant that possesses antiviral properties.

"We know that vitamin C stimulates and strengthens different aspects of the immune system," says Dr. Kowalsky. "It inhibits viruses and even cancer, so it's worthwhile to take it as a treatment for HIV and AIDS."

There is some concern, however, that doses of vitamin C greater than 1,000 milligrams taken three times a day may damage lymphocyte function. As a precaution, Dr. Kowalsky recommends starting with 500 milligrams three times a day and working your way up to three 1,000-milligram doses. To determine your tolerance, consult a naturopathic doctor.

Lipoic acid. This vitamin-like antioxidant is in a class by itself. Research shows that it can block the reproduction of HIV by reducing the activity of an enzyme called reverse transcriptase, which is responsible for manufacturing the virus from the genetic material of bloodborne cells.

"Lipoic acid can help treat HIV- and AIDS-related nerve damage," says Dr. Lichtenstein. "It can minimize the virus's attack on the brain and help the brain maintain its cognitive function. It reduces free radicals and removes toxic minerals from the body. It also raises levels of glutathione, vitamin C, and vitamin E, so people feel a lot better." This supplement is available in health food stores. Dr. Lichtenstein recommends 200 milligrams three times a day with food.

Help from B to Z(inc)

Along with getting additional antioxidants, people with HIV and AIDS can use help from zinc and some B vitamins, with your doctor's approval. Here's why.

The B vitamins. A deficiency of vitamin B_6 weakens the immune system. "It can lead to nerve damage and an impaired antibody response and affect how you metabolize amino acids," says Dr. Lichtenstein.

Low levels of vitamin B_{12} can cause nerve damage in the arms and legs. When you don't have enough vitamin B_{12}, you can also lose some muscle control and ease of motion, says Dr. Lichtenstein. Supplementation can prevent nerve damage, rid the body of toxins that can cause tissue damage, and stop the virus from replicating.

Dr. Lichenstein suggests taking 500 milligrams of vitamin B_6 twice a day and 1,000 micrograms of B_{12} once a day.

Zinc. By itself, zinc plays a vital role in maintaining a strong immune system. Unfortunately, it's scarce in people with HIV and AIDS. In studies of those taking AZT who also supplemented with zinc, researchers found that the supplement helped reduce the risk of other infections. What's more, zinc has been shown to increase the number of immunity-boosting T cells as well as blood levels of an important immune-system–regulating hormone called thymulin.

Not all experts agree on how much zinc to take. "Half of the studies say that you can take more than 35 milligrams, while others say you should take less," says Dr. Lichtenstein. "We recommend taking no more than 30 milligrams daily."

Deploying a Tough Herbal Defense

As part of an HIV and AIDS treatment plan, there is a variety of botanical medicines that have been shown to slow the spread of the virus in the body.

Licorice. Much attention is being given to licorice root as a potential additional treatment for HIV infection. Research shows that the herb's active ingredients, glycyrrhizin and glycyrrhetinic acid, can prevent a number of processes involved in viral replication, such as the virus's ability to penetrate cells and alter their genetic material.

Both compounds stimulate the release of the immune system chemical interferon, says Dr. Kowalsky. Interferon is your body's built-in virus fighter. It attaches to cell surfaces and prevents viral DNA and RNA from reproducing, she says. Shortly thereafter, white blood cells called macrophages and natural killer cells are summoned to the scene to mount an even stronger defense against the virus.

In a study, 16 HIV-positive participants received 150 to 225 milligrams of pure glycyrrhizin, daily for three to seven years. At the end of the study, researchers discovered that not one person who received the licorice developed AIDS or showed any signs of deterioration in their immune systems. Among those in a similar group who didn't receive the herb, two participants developed AIDS.

In another study, researchers gave 10 HIV-positive patients 150 to 225 milligrams of glycyrrhizin daily. After two years, not one had developed AIDS. Of the participants in the control group—people who took no supplements—three developed AIDS. "Licorice is definitely antiviral," says Dr. Kowalsky.

Under a doctor's supervision, you can take a daily dose of 1,500 milligrams of pure powdered licorice root that contains 5 percent glycyrrhetinic acid, says Dr. Kowalsky. There are reasons to be cautious, however. If you take high daily doses of powdered licorice root, which comes in capsules, or of glycyrrhizin for more than four to six weeks, the supplements may cause sodium and water retention, potassium depletion, and high blood pressure. Don't take licorice if you have high blood pressure or kidney problems.

Turmeric. Another herb that research shows can halt HIV replication in a variety of ways is turmeric, the spice that gives curry its pungent flavor. The active ingredient in this versatile antiviral herb is curcumin, which has a yellow pigment that gives turmeric its color.

Curcumin is an antioxidant that is 300 times more powerful than vitamin E. "Curcumin's antioxidant properties will protect your DNA from the ravages of the virus. It's also antimicrobial, so it will help prevent the many opportunistic illnesses associated with HIV and AIDS," says Dr. Kowalsky.

In a study at Harvard Medical School, researchers showed that turmeric prevented the reproduction of HIV by blocking a specific gene that activates the virus and causes it to spread. Another study showed that it can inhibit some of the steps that lead to the reproduction of HIV.

A group of 18 HIV-positive participants with T-cell counts ranging from 5 to 615 took an average of 2,000 milligrams of curcumin daily in a preliminary study. Researchers saw an increase in their T-cell counts compared with a control group that didn't take any curcumin. There's ongoing work in even larger studies that may tell us more about curcumin's effect on HIV. If your doctor is familiar with the benefits of turmeric, he may prescribe 2,000 milligrams daily, taken in 500-milligram doses four times a day.

St. John's wort. This herb, well-known for its use in treating mild to moderate depression, is also being studied to find out whether it can slow the progression of HIV to AIDS. The herb contains two antiviral compounds that have been shown in animal studies and in test tubes to inhibit the reproduction of HIV.

In a study, 18 HIV-positive participants were given two milligrams of hypericin, a substance found in St. John's wort, through weekly injections and oral supplements. Sixteen of the patients showed an increase in T-cell counts during the 40 months that they were observed. Only 2 of the 16 developed opportunistic infections during the study; the rest remained healthy.

Although St. John's wort looks promising, researchers must continue to study the herb to determine its effectiveness. Currently, it must be taken in very large doses in order to slow the spread of HIV in the body. Taken in such massive doses, however, it can cause severe sun sensitivity, cautions Dr. Lichtenstein.

If you are taking any medications, talk to your doctor before starting St. John's Wort.

The Case for Carnitine

Carnitine is a vital nutrient that's related to the B vitamins but is often referred to as an amino acid. Its main function is to transport fat to cells, where they are turned into energy. What's more, carnitine increases the effectiveness of the antioxidant vitamins E and C. It has also been shown to boost immune function, and it can help prevent side effects of AZT.

If you have HIV or AIDS, talk to your doctor about taking this supplement. If you don't supplement with carnitine, your health could be in jeopardy, says Dr. Lichtenstein. "Carnitine prevents key white blood cells from dying. It prevents the nerve damage associated with AIDS. It can prevent wasting syndrome, which is a breakdown in muscle and other body tissues that's marked by weight loss, weakness, fever, diarrhea, and an increase in cholesterol."

In a study, researchers gave AIDS patients who were being treated with AZT 6,000 milligrams of carnitine daily. By the end of the study, the participants showed a significant increase in white blood cell counts.

impotence

If you're like most men, the very word *impotence* suggests a whole range of emotions that you'd rather deny, situations you'd prefer to forget, and issues you'd rather not face. Translated, that means fear, anxiety, and humiliation.

Here's a less loaded term, then—*erectile dysfunction*. It means the same thing but doesn't have quite the same negative connotation that seemingly threatens the very fabric of manhood.

An estimated 10 to 15 million American men regularly suffer from erectile dysfunction, defined as the inability to achieve and maintain an erection long enough to have satisfactory sexual intercourse. Of those men, 15 to 25 percent are over age 65.

The most common cause of erectile dysfunction in men over 50 is clogged arteries in the penis. Frequently, what's behind this clogged-up situation is a buildup of cholesterol and fatty deposits inside artery walls. For other men, there are other possible causes. For those in their teens, twenties, and thirties, stress, depression, anger, fatigue, and performance anxiety are the most common triggers. Among the medical problems associated with erectile dysfunction are diabetes, thyroid problems, stroke, heart disease, and multiple sclerosis.

Otherwise helpful or beneficial medicines can also extract a hidden cost. Sometimes, erection problems are a reaction to blood pressure medications, tranquilizers, antidepressant drugs, or antihistamines.

Because erectile dysfunction could be a side effect of prescription drugs or a symptom of other health problems, see a doctor before you take any nutritional supplement. If you've been having trouble achieving or maintaining an erection during a period of more than 90 days, let your doctor know.

Alternative medicine practitioners believe that there are dietary and other natural measures that men can take to restore the ability to achieve erections. For starters, experts suggest that you get at least 30 minutes of aerobic exercise several days a week. Improving your heart health will boost your sexual virility.

Experts also say that you should eat a low-fat diet, including lots of fruits and vegetables, whole grains, and legumes. Moreover, they say that men who smoke will just have to quit. Puffing just two cigarettes a day causes blood vessels throughout your entire body to constrict, reducing blood flow to the penis.

Alcohol is another roadblock to satisfying sex. Drink no more than two alcoholic beverages a day, says E. Douglas Whitehead, M.D., associate clinical professor of urology at Albert Einstein College of Medicine in the Bronx and co-founder and director of the Association for Male Sexual Dysfunction in New York City.

Once you've adopted these changes, some practitioners believe that a combination of nutritional supplements can speed your progress toward sexual health and that certain herbs are potent enough to dramatically increase blood flow to the penis and boost your sex drive, says Thomas Kruzel, N.D., a naturopathic doctor in Portland, Oregon. Additionally, some vitamins and minerals provide the building blocks for sexual health.

Yohimbine: Charge Up Your Sex Life

For centuries, people have used yohimbe, the bark from a West African tree, to boost sex drive. It is said to increase blood flow to the penis, which makes it possible to attain and sustain an erection. The drug companies took notice. After finding a way to extract the active ingredient from yohimbe, they received approval for yohimbine (Yocon, Yohimex), which is now available by prescription.

In an unusual reversal, herbal experts recommend the prescription drug yohimbine over the over-the-counter herb yohimbe. "Yohimbe is not an herb that you want to mess around with," says James A. Duke, Ph.D., botanical consultant, former ethnobotanist with the U.S. Department of Agriculture who specializes in medicinal plants, and author of *The Green Pharmacy*. Just a few of its nasty side effects are anxiety, increased heart rate, and hallucinations.

In contrast, side effects of the prescription drug are mild, and one may even be pleasing. Men who have used it report having pleasant tingling sensations along their spines and in their genitals.

Yohimbine is powerful, concludes Ian Bier, N.D., a naturopathic doctor and licensed acupuncturist at the Institute for the Advancement of Natural Medicine in Portsmouth, New Hampshire. In a study conducted at the University of Exeter in England that analyzed results from several clinical trials measuring yohimbine's safety and effectiveness, researchers found that the benefits of using it far outweigh the risks. They concluded that serious side effects were infrequent and reversible and that yohimbine should be considered the first line of defense for the treatment of impotence.

You shouldn't take yohimbine if you have certain health conditions such as high blood pressure or heart disease or with certain foods and drugs. Be sure to discuss possible interactions and side effects with your doctor.

Other Herbs to Turn You On

Other herbal supplements are recommended by naturopathic doctors to treat erectile dysfunction. Ginkgo, a medicinal plant with a long tradition, is mainly used to improve blood circulation to the brain. It may also aid mental alertness and memory and even relieve depression. Because it can improve blood flow throughout arteries and veins, it's been successfully used to treat many men whose impotence is caused by poor blood circulation, says Dr. Kruzel.

In a study, 60 men with erectile dysfunction who didn't respond to injection treatments with a prescription medication were given 60 milligrams of ginkgo daily for 12 to 18 months. Every four weeks, penile blood flow was evaluated. The first signs of improvement in blood circulation occurred after six to eight weeks. When the men were evaluated again after a six-month period, 50 percent of those who took the ginkgo reported that they had regained potency.

"You can try 60 to 240 milligrams a day, but don't go any higher than that," says Dr. Duke. High amounts of ginkgo may cause side effects.

Asian ginseng, also called panax, Korean, or Chinese ginseng, tops the list of herbs used to restore vitality, boost energy, reduce fatigue, and improve physical performance. It protects the body from the negative effects of stress. Traditionally, it's been used as an aphrodisiac, and research seems to back up its reputation, showing that it can increase blood flow to the penis, says Dr. Kruzel.

In a study conducted in Korea, 90 men with erectile dysfunction were divided into three groups. Thirty men were given Korean red ginseng, 30 were given the drug trazodone (Desyrel), and 30 were given an inactive substance (placebo). Sixty percent of the men who took the ginseng experienced improvements in the rigidity of their erections and their sex drive, compared to improvement in only 30 percent of those who received the drug or placebo.

The amount of ginseng you should take for erectile dysfunction depends on the species you buy and how much of the active ingredients is in the product. Dr. Kruzel recommends that most of his patients take 500 milligrams daily, but he says that it's best to consult your doctor for the optimum dose.

For Prostate-Related Impotence

In rare cases, an enlarged prostate gland, known as benign prostatic hyperplasia (BPH), causes impotence. Located below the bladder and surrounding the urethra, the prostate gland is normally no bigger than a walnut. At some point in your late forties or fifties, it starts growing, and what was once walnut-size can balloon to the size of an orange, causing all sorts of problems.

If you've been diagnosed with BPH and it happens to be causing impotence, the herb horsetail may be what you need, says Dr. Kruzel. Although it hasn't been proven effective in clinical studies, he's seen it work in his practice.

Horsetail's anti-inflammatory properties can shrink the prostate gland to normal size and restore potency in some men, he says. "Horsetail is best used in men over age 60 who have BPH. For them, it can work very well," he comments. Saw palmetto is another herb exihibiting anti-inflammatory properties.

The amount of horsetail you should take depends on how much your prostate gland has enlarged. After a doctor examines you, he may prescribe a dose ranging from 400 to 800 milligrams of horsetail daily, Dr. Kruzel says. Be sure to take the prescribed amount, and ask your doctor about possible side effects. Horsetail may cause thiamin deficiency, and you shouldn't take it if you have heart or kidney problems.

Zinc and Other Vitamin Basics

The most important nutrient for overall sexual health is zinc. This trace mineral is vital for a number of functions. It enhances the production of testosterone, the male hormone that's required for sexual development and potency. It also influences sperm motility—that is, the speed and mobility of sperm—which can be a factor in fertility.

Zinc has antibacterial and antiviral properties, says Dr. Kruzel. "The prostate has the highest concentration of zinc of any tissue in the body. It's abundant in semen and in the thin, milky fluid that the prostate gland secretes into the urethra just before ejaculation to prevent infections," he says.

Certain forms of zinc are better-absorbed than others. Zinc picolinate, zinc citrate, and zinc monomethionine are the most absorbable. If you're experiencing impotence, Dr. Kruzel says that you can take 15 to 30 milligrams of zinc daily, but he advises that you talk to your doctor if you're considering taking more than 20 milligrams. If you don't see results after four to six weeks, Dr. Kruzel recommends that you see your doctor for a re-evaluation.

He also recommends taking a high-potency multivitamin and mineral supplement in addition to the zinc to help keep your urinary tract in good working order and to lay the foundation for sexual health. "Vitamins C and E are also found in high concentrations in the prostate gland, so they can help speed your recovery from impotence," says Dr. Kruzel. He recommends 2,000 to 4,000 milligrams of vitamin C with meals and 400 to 800 international units of vitamin E daily.

indigestion

Indigestion is a general descriptive term for discomfort in the gastrointestinal tract. Usually, you have a lot of gas, belching, and bloating after eating. Your stomach may be distended, and sometimes you may even have vomiting or diarrhea.

If you have frequent indigestion or if it's causing you a lot of discomfort, you should consult a physician to make sure that you don't have a condition that needs medical attention. It also helps to be tested for food allergies just to make sure that the symptoms aren't caused by what you're eating. Barring those problems, however, a few lifestyle changes can help. So can some supplements that aid digestion.

Eat Better, Eat Slowly, Add Fiber

Many people who have indigestion just don't eat well and tend to eat on the run, says Melissa Metcalfe, N.D., a naturopathic doctor in Los Angeles. She finds that their diets contain too much fat and refined food and too little fiber.

"Digestion starts with eating habits. People who eat fast or swallow a lot of air have problems with digestion. The solution is to just slow down and enjoy your food," she says. "Also, cut down on fat, eat more whole-grain foods, and include lots of fruits and vegetables." You can get more fiber by eating foods like prunes, apples, oat bran, carrots, kidney beans, and spinach.

In addition to getting that dietary fiber it's often helpful to take a fiber supplement that contains psyllium husks or seeds, says Dr. Metcalfe. Fiber absorbs water and helps move food and waste through the gastrointestinal tract more quickly. She recommends two tablespoons a day, usually at breakfast. A typical product is Solgar Psyllium Seed Husks Fiber supplement. Each tablespoon contains about six grams of psyllium husk fiber.

Some Hydrochloric Support

Hydrochloric acid is nasty, corrosive stuff. Nevertheless, it is one of the most important secretions in the stomach. It helps in the digestion of protein and the absorption of some minerals and vitamins.

Lack of this stomach acid is officially known as hypochlorhydria. It's more likely to occur as you age, says William Warnock, N.D., a naturopathic doctor in Shelburne, Vermont. Without it, you may have an upset stomach, a feeling of fullness, or a sense of discomfort or indigestion.

"The ability of the stomach to secrete acid declines with age," he says. "I believe that many older people have digestive problems because they just aren't producing enough hydrochloric acid."

Lack of acid may be the result of gluten intolerance, an intestinal problem. A low-acid condition is also commonly seen in people with chronic autoimmune disorders such as rheumatoid arthritis or lupus. Hypochlorhydria has also been associated with gastritis, a stomach inflammation, and with the skin disease psoriasis.

Some alternative practitioners believe that you can reverse hypochlorhydria by taking supplements of betaine hydrochloride as part of an enzyme combination, which is available at most health food stores, says Dr. Warnock. Typically, these supplements contain 10 grains, or about 600 milligrams, of betaine hydrochloride.

Usually, these supplements include other kinds of acids that help bind the ingredients together. Many formulas also contain pepsin, an impor-

"You should also be drinking lots of water as you're increasing your fiber intake," she says. The recommended minimum is usually eight full eight-ounce glasses daily.

A few people may experience more indigestion when they start upping their fiber intakes. "If your body isn't used to it, fiber can be really hard on the digestive system," she says. "Just introduce it gradually."

Build Up Your Acid

As we age, our bodies produce less hydrochloric acid, which is instrumental in the digestive process. We also produce less pepsin, an enzyme secreted by the stomach that aids in the digestion of protein. Older people

tant digestive enzyme secreted in the stomach. "The combination of hydrochloric acid and pepsin works together in the stomach. That's why you often find them together in digestive formulas," says Dr. Warnock.

To determine whether your stomach is producing enough hydrochloric acid, your doctor can perform a gastric analysis test. The results of that test will indicate whether your stomach acidity is normal or whether you need supplementation.

If you need to take supplements, start small and increase the dose gradually. For the first dose, take one 600-milligram capsule with a meal. If you feel no discomfort, you should increase the dose by one 600-milligram capsule at the next meal, suggests Dr. Warnock. If necessary, you can increase the dosage once more, for a maximum of three capsules at a meal, as long as you don't have an adverse reaction. With smaller meals, however, you should take less, especially if the meal has little or no protein in it.

"If you feel a slight burning or warmth in your stomach, back off the dosage and take a little less," says Dr. Warnock. When you feel that warmth, continue eating so that the food buffers the acid.

In Dr. Warnock's experience, most people continue the supplementation for a few weeks or months and then gradually wean themselves off it. Initially, the stomach is stimulated by the supplements, but after a while, it may produce an adequate amount of acid on its own, he says.

often have digestive problems because they aren't producing enough acid to break down the food in their stomachs, says William Warnock, N.D., a naturopathic physician in Shelburne, Vermont.

Dr. Warnock suggests taking supplements of betaine hydrochloride with each full-size meal. Take them for three months, then stop and see how you do without them. Before you take these supplements, consult your doctor to find out whether your level of stomach acid is too low and, if it is, get a diagnosis of the underlying cause. If the condition that's causing low acid is diagnosed and treated, he says, acid levels may increase without the help of supplements.

Several herbs known as bitters, including wormwood, turmeric, gentian, and ginger, are believed to stimulate the release of hydrochloric acid and gastric juices. "Bitters are really big in Europe for enhancing digestion," says Dr. Metcalfe.

In the United States, ginger and turmeric are the most recognized due to their kitchen use as spices. Ginger enhances digestive activity and settles the stomach, while turmeric has been shown in animal studies to stimulate the flow of bile and the breakdown of dietary fats.

Dr. Metcalfe recommends taking one or two 250-milligram capsules of ginger at mealtimes, or you can munch on a stick or two of candied ginger for a similar effect. Preserved, sugar-soaked ginger sticks are available in many health food stores, supermarkets, and Asian markets.

"It's quite amazing how quickly ginger works," she says. "If people have been having indigestion problems due to chronic stress, I often tell them to use it."

If you decide to try turmeric, a typical dose is one 300-milligram capsule up to three times daily.

Sowing Bacteria

Another cause of indigestion may be an overgrowth of yeast, or candida. Candida is a type of naturally occurring yeast that always grows in the gastrointestinal tract as part of what's called the gut's flora, or microorganisms. A bout of illness or a course of antibiotics can wipe out much of the other flora, however, leaving room for candida to thrive, says Dr. Warnock. When the normal amount of yeast increases, it may contribute to malabsorption due to the inflammation it causes in the intestine, he says.

One way to get rid of the excess yeast is to sow more good bacteria in the gut. You can do that by taking a supplement containing acidophilus, the digestive system's primary beneficial bacteria.

"Yeast is like a weed trying to invade the yard of your intestine," says Dr. Warnock. "Sometimes, you just have to plant more grass seed."

Supplement companies sell many different beneficial bacteria combinations. Look for a product that has one billion or more organisms per capsule and has been refrigerated in the store or is marked "heat-resistant," suggests Dr. Warnock. It should contain *Lactobacillus acidophilus*, *Bifidobacterium bifidum*, and *B. longum*. The suggested dosage is one capsule with meals twice daily for about a week.

Energize Your Enzymes

Digestion begins in your mouth, where enzymes in saliva begin the breakdown of starch as you chew. There are also digestive enzymes that break down carbohydrates, fats, and proteins as food moves through your digestive system.

Most of the nutrients are absorbed through the lining of your small intestine. If enzymes aren't doing all of their work, an excess of undigested food may make its way into your large intestine, making it more likely that bacteria can feed upon the food. The result may be bloating, gas, and intestinal pain, says Dr. Warnock. Some folks who are deficient in some types of digestive enzymes can benefit by taking digestive enzyme supplements. There are many products on the market, some containing up to 10 different enzymes. Dr. Warnock suggests looking for a supplement that contains amylase, lipase, and protease enzymes.

Typically, you would take a 500-milligram capsule three times a day with meals, says Dr. Warnock. Freeda, for instance, sells a product called Freeda Hi-Vegi-Lip Digestive Enzymes that contains all the enzymes. The dose is three pills a day.

Heal with Glutamine

Sometimes, indigestion is caused by inflammation along the gastrointestinal walls, perhaps from illness, a bacterial infection, or a condition such as irritable bowel syndrome. To help heal that inflammation, Dr. Metcalfe suggests taking a supplement of glutamine, an amino acid common to the body. It encourages the disposal of damaged cells and increases production of new cells along the gut wall. It's also an antioxidant. She recommends taking one 500-milligram capsule four times a day for about a month.

infertility

Conception is supposed to be a pretty simple process. The little egg leaves the ovary to travel down the fallopian tube on its way to the uterus. Somewhere along the way, it encounters a swarm of sperm. Through sheer diligence, one of the tail-flailing sperm manages to make its way into the egg. The fertilized egg then implants itself into the cushiony, blood-lined wall of the uterus. Nine months later, if all goes well, there's a baby.

It's not that easy, however, for the 5.3 million American women and their partners who try for 12 months or more to initiate this close encounter of the first kind. For them, the meeting of sperm and egg is a no-show. Often, it's not clear why the initiation ceremony doesn't quite come off. About 35 to 40 percent of the time, the problem lies with the male half of the process; about the same percentage of the time, it's with the female; and about 20 percent of all infertility goes unexplained.

If the infertility problem can be identified, it can sometimes be fixed with surgery. A surgeon can open up a blocked fallopian tube, clearing the way for sperm and egg to meet. A varicose vein in a testicle can also be surgically treated. Blood that backs up in the vein and creates excess heat can cause low sperm counts, but once the varicose vein has been removed and the temperature is regulated, the sperm count might climb back up to normal.

Stress, smoking, alcohol, and a poor diet can also make it difficult to conceive. Sometimes, however, the problem lies with hormone or metabolic imbalances.

Whatever the cause, it can't hurt to get your hormones and every cell of your body primed for conceiving a child—and that's where supplements may come in handy. "I'm not saying that if you take these supplements, you'll definitely conceive," says Jennifer Brett, N.D., a naturopathic doctor at the Wilton Naturopathic Center in Stratford, Connecticut. There's evidence, however, that taking them can improve your chances, she says.

Vitamin E for Men and Women

Vitamin E can be helpful for both sexes, says Liz Collins, N.D., a naturopathic doctor and co-owner of the Natural Childbirth and Family Clinic in Portland, Oregon. One study showed that giving just 100 to 200 international units (IU) of vitamin E a day to both partners increased fertility, she says.

Vitamin E may help balance hormones. A lot depends on this balance, and a lot can go wrong when hormones are out of sync with the reproductive cycle. When a fertilized egg sets out on its journey to the uterus, for instance, hormones prompt the welcoming committee. If the signals are straight, by the time the egg arrives at its destination, the uterus will be well-lined with blood to nourish the egg during its first growth stages. Lacking that important hormonal signal, the egg may arrive at an unprepared landing site, where it doesn't stand a chance of thriving. With vitamin E restoring the hormone balance, the fertilized egg may get the nourishment it needs upon arrival in the uterus.

Vitamin E is also a powerful antioxidant. This means that it helps control the damage caused by free-roaming, unstable molecules called free radicals. These unbalanced molecules steal electrons from healthy molecules. When they succeed, the molecule that was robbed is damaged, and damage spreads to the living cell.

Antioxidant vitamins such as E and C help stabilize free radicals and stop their chain of destruction. The vitamins sacrifice their own electrons to the free radicals, which helps prevent the cell-damaging chain reaction. While it's not entirely clear yet how that antioxidant function improves fertility in women, there are numerous reasons that stabilizing free radicals helps men.

For starters, 40 percent of infertile men have high levels of free radicals in their semen. Their damage causes abnormal sperm cells and low sperm counts.

Results from a study done by researchers from the department of clinical biochemistry at the King Saud University College of Medicine in Saudi Arabia suggest that vitamin E helps improve sperm motility. This means that sperm are better able to make the long swim from the vagina into the uterus and fallopian tube.

In her practice, Dr. Collins recommends that women take up to 500 IU of vitamin E twice a day and men take 200 to 400 IU daily. If you are considering taking amounts of vitamin E over 400 IU, discuss it

A Berry for Better Birthing

For centuries, women who were likely to have miscarriages took an herbal preventive that is also associated with a well-known fruit. Red raspberry leaf has the reputation of helping to relax the uterus. In addition to helping to prevent miscarriages, it is also recommended for infertility. "Raspberry works by helping the fertilized egg attach to the uterine lining and stay attached," says Jennifer Brett, N.D., a naturopathic doctor at the Wilton Naturopathic Center in Stratford, Connecticut.

Raspberry also seems to have a toning effect that helps women's reproductive systems function normally. Nowadays, herbalists capitalize on this benefit by recommending raspberry for a variety of women's problems, such as morning sickness, menstrual cramps, and heavy menstrual bleeding.

Compounds called tannins in the raspberry plant have an astringent quality—that is, they cause some constriction in cells that they come in contact with. When the tannins reach your intestine, they can help reduce inflammation, which is one way to reduce problems like diarrhea.

Raspberry also has some minerals that your body urgently needs to help incorporate liquids into your cells, so taking raspberry can be a good treatment for dehydration. It can give you a boost when thirst is making you feel exhausted.

If you want to give raspberry a try, it's available at most health food stores in a number of forms—as capsules, tincture, and often tea.

with your doctor, and be sure to stop taking it as soon as you become pregnant.

Supplements for Women

For women, the presence of yeast infections can reduce the chances of conception. Yeast infections may thicken vaginal mucus and make it impossible for sperm to get through to do their job, says Dr. Brett. Thus, taking measures against yeast infection is a first step in the right direction.

There's more. Women should also start taking a good multivitamin, says Dr. Collins. "So many of the nutrients in a multivitamin, especially the B vitamins, can help with infertility," she says. It's a good idea to see your gynecologist and have her recommend a prenatal vitamin for you, Dr. Collins says. That way you'll be sure to get all of the necessary nutrients, and if you do become pregnant, the baby will have a solid foundation to build from.

Your prenatal vitamin is sure to have folic acid in it, says Dr. Collins, and that's another building block. This B vitamin is instrumental in cell division. If an egg does become fertilized, it will need folic acid to start dividing and growing. Folic acid is also important in preventing birth defects of the brain and spinal column.

In one study by researchers in Budapest, Hungary, researchers who gave women 800 micrograms of folic acid a day found that the women conceived more quickly than women who did not take supplements.

If you are thinking about becoming pregnant, just 400 micrograms a day of folic acid should be adequate to prevent some birth defects. It is critically important during the first six weeks of pregnancy and should be taken at least through the first three months, says Aubrey Milunsky, M.D., professor of human genetics, pediatrics, and pathology and director of the center for human genetics at Boston University School of Medicine. It is safe to continue throughout pregnancy, he says.

Herbs for Conception

Apart from vitamins, there are a few herbs that a woman can take to help balance hormones so that conditions are just right for conception. Although they haven't been proven effective in clinical studies, chasteberry, red raspberry leaf, false unicorn, and red clover are among the herbs to consider if you're having trouble conceiving, says Dr. Brett. With any of these herbs, she recommends following the dosage directions on the packages. These or similar amounts are effective in helping to balance your hormones, she says. Be sure to stop taking them as soon as you think you might be pregnant, however, since these and other herbs are not recommended during pregnancy.

Of these four hormone-balancing herbs, some act like progesterone and others like estrogen—the two hormones that are essential to reproduction. "To keep the estrogen-to-progesterone balance in order, I usually recommend that women choose one of the herbs that act like progesterone and one that acts like estrogen," says Dr. Brett.

Calling on Unicorn

For many years, American Indians used a plant called false unicorn to make fertility formulas for both men and women. Today, we still have reason to call on its ability to strengthen and regulate the function of the reproductive system. According to herbalists, this herb can help treat infertility and may also help women prevent a wide range of problems, including miscarriage, morning sickness, and delayed menstruation.

Quickly becoming rare in the wild, false unicorn isn't something that you'll find alongside the average forest path. Fortunately, it's commercially cultivated, and herbalists advise that you stick with brands whose labels state that only the cultivated herb was used.

Perhaps legend can offer some insight into why false unicorn has become such a rarity. It seems that the devil became extremely angry because of the powers of this herb. In a rage, he tried to get rid of the species by biting off every plant at the roots.

Well, he didn't succeed. Today, false unicorn's star-shaped flowers still bloom every spring. He did leave his mark, however, because the plant's roots look as if they'd been chewed. It also bears the diabolical nickname of Devil's Bite.

A Boost from Two Berries

Chasteberry acts like a mild progesterone, says Dr. Collins. When you take it, you're lending support to half of the progesterone/estrogen team. If infertility is the result of the estrogen-to-progesterone ratio being out of balance, chasteberry might tip the scales just enough to improve your chances of success.

Chasteberry is especially good for women who are just coming off birth control pills, says Dr. Brett. The pills seriously change your hormone levels to prevent conception. With chasteberry, you can help restore the levels that encourage conception.

This herb is also recommended for women who have had repeated early miscarriages, notes Dr. Collins. Early miscarriages are often the result of a progesterone deficiency. By taking chasteberry to help boost progesterone levels, there's a chance that the herb can help prevent another miscarriage. She recommends the standard dosage, which is 175 to 225 milligrams a day.

Red raspberry leaf is another herb that can be used to increase progesterone levels, says Dr. Brett. It's a phytoprogesterone, she notes, which is a plant that acts like progesterone in the body. It is also often recommended to pregnant women to calm the uterus. Dosages vary depending on the concentration. For a 400-milligram supplement, a typical dose is one or two capsules two or three times daily at mealtimes.

The Estrogenic Herbs

False unicorn and red clover are herbal supplements for women that can act like weak estrogens in the body. Naturopathic doctors believe that they help balance hormone levels, either making up for a shortfall of estrogen or encouraging your body to excrete excess amounts.

The recommended dosages will vary with each of these herbal supplements, so Dr. Brett recommends following the directions on the packages.

False unicorn may be taken as a tincture or a tea. For either, follow the directions on the label. For tincture, that's typically 6 to 8 drops taken in a little water two or three times daily. Be aware that false unicorn may cause nausea and vomiting in doses higher than 5 to 15 drops of tincture, ½ cup of infusion, or 3 to 4 cups of tea blend per day.

For red clover, a typical dose for 430-milligram capsules is one or two capsules three times daily with water at mealtimes.

Remember that you should take only two of these four herbs at a time. One balancing pair, for example, is red raspberry leaf, which provides progesterone, and false unicorn, which supplies estrogen. Once you've made your choices, take both herbs every day until you know that you're pregnant, Dr. Brett says.

Supplements for Men

There are many supplements that men can take to improve both sperm counts and sperm motility and to reduce the number of abnormal sperm cells. Among them are the antioxidants vitamin C, vitamin E, and selenium and other nutrients such as zinc, arginine, and carnitine.

Selenium and vitamin C work in the same way that vitamin E does, by helping to stop free radical damage. In one small study, researchers in Canada gave selenium and vitamin E supplements to infertile men for six months. With supplementation, the men showed significant increases in sperm motility, percentage of live sperm, and percentage of normal sperm cells. The researchers concluded that these improvements were due to the supplements because all three benefits faded later when the men stopped taking them.

Vitamin C helps to keep sperm cells from clumping together. When sperm cells clump, they aren't able to move very well. Researchers have found that the chances of fertility are vastly reduced whenever more than 25 percent of sperm cells are stuck together. It's kind of like trying to make your way through a crowded room: The more dense the crowd, the harder it is to get to the other side.

Counting on C

Vitamin C may also play a role in increasing sperm counts. In one study, researchers selected 30 men who were infertile but had no other health problems and divided them into three groups of 10. One group received 200 milligrams of vitamin C a day, the second was given 1,000 milligrams of vitamin C a day, and the third received pills that looked like the other supplements but didn't contain vitamin C (placebos).

Researchers measured sperm count, motility, and sperm clumping every week. After one week, the 1,000-milligram group had a 140 percent increase in sperm count. The group getting 200 milligrams had a 112 percent increase. The sperm count of the group taking the placebo didn't increase at all.

Clumping was influenced, too. When the study began, all three groups of men had more than 25 percent of their sperm cells clumped. After three weeks, clumping was down to 11 percent in the two groups that were supplementing with vitamin C.

For those taking vitamin C, success soon followed. After 60 days, all of the men taking vitamin C had impregnated their wives. Among the group that took no supplements, by contrast, the fertility rate was still zero.

Dr. Brett recommends taking up to 5,000 milligrams of vitamin C in divided doses daily. Since too much vitamin C can cause diarrhea, she recommends starting with 1,000 milligrams a day and increasing the dosage by 1,000 milligrams each week, going all the way to 5,000 milligrams daily if you find that your body can tolerate that amount. Continue until your partner becomes pregnant.

Zinc Positive

Zinc is another good nutrient for infertile men because it can help increase sperm counts and improve sperm motility. Low levels of zinc can decrease production of the male hormone testosterone, which can lead to impaired fertility.

Studies show that most men get between 10 and 15 milligrams of zinc a day, but Dr. Brett recommends 25 milligrams a day for infertile men. With your doctor's okay, you can take this amount until your partner becomes pregnant, or up to six months.

Arginine and carnitine are two other nutrients to consider, says Dr. Collins. Arginine is an amino acid that your body needs in order to make sperm, while carnitine is a vitamin-like compound that helps sperm function properly.

In one study, researchers found that 74 percent of 178 men with low sperm counts had significantly higher counts and improved motility after taking 4,000 milligrams of arginine daily for at least three months. Dr. Brett recommends taking 1,000 milligrams of arginine twice a day until you know your partner is pregnant.

For carnitine, the optimum dose is 300 to 1,000 milligrams three times a day, Dr. Collins says. It may help improve sperm development, motility, and function. One clinical study in Bologna, Italy, found that 37 of 47 men who supplemented with 1,000 milligrams of carnitine three times a day for three months had improved sperm counts and motility. Since it's comparatively expensive, however, you might want to try other supplements first.

insomnia

Insomnia is something that many of us have experienced at one time or another. Anyone can have a sleepless night or two—or three. Before you reach for that over-the-counter sleeping pill or a prescription-strength remedy, however, consider some dietary and lifestyle changes to help catch up on your rest.

It's just common sense to eliminate caffeinated beverages and alcohol from your diet. Caffeine—whether from coffee, tea, or caffeinated soft drinks—is a nervous system stimulant that can keep you up at night. As for alcoholic drinks, they may seem like a shortcut to dreamland, but alcohol actually disrupts the chemical messengers that help initiate sleep.

Moderate aerobic exercise, as long as you time it right, is good for improving sleep. Try to get at least 20 minutes of exercise a day in the morning or afternoon, but not right before bedtime. This might be enough to help you quickly fall asleep and stay asleep throughout the night.

If you still have insomnia after taking these steps, you can try herbal and nutritional supplements. Herbal sedatives naturally calm your nervous system. Some relieve anxiety and serve as mild tranquilizers. Others, like magnesium and calcium, relax tense muscles and stimulate sleep-related brain chemicals. There is also a hormone supplement that works with your body's own natural sleep-wake cycles.

Valerian for Steady Sleep

Long before over-the-counter and prescription sleeping pills became available, herbal sedatives were widely used. One of nature's more popular herbal sedatives, used centuries ago and today, is valerian. This herb sends you off to dreamland more quickly. Once you nod off, the deep sleep stages are deepened. What's more, you won't wake up as often during the night, nor will you feel fatigued and drowsy in the morning.

Valerian's active ingredients, found in the roots, include a group of compounds called valepotriates. Research shows that these components attach to the same brain receptors as two types of pharmaceutical tranquilizers. Unlike the pharmaceuticals, however, valerian produces few side effects, and it doesn't carry the risk of dependency.

"Valerian root is a great herbal sleep aid because it sedates the central nervous system," says Chris Meletis, N.D., professor of natural pharmacology at the National College of Naturopathic Medicine in Portland, Oregon.

If anxiety, muscle tension, or muscle spasms leave you staring at the ceiling, valerian root can help relax these annoyances and send you off to la-la land, says Thomas Kruzel, N.D., a naturopathic physician in Portland, Oregon.

Dr. Meletis recommends taking 400 to 425 milligrams of valerian root one hour before bedtime. "That will give the valerian plenty of time to wind down your nervous system," he says.

In some people, however, valerian acts as a stimulant, causing nervousness and heart palpitations. If this is the case, simply stop using it, advises Dr. Meletis. Also avoid valerian if you're taking sleep-enhancing or mood-regulating medications such as diazepam (Valium) or amitriptyline (Elavil).

Snoozing with Kava

Kava kava, another time-honored herbal insomnia fighter and muscle relaxant, can put you fast asleep if stress has been keeping you awake. Kava relieves anxiety and acts as a tranquilizer, says Kristy Fassler, N.D., a naturopathic doctor in Portsmouth, New Hampshire.

"Kava helps shift the body into the parasympathetic nervous system, a state of total relaxation, which is required for sleep," says Dr. Fassler. "Normally, people are in the sympathetic nervous system, or the fight-or-flight response mode—rushing here and rushing there."

Kava's active ingredients are a group of chemicals called kavalactones. Animal studies show that these ingredients act on your limbic system, the part of the brain that is the center of your emotions. People who have taken kava for insomnia say that it continues to be effective over time, and it's not addictive. Also, it doesn't leave you feeling spaced-out or groggy the next morning as many of the prescription drugs do, says Dr. Fassler.

5-HTP: A Natural Serotonin Booster

Considering the many people who would love to find a shortcut to sounder sleep, it's hardly surprising that the promise of another natural sleep aid has grabbed the attention of consumers. The pill is 5-hydroxy-tryptophan, or 5-HTP for short.

Actually, 5-HTP started its reign of popularity as a substitute for another sleep aid, l-tryptophan. An over-the-counter product, l-tryptophan was taken off the market because of a product contamination scare in the late 1980s.

Since it was introduced to the market, 5-HTP has been called one of the next best alternatives to the hormone supplement melatonin.

This substance is an immediate precursor of serotonin, a vital brain chemical that regulates our moods, behavior, appetite, and sleep patterns. When you pop a supplement, the 5-HTP is absorbed from your gastrointestinal tract and travels to your brain, where it's converted into serotonin, says Ray Sahelian, M.D., a physician in Marina del Rey, California, and author of *5-HTP: Nature's Serotonin Solution*. The serotonin is then converted into melatonin, which is stored in your brain's pineal gland. At night, when it's secreted by the gland, the extra melatonin helps promote restful sleep, says Dr. Sahelian.

Studies show that 5-HTP can shorten the time it takes to nod off and reduce middle-of-the-night awakenings. It is reported to increase the time you spend in REM sleep (the dream state) and in the deep sleep stages that you need to feel fully rested in the morning.

To fall asleep shortly after your head hits the pillow, take 25 to 50 milligrams of 5-HTP one hour before bedtime on an empty stomach or at least two hours after dinner, says Chris Meletis, N.D., professor of natural pharmacology at the National College of Naturopathic Medicine in Portland, Oregon.

Because 5-HTP may lose its effectiveness over time if you use it every night, Dr. Sahelian suggests that you take it only once or twice a week. It's advisable to consult your doctor before taking it, especially if you're taking prescription antidepressants, some of which interact with 5-HTP. The supplement has sedative effects that could be dangerous if you drive or operate heavy machinery, and high doses can cause nausea in some people. Women who are pregnant or trying to conceive should not take 5-HTP.

A 125-pound person should take two 150-milligram capsules, says Dr. Fassler. For each additional 30 pounds of body weight, add another 75 milligrams of kava, she advises. Kava begins working its magic pretty quickly, so take it about 20 minutes before bedtime. Do not take it if you are pregnant, breastfeeding, or trying to conceive.

Magnesium and Calcium: A Snoozer's Duo

If tense muscles are keeping you up, pop some magnesium and calcium. Taken together, these two minerals act as mild muscle relaxants, says Dr. Meletis.

"Magnesium and calcium are minerals that are used in every muscle movement we make, so taking them together will relax your muscles and help promote sleep," says Dr. Fassler.

Some research suggests that people who get less than 200 milligrams a day of magnesium can have shallow sleep patterns and more nighttime awakenings. These patterns of insomnia sometimes show up among people who have reduced their calorie intakes or have started on weight-loss diets.

Even if your magnesium intake is normal, certain medications such as diuretics for high blood pressure, which reduce water retention, cause the kidneys to excrete excessive amounts of the mineral. The Daily Value for magnesium is 400 milligrams from food and supplements, and this amount should be enough to prevent sleep problems. If you still have trouble sleeping, take 500 milligrams of magnesium and 500 milligrams of calcium, along with a carbohydrate like bread, within one hour of bedtime, says Dr. Kruzel.

Doze Off with Melatonin

Trumpeted as a panacea for jet lag, cancer, and depression, melatonin has been widely accepted for treating insomnia. This hormone is secreted by the pineal gland, a pea-size gland in your brain that helps control periods of sleepiness and wakefulness.

The pineal gland releases melatonin into the bloodstream. At night, your body produces more melatonin, while the stimulus of light inhibits production. Between 2:00 and 4:00 A.M., production hits a peak. Then, toward dawn, it tapers off.

Before taking supplemental melatonin, have your doctor check your natural levels of melatonin. If they are low, take up to one milligram at least two hours before you go to bed, suggests Dr. Meletis. If you don't respond to this dosage, two to three milligrams may do the trick.

This supplement is for short-term use only. "Although melatonin works very well as a sleep aid, you shouldn't take it indiscriminately," Dr. Meletis says.

There hasn't been enough research to show whether there are long-term side effects from melatonin, he notes. It's possible that even at the recommended dosages, melatonin could disrupt your normal cycles of sleeping and waking, and other risks have also been associated with this supplement.

intermittent claudication

If the arteries in your legs are clogged by cholesterol deposits, chances are good that your legs will eventually seize up when you walk. When your leg muscles don't get enough oxygen-rich blood for the amount of activity they're being asked to do, the result is pain and muscle spasms. That condition is called intermittent claudication.

The pain of intermittent claudication is severe when you walk. In addition, poor circulation in your legs can cause related problems, such as skin breakdown and poor wound healing.

Treatment for intermittent claudication addresses the cause: poor circulation. Your doctor will advise you to stop smoking (if you do) and lose weight (if you need to). For people who have high cholesterol, high blood pressure, or diabetes, it's necessary to get those conditions under control as well in order to improve leg circulation.

You'll probably need a controlled walking program or some other form of exercise that gradually trains your leg muscles to make the most of their limited oxygen supply. "I also find that older people really benefit from yoga or tai chi for this problem," says Decker Weiss, N.M.D., a naturopathic doctor at the Arizona Heart Institute in Phoenix.

In addition, Dr. Weiss and other alternative medicine doctors use herbs and nutritional supplements. If you've been diagnosed with intermittent claudication, talk with your doctor about trying these remedies.

Arginine and Magnesium Can Open Up Arteries

The amino acid arginine is involved in the production of nitric oxide, a chemical released by the cells lining the artery walls. Nitric oxide allows blood vessels to relax and open up, Dr. Weiss says.

A standard dose is 500 milligrams up to three times a day. If you've been infected by the herpesvirus, though, you should use arginine only with medical supervision, Dr. Weiss says. "In people harboring the virus, high doses of arginine can cause severe outbreaks."

Along with arginine, Dr. Weiss recommends magnesium, an essential mineral. Magnesium is known for its ability to relax the muscles that wrap around blood vessels, so it can help dilate arteries that have been clogged by cholesterol deposits.

You might have a deficiency of magnesium if you are taking drugs meant to help heart problems, such as diuretics. Some people have deficiencies if they're taking commonly prescribed digitalis heart medications such as digitoxin (Crystodigin) or digoxin (Lanoxin). Signs of magnesium deficiency include muscle weakness, nausea, and irritability.

Most people can safely take up to 350 milligrams of supplemental magnesium, Dr. Weiss says. He recommends it in the form of magnesium orotate or glycinate.

B Vitamins Give You a Leg to Stand On

Researchers now realize that an amino acid by-product, homocysteine, can harm the insides of blood vessels, setting the stage for the cholesterol deposits that cause intermittent claudication. In one study, researchers were able to reduce high homocysteine levels using 5 milligrams of folic acid, 400 micrograms of vitamin B_{12}, and 50 milligrams of B_6. "I recommend these B vitamins to all my patients with heart or circulatory problems as part of a high-potency multivitamin or, if they have absorption problems, as injections or under-the-tongue supplements," Dr. Weiss says. This therapy should be done only under a doctor's supervision, he adds.

Ginkgo Gets You Going

Ginkgo has a reputation for improving circulation in the brain, but it also has body-wide effects that make it useful for all sorts of circulatory problems, including intermittent claudication, Dr. Weiss says. It helps to stimulate growth of new blood vessels and improves the use of oxygen and blood sugar (glucose), the main form of energy for muscle cells.

Ginkgo also helps to reduce the stickiness of clotting components, called platelets, in the blood. When the platelets become less sticky, harmful clots are less likely to form, especially in areas where blood flow is hindered.

Ginkgo has been tested in several studies of intermittent claudication, and it has worked at least as well as pentoxifylline (Trental), a drug that is commonly prescribed for this problem. Many people in the studies found that they could walk much farther without experiencing pain when they were taking ginkgo. The supplement also improved blood flow to the limbs, which was measured using a noninvasive technique called Doppler ultrasound.

Herbalists often recommend 120 milligrams of ginkgo in divided doses of 40 milligrams three times a day. In some studies, however, people have used 160 milligrams a day with good results.

Dr. Weiss's recommendation is lower. He prefers to use a standardized liquid extract of ginkgo, prescribing 20 drops four times a day for at least six months.

Antioxidants Act on Arteries

People with intermittent claudication usually do better in general if they are taking antioxidant nutrients such as vitamins E and C, which may help prevent the early stages of atherosclerosis (hardening of the arteries), Dr. Weiss says.

Vitamin E has a long history of use for intermittent claudication. In one study, conducted in Sweden, researchers found that they could reduce symptoms if they gave people supplementation with 300 international units (IU) a day.

For smokers, however, supplementation with vitamin E doesn't seem to reduce the symptoms of intermittent claudication. It's quite possible that the vitamin can't entirely overcome the harmful effects that smoking has on your circulatory system, Dr. Weiss says. Breaking the habit comes first: Often, when people stop smoking, intermittent claudication disappears with time.

Dr. Weiss gives many of his patients with atherosclerosis 400 to 800 IU of vitamin E and 1,000 to 3,000 grams of vitamin C a day. Vitamin E helps prevent the oxidation of harmful LDL cholesterol, a first step in cholesterol blockage. Vitamin C regenerates vitamin E and also helps the cells lining the blood vessel walls to produce nitric oxide, which keeps blood vessels open and dilated.

For vitamin E, you should use natural d-alpha-tocopherol and mixed tocopherols, says Dr. Weiss.

Take Ginger and Pineapple

"Ginger can be a wonderful addition to a treatment program for intermittent claudication, especially if you also have arthralgia, or pain in your joints," Dr. Weiss says. Like ginkgo, ginger helps keep platelets from getting too sticky, so it keeps your blood flowing smoothly. "It's also a slight vasodilator and a warming herb," Dr. Weiss says, so if you have cold feet, it might provide additional benefits.

Most research studies with ginger use about 1,000 milligrams a day of powdered gingerroot, which is about what you'd get from a ¼-inch slice of fresh root. Ginger is safe to take long-term, Dr. Weiss says.

Another common food—pineapple—also offers some relief in supplement form. The same ingredient in pineapple that prevents gelatin from setting can help the arteries in your legs stay open, Dr. Weiss says. It's an enzyme called bromelain, which helps keep blood from clotting too readily and may also help existing clots dissolve.

"I might use this if someone with circulatory problems also has had clotting problems in their legs, such as thrombophlebitis," Dr. Weiss says. "Since bromelain also helps to reduce inflammation, I find it's good to use after surgery or injuries," he adds.

Take bromelain between meals; otherwise, it will be used up digesting your meal. A common daily dose used in studies ranges from 60 to 160 milligrams. Dr. Weiss usually recommends much more to his patients—500 milligrams twice a day, as long as needed. With your doctor's supervision, take note of how your body reacts.

irritable bowel syndrome

In the scary world of intestinal tracts, the most common ghost—unfortunately—is a mysterious disease that travels under the code name IBS. These three sinister initials are shorthand for irritable bowel syndrome.

People with IBS tend to have alternating constipation and diarrhea, bloating, unformed stools, gas, and sometimes, cramps followed by an urgent need to have a bowel movement. As the discomfort goes on, though, the root causes are frustratingly elusive.

IBS is not a disease, and rarely is there any inflammation of the bowel. Doctors who have studied the problem say that it's probably related to stress and food intolerances.

"In my practice, I find that there are two kinds of people who get IBS. First are go-getters who are really stressed; they are hard-wired for stress to stimulate their colons. And then there are the folks who have an intolerance to certain foods," says Leon Hecht, N.D., a naturopathic physician at North Coast Family Health Center in Portsmouth, New Hampshire.

Since the causes are elusive, finding an appropriate remedy can pose a real challenge. Some supplements, however, seem to make the symptoms of IBS more tolerable and possibly less likely to occur, says Dr. Hecht. These treatments—combined with lifestyle and diet changes and stress reduction—may be sufficient for some folks, he says.

Hydrate with Fiber and Water

To start, you need to get enough water, and that may be a good bit more than you're accustomed to drinking. Some people with IBS have small, hard stools that are difficult to pass. By drinking water, they can add soft bulk to the stool and ease its passage through the bowel, says Melissa Metcalfe, N.D., a naturopathic doctor in Los Angeles.

"You should drink eight 12-ounce glasses of water a day, and more if you're an active person," says Dr. Metcalfe.

519

While you're emptying your water bottle, also increase the amount of fiber in your diet, Dr. Metcalfe advises. Fiber absorbs water and helps move food and waste through the gastrointestinal tract more quickly. Some excellent sources of fiber are foods like prunes, apples, oat bran, and carrots.

If you need more fiber, you can benefit from a supplement. In a study published in a British medical journal aptly named *Gut*, 80 patients with irritable bowel syndrome were given either a supplement containing psyllium or a harmless, inactive substitute (a placebo). More than 80 percent of the group taking psyllium experienced relief from their constipation, while those in the placebo group noticed no change.

Dr. Metcalfe recommends taking two tablespoons daily—in two separate doses—of a fiber/nutritional supplement that contains psyllium husks. Fiber supplements like Metamucil come in a wide range of textures, and some are flavored to make them more palatable. Take them before meals, or take one tablespoon in the morning and another before you go to bed. Just make sure that you mix each tablespoon dose with at least two eight-ounce glasses of water, says Dr. Metcalfe.

Calming the Colon

Irritable bowel syndrome isn't just irritating; it can be downright painful. When you're having an attack, you can calm your aching colon by taking peppermint oil extract, an herbal medicine long used for digestive problems, says Dr. Hecht. To decrease the severity of your IBS symptoms, you can take it every day.

Peppermint oil extract relaxes the smooth muscles that line the intestines and other internal organs. The herb calms overactive peristalsis, the muscular contraction that moves food through the gastrointestinal tract, and relieves cramping. It also helps you belch and relieve gas buildup, according to Dr. Hecht.

In one German study, doctors combined peppermint oil extract with caraway oil and gave the mixture to 54 patients with IBS. Some patients were given 90 milligrams of peppermint oil extract combined with 50 milligrams of caraway, while others received a placebo. After four weeks of taking one capsule before meals, 63 percent of the patients given the oils found that they were pain-free. Only 25 percent of the placebo group noticed any improvement.

Dr. Hecht has found that even peppermint oil extracts alone are effective for some of his patients with IBS. To get the medicine to the intestines where you need it, look for a peppermint oil capsule or pill that's enteric coated. The coating protects the extract from the acid of the stomach and enables it to release its therapeutic benefits in the small intestine, explains Dr. Hecht.

He suggests a supplement that contains 0.2 milliliters of peppermint oil extract. "Take one capsule between meals three times a day," he says, but he advises that you not take the capsule immediately after a meal.

You may have some discomfort if you take too much peppermint oil, since it can cause some burning at the anus. "If that happens, just back off on the dosage and take less," suggests Dr. Hecht.

Diet Detection and Bacteria Banishment

Food intolerance is often a contributing factor to IBS, but the reactions can happen hours after a meal, so people don't always connect what they ate with how they feel, says Dr. Hecht.

Many naturopathic doctors suggest that their patients try to find out what's causing the problem by a process of elimination. This is called, logically, an elimination diet. The first step is to cut out the foods that are most likely to be irritants. Many people, for example, have adverse reactions to sugar, wheat, and corn. Milk and other dairy products are common culprits. Chocolate may also be a problem, and a high-carbohydrate diet is involved in 30 to 50 percent of Dr. Hecht's cases. Sometimes, blood testing or allergy testing can provide clues as well, he notes.

For many people, refined sugar is the culprit, says Dr. Hecht. He compares it to a fertilizer for yeast. Although yeast is always present in the body, dietary sugar can lead to an overgrowth in the intestinal tract, resulting in gas, bloating, and pain and triggering cramps and other symptoms of IBS.

In the meantime, if bad microorganisms in your intestinal tract start to crowd out the good ones, any problems that you have with food sensitivities or with indigestion may be intensified. One way to combat the problem is to repopulate the gut with good bacteria. Usually, that means that you need to take acidophilus, says Michael Gazsi, N.D., a naturopathic doctor in Ridgefield, Connecticut. It is also a good idea to have a stool microbiology test to assess the good and bad bacterial levels as well as fungal levels.

Acidophilus supplements come in various dosages, depending on the manufacturer, says Dr. Gazsi. Your best bet is to follow the directions on the label of the supplement and then observe any changes in your condition. A typical dose is one capsule with a meal twice daily.

Some Mint for Movement

Here's a medicine that's good for you, and it tastes good, too. Peppermint has been a popular flavoring agent in candies for centuries, but it has important healing properties as well. It stimulates digestion, relieves gas and bloating, and makes you burp.

The herb's therapeutic qualities are related to its menthol content. Peppermint oil extract contains 50 to 70 percent free menthol, a compound that stimulates bile flow and other gastric secretions in the digestive system. The herb's active oils also have an effect on the sphincter muscle at the lower end of your esophagus. By temporarily changing the behavior of that muscle, peppermint oil extract promotes belching.

Strangely, peppermint also inhibits hunger pangs in the stomach by suppressing peristalsis, the muscular contraction that moves food through the gastrointestinal tract. When the effects of the herb begin to subside, however, the peristaltic movements come back even more strongly.

With more gastric secretions and stronger stomach movements induced by peppermint, food spends less time in your stomach. It is passed along to the small intestine more rapidly, and that means digestion improves.

As a supplement, peppermint oil extract usually comes in capsules. You can also drink peppermint tea.

"If the bowel continues to feel really irritated, I'd back off the dosage a bit or try a different brand," says Dr. Gazsi. "Unfortunately, there's not a lot of quality control with some of these supplements. There's no way of knowing if you're getting enough or too many of the bacteria. You just have to see how you're reacting and adjust accordingly."

Eventually, the good bacteria should re-establish themselves, and you can forgo the acidophilus supplement. Or you can continue taking it. "It's one of those things that you can take indefinitely," says Dr. Gazsi.

Bring On the Enzymes

Bacteria aren't the only players in digestion. You also need plenty of digestive enzymes, specialized proteins that break down the food chemically and make it available for use by the body. If enzymes don't do their work properly or are in short supply in the gastrointestinal tract, food passes undigested through the small intestine. As that undigested food reaches the bowel, it may be attacked and consumed by bad bacteria, which in turn causes gas and bloating.

If you're having an irritable bowel problem partly because you lack enough digestive enzymes, you may benefit from taking a supplement to make up the shortage, says Dr. Gazsi. There are several types on the market. Look for a product that contains plant-derived enzymes and follow the dosage recommendations on the bottle.

Another way to get your enzymes is to eat more fresh, uncooked vegetables and fruit. You don't get the enzymes from canned, processed, or cooked food, since many of the natural plant enzymes are destroyed by cooking and processing, according to Dr. Gazsi.

"You don't want to eat too much raw food all at once, though," he says. "Some people try to change their diets too quickly, which may make their irritable bowels even worse."

Coat and Soothe

Although the exact cause of IBS isn't known, herbs that are generally soothing and healing to the digestive tract can be helpful. These herbs, known as demulcents, have the ability to coat mucous membranes.

By direct contact, the demulcents help relieve inflammation and are therefore very soothing, explains Pamela Taylor, N.D., a naturopathic doctor in Moline, Illinois.

A good example is slippery elm. When a dose of one to two tablespoons of liquid extract is dissolved in water or juice or added to a cooked cereal as a demulcent, it forms a soothing coating that bathes the intestinal walls. "Demulcents such as slippery elm also have a wound-healing effect," she says.

Supplement combinations of demulcent herbs usually include slippery elm, marshmallow root, echinacea, goldenseal, and geranium. This combination is commonly known as Robert's Formula and is often recommended by naturopathic physicians, says Dr. Taylor.

kidney stones

The pain of passing a kidney stone has been compared to the pain of childbirth. With childbirth, there's a sweet reward. With a kidney stone, there's nothing but the production of a granular object.

Men are more likely than women to get calcium stones, and genes play a role as well. Because of that genetic factor, if your parents or grandparents had kidney stones, you're at higher risk for getting them yourself.

Some people have a tendency to excrete high levels of calcium oxalate and calcium phosphate. If all goes well, you get rid of these calcium salts every time you urinate. But sometimes, however, the salts hang around the kidneys like bad leftovers. Eighty percent of all kidney stones are composed of these calcium salts.

Diet is important if you're trying to avoid kidney stones. Stay away from foods such as spinach, beans, parsley, tea, and coffee. Although some of these items are normally thought of as healthy foods, they are rich in oxalates, says Anne McClenon, N.D., a naturopathic doctor at the Compass Family Health Center in Plymouth, Massachusetts. If you have a problem turning oxalates into a form that your body can use, they remain in your urine. "They may precipitate as a stone," she says.

The stones can't be ignored, and there's no way to treat them yourself. If you have a stone, you may have severe pain, blood in the urine, and fever. Any of these symptoms should tell you to see a doctor as soon as possible. "It can be a medical emergency. The pain can be excruciating," says Dr. McClenon.

Sometimes, a small stone will pass on its own—with that childbirth-type pain mentioned earlier. If you have a stone that's too big to pass, your doctor will probably recommend an ultrasound procedure that breaks it up without surgery.

There are a few strategies and supplements that might help you avoid forming another kidney stone from calcium salts. First, however, you should see your doctor and have a blood test and chemical analysis of your urine and stones to determine if calcium is really your problem. There are other types of stones, which can form because of a urinary tract infection, gout, or a hereditary kidney disorder.

If you're prone to getting calcium stones, here are some tactics and some supplements to help prevent them.

Drink Up

Water, that is. It's a simple bit of advice, but it makes a lot of sense when you consider that stones come from dissolved solids, says Leon Hecht, N.D., a naturopathic doctor at North Coast Family Health in Portsmouth, New Hampshire.

It's similar to the rationale behind adding more and more water to soup that's too salty. The objective is to keep the saltwater solution in the kidneys extremely diluted so that a concentration of stone-forming salts doesn't get stuck there. Water causes the concentration of chemicals in the urine to decrease, making them more soluble and less likely to form stones.

Drink at least 8 to 10 full 12-ounce glasses of water each day. Not juice or soda or milk—just water, says Dr. Hecht. (Salt and sugar can raise the level of calcium in your urine.) "You should drink enough so that you're urinating every couple of hours," he adds.

Stonewall with Magnesium

Having high levels of calcium oxalate and calcium phosphate in your urine isn't a problem as long at you excrete those salts. For that to happen efficiently, they need to hook up with other essential chemicals in the urine. Otherwise, they'll clump together, form crystals, and precipitate out like sugar settling to the bottom of a glass of iced tea.

That's where magnesium comes in. It binds with the calcium salts so they stay dissolved in the urine.

Magnesium is a regulator of calcium, says Michael Gazsi, N.D., a naturopathic doctor in Ridgefield, Connecticut. "You excrete it rather than having it settle out in the kidney," he explains. "If you keep the magnesium ratio in the urine high, there's less chance of forming a stone."

If you have a predisposition to calcium stones, Dr. Gazsi suggests that you take 500 to 1,000 milligrams of magnesium a day. "It's the single best thing you can do to prevent these types of stones," he says.

B₆ Boosts Protection

For added insurance, you can take a vitamin B$_6$ supplement, since B$_6$ reduces the production of oxalate, says Dr. Hecht.

He recommends taking 25 to 50 milligrams of vitamin B$_6$ daily along with a magnesium supplement. "Magnesium alone decreases the likelihood of kidney stones, but when you put it with vitamin B$_6$, it has an even greater effect," he says.

Keep Your Cs Low

Vitamin C is good for protecting your cells and boosting immunity, but high doses may be a problem for people with a tendency toward oxalate-type kidney stones, says Dr. McClenon. That's because one by-product of vitamin C is oxalate.

While this doesn't mean that you should avoid vitamin C entirely, it's probably a good idea to limit your dosage to no more than 2,000 milligrams a day, says Dr. McClenon.

Some research suggests, however, that for the average person, vitamin C does not promote kidney stones. It may even have a mild protective effect, according to Alan Gaby, M.D., professor of nutrition at Bastyr University in Bothell, Washington.

leg cramps

Baseball players coined the term *charley horse* more than 100 years ago for the cramps they got in their tired, overworked leg muscles.

Whether you're running the bases or lying in bed, nerves send signals to the muscles to tell them when to contract and relax. When these signals get scrambled, the muscle responds by cramping.

What mixes up the messages? The first suspected cause is a mineral imbalance, says Jacqueline Jacques, N.D., a naturopathic doctor and specialist in pain management in Portland, Oregon. That's not the only possibility, though. Cramps can also be caused by strenuous exercise, excess salt loss from sweating, or sitting or standing too long.

When you get a cramp, stretch and gently massage the muscle immediately. This should relax the muscle and provide you with some much-needed relief. If you find that you're having muscle cramps every night, your doctor is likely to prescribe quinine, but only for a limited time. This often-used treatment for leg cramps can quickly build to toxic levels in the blood and can cause nausea, vomiting, ringing in the ears (tinnitus), and deafness. It can even damage your eyesight.

A safer way to eliminate that knot of pain in your muscles is to try a combination of vitamin, mineral, and herbal supplements, say natural healers.

A Trio of Supplements for Nighttime Cramps

If you're getting a nightly wake-up call from your leg muscles, you probably need to get more magnesium and calcium, says Mark Stengler, N.D., a naturopathic doctor in Beaverton, Oregon, and author of *The Natural Physician: Your Health Guide for Common Ailments*. Both of these minerals are involved in relaxing nerve impulses and regulating muscle activity. Calcium is needed to contract the muscle, and magnesium is needed to relax it. An imbalance in this dynamic duo can irritate and confuse the muscle.

Since the calcium in bone provides a nearly inexhaustible mineral supply to replenish the relatively tiny amount that you need in your blood, you're more likely to be low on magnesium, says Dr. Jacques. If you're like most people, you probably get only 75 percent of the Daily Value (DV) for magnesium, which is 400 milligrams from food and supplements.

Mix In Magnesium

Start with a dose of 250 milligrams of magnesium glycinate or chelated magnesium twice a day, says Dr. Jacques. These amino acid–based mineral supplements are easier to absorb than magnesium oxide. The more you absorb, the less likely it is that you'll have diarrhea, a common problem with magnesium supplements.

Dr. Jacques is definitely not an advocate of magnesium oxide supplements. "Magnesium oxide is basically a rock," she says. "The reason it causes diarrhea is that it stays in the gut. We even see it occasionally on x-rays, where it shows up like little bone chips."

To help relieve cramps that interrupt your nightly Zzzs, take your second dose of magnesium right before you go to bed. If you don't get relief in three to five days, increase the dose to 500 milligrams twice a day, says Dr. Jacques. Stay at that level for another week to allow the tissue levels of the mineral to build up.

A Time for Calcium

If cramps are still a problem at that dosage, it's time to add 500 milligrams of calcium to the regimen. The average adult absorbs only about 30 percent of the calcium consumed.

To maximize absorption, Dr. Jacques gives her patients calcium citrate instead of calcium carbonate, the form commonly found in antacid tablets. It helps to take it with a glass of milk since vitamin D is necessary for calcium absorption. If you are unable to drink milk, you can take a calcium supplement that also contains vitamin D.

If you're taking both calcium and magnesium, keep in mind that they work best when they are taken in certain ratios. The two ratios recommended by naturopathic doctors are either equal doses of calcium and magnesium or twice as much calcium as magnesium. "A lot of it is a guessing game, particularly with something like leg cramps," says Dr. Jacques. "You have to find out what ratio works best for you."

Try the one-to-one ratio first, taking 500 milligrams of calcium and 500 milligrams of magnesium twice a day, Dr. Jacques says. If that doesn't give you the results you want, shift the ratio to 2:1 by reducing the magnesium to 250 milligrams.

The E Potential

Some patients with nighttime cramping have success with vitamin E, says Dr. Stengler. Although it has had mixed results in clinical trials, early studies suggest that you'll improve arterial blood flow and reduce leg cramping at night if you take vitamin E.

In one of the largest studies, 123 of 125 people who suffered from nighttime leg and foot cramps reported complete relief after taking vitamin E supplements. To see if it works for you, take 400 to 800 international units (IU) a day, says Dr. Jacques.

Are You Lacking Potassium?

Potassium is another mineral that helps regulate muscle contraction, says Dr. Stengler. Deficiencies of this crucial electrolyte aren't normally a problem if you eat a variety of fruits and vegetables. If you change your diet drastically, however, you might become deficient. This is a potential problem, if you go on one of the high-protein weight-loss diets that some experts advocate.

"When people go on high-protein diets, they begin to develop leg cramps. I see it repeatedly," says Dr. Jacques. She believes that such diets are related to potassium deficiency.

When protein makes up more than 30 percent of your daily calories, potassium levels may fall far short of the DV of 3,500 milligrams, according to Dr. Jacques. If you're eating eight or nine servings of fruits and vegetables, you'll get enough potassium to meet the DV, but the shift to a high-protein diet makes this significantly more of a challenge.

Cramps are more prevalent when you first start a high-protein diet, Dr. Jacques has observed. After a few months, they normally disappear on their own. To make them go away sooner, you can take one 99-milligram tablet of potassium a day, she suggests. This doesn't amount to much more than a bite or two of banana, but it can make your legs feel better, she says.

A word of caution, though: Don't take more than one tablet. It's easy to get too much potassium this way, which can upset the balance of other minerals in your body and cause heart and kidney problems. That's why Food and Drug Administration regulations don't allow more than 99 milligrams per tablet in over-the-counter supplements.

Little Players That Loosen Your Legs

When you get leg cramps, the first suspects are naturally the big minerals that we've already discussed—calcium, magnesium, and potassium. But maybe those cramps are due to an imbalance of trace minerals, especially if the pain is triggered by overexertion, says Dr. Jacques. "Muscle and nerve function are electrical, and we need the right mix of minerals for that to happen. There are a lot of little players in there."

You can deplete levels of trace minerals as you perspire. Electrolyte drinks work well to help restore these depleted minerals. You can also take a trace mineral supplement that contains copper, manganese, zinc, selenium, and chromium, says Dr. Jacques.

Although trace mineral supplements vary in content, don't exceed the dosage guidelines on the bottle, she says. "Trace minerals should be taken in small doses because that's how they are found in your body. More is not better."

If you get leg cramps when you walk, see your doctor to rule out other conditions such as intermittent claudication, which is caused by poor blood flow to the legs.

Soothing Spasms

Herbal extracts offer a natural way to soothe and relax spastic muscles. One of the most valuable is black cohosh, says Dr. Stengler. Also known as black snakeroot and bugbane, black cohosh root contains active substances called triterpene glycosides, antispasmodics that act as natural muscle relaxants.

When muscles seize up with pain, take a 500-milligram capsule of the root powder or 30 to 60 drops of tincture in warm water every one to two hours.

For acute cramps, two or three doses should be sufficient for a therapeutic effect, says Dr. Stengler. Don't use black cohosh during pregnancy,
though, or for more than six months at a time.

Bilberry contains chemicals called anthocyanins, a type of flavonoids
that have muscle-relaxant properties. Bilberry also helps to improve circulation in the extremities. To reduce muscle cramping, take 80 milligrams
three times a day of an extract standardized to contain 25 percent anthocyanidin. You should take it for at least a couple of months, but you can
continue indefinitely if necessary, says Dr. Stengler.

"Ginkgo is also useful, since it improves circulation through the extremities by dilating the arteries that feed the leg tissue," he says. While
cramps are a problem, Dr. Stengler gives patients 60 milligrams three times
a day of an extract containing 24 percent ginkgoflavoglycosides and 6 percent terpenelactones. If you have circulation problems, you can probably
use ginkgo on a long-term basis.

lupus

A painful and potentially life-threatening illness, lupus occurs when your immune system turns renegade and attacks your body's own tissues, causing inflammation and damage. The skin, kidneys, blood vessels, eyes, lungs, nerves, joints—just about any part of the body—can be involved. At the same time, your immune system sometimes ignores its normal duties of fighting infection, so you end up being prone to all sorts of illnesses.

The exact causes of lupus aren't known for sure, but research has shown that genetic and environmental factors are involved. There is no cure. Conventional treatment generally involves controlling the symptoms with drugs, including anti-inflammatories such as ibuprofen, analgesics such as acetaminophen, and corticosteroids (hormones) such as prednisone. Some people are also treated with immune suppressants—that is, medications that suppress the action of the immune system.

Alternative practitioners believe that their treatments can reduce inflammation, increase the body's production of certain hormones, and strengthen immunity. Naturopathic doctors may also treat what they think are possible underlying causes of lupus. They believe that diseases of this kind, called autoimmune diseases, may be associated with digestion problems, food allergies, and weakness of the adrenal glands.

A naturopathic doctor will usually do tests to determine if any of these underlying problems exist, says Jody Noé, N.D., a naturopathic doctor at the Brattleboro Naturopathic Clinic in Vermont. Once the possible causes are identified, there are a number of alternative treatments that may help.

"It's important to try to figure out the cause of this disorder," she says, "and to work out a treatment plan based on each person's symptoms." Supplements often play a role in alternative treatments, but you should get your doctor's approval before taking supplements to treat lupus. You'll also need to consult a holistic physician or naturopath to determine the dosages best suited to you.

Knocking Out Free Radicals

When inflammation occurs, the body produces more free radicals, the unstable molecules that can harm cells. One of the first lines of defense that a naturopathic doctor uses against inflammation is extra amounts of nutrients that neutralize the radicals. These nutrients, called antioxidants, are vitamins E and C, beta-carotene, and selenium. They also include zinc, which has antioxidant activity, and phytochemicals such as bioflavonoids, which are found in plants and herbs, Dr. Noé says.

Dr. Noé recommends that her patients take a mixture of antioxidant nutrients daily with food. She suggests 1,000 to 3,000 milligrams of vitamin C in divided doses, 400 to 600 international units (IU) of vitamin E, 200 to 400 micrograms of selenium, and 15 to 30 milligrams of zinc in the form of zinc picolinate or citrate.

She also recommends 1 to 2 milligrams a day of copper and 5 to 15 milligrams of manganese. Both help the body make its own antioxidants. These trace minerals should be taken only in these recommended doses to avoid getting toxic amounts.

Essential Fatty Acids Fight Inflammation

You can reduce levels of inflammation-generating biochemicals in your body by changing the kinds of fats you eat, Dr. Noé says. Meat and other animal products provide your body with something called arachidonic acid, which is used to make pro-inflammatory biochemicals. On the other hand, fish oils, which contain eicosapentaenoic acid (EPA) and docosahexaenoic acid (DHA), and certain plant oils, which contain gamma-linolenic acid (GLA), follow a biochemical pathway that reduces production of these biochemicals.

In studies of animals that spontaneously develop a lupuslike syndrome, diets high in fish oil reduced inflammation and improved kidney function and immunity. In human studies, results have been inconclusive, perhaps because the studies were not long enough or because people started taking fish oil too late in the course of the disease. Still, a study from India showed that people had lower levels of free radicals in their blood when they were taking fish oil than they did prior to taking it.

One study found that people with the most common type of lupus showed a reduction of free radical chemical "markers" and increased amounts of antioxidants in their blood after undergoing therapy with the omega-3 fatty acids EPA and DHA. Researchers surmise that fish oil, which is high in omega-3's, might be helpful for people with lupus.

"In my practice, I've seen that most people with an autoimmune disease benefit from getting essential fatty acids," Dr. Noé says. "These oils are good for everyone with chronic inflammation."

Dr. Noé recommends that people with lupus take 1,000 to 1,500 milligrams a day of EPA and 500 to 700 milligrams of DHA. She also recommends 500 to 1,000 milligrams of GLA from evening primrose, borage, or black currant oil. Since borage oil is the most potent and most economical, some specialists feel that it may be your best buy. These supplements are all available at health food stores. You can take them for as long as you like, but it is best to take them with food, says Dr. Noé.

DHEA—And What Sex Has to Do with It

Lupus is influenced by hormone fluctuations in the body. In some people, an imbalance of the estrogenic (female) and androgenic (male) hormones can make lupus symptoms worse. While scientists don't quite understand why this happens, they do have some clues, says Philip Mease, M.D., a rheumatologist at Minor and James Medical Center and clinical associate professor of medicine at the University of Washington Medical School, both in Seattle. Lupus may first appear during pregnancy, for instance, when there are changes in the hormone balance, according to Dr. Mease.

Animal studies also indicate a link between the balance of male and female hormones and lupus. Female mice with lupus tend to have more severe symptoms than male mice, according to Dr. Mease. Scientists found that the female mice's symptoms improved considerably when they were given male hormones.

In two studies at Stanford University Medical Center, researchers looked closely at the effect of DHEA to find out whether it could be helpful in treating lupus. DHEA—short for dehydroepiandrosterone—is a hormone that sets off a chain reaction when it arrives in certain tissues. At the end of that chain reaction, the body produces sex hormones, either testosterone (in male organs) or estrogen (in female organs). Thus, when taken as a supplement, DHEA leads to increased production of sex hormones.

The Hormone in Action

One study of DHEA involved 28 women who had mild to moderate lupus. Most of the participants were already taking doses of prednisone, a corticosteroid drug, to relieve their symptoms. Fourteen of the women were given pills that contained 200 milligrams of DHEA. The other 14 took pills that looked exactly the same but were inactive (placebos). At the end of a three-month trial period, the women who were receiving DHEA showed a marked improvement and were able to reduce their dosages of the prednisone. Women in the placebo group showed little improvement.

In another study, 10 women with lupus were given 200 milligrams of DHEA for three to six months. Three of the women had protein in their urine, which is a sign of kidney damage resulting from lupus. At the end of the trial period, 8 of the 10 women felt that their overall well-being had improved, and those with signs of kidney damage had less protein in their urine, indicating that they were getting some protection.

Some pharmacies can make up either a tincture or capsule of DHEA, Dr. Mease says. If you can get the tincture, take it as drops under the tongue as directed by your pharmacist, he says. Fifteen to 20 milligrams of DHEA twice a day will replace physiologic levels. Lower doses may be helpful with a comprehensive nutritional program.

Whatever you do, work with your doctor if you want to take DHEA, Dr. Mease advises. DHEA can cause acne, male-pattern baldness and facial hair, and its long term effects are unknown.

"People who need to take corticosteroid drugs, namely prednisone, to control their symptoms can usually reduce their drug dosage if they take DHEA," Dr. Mease says. Being able to reduce the dosage of steroid drugs is a benefit because these drugs cause bone loss, suppress immunity, and have other side effects, he adds.

Plugging a Leaky Gut

Some alternative doctors and practitioners who have studied cases of autoimmune diseases, especially certain types of arthritis, believe that these conditions might be associated with a special kind of intestinal problem. They call the condition increased permeability or, more commonly, leaky gut.

The theory proposes that if the walls of the intestines are leaky, molecules derived from incompletely digested foods or from bacteria are able to seep through the intestinal lining and get into the bloodstream. There, they set off an immune response that can result in immune cells going haywire, ultimately triggering attacks on the body's own cells. Whether or not this happens in some cases of lupus isn't certain, says Dr. Noé.

Tests are available that some experts claim can detect a leaky gut. Dr. Noé says that she orders certain blood, urine, and saliva tests, for instance, to reveal if someone is having an immune reaction that could cause lupus.

Enzymes to the Rescue

In addition to eliminating foods identified as contributing to the problem, such as wheat gluten, corn, and dairy products, Dr. Noé recommends nutritional supplements that nourish and rebuild the intestinal lining and restore good bacteria to the bowel. If there are enough good bacteria there, they will crowd out the bad types that can contribute to digestive problems.

"I also may recommend enzymes that help break down food for proper digestion if tests suggest that someone's pancreas is not producing enough for normal digestion," she says. The following supplements are among those that Dr. Noé recommends.

- 500 to 750 milligrams of the amino acid glutamine
- 100 to 300 milligrams of gamma-oryzanol, a component of rice bran oil
- 50 to 150 milligrams of butyrate
- 50 to 100 milligrams of fructooligosaccharides (FOS), naturally occurring sugars that promote the growth of friendly bacteria in the intestines

She suggests taking all of these two or three times a day between meals. She notes that these substances are safe to take on a continuous basis as long as you remain under a doctor's supervision while taking them.

All of these supplements except FOS are broken-down forms of amino acids, fats, or sugars that can be absorbed directly by the intestinal cells, bypassing digestion. FOS are used as food for intestinal bacteria in order to promote more friendly flora. Although there are no studies to show that supplements are effective for lupus, some alternative doctors use them in an attempt to decrease intestinal permeability.

To restore friendly bacteria and improve digestion, Dr. Noé suggests the following supplements.

• One or two capsules two or three times a day of a product that contains various forms of lactobacillus and other so-called friendly bacteria—*Lactobacillus acidophilus*, *L. rhamnosus*, *L. casei*, *L. plantarum*, *Bifidobacterium bifidum*, *B. longum*, and *B. breve*—with two to five billion active organisms in each capsule. (If you can't find some of these bacteria in supplements at a health food store, you may need to ask a naturopathic or holistic doctor to get them for you.)

• 500 to 1,000 milligrams of 10X U.S.P. of digestive enzymes. (10X U.S.P. is a measure of strength and is listed on the bottle.)

• A mixture of other enzymes derived from plants, including 12,500 to 18,000 U.S.P. of protease, 2,675 U.S.P. of lipase, 12,000 to 27,000 U.S.P. of amylase, and 175 CU(2) of cellulase.

Dr. Noé says that these supplements are safe to take on a continuous basis as long as you get your doctor's approval to take them and remain under medical supervision.

Indian Spice Eases Aches

Turmeric, an Indian spice used in traditional Ayurvedic medicine, contains an anti-inflammatory and antioxidant compound called curcumin that might be helpful for people with conditions, such as lupus, that involve inflammation, says Andrew Rubman, N.D., director of the Southbury Clinic for Traditional Medicine in Connecticut and consultant to the Office of Complementary and Alternative Medicine at the National Institutes of Health.

"In animals, curcumin has excellent anti-inflammatory and antioxidant effects, without any toxicity," Dr. Rubman says. When curcumin is present, the body is much less likely to form the compounds that are instrumental in causing inflammation, he explains. "Plus," he adds, "it may stimulate the body's own anti-inflammatory mechanisms by interacting with the adrenal glands and preventing the breakdown of cortisone in the body." Although research with humans is still sketchy, preliminary studies suggest that curcumin does have some benefits.

In one study, 1,200 milligrams a day of curcumin relieved morning stiffness and joint swelling in people with rheumatoid arthritis, which, like lupus, is an autoimmune disease. With curcumin supplementation, people with rheumatoid arthritis also found that they could walk faster. Moreover, the supplements didn't seem to cause any side effects.

Although no studies have established a similar connection between curcumin and lupus, Dr. Rubman observes that "lupus has enough in common with rheumatoid arthritis to make me believe that it is worth a try." It can be used initially to bring inflammation under control. "If it is going to work for you, you should feel less sensitive and have fewer aches within 24 to 48 hours," he says. You can also use it if you feel that a flare-up is coming on, he notes.

The recommended dosage of curcumin for treatment of rheumatoid arthritis is 400 to 600 milligrams three times a day, with or without food. Dr. Rubman advises using the same dosage range for lupus. If you don't notice some relief within 10 days, stop taking it. It is safe to take indefinitely, but for best results, he recommends seeking the advice of a naturopathic doctor.

Enzyme Adds Anti-Inflammatory Action

To enhance absorption of curcumin, supplement manufacturers sometimes mix it with the natural enzyme bromelain, Dr. Rubman says.

In addition to its ability to enhance absorption, bromelain has been shown to have anti-inflammatory action of its own and is frequently used for inflammatory conditions like lupus. "Bromelain can activate compounds that break down fibrin," says Dr. Rubman. Fibrin is a tissue that blocks off areas of inflammation, interrupting blood flow. The results are inadequate tissue drainage and swelling, Dr. Rubman says. Bromelain also blocks the production of certain compounds that increase swelling and cause pain when tissues are inflamed.

If you take bromelain separately, the usual dosage is 400 to 600 milligrams three times a day, says Dr. Rubman. He advises taking it at the same time that you take curcumin, and you should take them on an empty stomach. If you take bromelain with food, it will be enlisted for digestion rather than being absorbed by your body.

You can find special mixtures of bromelain and curcumin at some health food stores or obtain them from a naturopathic doctor. They're premixed in a ratio designed to reduce inflammation.

macular degeneration

What would life be like if you had macular degeneration? Well, for one thing, reading these words would be difficult or even impossible, because macular degeneration affects the macula, a tiny part of the back wall of the eye that's responsible for clear straight-ahead vision.

Loss of sight due to this disease affects more than 1.5 million Americans. Officially, it's called age-related macular degeneration because your risk for developing macular degeneration rises substantially after your sixtieth birthday. In fact, it is the number one cause of blindness in people age 60 and older.

One form of the disease, known as wet macular degeneration, makes vision deteriorate rapidly because tiny, delicate blood vessels start to grow under the macula, all the while leaking blood and fluid. For some lucky people with this type, laser treatment can destroy the new blood vessels. They won't recover the vision they've lost, but at least the deterioration won't get any worse.

The dry form is more common, affecting 90 percent of those with macular degeneration. In this type, light-sensing cells in the eye are slowly broken down. Scientists still don't know what causes this breakdown, although the free-roaming, unstable molecules called free radicals are partially to blame. There's a lot of chemical activity among oxygen molecules in the eye, and wherever those oxidative processes occur, cells are damaged by free radical action.

Even though sight loss is slower with the dry type than with the wet type, it seems to be an irreversible process. As of now, there's no medical treatment that can help.

Supplements may help slow the progression of dry macular degeneration. In ongoing research, the National Institutes of Health has undertaken an Age-Related Eye Disease Study to look at just this possibility. Among other things, the study is examining the potential role of certain vitamins and minerals in treating the disease.

Bilberry for Night Blindness

Macular degeneration isn't the only eye problem that can alter your vision for the worse. If you find that your day vision is about the same but you're having more trouble seeing at night, you may have a condition that's called, logically, night blindness.

As the name suggests, night blindness primarily affects vision in situations of low light. When you're driving after dark, for instance, you may find that you're momentarily blinded by the glare from headlights, or you may find that your eyes are slow to adjust when you move from a brightly lit room into a dim one.

Blame these difficulties on a chemical called rhodopsin. Produced in the rods of the eye—the photo receptors that help us see in low light—rhodopsin is necessary for distinguishing things that are poorly lit. If you lack rhodopsin, your night sight will be less than perfect.

As the story goes, British pilots during World War II began eating bilberry jam—made from a type of northern European blueberry—to help counteract night blindness. Searching for the active component in these dark berries, scientists found chemical substances called anthocyanins. "Blueberries, elderberries, huckleberries, and red grapes also contain this pigment," says Robert Abel Jr., M.D., clinical professor of ophthalmology at Thomas Jefferson University in Philadelphia and author of *The Eyecare Revolution*. In the body, Dr. Abel says, anthocyanins benefit the eyes by converting to rhodopsin.

You probably won't be able to find bilberries or bilberry jam in your local supermarket. You should be able to locate bilberry capsules at your local health food store or drugstore, though. Take 100 to 500 milligrams of bilberry twice a day. "Try it right before you go out at night," says Dr. Abel. "You should notice an effect within 20 minutes or so." You may take this for a month or two and see how it works for you. If you find that it's working, you can continue to take one dose of 100 milligrams before you go out at night.

While the official word isn't out yet, some practitioners already believe that it's wise and safe to take supplements for macular degeneration, particularly if you've already been diagnosed with it. Plus, since vitamins and minerals may also play a role in prevention, starting now could be your best bet to maintain healthy eyes. Be sure to get your doctor's approval, though, before you take supplements to treat this condition.

Save Your Sight with Carotenoids

Lutein and zeaxanthin are naturally occurring pigments that have a special association with the macula. In fact, these carotenoids, as they are called, actually form the visible yellow color that your doctor can detect when he examines your eyes with an ophthalmoscope.

"There is lutein actually present within the eye," says Robert Abel Jr., M.D., clinical professor of ophthalmology at Thomas Jefferson University in Philadelphia and author of *The Eyecare Revolution*. Eyes affected by macular degeneration may be lacking this lemon-colored luster.

If you eat lots of fruits and vegetables, you're already taking the right step to help lower your risk of developing macular degeneration. Fresh produce contains high amounts of yellow carotenoids, and since carotenoids are antioxidants, they can help protect the retina against oxidative damage that can lead to macular degeneration.

When you choose a carotenoid supplement, you should mimic a varied diet of fresh produce, with many healthful pigments, by looking for capsules in combination or mixed form. Also, check the label to be sure that the carotenoids come from natural sources instead of being synthetically produced, says Mark Lamden, N.D., a naturopathic doctor and adjunct faculty member at Bastyr University in Bothell, Washington. He notes that the natural types may be a little harder to find, but they may be safer than synthetics.

In addition to five or more servings of vegetables and fruits a day, people with macular degeneration should take a supplement containing 6 to 12 milligrams of lutein, recommends Dr. Abel. For best absorption, he says, be sure to take it with a meal that contains a little fat.

Try an Herbal Antioxidant

Antioxidants of all kinds, including vitamins C and E, are very effective at protecting cells from free radical damage. When it comes to macular degeneration in particular, however, there is an herbal source of antioxidants that stands out. Ginkgo, besides improving blood flow to the brain, is a macula-protecting antioxidant. Look for capsules containing standardized ginkgo extract and take 40 milligrams three times a day, says Dr. Lamden.

menopausal
changes

The changes that arise around the time of menopause may be predictable, but that certainly doesn't make them comfortable. Hot flashes and night sweats are just the beginning. Women may also experience vaginal dryness, loss of sex drive, mood swings, depression, and a host of related problems.

If you're experiencing uncomfortable menopausal changes that prompt you to see a conventional doctor, he may recommend hormone replacement therapy (HRT). Many women, however, fear the increased risks of breast cancer that go along with the therapy or find that they can't tolerate the side effects, says Lauri Aesoph, N.D., a health-care consultant in Sioux Falls, South Dakota.

If you fall into this group, you should discuss your menopausal changes with your regular doctor. In addition, there are lifestyle alterations that you can make to ensure a smoother transition and help reduce the risks of heart disease and osteoporosis that increase after menopause. Among these strategies are exercising (including weight training); keeping coffee, alcohol, sugar, and salt consumption to a minimum; eating lots of fruits, vegetables, and soy-based foods; and cutting down on stress, suggests Dr. Aesoph.

Many alternative practitioners will endorse these suggestions, and they may have others that involve diet, exercise, and lifestyle. They're also likely to recommend a number of supplements. Some address the whole range of discomforts, while others take aim at specific problems such as vaginal dryness or low sex drive. Here's an overview of what these many supplements can do and what we know about how they work.

The Estrogen Mimics

Menopause is kind of like puberty in reverse. With puberty, your body started producing larger quantities of the hormones estrogen and progesterone, among others, and you started to menstruate. In menopause, your body produces fewer of these hormones, so you stop menstruating.

By the time you get to this time of life, your body has gotten used to higher hormone levels. Thus, for some women, menopause is like going through some kind of withdrawal. To help take the pain out of the process, you can give your body a little of what it may be lacking: estrogen.

There are 300 to 400 plants, called phytoestrogens, that have estrogenic characteristics, says Dr. Aesoph. The most well researched phytoestrogen is soy, but there are also two widely used estrogen-mimicking herbs: black cohosh, and licorice.

Phytoestrogens are weaker than the body's own form of estrogen. Nevertheless, they are often powerful enough to provide some relief from hot flashes, vaginal dryness, and depression, says Willow Moore, D.C., N.D., a chiropractor and naturopathic doctor in Owings Mills, Maryland.

Getting Your Balance

Plant estrogens have a balancing effect on your body's hormones, says Dr. Aesoph. When levels are low, as they are during menopause, the phytoestrogen attaches to little cell receptors that would normally be occupied by the body's estrogen. The cell reacts as if it were receiving estrogen, and problems like hot flashes and mood swings are minimized.

"During menopause, your hormones can fluctuate dramatically," says Dr. Moore. Hot flashes and night sweats, for example, occur when estrogen levels go down and then come back up. These big swings cause your blood vessels to dilate, which in turn makes your body flush and sometimes even sweat profusely. "Women who are prone to hot flashes would probably find great relief from having balanced hormone levels," Dr. Moore says.

One way to achieve hormone balance is to eat a lot of foods that contain soy, such as tofu, soy milk, soy cheese, miso, and foods made with soy flour, says Dr. Aesoph.

Soy contains a class of phytoestrogens called isoflavones, and there are also supplements that contain these compounds. "As we learn more about the biochemistry of soy, supplement manufacturers are rushing forward to offer isoflavones in pill form. But you're still probably better off if you get your isoflavones from soy foods," says Dr. Aesoph.

Genistein is a soy isoflavone that seems to provide a benefit in addition to helping menopausal discomforts. One study suggests that it has value for helping to improve cardiac health, which often declines with the onset of menopause.

At the Baker Medical Research Institute in Melbourne, Australia, women who took 45 milligrams a day of genistein over 5- to 10-week periods had improved elasticity of their arteries—a primary indicator of cardiac health. The degree of this improvement was on a par with that of women who took conventional hormone replacement therapy.

Herbs to the Rescue

Black cohosh has a long history of use for menopausal discomfort, says Dr. Moore. A good dose to take is 40 milligrams twice a day of the standardized extract, she says. You probably won't feel relief until about two to four weeks after you start taking it. Also, you should continue taking black cohosh even after menopause ends, says Dr. Moore. She recommends taking it for six-month periods, with a month off in between.

Like other estrogenic herbs, licorice has an active ingredient that seems to increase levels of estrogen when they are low and decrease them when they are high. A safe daily dose of licorice is 5,000 milligrams, or less than ¼ ounce of powdered root, in divided doses, says Dr. Aesoph. Since taking high doses of licorice for more than four to six weeks can result in health problems, talk to your doctor before taking it.

A Chinese Remedy

Dong quai is yet another great all-around supplement to take for menopausal problems. "Many women in China and Japan who take a dose of dong quai every day, from the time they start menstruating all the way through menopause, have a reduced incidence of menstrual problems," says Dr. Moore.

Dong quai is thought to be good for relieving all kinds of female troubles, from premenstrual syndrome to heavy periods to menopausal problems, says Dr. Moore. For best results during menopause, follow the dosage directions on the package you buy, she says. The instructions for a product from Gaia Herbs, for example, are to put 30 to 40 drops in a small amount of warm water and take it three or four times a day between meals.

Dong Quai: A Versatile Helper

Dong quai is an herb that has been used for centuries in China. In fact, it is Chinese medicine's leading remedy for gynecological ailments, including hot flashes and vaginal dryness during menopause.

While no scientific studies have proven its effectiveness, dong quai has gotten a lot of mileage out of tradition and word-of-mouth recommendations. In addition to its gynecological powers, it has been used for other health problems.

It's said by Chinese herbal practitioners to improve liver function in people who have cirrhosis, relieve the back pain and inflammation of sciatica, and lessen the residual pain of shingles, a skin condition. It's also considered a mild sedative, and according to Chinese practitioners, it has anti-inflammatory and pain-relieving properties as well.

Because of this herb's increasing popularity, it is available alone or in combination with other herbs used to reduce common symptoms of women's ailments. You can find it at most health food stores.

Replenishing Progesterone

The most effective way, by far, to impact progesterone levels is to supplement with a natural form of the hormone, says Samantha Brody, N.D., a naturopathic doctor specializing in women's health in Portland, Oregon. "In addition to changing a woman's diet and exercise patterns, this is one of the best things I've found to help with menopausal discomforts," she says.

Progesterone is the hormone that affects the endometrial lining—that is, the tissue that lines the inside of the uterus. Before menopause, this hormone plays a role during ovulation, helping to prepare the endometrial lining to receive the egg. If there's no egg, progesterone helps shed the lining, which is important because more rapid shedding helps lower the risk of endometrial cancer.

Natural progesterone is usually derived from wild yam and is available over the counter as a body cream. You have to be careful, though, since wild yam must be chemically altered in the laboratory for it to be effective. Some products on the market have not been altered, so they won't be as beneficial, Dr. Brody says. "A company by the name of Emerita

Hormone Replacement Therapy— The Natural Way

In conventional hormone replacement therapy (HRT), the estrogen that's given to menopausal women is often collected from the urine of a pregnant horse. That fact alone might prompt you to go another route. You might want to try natural hormones that are manufactured from soybeans and wild yam in the laboratory and are identical to the estrogen and progesterone in the body, says Lauri Aesoph, N.D., a health-care consultant in Sioux Falls, South Dakota, who specializes in helping doctors and their patients find safe and effective ways to use and integrate natural therapies.

Plant-derived hormones have actually been around and in use for a long time. When compared to HRT, the hormones used in natural hormone replacement (NHR) offer similar relief from symptoms, says Dr. Aesoph. She notes as well that the number and severity of side effects is often lower with the natural hormones.

When a woman uses NHR as opposed to conventional HRT, she usually takes two or three types of estrogen. These are the same two or three estrogens that a woman's body makes on its own. The working names for these combinations are Bi-est and Tri-est.

Both the combinations and the estrogens used to mix them are prescription items that are prepared by a compounding pharmacist—that is, they are mixed in much the same way that old-fashioned pharmacists once for-

makes a natural progesterone cream that I recommend to my patients," she says. The product is Pro-Gest Body Cream, and it can be found in health food stores.

Natural progesterone is also available as an oil that can be absorbed under the tongue, in pill form, and as vaginal suppositories, but these are not available over the counter.

Treating the Discomforts

Some studies have found vitamin E to be effective for relieving hot flashes and vaginal complaints in menopausal women. In one, researchers found that vitamin E supplements relieved discomfort and also improved

mulated medications. If you can't locate a compounding pharmacist in your area, your doctor or practitioner can call in a prescription to one of several mail-order pharmacies. The hormones come in many different forms but are most commonly in capsules or drops.

Natural hormones are not as strong as the hormones used in HRT, so the dosages prescribed will be stronger. Dr. Aesoph advises that you work closely with your doctor for the first few months, making adjustments as necessary until you find the dose that's right for you. Also be aware that like any custom-designed product, NHR prescriptions can vary from pharmacy to pharmacy.

Hormones taken by mouth lose some of their effectiveness because they pass through the digestive system, says Dr. Aesoph. A special type of progesterone, called oral-micronized progesterone, solves this problem. Prometrium (a natural oral progesterone pill) is one brand. Some doctors also use natural estrogen or progesterone drops placed under the tongue, which is another way to bypass the digestive tract.

"Many women tolerate and like natural hormones better," says Dr. Aesoph, "so they stick with them, which is just one way that these hormones can be more effective than conventional therapy."

vaginal blood supply when taken for four weeks or longer, but supporting research is lacking, so we really don't know how it might work.

Despite this, anecdotal evidence suggests that it's worth a try. You can take vitamin E capsules orally or use vitamin E oil topically inside your vagina once a day, says Dr. Aesoph. The combination of topical and oral vitamin E, including what may be in your multivitamin, should not exceed 1,200 international units (IU) a day, she says. Take 800 IU a day orally in two separate doses until your discomfort starts to decrease, then scale back to 400 IU a day, which you can take every day for the rest of your life. You should discuss taking this amount with your doctor first, though.

You may also need vitamin C, which is important during menopause because it helps boost adrenal gland function, says Dr. Moore. Your adrenal glands, located above your kidneys, pretty much take over most of the estrogen production when your reproductive system stops, she adds. If your adrenal function is good, you might make enough estrogen to satisfy your body during menopause, which might make menopause a breeze, she says.

Experts suggest taking vitamin C along with bioflavonoids, which help strengthen veins. The recommended dose is 1,200 milligrams a day of vitamin C with hesperidin once a day during menopause. Together, these nutrients can help relieve hot flashes, regulate heavy bleeding, and reduce constipation, say herbal experts. Vitamin C and flavonoids can help put menopause in its place, adds Dr. Aesoph.

Researchers gave 94 women who had hot flashes a formula of 900 milligrams of hesperidin, 300 milligrams of hesperidin methyl chalcone (another citrus flavonoid), and 1,200 milligrams of vitamin C a day. After one month, hot flashes were reduced or relieved in 87 percent of the women. The reviews weren't entirely favorable, however, as the women reported a slightly increased body odor and sweat that discolored their clothing.

You can find vitamin C supplements with hesperidin at health food stores and drugstores.

Other Forms of Assistance

Another adrenal function booster is pantothenic acid, a B vitamin, says Dr. Moore. Taking 500 milligrams a day can help reduce depression, fatigue, and insomnia, she suggests. Continue to take it until you feel relief.

For low sex drive, you might want to try the herb Siberian ginseng, says Dr. Brody. It has been shown in some animal studies to block stress-induced decreases in sexual activity, she says. Since recommendations vary, you should talk to your doctor about how much Siberian ginseng is right for you.

Some women experience anxiety with menopause. If you are one of them, the first thing you should do is avoid caffeine and sugar, says Dr. Brody. Then, if you still find yourself wrestling with nervous tension, you might want to try kava kava, she suggests. For depression try St. John's wort, which has been shown in many studies to have a significantly positive impact for many women. Both herbs have few side effects and are safe to take for an extended period if you follow the dosage directions on the packages.

mitral valve prolapse

Things react differently to pressure, but they always react. Squeeze a toothpaste tube, and toothpaste squirts out. Put pressure on a balloon, and it pops. Push hard against a mitral valve, and you've got a case of mitral valve prolapse. This is not due to high blood pressure, however. It happens because there is something wrong with the connective tissue of the valve.

The mitral valve is located between the two left chambers of the heart. Usually it works fine, letting blood flow from chamber to chamber when the heart compresses, then shutting off like a clever trapdoor when the heart muscle expands. In some people, however, misshapen connective tissue causes real problems. When the heart compresses, the valve pops upward, almost like a parachute being snapped in the wind.

Although you may not feel the difference, a doctor can detect that slight popping sound with a stethoscope. It means that one of the fibrous cords holding the valve in place has stretched too far or that one of the two leaflets that make up the valve has become elongated, thickened, or floppy. Often it's an inherited disorder.

The valve problem may be accompanied by mood and body changes such as jumpiness, irritability, and muscle stiffness. These symptoms seem to be associated with hyperactivity in the body's autonomic nervous system, says Sidney M. Baker, M.D., a physician in Weston, Connecticut. The autonomic nervous system works without conscious control and governs the glands, the heart muscle, and the tone of smooth muscles, such as those of the digestive system, the respiratory system, and the skin, Dr. Baker says. "People with mitral valve prolapse may have a hard time adjusting to changes in their environment. They may be sensitive to noise and light, for instance."

To treat mitral valve prolapse, doctors want to reduce pressure on the valve, which is best done by keeping blood pressure normal or slightly below normal, says Decker Weiss, N.M.D., a naturopathic doctor at the Arizona Heart Institute in Phoenix. They also caution people to avoid stress as a way to help the heart work as efficiently as possible. Treatment may also relieve symptoms of irritability and anxiety.

Pharmaceutical drugs can help with all of these approaches, but natural remedies can have fewer side effects, Dr. Weiss says. If you've been diagnosed with mitral valve prolapse and want to try supplements, talk to your doctor about the following treatment options.

Magnesium—A Mineral for All Symptoms

Several studies indicate that many people with mitral valve prolapse are low in magnesium. Moreover, in one study by researchers at the University of Alabama School of Medicine in Birmingham, people with mitral valve prolapse who took 250 to 1,000 milligrams of magnesium daily had a 90 percent decrease in muscle cramps, a 47 percent decrease in chest pain, and a definite decrease in blood vessel spasms.

This study revealed other benefits, too. People had fewer heart palpitations, the rapid or irregular heartbeat that's accompanied by a fluttering sensation. Magnesium also helped to regulate heartbeat in those with a type of arrhythmia called premature ventricular contraction. People taking magnesium also reported fewer migraines and less fatigue.

It's reasonable for people to take 350 milligrams a day of magnesium, Dr. Weiss says. You have your choice of mixtures. If magnesium citrate or gluconate tends to cause diarrhea, you can take the glycinate or orotate form instead. "I've recommended as much as 1,500 to 2,000 milligrams a day to some people with severe symptoms" he says.

Magnesium has a body-wide calming effect, Dr. Weiss says. "In addition to being jumpy and irritable and nervous, many people with mitral valve prolapse also have muscle fatigue and stiffness throughout the body, and magnesium helps with all those things."

People who are going to respond to magnesium generally do so fairly quickly, within a week or less. If you have heart or kidney problems, check with your doctor before taking supplemental magnesium.

More Pump Power with CoQ$_{10}$

Along with magnesium, Dr. Weiss always recommends coenzyme Q$_{10}$ (coQ$_{10}$) for mitral valve prolapse. This vitamin-like substance is made in the body, particularly in the cells of the heart muscle. It provides an energy boost to the muscle.

If you get additional coQ_{10}, it seems to pour even more energy into the muscle cells. That means that the heart contracts more effectively, Dr. Weiss says.

CoQ_{10} also seems to help reduce stiffening of the muscle, says Peter Langsjoen, M.D., a Tyler, Texas, cardiologist who has been using the substance in his private practice to treat heart disease since 1985.

The diastolic, or filling, phase of the cardiac cycle actually requires more energy than the systolic, or contraction, phase, Dr. Langsjoen notes. "This stiffening of the heart muscle returns to normal with supplemental coQ_{10}, and many of my patients have less fatigue, irregular heart rhythm, and chest pain."

How much you need to take depends on your symptoms. Dr. Weiss starts with a minimum dose of 120 milligrams a day, divided into three 40-milligram doses. To aid absorption, he suggests taking coQ_{10} with omega-3 and omega-6 fatty acids. (For the doses of these fatty acids, see page 552.)

Dr. Langsjoen starts people on twice that much, 240 milligrams a day, and he may go as high as 360 milligrams a day divided into three doses if symptoms are severe. CoQ_{10} is expensive, so you'll want to stay with the lowest dose that relieves your symptoms, but there are no apparent side effects or toxicity related to the supplement, says Dr. Langsjoen.

Because blood and tissue levels build slowly, it takes about four to six weeks to notice improvements. "In a month, most people can tell if they're wasting their money or not," says Dr. Langsjoen. "Improvement in stamina is usually very obvious to the person and does not require any fancy testing or blood work."

CoQ_{10} is a fat-soluble supplement, and gel caps are more easily absorbed than tablets. If you do opt for the tablets, chew them with a fat-containing food such as peanut butter or essential fatty acids to maximize absorption.

Heart-Smart Fats

Dr. Weiss recommends that you cut back on the fats that can harm your heart—saturated and hydrogenated fats—and get more of two essential fatty acids that help to protect your heart. You'll need some omega-3 and omega-6 fatty acids, which are found in various proportions in fish oil, flaxseed oil, borage oil, and cold-pressed safflower or sunflower oil.

People with mitral valve prolapse should get 1,000 to 3,000 milligrams a day of a mixture of these two fats, says Dr. Weiss, which are available as gel caps.

Herbal Heart Helper

When someone's heart is additionally weakened by cardiovascular disease or congestive heart failure, Dr. Weiss may add hawthorn, an herb long known for its heart-strengthening effects. Hawthorn contains bioflavonoids, compounds that, like vitamins C and E, act as heart-protective antioxidants.

Although hawthorn is relatively safe, you should take it with medical supervision, especially if you have low blood pressure or are under doctor's orders to take other heart medications, Dr. Weiss says. The amount you'll need depends on your symptoms and the type of hawthorn you're using. For capsules, a typical dose would be 150 milligrams three times a day.

Kava Calms Jittery Nerves

If anxiety and irritability continue to be a problem even after someone has been taking magnesium for a few weeks, Dr. Weiss recommends kava, a South Seas herb. Kava eases anxiety but doesn't leave you feeling spaced-out or produce a hangover effect, he says.

Kava's talents shine in several European studies. In one, people taking 100 milligrams of kava extract three times a day for four weeks had fewer signs of nervousness. They were also less likely to report symptoms of heart palpitations, chest pain, headaches, and dizziness than people taking an inactive substance (placebo).

Dr. Weiss recommends 100 milligrams two or three times a day. Take one dose before bed to help you sleep, he suggests. See page 239 for important information about kava.

morning sickness

Not every expectant mother goes through morning sickness, of course, but those who do tend to list it among their worst experiences. Not only do they have to endure the daily bouts of nausea, they have to be very protective of the fetus that's prompting the disturbance. That means that they can't do much, particularly in the way of pharmaceuticals, to quell the nausea.

For women in this pickle, doctors may recommend some very basic procedures to settle their stomachs. For starters, eat five or six frequent meals that combine carbohydrates and proteins, says Barbara Silbert, D.C., N.D., a chiropractor and naturopathic doctor in Newburyport, Massachusetts.

For breakfast, for example, she recommends plain crackers or toast rather than a sugar-laden doughnut. Combine your plain carbs with protein such as cheese, peanut butter, or yogurt. She also recommends kefir (a type of liquid yogurt usually found in health food stores). "The key here is to always have easily digestible food in your stomach," she says.

Chewing gum might also help quell feelings of nausea, says Willow Moore, D.C., N.D., a chiropractor and naturopathic doctor in Owings Mills, Maryland.

If you still need some extra help sparing your stomach while you nurture your baby, reach for some safe, time-tested natural remedies.

A Vitamin to Settle Your Stomach

"Vitamin B_6 is the primary supplement I suggest for morning sickness," says Dr. Moore. Studies from as early as the 1940s suggest that B_6 provides effective morning sickness relief. In studies since then, researchers have found that pregnant women who take between 10 and 25 milligrams every eight hours get varying degrees of relief from their morning sickness.

In a more recent study, researchers from Columbia University's department of obstetrics and gynecology and the university's Center for Complementary and Alternative Medicine Research in Women's Health evaluated all available evidence for every type of alternative remedy for morning sickness. They concluded that acupressure, vitamin B_6, and ginger are currently the most effective.

Try taking 50 milligrams of B_6 twice a day, says Dr. Silbert. "I think the activated form of vitamin B_6, called P5P, works best." Take the supplement first thing in the morning, even before you get out of bed. Then take a second dose around lunchtime, Dr. Silbert advises. You should feel relief after the first few doses.

It might seem logical to take the vitamin as a preventive before you go to bed, but Dr. Silbert warns against it. "Several of my patients have complained of having nightmares when they took a dose of B_6 before going to bed," she says. "Just to be on the safe side, get your two doses in before the sun goes down."

Some women's nausea is so bad that they can't keep the capsule down, says Dr. Moore. Such women may need a vitamin B_6 injection. The injection has to be given by a doctor, of course, but you may not have to go back repeatedly. One injection is usually sufficient to get things under control enough so that you can start taking the supplement orally, Dr. Moore says.

The Ginger Cure

Ginger is another great nausea fighter. One study showed that 940 milligrams (about ½ teaspoon) of ginger worked as well for relieving motion sickness as the common over-the-counter remedy dimenhydrinate (Dramamine). The results of a British study suggest that ginger works as well as drugs for relieving the nausea and vomiting sometimes induced by general anesthesia and showed that it didn't have as many side effects as anti-nausea drugs.

One theory is that ginger works to prevent the gastrointestinal tract from relaying messages to the brain that trigger nausea and vomiting. Whatever the reason, it's worth a try.

While ginger ale or ginger tea might help, the most effective form of ginger is the powder in a supplement capsule, says Dr. Silbert. You can follow the dosage directions on the bottle but limit the dosage to 250 milligrams four times a day. Ginger contains some mutation-causing compounds and may not be safe at dosages higher than 1,000 milligrams a day.

multiple sclerosis

In multiple sclerosis (literally, "many scars"), the immune system acts like a troublemaking mouse living in the walls of your home. For reasons that are unknown, the immune system will attack various spots on the covering of nerve cells in the brain and spinal cord, like a mindless mouse chewing away at the vinyl coating on electrical wire.

When the fatty material that normally protects nerve endings (called myelin) is damaged or completely worn away, nerve signals sputter and sometimes go dead. Depending on where the random damage occurs, multiple sclerosis (MS) can lead to various symptoms, including blurred vision, fatigue, loss of movement, memory problems, numbness, and trouble with bowel, bladder, and sexual functions.

The standard medical approach is to give a person with MS drugs that suppress the over-revved immune system. According to some experts, however, taking certain supplements in addition to medication, under the supervision of a doctor using traditional medical therapies, may help naturally regulate a self-destructive immune response. None of these supplements promises to provide a cure, but in some cases, they seem to help control the symptoms of MS. Quite possibly, they can also help heal damaged and inflamed myelin.

Fatty Acids and Vitamin E: Truly Essential Oils

The most important nutritional strategy for dealing with MS is to get enough of the right fats in your diet while avoiding the wrong ones, says David Perlmutter, M.D., a neurologist in Naples, Florida, and author of *Lifeguide*. "This is critical in any neurological problem," he says.

Our bodies use essential fatty acids—omega-3 and omega-6—to create a trio of influential chemicals called prostaglandins. Prostaglandin 1 and prostaglandin 3 calm down the immune system. Prostaglandin 2 is more activating: It stimulates cells called lymphocytes to send up an immune response.

Normally, harmony rules in this process of creating and balancing prostaglandins. Prostaglandins 1 and 3 keep prostaglandin 2 in check. In MS, lymphocytes get too strong a message from prostaglandin 2 and react by launching attacks on the body's own nerve tissue.

From our understanding of biochemistry, it appears that you can partially control an overactive immune system by helping your body generate more of the "good" prostaglandins—numbers 1 and 3, the kind that calm down the system, Dr. Perlmutter believes. To do that, you need to start with the the essential fatty acids. Prostaglandin 1 comes from the omega-6's, which are found in evening primrose oil and borage oil. Prostaglandin 3 is made from the omega-3's, which are present in fish oil and flaxseed oil.

You can downplay the inflammatory prostaglandin 2 by avoiding saturated fat and cholesterol in your daily diet, says Dr. Perlmutter. He recommends sticking to a low-fat diet overall, so you get less than 18 percent of your calories from fat. This means that if your average daily diet provides about 2,000 calories, you should get about 40 grams of fat a day. With prostaglandin 2 discouraged by this low-fat diet, you can help the supplemental omega-3's and omega-6's do their job better. "That way, the less acceptable, less helpful fats won't be competing for absorption with the quality essential fatty acids," says Dr. Perlmutter.

By controlling this inflammation, you may be able to reduce the severity of MS, since it is an inflammatory condition.

Dr. Perlmutter suggests taking 2,000 milligrams of evening primrose or borage oil along with 400 to 500 milligrams of eicosapentaenoic acid (EPA) and 300 to 400 milligrams of docosahexaenoic acid (DHA) from fish oil each day.

When supplementing with essential fatty acids, it's important to include vitamin E, says Dr. Perlmutter. As part of your healthy oil regimen, he recommends 800 international units (IU) once a day of the vitamin E supplement that's labeled d-alpha tocopherol.

B_{12} Prevents Breakdown

Vitamin B_{12} has been used by some doctors to treat patients with MS. Although the symptoms of B_{12} deficiency mimic those of MS, the amount of the vitamin used to treat MS is far greater than the amount required simply to correct a deficiency.

The question, however, is how to take it and how much to take. Dr. Perlmutter believes that injections are necessary. "In order to achieve therapeutic blood levels, our patients are trained to self-administer 1,000 micrograms once a week," he says.

But injections might not be the only way. At least one other expert, however, says that you can get benefits from taking the supplement in pill or capsule form. Carl Germano, R.D., a registered/certified nutritionist in New York City and co-author of *The Brain Wellness Plan*, recommends 1,000 micrograms of B_{12} taken sublingually (under the tongue) once a day.

The Daily Value for B_{12} is just 6 micrograms a day—hardly one-half of 1 percent of these megadoses. Vitamin B_{12} supplements are considered very safe, Germano says. If you take amounts that are more than your system can handle, the excess is simply excreted in your urine.

Vitamin D: The Key to Prevention?

It has long been observed that MS has a strange affinity for higher latitudes, in both the northern and southern hemispheres. In the United States, people living in the north have much higher rates of the disease than those who are closer to the sunbelt.

Several studies show evidence that sun exposure might have a protective effect against the disease. The question is, Why? What is it about that big bright ball in the sky that seems to ward off an autoimmune disease like MS?

Researchers speculate that vitamin D may be the mysterious substance affecting MS risk. When skin is exposed to sunlight, the body is able to synthesize its own vitamin D. Living in a place without enough sunshine—in a far northern clime or a smog-filled city—may make it harder to get enough vitamin D from the sun alone.

The most interesting vitamin D studies involve a protein that causes a deadly, MS-like disease in mice. In one case, mice that were given high doses of vitamin D after being injected with the protein were able to resist developing the paralyzing disease.

In another test, mice that already had the MS-type disease were either injected with vitamin D or left untreated. The treated mice showed hardly any disease progression, while the untreated mice went on to become completely paralyzed. Researchers speculate that the vitamin may work by regulating immune function.

"I think vitamin D is worthy of further study for autoimmune disease," says Jay Lombard, M.D., assistant clinical professor of neurology at Weill Medical College of Cornell University in New York City and co-author (with Germano) of *The Brain Wellness Plan.* From what he's observed, says Dr. Lombard, vitamin D definitely can suppress an overactive immune system. Since that overactivity is precisely the problem when someone has MS, he sees an interesting connection.

Some Options in D

More research is needed to say whether vitamin D can actually prevent or stall MS progression in humans. Moreover, we don't know how much vitamin D would be needed to be most effective.

This vitamin is important for other reasons, however. Optimal amounts of vitamin D help make and maintain bone and may also benefit other parts of the body, including the skin and the reproductive organs.

The recommended daily amounts are 200 international units (IU) for people ages 31 to 50, 400 IU for people ages 51 to 70, and 600 IU for those over 70. The safe upper limit for vitamin D is 2,000 IU per day, but don't take this much or more without your doctor's okay.

For an additional source of vitamin D, you might consider cod-liver oil, says Alan Gaby, M.D., professor of nutrition at Bastyr University in Bothell, Washington. Anyone with MS is really getting two benefits from one source with this oil, since it has good amounts of vitamin D and is also recommended because of its fatty acid content.

muscle soreness

In a classic episode of the venerable *I Love Lucy*, Lucy had a chance to meet a slew of British royalty, including the Queen. In conscientious preparation, Lucy set out to learn a perfect curtsy. After an afternoon's practice—half deep-knee bends and half forward lunges—her over-worked muscles were frozen in curtsy position. When the moment finally came, Lucy had to be toted like a doubled-up curtsy doll to meet Her Majesty.

Very funny—right?

If you recall experiencing that kind of overstrained pain, you probably found it no laughing matter.

One culprit, whether you're practicing curtsies or working out, is lactic acid. As it builds up in muscles, lactic acid creates the soreness that we associate with overexertion. If your body's in good working order, however, it quickly purges this excess waste product, usually within an hour.

Soreness that comes a day or two after you exercise has a different source. The delayed ache is caused by tiny tears in the muscle that become inflamed. Fitness experts call it delayed-onset muscle soreness, but you probably know it as plain old pain. It's a signal from your body to slow down and take a rest. It's also part of the recovery process that actually re-sults in stronger muscles.

You can prevent sore muscles by warming up before you exercise and cooling down afterward, advises Jacob Schor, N.D., a naturopathic doctor in Denver and president of the Colorado Association of Naturo-pathic Doctors. Include at least a few minutes of movement with each of the major muscle groups—the calves, thighs, hips, back, abdomen, chest, and arms.

Once the damage is done, says Dr. Schor, you can treat the muscle with alternating hot and cold packs after the first 24 hours. The contrast in tem-peratures works like a pump to increase the flow of oxygen and nutrients

559

in the muscle. It also provides a flushing action to remove the tiny fragments of protein generated by the torn muscle.

While popping an aspirin or rubbing on a topical cream will help mask the pain, you may need much more to speed healing and help soothe the inflammation. Fortunately, Mother Nature provides an array of possibilities, and many of these natural pain soothers are in supplement form.

Do Some Damage Control

Even before your muscles seize up, you can get a jump on the healing process with bromelain, an enzyme derived from pineapple, says Dr. Schor. "If I know I'm going to be sore tomorrow—that I'm not going to want to get out of bed in the morning—I take bromelain."

Like the clean-up crew the morning after a big bash, bromelain goes in and picks up all the debris floating around your damaged muscle. When you overwork a muscle enough to cause pain, bits of muscle fiber actually break off. These tiny scraps of protein may clog the muscle and cause pain and inflammation. The body has to clean house.

Because it's an enzyme, bromelain helps by breaking down these proteins and digesting them. Once the waste products are eliminated, pain and stiffness go away, says Dr. Schor.

In an early study of the enzyme's ability to speed healing of soft tissue injuries, researchers studied the recovery process of 146 boxers. Bromelain was given to 74 of the boxers four times a day, while the remaining 72 took an inactive substance (placebo). Among 58 of the boxers who took bromelain, all signs of bruising disappeared in four days. In the control group—those who were getting the placebos—only 10 healed completely in four days.

To speed up your muscle-repair work, take 500 milligrams of bromelain three times a day between meals until the pain goes away, says Dr. Schor. If you take it with meals, bromelain's protein-digesting powers will work on your food, not on the muscle debris that's prompting your pain and inflammation.

Be sure to check the product label to make sure that it specifies a strength of to 1,800 to 2,400 milk-clotting units (mcu). "When it's not on the label, it makes me suspicious," cautions Dr. Schor. "The company may not know what it's doing, or it may have a very weak product and not want anyone to know." Bromelain is also sometimes measured in gelatin-dissolving units (gdu). Look for a range of 1,080 to 1,440 gdu.

Home-Style Ibuprofen

For all-over muscle pain, take ginger, says Dr. Schor. "It's kind of like a home-style ibuprofen."

Ginger is well-known for its anti-inflammatory properties. Like bromelain, it also contains an enzyme that can break down protein, says Dr. Schor. In ginger, this enzyme is zingibain.

Ginger has more, including various antioxidants, which help neutralize the free-roaming, unstable molecules called free radicals that play a role in causing inflammation. As a supplement, you can take ginger in tincture or capsule form. If you're in acute pain, take six 500-milligram capsules of the concentrated extract per day, says Dr. Schor.

Power Up with Antioxidants

Because your muscles produce more free radicals when you exercise, you should take supplements of vitamins C and E, says Mark Stengler, N.D., a naturopathic doctor and author of *The Natural Physician: Your Health Guide for Common Ailments*. A healthy supply of these nutrients will help minimize pain the day after your workout and will speed the healing process as your body rebuilds its muscle tissue.

To test the effects of vitamin C in preventing muscle soreness, researchers at Western States Chiropractic College gave 3,000 milligrams of vitamin C to a group of students. Another group of students received placebos. After both groups had been taking pills for three days, the students who took vitamin C developed significantly less muscle soreness after exercising than the group that took the placebos.

Vitamin C is also needed to help make collagen, the "glue" that holds muscle cells together. Following an injury, even a minor one like a sore muscle, the body needs to make more collagen to repair the damaged tissue.

Vitamin E helps reduce muscle soreness, prevent cellular damage, and repair muscle tissue.

To get your dose of pain prevention, take 2,000 milligrams of vitamin

C in divided doses each day, along with 400 international units of vitamin E, says Dr. Stengler.

Train without Pain

Siberian ginseng, an herb used by Russian cosmonauts and Asian Olympic athletes, can help you train for your next marathon—or your next curtsy before the Queen. "It's classified as an adaptogen, meaning that it helps the body adapt and recover from physical stress," says Dr. Stengler.

The herb helps the adrenal glands produce more stress hormones. Those stress hormones, in turn, help your body recover more quickly from the effects of strenuous or muscle-straining exercise.

The name Siberian ginseng is really a misnomer, since the plant is not even in the same genus as true ginseng. Still, its stimulant and tonic effects are similar to those of true ginseng. Although you may have to take Siberian ginseng regularly for a month before it begins to yield benefits, clinical studies do suggest that ginseng improves athletic performance, says James A. Duke, Ph.D., botanical consultant, former ethnobotanist with the U.S. Department of Agriculture who specializes in medicinal plants, and author of *The Green Pharmacy*.

In your quest for peak performance, take 250 milligrams of Siberian ginseng three times a day, says Dr. Stengler. While you are training, take the ginseng for four weeks, then take a break for one week. Look for a standardized extract containing 0.4 percent eleutherosides.

osteoarthritis

Just like age, osteoarthritis can creep up on you. It starts out quietly, with some occasional stiffness. Later, you may begin to feel some occasional joint pain. Human nature tells you to ignore it, but maybe you shouldn't. If you try some alternative therapies, you may be able to slow the disease before it does too much damage.

What's going on is ordinary wear and tear for the most part. Take a look at the tread on a pair of tires after you've racked up about 50,000 miles. The tires are worn, their surfaces uneven. The steel belts may even be peeking through in places.

Inside your body, it's the smooth, rubbery cushioning called cartilage that starts to erode. The gliding surface that normally acts as a shock absorber between your bones can become compressed and irregular. As the underlying cartilage and bone disintegrate, painful bone spurs can form in the joint. Ordinary movements can produce a grinding symphony of creaks and crackles.

While no one really knows what makes cartilage break down, heavy use of the joint seems to be a contributing factor. That's why osteoarthritis typically strikes the fingers, back, hips, or knees. Moreover, a joint injured in the past tends to develop arthritis sooner than one that's led a relatively pampered existence.

Scientists suspect that the damage from osteoarthritis may be due to an imbalance of enzymes in the joints. The right balance of enzymes allows for the natural breakdown and regeneration of cartilage. Too many enzymes, however, can cause the joint cartilage to break down faster than it can be rebuilt.

Among most people over age 60, signs of osteoarthritis show up in x-rays. But only about a third show any of the typical symptoms of pain, stiffness, limited range of motion, or inflammation. That's one of the puzzling things about osteoarthritis. There doesn't seem to be a relationship between the amount of pain and the degree of joint damage. Some people never have more than a mild ache. Others develop crippling pain.

Molecules on the Bestseller List

Glucosamine is a word that's pasted together from two other words that may be familiar from biology or chemistry—glucose and amine. Glucose is just blood sugar, the energizing "food" that your body uses in its cells. As for amine—well, it's not an everyday word, but in chemistry it means that nitrogen and hydrogen are glued together in the same molecule. Put it all together, and you have a word that describes a simple molecule, one that combines the stuff of blood sugar, nitrogen, and hydrogen.

Despite its simple components, this molecule is a complex contributor to your body's health, especially joint health. That's where the osteoarthritis connection comes in. One theory holds that osteoarthritis results from the body's inability as we age to make enough glycosaminoglycans, the major molecules that give cartilage its ability to bear weight, notes Amal Das, M.D., an orthopedic surgeon at Hendersonville Orthopedic Associates in North Carolina. "Your body has a hard time making glucosamine," says Dr. Das. "It would be a lot easier if your body could get that glucosamine somewhere else—say, in a supplement."

The second substance that may play a role, chondroitin sulfate, is actually built up from glucosamine. "If glucosamine is the two-by-four used

Still, arthritis is the leading cause of disability among Americans over age 15. Osteoarthritis, the most common form, affects 20.7 million people. While there aren't any miracle cures, there's a lot you can do to minimize the damage.

The Basics of Care

First, maintain a healthy weight, doctors suggest, since people with osteoarthritis are more likely to be overweight. Research shows that losing weight can significantly reduce the risk of developing it. In a large study done in Framingham, Massachusetts, women who lost an average of 11 pounds were much less likely to get arthritis of the knee over the next 10 years than women who didn't shed the pounds.

Exercise is another essential. Low-impact activities like brisk walking,

to build a house of cartilage, then chondroitin sulfate is an entire wall," says Dr. Das.

Chondroitin sulfate is a long chain of glucosamine molecules. According to Dr. Das, it helps promote water retention in the cartilage, which is necessary for shock absorption. There's a big difference in the way your body absorbs chondroitin sulfate, however. Studies show that if you take a supplement of chondroitin, your body absorbs less than 8 percent of it. By comparison, you absorb about 90 percent of glucosamine sulfate from a pill or capsule.

Although we produce our own supplies of glucosamine and chondroitin sulfate, our aging bodies can always use some help from supplements, says Dr. Das. The glucosamine in supplements comes from chitin, a compound that forms crab shells. Chondroitin sulfate is found in cartilage. Although cow cartilage is usually the source, it doesn't matter what animal the cartilage is from.

Apart from their absorption rates, another difference between glucosamine and chondroitin sulfate may lie in how they go about the business of saving cartilage from destruction. Whereas glucosamine may help with the rebuilding of cartilage to keep up with its breakdown, chondroitin may actually decrease the breakdown, says Dr. Das.

swimming, and biking are best at strengthening muscles and are easy on your joints. Stronger muscles help protect the joints by providing support and added stability.

Exercise also helps the joints absorb fluid and needed nutrients. Unlike muscle or bone, cartilage doesn't get its nutrients from blood. It soaks them up like a sponge from the fluid surrounding the joint. The more you exercise, the more you force fluid in and out of the joint.

Aspirin and other similar drugs called nonsteroidal anti-inflammatory drugs (NSAIDs) focus on nursing arthritis pain, but that pain relief isn't in your long-term interest, according to doctors. While NSAIDs are easing the pain, they can actually speed up joint deterioration. Natural measures attempt to slow the progression of the disease and preserve cartilage and bone by providing the proper nutrients in the right amounts.

A Steady Supply of Building Materials

One of the arthritis treatments that has hit the spotlight is the supplement combo glucosamine and chondroitin, two substances that your body makes to help build and protect cartilage. In studies, these supplements do appear to slow the progression of the disease and help to relieve pain. But researchers haven't found evidence that they rebuild lost cartilage.

Remember that worn tire? The way that glucosamine and chondroitin work is similar to pumping air into a punctured tire. If you can pump air into the tire as quickly as it leaks out, you can keep it from going flat, says Amal Das, M.D. an orthopedic surgeon with Hendersonville Orthopedic Associates in North Carolina.

When taken together, glucosamine and chondroitin seem to slow the loss of cartilage from the joint by pumping more cartilage-generating nutrients into the body, says Dr. Das. They don't fix the hole in the tire, however, and they don't work if the tire is already flat—that is, if there's no cartilage left in the joint.

In a study conducted by Dr. Das, people with osteoarthritis were given two tablets containing 500 milligrams of glucosamine hydrochloride and 400 milligrams of chondroitin sulfate in the morning and evening. For people with mild to moderate arthritis, the supplements decreased pain and allowed them to decrease the amount of anti-inflammatory medication they used. They did not help people who already had severe arthritis in a joint—that is, bone rubbing on bone.

Scientists believe that glucosamine somehow stimulates the cartilage cells to produce two important compounds that are the building blocks of cartilage. Once you have taken it for eight weeks, the supplement seems to provide pain relief comparable to that of ibuprofen, but without side effects.

In a study done in Europe, 200 people with active osteoarthritis of the knee took either 400 milligrams of ibuprofen or 500 milligrams of glucosamine sulfate twice a day. Although the people in the ibuprofen group got immediate pain relief, 35 percent of them experienced adverse reactions such as upset stomachs. Glucosamine took a little longer to work—about two weeks—but none of the group reported any side effects.

While the research seems to paint a clear picture of the role of glucosamine supplements, the image is still fuzzy when it comes to chondroitin, says Lauri Aesoph, N.D., a health-care consultant in Sioux Falls, South Dakota, and author of *How to Eat Away Arthritis*. Glucosamine is a small molecule that is readily absorbed. Chondroitin is huge by comparison. Ranging from 50 to 300 times larger, it is unable to pass through the intestinal wall intact. Thus, the question arises: If it's that much harder to absorb, why should you take it?

Apparently, they seem to make a good team. Although researchers aren't sure, the two supplements seem to work best together, says Dr. Das. "Chondroitin inhibits the enzyme that breaks down cartilage. We're really excited about it, because it may be the first disease-modifying agent for arthritis. It's the first medicine to give us hope."

Two to the Rescue

Because the pair works best by preserving the cartilage you have left, don't wait until you're in agonizing pain to start on a supplement program, advises Dr. Das. If you've been diagnosed with arthritis, get your doctor's approval first, then take 500 milligrams of glucosamine and 400 milligrams of chondroitin sulfate twice a day, says Dr. Das. From the time you start the double dose, allow from two weeks to four months to let the supplements do their work. You can continue to take them indefinitely.

Although the patients in Dr. Das's study took glucosamine hydrochloride, many naturopathic physicians typically recommend taking glucosamine sulfate because it is the type that has been tested most thoroughly in clinical trials.

You might see a third form of glucosamine on store shelves called N-acetylglucosamine, commonly referred to as NAG. While the label may state that NAG is better-utilized and therefore more effective than glucosamine sulfate, research has not yet been conducted that would prove or disprove that claim, says Dr. Aesoph.

"The big argument now is what form to use," she explains. "We need studies where these different forms are compared head-to-head." In the meantime, glucosamine sulfate is the supplement of choice. "The bulk of the research is on glucosamine sulfate," says Dr. Aesoph, "so we know that works."

Antioxidant Relief

Antioxidants—especially vitamin C, vitamin E, and beta-carotene—are another means of preventing your cartilage from wearing away.

"Arthritis is known to increase free radical production, so your need for antioxidant nutrients increases," says Dr. Aesoph. Those free radicals are free-roaming, unstable molecules that can set off a chain reaction in the body, aging cells prematurely and sometimes harming the genetic material. While the healing powers of antioxidants may seem somewhat mysterious, the process is crucial when it comes to protecting your joints.

If you have arthritis, antioxidants can protect joints from damage caused by oxidative stress, a process that speeds up cartilage breakdown. Joints damaged by osteoarthritis release the unstable free radical molecules that are missing an electron. Like scavengers, these highly reactive compounds look for a place from which to snatch an electron in order to stabilize themselves. They usually attack the nearest healthy molecule, which then becomes a free radical itself.

Antioxidants help break this chain reaction and stop cell damage by offering up their own extra electrons. No one is sure exactly how this process occurs in the joints, but research has shown that diets high in antioxidants help reduce pain and cartilage deterioration.

Three Protectors

Researchers in the Framingham osteoarthritis study evaluated the diets of 640 people to see if there was a link between their osteoarthritis and their intake of vitamins C and E and beta-carotene, the highly pigmented component that is converted to vitamin A in the body. The results showed that the trio of antioxidant nutrients won't prevent you from getting osteoarthritis, but it may keep it from getting worse.

After reviewing knee x-rays of the participants over a 10-year period, researchers concluded that people who had the most vitamin C in their diets were three times less likely to experience progressive deterioration of the joint. They also were less likely to develop knee pain. Vitamin E and beta-carotene also helped ailing joints stay healthier.

The benefits of vitamins C and E extend beyond their antioxidant properties. Together, they enhance the stability of components called proteoglycans that help to protect your cartilage, according to Jody Noé, N.D., a naturopathic doctor at the Brattleboro Naturopathic Clinic in Vermont. Vitamin C helps to form the structural protein known as collagen, the single most important protein in connective tissues.

To protect your cartilage and quell those aches and pains, take 1,000 milligrams of buffered vitamin C three times a day, says Ruth Bar-Shalom, a naturopathic doctor in Fairbanks, Alaska.

Studies show that vitamin E offers relief from inflammation. In research conducted by German scientists, people with osteoarthritis who took 600 international units (IU) of vitamin E every day for six weeks had significantly less pain. They also had better range of movement and were able to take fewer pain relievers. To get these benefits, include 600 IU of vitamin E and 10,000 IU of beta-carotene in your daily antioxidant regimen, says Dr. Bar-Shalom.

Crucial Cartilage Nutrients

If you're not getting the right nutrients, your body cannot make and maintain cartilage. In addition to antioxidants, five key players in the production process are pantothenic acid, manganese, zinc, copper, and vitamin D. A deficiency of any one of these can cause accelerated joint degeneration, says Sam Russo, N.D., from Brattleboro Naturopathic Clinic in Vermont.

Although many mainstream doctors view osteoarthritis as an inevitable part of growing older, naturopathic doctors contend that it is a metabolic disorder brought on by the body's inability to regenerate bone and cartilage. Taking a holistic approach to treating arthritis, a naturopathic doctor looks at imbalances that may be occurring in the whole body, then attempts to correct those imbalances. Among the factors that play a part are diet, exercise, and regular bowel movements to eliminate inflammation-producing toxins from the body.

"Permanent relief will always require lifestyle changes," says Dr. Bar-Shalom. "Just taking natural pills will not make someone healthy. It's the same as going into a really dirty house and just hanging a few pictures to try to make it look better. You've got to clean house."

Dr. Bar-Shalom customizes the diet plan for each of her patients, but in general, she suggests starting with a low-fat diet that is high in fiber and complex carbohydrates and drinking at least eight full eight-ounce glasses of water a day. Then you're ready to supplement a healthy diet with other crucial cartilage nutrients.

Pantothenic acid is one of those nutrients, according to Dr. Bar-Shalom. Without pantothenic acid, cartilage can't grow. Studies have found that supplements of this B vitamin relieved arthritis symptoms, and research with

animals has shown that if animals have a profound deficiency of pantothenic acid, their cartilage will stop growing.

Pantothenic acid is found in foods such as whole grains, legumes, fish,
and poultry. The Daily Value is 10 milligrams, but Dr. Bar-Shalom recommends 12.5 milligrams of pantothenic acid plus 50 milligrams of vitamin B_6 daily to encourage your body's ability to regenerate cartilage as it's
being lost.

Add Zinc and D

Zinc is another of the body's much-needed resources. While virtually
all cells contain zinc, some of the highest concentrations are in bone. If you
have a deficiency, your body's ability to make collagen—the "glue" for your
connective tissues—is seriously impaired.

To promote tissue repair, Dr. Bar-Shalom recommends a daily dose of
45 milligrams of zinc. Doses above 20 milligrams must be taken under medical supervision. When zinc intake is high, it can interfere with your absorption of copper, so Dr. Bar-Shalom adds 1 milligram of copper to the
daily supplement regimen.

Underneath degenerating cartilage, bone also deteriorates. Vitamin D,
a necessary nutrient for absorption of calcium, can help preserve bone and
slow the loss of cartilage, says Dr. Aesoph.

In the Framingham research, doctors also examined the influence of vitamin D levels on osteoarthritis. They found that people who had low levels
of vitamin D were three to four times more likely to experience progressive
joint damage. You can get vitamin D from exposure to sunlight or from fortified milk. If you're over 50 or have osteoarthritis, you should supplement
with 400 IU of vitamin D daily.

Turn Off Inflammation

The word *arthritis*, derived from Greek, literally means "inflammation
of the joint." While this definition certainly applies to another kind of
arthritis—rheumatoid arthritis—the term is somewhat contradictory in referring to osteoarthritis. People with osteoarthritis generally have very little
inflammation.

Nevertheless, doctors do recommend anti-inflammatory medicines such
as aspirin and ibuprofen for pain relief. Are they effective?

A Devilish Pain Reliever

Devil's claw gets its odd name from the woody fruits of the plant, which look like a clawlike hand. The active substance, a compound called harpagoside, is found in the tuberous roots. The bitter compound is used primarily by herbalists as an appetite stimulant and as a supplemental treatment for arthritis and rheumatism.

The plant grows in the savannas of southern Africa, where it is used in traditional folk medicine to treat indigestion and fevers and as a laxative. Externally, devil's claw is used to help heal sores, boils, and other skin lesions.

The herbal drug was introduced in Europe in 1953, where it has been used to treat a wide variety of conditions, including diseases of the liver, kidneys, and bladder; headache; allergies; and digestive disorders.

Extracts of the root are available in supplement form as capsules, tablets, tinctures, and ointments.

While they do relieve pain, these over-the-counter drugs, along with many prescription-strength pain relievers, take a toll on your body, says Dr. Aesoph. Their long-term use has been associated with ulcers and gastrointestinal bleeding.

"The side effect that is often overlooked is that they prevent cartilage repair," says Dr. Noé. Those pain relievers actually interfere with the way the body creates new tissue around the joints, she notes. They actually accelerate the destruction of cartilage.

Given those side effects, it certainly makes sense to look for an alternative way to stop pain and inflammation. For drug-free relief, take one tablespoon of flaxseed oil and 500 milligrams of black currant oil (or three capsules of evening primrose oil) every day, says David Perlmutter, M.D., a neurologist in Naples, Florida, and author of *Lifeguide*.

Studies show that these two supplements switch on your body's natural inflammation-fighting powers. Rich in omega-3 and omega-6 essential fatty acids, they also generate some hormonelike substances that have a beneficial effect.

"The entire process of turning inflammation on and off is controlled by a group of hormones called prostaglandins," says Dr. Perlmutter. "Basically,

Soothe with Yucca

Natives of the desert, yucca plants now dot the landscape of thousands of suburban lawns in the southwestern part of the United States. Clusters of spiny, swordlike leaves stick up from the manicured green lawns like the quills on a porcupine's back—and they can hurt just as much.

Before it became an ornamental cactus, yucca was used for centuries by the native people of North and South America to treat everything from hair loss to constipation. For those who had to contend with the limited vegetation resources of the desert, yucca provided valuable raw materials for basic household necessities like baskets, paint brushes, and soap. It was also a rich source of herbal remedies.

For birth control, Navajo women drank suds from the rotten root. The water-filled leaves from the plant were used for their laxative and sedative effects. Several tribes used the crushed root to make a shampoo to cure baldness.

Modern herbalists use yucca root primarily as an anti-inflammatory to treat arthritis. The plant contains large quantities of saponins, bitter substances that are known for their ability to foam when mixed with water. In animal studies, saponins have demonstrated an ability to reduce inflammation.

Yucca root is available in 500-milligram capsules or as a liquid.

there are two groups of prostaglandins. One group starts inflammation, and one group reduces the inflammation." By adding the right essential fatty acids to your diet, you can stimulate your body to produce increased levels of good prostaglandins and reduce inflammation, he says.

Gentle Pain Relief

Supplementing with the herb devil's claw can sometimes relieve joint pain, says Dr. Bar-Shalom. Studies have shown that this herb provides some relief from pain and inflammation.

In a German study of 54 people with chronic back pain, 9 became completely pain-free after taking 800 milligrams of extract three times a day for one month. In a comparable group that didn't take the extract, just 1 person showed the same recovery. The study suggests that devil's claw may work when traditional pain relievers fail. Most of the people had experienced back pain for 15 years even while taking conventional painkillers.

The active substance at work is harpagoside, a compound found in the tuberous roots of the plant. It reduces inflammation in the joints and helps stimulate cortisol, your body's natural version of pain-relieving cortisone. A sensible dose to start with is 400 milligrams of dry standardized extract three times a day, says Dr. Noé. Do not use devil's claw, however, if you have gastric or duodenal ulcers.

Although better known for its power to defuse migraines, feverfew also inhibits an enzyme that causes inflammation, says Betzy Bancroft, a professional member of the American Herbalists Guild in Washington, New Jersey.

To control joint pain, take 125 milligrams of standardized extract containing at least 0.2 percent parthenolide or one to three milliliters of tincture daily, says Dr. Noé.

Maybe It's All in Your Gut

Yucca, an herb with more than 40 species, is recommended for relief of joint pain, by Jill Stansbury, N.D., assistant professor of botanical medicine and chair of the botanical medicine department at the National College of Naturopathic Medicine in Portland, Oregon.

In treating arthritis, herbalists believe that yucca works best when it is used with other herbs that fight inflammation, such as ginger, turmeric, devil's claw, angelica, and willow bark.

Another theory is that the plant eases arthritis pain by reducing the absorption of wastes produced by bacteria in the intestine. "We think that arthritis might have its roots in the digestive process," says Dr. Stansbury.

A link between the gut and sore joints may sound far-fetched, but an animal study has shown that an accumulation of bacterial wastes in the intestine can impair cartilage growth. When your food is not broken down properly during digestion, undesirable bacteria can multiply rapidly and produce toxic substances called endotoxins. If absorbed through the walls of the intestine, these toxins can travel through your body and inflame the connective tissue, says Dr. Stansbury.

Naturopathic physicians believe that yucca may decrease absorption of endotoxins in the intestine. It works very gradually, however, and sometimes takes up to three months before providing signs of improvement, says Dr. Stansbury.

Yucca may be difficult to find in your local health food store. You're more likely to find it as part of an herbal arthritis formula. Dosage recommendations on the package tend to be on the low side, says Dr. Stansbury. If the formula gives a dosage range such as ½ to 1 teaspoon of liquid two to five times a day or one or two capsules two to four times a day, she recommends aiming for the high end.

Try Niacinamide—With Caution

Since the 1940s, some doctors have recommended niacinamide, a form of niacin, to treat osteoarthritis. There is growing evidence that large doses of this B-complex vitamin can improve joint flexibility and reduce inflammation.

A study of 72 people with osteoarthritis at DeWitt Army Community Hospital in Fort Belvoir, Virginia, confirmed what early research showed. After 12 weeks, symptoms improved in the group that took 500 milligrams of niacinamide six times a day. They were also able to reduce the amount of pain medication that they were taking.

The niacinamide form of the vitamin is used because it produces fewer side effects, such as the uncomfortable flushing and rash associated with niacin. How it works is still uncertain. Doctors and researchers think that large amounts of extra niacinamide somehow improve the ability of the cartilage to repair itself.

Before you stock up on this supplement, check with your doctor. The 3,000-milligram daily dose used in the study is 150 times the Daily Value of 20 milligrams. "At high doses there is a significant risk for liver damage," says Dr. Noé. "You need to be monitored by a health-care professional when you're taking high-range doses."

Anyone taking more than 1,500 milligrams of niacinamide a day should have a blood test for liver enzymes after three months of treatment, Dr. Noé advises. If the levels are elevated, the dosage will have to be reduced. Nausea is an early warning sign of stress on the liver.

osteoporosis

For some people, especially women, osteoporosis is just one of the tolls you may expect to pay for living a good long life. Gradual bone loss, which proceeds at an accelerated pace among women after the age of menopause, is a silent, unseen process. Unless you have a bone density test, you may not even be aware that it's going on. But when bones are weakened, they fracture more easily, which is often the result of osteoporosis.

We're all at risk for bone loss as we age, but women are hit the hardest. That's because bone density is strongly influenced by the amount of estrogen in a woman's body.

For about the first five years after menopause, when a woman's body stops producing as much estrogen, the rate of bone loss may be as high as 2 to 5 percent a year. The people who are most at risk are thin, small-boned women who are fair-skinned and of northern European or Asian descent, says Lorilee Schoenbeck, N.D., a naturopathic doctor with the Champlain Centers for Natural Medicine in Shelburne and Middlebury, Vermont.

Whatever your risk of osteoporosis, there's no reason to wait for a bone density test to bring you the bad news. Early steps to save your skeleton can have a big payoff in later years. The best defense you can mount is one of prevention, says Dr. Schoenbeck.

"A balanced diet and regular, weight-bearing exercise can go a long way in preventing osteoporosis," she notes. Most women don't get enough of the nutrients they need to prevent osteoporosis from diet alone, she says. That's where supplements come in.

The specific nutrients that you should consider supplementing are the minerals calcium, magnesium, and boron, plus vitamins D and K. "I always recommend that people keep a food diary for a few days so we can get an idea of their intake of calcium and other nutrients," Dr. Schoenbeck says.

Calcium: The Nonnegotiable Nutrient

Most women get about 500 milligrams of calcium a day from food, says Dr. Schoenbeck. Much of that comes from dairy sources. If you happen to be lactose intolerant and therefore avoid most dairy products, you're probably getting even less than the average. In any case, you should probably have two or three times as much calcium as you're getting from food.

"Calcium is a nonnegotiable part of every regimen I set up to help women avoid or slow the rate of osteoporosis," says Dr. Schoenbeck.

Almost every bit of calcium in your body is stored in your bones. There is also some in your blood that's used to regulate your heartbeat and keep muscle and nerve function and blood clotting at optimal levels. Your body's top priority is to maintain adequate levels of blood calcium. When these levels decline, your body will begin mining calcium from the next available source—your bones.

Knowing this, researchers have been probing to discover the optimal amount of calcium supplementation that most women need. At University Hospital in Ghent, Belgium, doctors found that a calcium intake of 1,500 milligrams a day helped protect postmenopausal women from bone loss. Another study, at Winthrop-University Hospital in Mineola, New York, showed that giving 1,700 milligrams a day of calcium to women who were past menopause significantly slowed their rate of bone loss. Other studies show calcium's protective role against osteoporosis, but there are varying estimates of how much you need to take.

Dr. Schoenbeck recommends 1,000 milligrams a day for women who haven't gone through menopause and for men of all ages. Women who are pregnant should plan on taking around 1,200 milligrams a day. Women who are in menopause or have passed through it should take 1,500 milligrams every day.

Whatever the amount you're taking, you want a supplement that provides the most easily absorbed form. Your body is better able to absorb and use calcium if it's in the form of citrate or aspartate, says Samantha Brody, N.D., a naturopathic doctor specializing in women's health in Portland, Oregon.

While some doctors say that you can get what you need from antacid tablets, Dr. Schoenbeck notes that the calcium in antacids is less absorbable than calcium citrate. Another form you'll see on drugstore shelves is calcium carbonate, but that's the least absorbable, she says.

Nutrient Combos

"Taking a calcium supplement is good, but it's not as good as taking a supplement that combines calcium with all of the other nutrients that help your body absorb and use it," says Dr. Schoenbeck. Those other valuable nutrients include vitamin D, magnesium, vitamin K, and boron.

Vitamin D helps your body absorb calcium. A deficiency of D can lead to soft bones, which in turn could lead to fractures. Studies suggest that vitamin D is related to bone mineral density. Researchers at the Institute for Research in Extramural Medicine in Amsterdam studied 81 women age 70 or older. They found that women who were given 400 international units (IU) of vitamin D for at least two years had significantly higher bone mineral densities than women who were not given any.

Research at the Jean Mayer USDA Human Nutrition Research Center on Aging at Tufts University in Boston showed that vitamin D enhances the effectiveness of supplemental calcium. Researchers in this study concluded that anywhere from 400 to 800 IU of vitamin D a day (taken with 1,000 to 1,500 milligrams of calcium) is necessary to minimize bone loss. "I recommend 400 IU a day of vitamin D to address osteoporosis concerns," Dr. Schoenbeck says.

Magnesium serves a different function than vitamin D. This mineral is important because it transports calcium to the bones. It also helps convert vitamin D to its active form in the body.

A study from Israel found that 22 of 31 postmenopausal women who were given anywhere from 250 to 750 milligrams of magnesium for 6 months, then 250 milligrams a day for 18 months, increased their bone density by 1 to 8 percent. Comparatively, a group of women who didn't receive any supplementation over the same period had rapid loss of bone density.

To figure out how much magnesium you need, just take your calcium dose and divide it in half, suggests Dr. Schoenbeck. If you're taking 1,000 milligrams of calcium, for instance, you should take about 500 milligrams of magnesium.

The least absorbable form of magnesium is magnesium oxide, says Dr. Brody. You'll do better with magnesium aspartate, she says.

Add K and Boron

Vitamin K is a bit of a forgotten vitamin. It certainly doesn't get much mention in the media, but it's very important for maintaining bone health.

It helps reduce the amount of calcium you lose through urine, says Dr. Schoenbeck.

Vitamin K is also crucial to the formation of osteocalcin, a protein that is the matrix upon which calcium is put into the bone. "Vitamin K is kind of like the foundation that calcium builds on," Dr. Schoenbeck says.

The Daily Value for vitamin K is 80 micrograms. Since this vitamin is abundant in green leafy vegetables and whole grains, a diet rich in these foods may supply you with your daily quota.

Boron, a trace mineral that is found in many vegetables and fruits, helps reduce the amount of calcium and possibly magnesium that you excrete in your urine. It may also help to slightly raise estrogen levels, which could prevent bone loss as well, says Dr. Schoenbeck. Because of that same estrogen-increasing property, however, women with breast cancer should avoid it, she says. A safe daily amount for women with no breast cancer history is three milligrams, says Dr. Schoenbeck.

overweight

If you're like many people, you're embroiled in a never-ending battle to lose weight and keep it off. The battle is often so tiresome and frustrating that advertisements about the latest magic pill that promises to melt away the fat and make you slim start to sound really good. And why shouldn't they? You think, "I'll finally be able to slip into that little black dress or designer suit that used to fit like a glove in the old days."

Unfortunately, there's no such thing as a miracle weight-loss pill. If there were, we'd all be showing off our new-found physiques. Ninety-seven million American adults are overweight or obese, and carrying around these extra pounds is putting us at risk for developing diabetes, heart disease, and cancers of the breast, ovaries, uterus, prostate, and colon. The added weight is also affecting our emotional health.

To avoid these health problems, experts say that the best action plan is to achieve a healthy weight that's right for your age and build. The fact still remains that in order to lose weight, you must burn more calories than you consume. You can do that by eating healthfully and exercising regularly. That means eating lots of fruits, vegetables, legumes, and whole grains so that your diet derives 30 percent or less of its calories from fat.

For optimal weight control, you should also get 30 minutes or more of moderate-intensity aerobic exercise such as walking, jogging, or cycling five to seven days a week. Strength training or resistance training helps, too, whether you use hand weights or exercise machines. Working with any kinds of weights increases lean muscle mass, which burns more calories than fat does and speeds up your metabolism.

None of these measures is the equivalent of a magic potion, but taken together, they're reliable weight-loss strategies. Once you adopt them, however, you may find that supplements can also work in your favor. Some nutritional and herbal supplements can help suppress your appetite, alternative medicine experts say. There are also some supplements that will help increase the rate at which you burn calories.

Fill Up with Fiber

Just as fiber-rich fruits and vegetables can help you achieve that slender waistline, so can fiber supplements. "Once you take a fiber supplement, it expands in your stomach dramatically, filling you up," says Jennifer Brett, N.D., a naturopathic doctor at the Wilton Naturopathic Center in Stratford, Connecticut. "When your stomach feels full, it sends a signal to your brain, telling it that you don't need to eat as much. The supplements diminish those hunger pangs." The best fiber supplements for weight loss are psyllium and glucomannan because they are rich in soluble fiber, says Dr. Brett.

What's more, these supplements have been shown to reduce the number of calories that your body absorbs from food each day, says Liz Collins, N.D., a naturopathic doctor and co-owner of the Natural Childbirth and Family Clinic in Portland, Oregon.

Several studies on weight loss have shown that fiber supplements can reduce the number of calories absorbed by the body each day by 30 to 180 calories. That adds up to approximately 3 to 18 fewer pounds a year.

Dr. Brett says that glucomannan is the best fiber supplement you can buy because it has more fiber in each pill than psyllium. Take one glucomannan pill 20 minutes before each meal, she says, or two or three capsules of psyllium or two chitin supplements before meals. Drink at least eight ounces of water with each dose to prevent constipation.

Get Lean with Chromium

Research shows that chromium picolinate, a supplemental form of chromium, can build muscle mass and reduce fat in people who exercise. The more muscle you gain, the more calories you'll burn each day.

Chromium also helps your body turn carbohydrates and fats into energy. Moreover, it improves the effectiveness of insulin, the hormone that allows cells to pick up blood sugar that your body needs for fuel from the bloodstream. As a result, blood sugar levels are kept under control. Your energy soars, you crave fewer sweets, and your body's sensitivity to insulin increases, which is key for successful weight loss, says Dr. Brett.

In a study at the University of Texas Health Science Center, 154 participants were asked to drink two servings daily of a protein/carbohydrate drink. Fifty-five received plain drinks, 33 received drinks containing 200 micrograms of chromium picolinate, and 66 received drinks containing 400 micrograms of the mineral. Body composition was measured before and after the study.

The study continued for two-and-a-half months. In the end, researchers found no significant changes in body composition in those who received the plain drinks. Participants who received 200 or 400 micrograms of chromium picolinate daily showed significant increases in muscle mass and reductions in body fat.

Although this study suggests that chromium picolinate can be helpful as a weight-loss aid, other studies suggest that you also need to exercise regularly while taking the supplement if you want to reduce fat and improve muscle tone. Dr. Brett suggests taking 200 to 400 micrograms of chromium picolinate daily, but doses this high must be taken under medical supervision.

An Herbal Fat Burner

In health food stores, you'll find several herbs that claim to be the answer to all your weight-loss problems. The truth is, many don't live up to their claims, and some are downright dangerous. Kelp is one herb, however, that may actually help whittle away extra pounds when combined with a low-fat diet and daily aerobic exercise, says Ellen Evert Hopman, a professional member of the American Herbalists Guild, a lay homeopath in Amherst, Massachusetts, and author of *Tree Medicine, Tree Magic*.

Kelp is a type of seaweed that's rich in antioxidant vitamins and iodine. It is believed to stimulate a hormone produced by the thyroid gland that's responsible for boosting metabolism, so you'll burn more calories by the hour, says Hopman. You can also get other kinds of seaweed in your diet by adding them to soups and salads, she says.

If you take kelp, just follow the instructions on the bottle. While it's completely safe for most people, you should check with your doctor before taking it if you have a thyroid disorder, high blood pressure, or heart problems, says Hopman.

Parkinson's disease

When doctors describe Parkinson's disease in clinical terms, they talk about symptoms like tremor, slowed movement, and muscle rigidity. These symptoms are far more than minor inconveniences. With Parkinson's, all of the little details that make us who we are—a jaunty gait, a sarcastically raised eyebrow—are slowly stripped away. Even a signature changes, since it becomes impossible to write with the usual flourish.

We don't know for sure what causes Parkinson's disease to affect some people and not others. It's clear, though, that symptoms are due to progressive destruction of cells deep inside the part of the brain called the substantia nigra, the area that controls movement. These cells normally produce dopamine, a chemical that transmits nerve signals to muscles. The death of these cells causes reduced dopamine levels, which in turn lead to the faulty muscle control that's characteristic of Parkinson's.

Many experts believe that Parkinson's disease comes from a combination of two malevolent forces—poor genes and a toxic environment. In some people, genetic messages carried from generation to generation allow them to detoxify cells—that is, dispose of any harmful components that might damage the cells. In someone who has a less-than-perfect ability to detoxify cells, nerve cells could be easily damaged.

Maybe that's not the whole story, however. There's also the possibility that certain toxins in the environment contribute to the problem. If we are overexposed to those toxins and they make their way to the cells, it's a recipe for progressive cell damage that leads to cell death.

Could the toxins contained in pesticides be adding to our susceptibility to Parkinson's? "The incidence of this disease is dramatically higher in farmers and other people who've had pesticide exposure," says David Perlmutter, M.D., a neurologist in Naples, Florida, and author of *Lifeguide*. He has noted that in general, rates of Parkinson's are rising with rates of pesticide use around the globe.

You can reduce your risk for Parkinson's as well as slow its progression in two basic steps, Dr. Perlmutter believes. First, protect your brain cells from damage by taking antioxidants, then boost your body's ability to dispose of toxins. That can be done by taking supplements that target the liver and intestines as well as the brain, he says.

If you've already been diagnosed with Parkinson's, you should know that none of the remedies that follow are substitutes for any medication your doctor may prescribe. If they are started early enough, however, Dr. Perlmutter believes that they can help prolong the time before medication becomes necessary. If you're already taking prescription drugs, adding supplements like these is a safe and effective way to help keep your symptoms from getting worse, he says. Even so, be sure to inform your doctor about any supplements that you're taking, since some can interact with prescription medicines.

Antioxidants Are a Must

Free radicals—the free-roaming, unstable molecules that harm cells—and the damage they do are associated with Parkinson's in two ways. Excess free radicals may contribute to development of the disease in the first place. Then, once Parkinson's is under way, experts believe that the disease progression generates a wave of one kind of highly toxic free radical known as peroxynitrite.

Also, research has shown that Parkinson's symptoms are likely to be worse when there are not enough antioxidant nutrients in the body. "Studies on this topic have been done since 1984," says Dr. Perlmutter. "Using antioxidants to treat this disease is not new."

One study on antioxidants and people with early Parkinson's showed the result of high-dose supplementation with the high-powered antioxidants vitamin E and vitamin C. When people with early Parkinson's took those vitamins, their need for medication was delayed for up to two-and-a-half years.

Another study published two years later looked at the effects of vitamin E alone, but this time, there was no benefit from supplementation. Researchers believe they can explain the apparently contradictory results by the fact that antioxidants, particularly vitamins C and E, work much better in tandem.

Experts who recommend supplements for Parkinson's agree that higher-than-normal amounts of these nutrients are often needed. Dr. Perlmutter

Lipoic Acid Boosts Vitamin Power

When you're battling Parkinson's disease, you need to call in the big guns. According to Carl Germano, R.D., a registered/certified nutritionist in New York City and co-author of *The Brain Wellness Plan*, lipoic acid is just the weapon for the job.

Lipoic acid is a unique substance. It isn't really considered a vitamin because the body usually makes enough on its own, and what the body doesn't make, it can get from food. In certain crisis situations, however, supplements of this special antioxidant can add some power.

The other supernova antioxidant stars are vitamins E and C. Vitamin E is fat-soluble, while vitamin C is water-soluble. In other words, vitamin E travels in a medium of fat molecules, while vitamin C needs a water medium to move about. Because of that exclusivity, each of these vitamins has a limited way to travel, which in turn limits the tissues on which either of them alone can have an effect. Lipoic acid, on the other hand, is both fat- and water-soluble, giving it an edge when it comes to protecting brain tissue, which is made up of both fatty and nonfatty tissue, says Germano.

That's not all. Lipoic acid is also a "recycler" that keeps vitamins E and C in their active forms. It may also help raise levels of glutathione, according to a study by researchers at the University of California at Berkeley. This important substance is produced throughout the body, but people who have Parkinson's often have a shortfall.

The dose of lipoic acid that Germano recommends for people who have Parkinson's, 200 milligrams daily, appears to be completely safe. In studies, no harmful effects showed up in people who took as much as 800 milligrams daily for four months. This supplement can be dangerous for people who are thiamin deficient, however. If your doctor determines that you have a thiamin deficiency, you should take a B-complex vitamin that contains thiamin whenever you begin taking doses of lipoic acid.

recommends 4,000 milligrams of vitamin C a day. Since this vitamin doesn't stay in the body very long, you should take it in two separate doses of 2,000 milligrams each. Combine that with a once-daily dose of 800 international units of oil-based vitamin E, he suggests.

Another antioxidant supplement to consider is lipoic acid. Although your body makes lipoic acid and you get some from food, there's evidence that some people have a shortage of it. Having enough lipoic acid is important because it helps prolong the effectiveness of vitamins E and C. To help mount your defense against Parkinson's disease, take 200 milligrams of lipoic acid daily with a meal, recommends Carl Germano, R.D., a registered/certified nutritionist in New York City and co-author of *The Brain Wellness Plan*.

Put Ginkgo on Guard

Ginkgo, the popular "memory herb," boosts blood circulation to the brain, but it appears to have additional positive effects on gray matter. In particular, it may offer hope for people with Parkinson's.

Studies have shown that animals exposed to a neurotoxin called MPTP will develop symptoms that are identical to those of Parkinson's disease. When they are pretreated with ginkgo extract, however, they don't develop the symptoms, says Dr. Perlmutter.

Ginkgo performs its guardian gig through a process of membrane stabilization. By stabilizing nerve cell membranes, it helps prevent a breakdown of communication between the nerve cells. "It allows neurons to communicate with each other more readily," concludes Dr. Perlmutter.

Ginkgo has antioxidant properties that come in quite handy as well. "Ginkgo blocks the formation of free radicals that would otherwise be stimulated into destroying brain cells," says Dr. Perlmutter. Take 60 milligrams of ginkgo extract twice a day, he suggests.

Call on Coenzyme Q_{10}

Coenzyme Q_{10} (coQ_{10}) is a chemical with a dual personality. Not only does it help generate energy inside the microscopic cell bodies called mitochondria, it also functions as a powerful antioxidant.

CoQ_{10} is most often associated with treating heart disease, but people with Parkinson's should take note as well, says Germano. A study by Harvard Medical School researchers showed that coQ_{10} protects certain neurons in the brain from the substance that produces Parkinson's damage, according to Germano.

In terms of its antioxidant ability, coQ_{10} gives superhero vitamin E a run for its money. In fact, coQ_{10} appears to go one step farther than E, protecting not only the outer membranes of cells but their inner components as well. In this way, it may be able to defend vulnerable DNA (cell genetic blueprints) from the oxidative damage that seems to cause Parkinson's, says Germano. He recommends taking 200 milligrams of coQ_{10} once a day with a meal.

Lift Liver Function with a Helpful Herb

Parkinson's disease is often regarded as strictly a brain disorder, but addressing only the brain may mean missing out on other ways to ease the disease. "You need to look at the entire picture," says Germano. "There are many pathways to this disease." That means that there are many paths to healing as well.

When the body is dealing with the negative effects of a possible overload of toxins such as pesticides, liver function is crucial. In fact, Dr. Perlmutter believes that healing the liver can bring dramatic improvement to people who have Parkinson's. "I have patients diagnosed with this disease in their thirties who respond beautifully to liver detoxification," he says.

One herb that's linked to liver health is milk thistle. This herb, and the extract it yields, silymarin, are said to be powerful liver protectors. For anyone who regularly deals with pollutants like pesticides and who may thus be at higher risk for Parkinson's, milk thistle is one of several herbs recommended by Germano. Take up to 300 milligrams of standardized milk thistle extract daily, he says.

Be Free of Dangerous Debris with Fiber

The liver isn't the only body organ that processes toxins. Properly functioning intestines are also very important for whisking unwanted, potentially dangerous substances out of the body, says Dr. Perlmutter.

Unfortunately, many people who have Parkinson's—who may have impaired detoxification abilities to begin with—also show signs of constipation, according to Jay Lombard, M.D., assistant clinical professor of neurology at Weill Medical College of Cornell University in New York City and co-author (with Germano) of *The Brain Wellness Plan.*

You could say that dietary fiber comes from the whisk in the whisk broom, since it's the indigestible rough part of fruits, vegetables, beans, and whole grains—and it does a pretty fair broom imitation. Ample fiber in your diet cleans out the colon. Waste products—and possibly pesticide residues—have less time to corrupt sensitive intestinal walls.

The Daily Value for fiber is 25 grams. To reach that amount, make it a point to eat more unprocessed foods, including fresh produce and whole grains. You may need to go one step farther, though. "Almost every one of my Parkinson's patients is on some form of supplemental fiber," says Dr. Lombard. If you've increased your dietary fiber but are still experiencing constipation problems, ask your doctor about healthy fiber supplements like Metamucil or Citrucel.

phlebitis

Phlebitis is inflammation of a vein, usually caused by a clot that forms in the vein due to poor circulation. When the clot forms, blood flow is blocked, causing pain and swelling.

Often, someone who has phlebitis can actually feel a lump under the surface of the skin where the blood-distended vein is bulging. It may feel like a hard, painful knot or a sore, bruised spot. If the clot occurs very close to the surface of the skin, a red streak may be visible.

If you suspect that you have phlebitis, you need to get a medical diagnosis, followed by appropriate treatment. With the type called deep-vein phlebitis, there is a risk that the clot will dislodge and move to your heart, brain, or lung, where it can do extensive damage. Don't delay having it diagnosed, monitored, and treated by your doctor.

If you've had phlebitis in the past, however, there are ways to prevent a recurrence. Just moving around can help. So can elevating your legs when you sit down to rest, getting regular exercise, and wearing surgical pressure stockings.

If you're prone to phlebitis, you don't want to sit anywhere for very long. Sitting still for more than a couple of hours at a time can cause phlebitis in someone who's susceptible to the problem.

Along with those precautions, some supplements may help prevent phlebitis. They can reduce the tendency of your blood to clot, improve blood circulation in your legs, and help keep your legs from swelling with fluid. Just be sure to check with your doctor before trying these remedies.

Take Bromelain to Stop Clots

The blood-thinning and anti-inflammatory properties of bromelain, an enzyme derived from pineapple, work together to help prevent a recurrence of phlebitis, says Decker Weiss, N.M.D., a naturopathic doctor at the Arizona Heart Institute in Phoenix. In a study of 73 people with a severe kind of phlebitis who took bromelain along with a pain reliever, researchers found that all symptoms of inflammation decreased, including pain, swelling, and elevated skin temperature.

"Bromelain is a potent inhibitor of platelets, components in blood that promote clotting," Dr. Weiss says. The enzyme prevents platelets from sticking together and also helps keep them from adhering to the sides of blood vessels.

Bromelain also declares war on fibrin, which is a protein at the core of the clotting process. By breaking down fibrin, the enzyme counteracts clot formation.

Dosages of bromelain typically range from 500 to 1,000 milligrams a day, says Dr. Weiss. To get the best effect, take a divided dose four times a day on an empty stomach, he advises. If it's taken with food, bromelain will simply act as a digestive enzyme rather than helping to prevent clotting.

Spices and Herbs as Add-Ons

Curcumin, a yellow pigment that comes from the Indian spice turmeric, acts as a strong natural anti-inflammatory and anti-clotting agent, says Dr. Weiss. Its anti-clotting properties resemble those of aspirin, which is commonly prescribed to help thin the blood and improve blood flow. "I like to use a mixture of curcumin and bromelain instead of aspirin with my patients," he says.

Dr. Weiss first prescribes a mixture of bromelain and curcumin, along with anticoagulants (blood thinners), to dissolve a clot. Once the clot is dissolved, he advises people to continue taking bromelain and curcumin. At the same time, he keeps them on an exercise program that includes yoga, and he prescribes hot and cold packs after the blood thinners have been discontinued. Usual doses of curcumin are 400 to 600 milligrams a day, which can be taken for up to three months without adverse effects, says Dr. Weiss. Do not take curcumin supplements if you are pregnant, however.

Ginger is another spice that can help prevent a recurrence of phlebitis. It also has strong anti-clotting and anti-inflammatory powers, Dr. Weiss says. You can buy ginger in capsules. To reduce inflammation, you may need to take about 2,000 milligrams a day of dry powdered gingerroot, he says.

Vitamins to Help the Flow

Researchers now realize that an amino acid by-product called homo-cysteine can harm the insides of blood vessels, increasing the risk of athero-sclerosis (hardening of the arteries). Homocysteine can also raise your chances of developing a blood clot, according to research.

In one study, researchers were able to reduce high homocysteine levels using 5 milligrams of folic acid, 400 micrograms of vitamin B_{12}, and 50 milligrams of vitamin B_6. "I recommend B vitamins to all my patients with heart or circulatory problems as part of a high-potency multivitamin," Dr. Weiss says.

The same antioxidant nutrients that are recommended to help prevent heart disease are also good if you have phlebitis, he adds. Vitamin E helps to reduce platelet stickiness, which means that you'll be less likely to have clotting. Studies suggest that reducing platelet stickiness with vitamin E could help treat people who have traveling blood clots, particularly those who have type 1 (insulin-dependent) diabetes and thus are at higher risk for clotting problems.

Vitamin C is essential because it helps to regenerate vitamin E, and both vitamins also help to reduce inflammation. Dr. Weiss recommends 400 to 800 international units a day of vitamin E and 1,000 to 3,000 milligrams a day of vitamin C in divided doses. Before you take that much vitamin E, however, you should check with your doctor, particularly if you are taking anticoagulants or aspirin.

PMS and menstrual problems

For many women, monthly periods mean monthly discomfort. As their periods approach, they regularly experience mood swings, headaches, cramping, diarrhea or constipation, acne, and fatigue. Many of these signs point in one direction—to the notorious problem known as premenstrual syndrome (PMS).

If you have PMS, you can almost count on feeling bloated, sore, and headachy every month, plus you're likely to have predictable cramping. During your period itself, you might have cramping and heavy bleeding. For many of these problems, alternative practitioners recommend some lifestyle changes, along with herbs, minerals, and other supplements.

Defense Tactics

To help defuse PMS symptoms, cut down on or steer clear of coffee, chocolate, soda, and sugar-laden foods, says Barbara Silbert, D.C., N.D., a chiropractor and naturopathic doctor in Newburyport, Massachusetts. Instead, experts recommend that you go for a diet that's full of fruits, vegetables, and fiber.

Foods that contain soy, such as tofu, miso, and soy milk, can help your body deal with the hormonal shifts during the menstrual cycle, says Samantha Brody, N.D., a naturopathic doctor specializing in women's health in Portland, Oregon. Regular exercise can also go a long way toward curbing PMS.

If you're having any kind of menstrual problems, it's always important to keep your physician informed, says Dr. Silbert. She cautions that supplements can't take the place of a doctor's care. If your cramps or blood flow are excessive enough to disrupt your life, be sure that your doctor knows about your symptoms before you start taking supplements.

A Hormonal Balancing Act

One possible cause of cramps and heavy bleeding during periods is an unbalanced ratio of estrogen to progesterone, says Willow Moore, D.C., N.D., a chiropractor and naturopathic doctor in Owings Mills, Maryland. These are the two hormones that play the biggest part in regulating the female reproductive system. Usually, women who experience problems with their periods have too much estrogen and not enough progesterone in the one to two weeks before their periods. This imbalance can set the stage for painful cramping and heavy flow, along with other unwelcome symptoms such as headaches and mood swings.

Supplements that balance estrogen and progesterone can make a big difference in how you feel before and during your period, says Dr. Moore. Along with soy foods, an herb that is believed to have a positive effect on hormone balance is chasteberry. In two surveys of doctors in Germany, chasteberry was rated as "very good" or "good" for treating PMS symptoms, from bloating and cramping to mood swings. Of the 1,500 women included in the studies, one-third reported having no PMS symptoms after being on chasteberry extract for an average of 166 days. Another 57 percent said they had significant improvement.

A Chasteberry Boost

Chasteberry seems to help by stimulating progesterone production. When that happens, your hormone levels start to stabilize and you begin to feel a lot better, says Lauri Aesoph, N.D., a health-care consultant in Sioux Falls, South Dakota.

Chasteberry comes in capsules. A normal dose is 175 to 225 milligrams a day. Be patient, though, advises Dr. Aesoph, since it may take about three months to work. If you are taking birth control pills, she suggests that you try a different remedy, since chasteberry may counteract the effectiveness of oral contraceptives.

More Herbal Help

Licorice works to balance estrogen, says Dr. Aesoph. It can also increase progesterone by inhibiting its breakdown, and it may help prevent bloating. Since high levels of estrogen can cause many menstrual problems, licorice often helps by decreasing the amount of estrogen in your body, says Dr. Moore. Alternative practitioners believe that when your estrogen levels are

Chase PMS with Chasteberry

Chasteberry has been used since Greco-Roman times, most frequently to treat women's ailments. The berries come from a tree that is native to the Mediterranean region. As you might guess from its name, it was also once used to suppress sexual urges.

Today, chasteberry extract is popularly used to help relieve symptoms of PMS, along with menopausal discomforts and certain menstrual problems such as the absence of periods.

Chasteberry isn't for everyone, however. If you experience depression, you may want to avoid chasteberry because it could worsen depression, says James A. Duke, Ph.D., botanical consultant, former ethnobotanist with the U.S. Department of Agriculture who specializes in medicinal plants, and author of *The Green Pharmacy*.

Chasteberry has been approved in Germany for treating menstrual problems, PMS, and breast tenderness. The fresh herb is available, and you can also find it in tinctures and capsules.

---

too high, the weaker form of plant estrogen found in an herb such as hops and in soy isoflavones takes up receptors that would normally be occupied by your body's much stronger estrogen. When these sites are occupied by plant estrogen, some of your body's estrogen has nowhere to go, so it is excreted as waste.

If you want to try licorice, follow the directions on the package, says Dr. Aesoph. A typical dose for PMS is 250 to 500 milligrams once a day, beginning 14 days after the first day of your period and continuing until your next period begins—essentially the two weeks prior to the start of your period. Since licorice can have some side effects, check with your doctor before taking it.

Black cohosh is another hormone-regulating herb that's often used for women's health problems, says Dr. Aesoph. In one study, researchers analyzed the effects of a standardized black cohosh extract that's been used in Germany for more than 40 years. They found that it reduced depression, anxiety, and mood swings in women with PMS.

If you take black cohosh, follow the dosage directions on the package you buy, says Dr. Aesoph. A typical dose would be 20 milligrams in the morning and 20 milligrams in the evening.

The Chinese Solution

Dong quai is an herb that's long been used in Chinese medicine for various women's ailments. One of its primary benefits is its ability to relieve cramps by helping the uterus relax. Dong quai can also help reduce menstrual blood flow, says Dr. Moore.

If you'd like to try dong quai, it's available in most health food stores. Just follow the dosage directions on the package you buy. (A typical dose might be one or two 550-milligram capsules twice a day.) Practitioners usually recommend taking it from 14 days after a period begins until the start of your next period. Do not take dong quai while menstruating, as it can increase blood loss.

Clearing Up Cramps

"Cramps are very common among menstruating women," says Samantha Brody, N.D., a naturopathic doctor specializing in women's health in Portland, Oregon. Fortunately, you may not have to resort to over-the-counter pain relievers to get them under control.

One of the first things you should do is back off on consuming chocolate, coffee, soda, and anything else with caffeine, says Dr. Silbert. These types of foods can lead to cramps.

Menstrual cramps have also been associated with sugar and refined carbohydrates, adds Dr. Brody. After making these dietary changes, consider trying some of the best cramp relievers around—magnesium, calcium, vitamin B_6, and feverfew.

Calcium works wonderfully to relieve some women's cramps. According to a study at Metropolitan Hospital in New York City, 73 percent of women who took 1,000 milligrams of calcium a day for at least a month experienced fewer PMS symptoms than they had previously. The research suggests that the calcium helped reduce breast tenderness, headaches, and abdominal cramps. Researchers think that these benefits stem from calcium's ability to relieve muscle contractions. A good daily dose is 1,000 milligrams, says Dr. Moore.

Like calcium, magnesium helps relieve muscle contractions, says Dr. Moore. Some studies have found lower levels of magnesium in women who have PMS. Other studies suggest that increasing magnesium can ease or eliminate PMS symptoms.

Taking 500 milligrams of magnesium a day may help ease the pain, says

Dr. Brody. Too much magnesium, though, can cause diarrhea. If that happens, reduce your intake to a level that your body can tolerate.

Do You Need B₆?

Vitamin B_6 is a good supplement to take because it helps your body retain the cramp-relieving magnesium, but that's not the only reason you should consider it. Some research suggests that vitamin B_6 supplementation can also decrease cramps if you're deficient in it, says Dr. Silbert.

Best of all, there's a little test that you can do to see if you may be lacking this vitamin, says Dr. Moore. Before you get out of bed, try to curl your fingers down to touch your palm where your fingers join. Your fingers should be as curled up as you can get them in this position, she says. If you can't bend your fingers enough to make them touch your palm, you should probably consider taking B_6, she says.

Taking 50 milligrams of B_6 twice a day should help, says Dr. Silbert. "I recommend taking a dose with breakfast and another with lunch. Whatever you do, though, don't take it near bedtime. It seems to cause nightmares in some women."

Many women's bodies have trouble converting this vitamin into a usable form, says Dr. Silbert. She often recommends P5P, which is short for pyridoxal-5-phosphate, because it is easier to convert. Dr. Silbert suggests taking 50 milligrams of P5P instead of straight B_6.

Many antispasmodic and anti-inflammatory herbs are also used to relieve cramps, says Dr. Silbert. She often recommends feverfew. Some research suggests that this herb helps lessen pain by preventing the formation of prostaglandins, chemicals that are a critical part of the chain that creates the sensation of pain.

Take the amount indicated on the package on the days that you experience cramping, says Dr. Silbert. A typical dosage of feverfew is 125 milligrams three times a day.

Supplements for Heavy Bleeding

Life is busy enough without having to worry about embarrassing accidents. Luckily, there are a lot of supplements that you can try individually or in combination to stem heavy menstrual flow. A few of these are yarrow, shepherd's purse, iron, vitamin C, and bioflavonoids.

Shepherd's Purse Helps with Heavy Flow

The herb called shepherd's purse has strong astringents, which are compounds that constrict blood vessels. That astringent action can help to stanch the flow of blood by encouraging blood clots to form, says Matthew Wood, a professional member of the American Herbalists Guild in Minnetrista, Minnesota, and author of *The Book of Herbal Wisdom*.

From the time of Hippocrates until World War I, shepherd's purse was used to close bleeding arteries. It has also been used by midwives around the world from antiquity to the present to slow or stop blood loss from labor and childbirth.

A relative of the mustard plant, shepherd's purse is safe to take for long periods. With the consent of a doctor, women can take it during labor and delivery, says Wood.

Other uses of shepherd's purse also relate to bleeding. Some practitioners recommend it for chronic internal bleeding problems, such as blood in urine or stools, and for mild bladder infections, midcycle bleeding, and heavy menstrual bleeding. (If you notice blood in your urine or stools, however, see your doctor.) The French take it orally or put it into their baths to treat varicose veins and hemorrhoids. You can purchase it in tincture form or use the fresh herb for tea.

Yarrow and shepherd's purse are two herbs that can help stem bleeding. But how do you decide which one to take?

Yarrow works best for women who have bright red blood flow, says Matthew Wood, a professional member of the American Herbalists Guild in Minnetrista, Minnesota, and author of *The Book of Herbal Wisdom*. It also tends to be more effective in women who have strong, robust constitutions, he says. Shepherd's purse, on the other hand, is best-suited for women whose flow is more clotted and who have milder temperaments.

Both are astringents that promote rapid blood clotting to slow or stop excess blood loss. Two clinical studies suggest that shepherd's purse is an effective remedy for heavy menstrual bleeding. Whichever remedy you decide to try, you'll need to take it every day, says Wood. But he cautions against using shepherd's purse if you have kidney stones.

"You'll know within six weeks if it's working," he says. If you don't see any results in that time, switch to another remedy or consider seeing a doctor. Since concentrations vary by product, Wood recommends using a tincture and following the dosage instructions on the label.

Iron Things Out

Iron is probably the most important mineral you can take to help control menstrual blood loss, says Dr. Brody. Heavy menstrual flow can deplete your body's iron stores, and some researchers also believe that chronic iron deficiency may cause heavy bleeding.

In one study, 75 percent of women who supplemented with iron had decreased menstrual blood flow compared with only about 33 percent in a group that took inactive substances (placebos). Thus, iron might just be the answer to your heavy bleeding problems. Do not take more than the Daily Value of iron (18 milligrams) on your own, though, says Dr. Brody. You must be tested for iron deficiency before supplementing with higher doses.

Get a C-Plus

Two other supplements for heavy bleeding are vitamin C and bioflavonoids, says Liz Collins, N.D., a naturopathic doctor and co-owner of the Natural Childbirth and Family Clinic in Portland, Oregon. Vitamin C can significantly increase iron absorption, so it goes in tandem with an iron supplement, but the combination of vitamin C and bioflavonoids is better yet, according to Dr. Collins.

If you're prone to excessive menstrual bleeding, it might be the result of fragile blood vessels. Vitamin C and bioflavonoids may strengthen those blood vessels and make them less susceptible to damage. In one study, for example, 14 out of 16 women who supplemented with 200 milligrams of vitamin C three times a day along with bioflavonoids found relief from heavy bleeding.

Dr. Collins recommends taking 500 to 1,000 milligrams of vitamin C three times a day and 500 to 1,000 milligrams of bioflavonoids once a day.

prostate problems

If you're the kind of guy who never gives your prostate gland much thought, chances are that you will by the time you reach your late forties or early fifties.

Due to a variety of hormonal changes associated with aging, the walnut-size gland that lies below the bladder may decide to start growing in ways that aren't exactly comfortable. The gland surrounds the urethra, the tube that carries urine from the bladder to the penis, so the prostate's little uninvited growth spurt puts some pressure where you don't want it.

As the prostate balloons in size, it puts pressure on the urethra. You may feel the urge to urinate more often, your bladder may still feel full after you've finished urinating, your stream may be weak, or you may find it difficult to get things going and keep things flowing.

The sum of all these annoyances is a condition called benign prostatic hyperplasia (BPH). Like it or not, men have more than a 50 percent chance of developing BPH in their lifetimes.

Fortunately, BPH isn't a sign of cancer, nor does it indicate that you'll develop cancer somewhere down the road. In fact, BPH is treatable. Not only that, there are things you can do to help minimize the problems it causes if you're willing to make a few adjustments in your diet and lifestyle.

Foods to Favor

Eating less red meat and increasing your consumption of fruits, vegetables, and soy foods are good ways to start. Soy foods such as soybeans, tofu, soy milk, tempeh, roasted soy nuts, and roasted soy nut butter are rich in plant compounds called phytosterols, which studies have shown to lower the risk of prostate enlargement.

While you're getting more of these soy foods, you should also try to lower your intake of high-fat foods and alcohol. A diet high in saturated fats and low in plant foods can contribute to an enlarged prostate, and alcohol increases urine production, which can create more congestion in the prostate.

To strengthen your protection against BPH, there is a variety of nutritional supplements that may be helpful. Certain herbs and the trace mineral zinc can significantly relieve those nagging symptoms. Also, supplementing with essential fatty acids and some amino acids can give you some much-needed relief.

At the same time, it's important to keep in mind that prostate gland disorders are serious and should only be diagnosed by your doctor. If you are experiencing any BPH symptoms, you should visit your doctor immediately for proper diagnosis and treatment. If your symptoms are mild or moderate, you can talk to a practitioner of alternative medicine to find out which of the following supplements might be right for you. Before you take these supplements, though, discuss them with your doctor to make sure that they won't interfere with any other medications that you may already be taking.

Saw Palmetto to Shrink Your Prostate

One of the most widespread herbal medicines used to reduce the size and irritating symptoms of an enlarged prostate is an extract of the berries of saw palmetto. Studies show that up to 60 percent of men with mild to moderate BPH experience some relief from all major symptoms within the first four to six weeks of treatment with this herb.

In a study, 305 men who had mild to moderate BPH were given 160 milligrams of saw palmetto extract two times a day for a period of three months. After 45 days, there was a significant improvement in symptoms. After 90 days, 88 percent of the participants reported that the treatment was successful.

Researchers speculate that saw palmetto improves the symptoms of prostate enlargement in a number of ways. For one thing, it might block the effect of dihydrotestosterone (DHT) on prostate tissue, says Ray Sahelian, M.D., a physician in Marina del Rey, California, and author of *Saw Palmetto: Nature's Prostate Healer*. DHT is known to be a powerful stimulator of prostate gland growth. By blocking its actions, saw palmetto may interfere with this process, says Dr. Sahelian.

If you have mild to moderate BPH, take 160 milligrams twice a day with meals until your symptoms improve, says Thomas Kruzel, N.D., a naturopathic doctor in Portland, Oregon. Then, he suggests, continue taking at least 160 milligrams daily as a maintenance dose. The capsules should contain 85 to 95 percent liposterolic extract.

Studies show that saw palmetto is well-tolerated by most men, but you should talk to your doctor before taking it.

Help from Tree and Weed

Two other botanical medicines that are widely used to treat prostate enlargement are *Pygeum africanum* and nettle. Although neither has been as widely studied as saw palmetto, they are considered good choices.

P. africanum is an evergreen tree native to Africa that contains compounds that have anti-inflammatory properties. Several clinical trials involving more than 600 men have shown that pygeum extract is effective in reducing BPH symptoms.

In a study in which 263 men were given 50 milligrams of pygeum in the morning and evening for 60 days, researchers got some noteworthy results. By the end of the study, 66 percent of the men reported that they had fewer problems urinating. During the same study, a similar group of men with similar problems was given pills that contained no pygeum (placebos); among that group, only 31 percent showed any improvement.

As for nettle, this herbal supplement is best used during the early stages of BPH, says Dr. Kruzel. Researchers believe that extracts of nettle root reduce BPH symptoms by blocking inflammatory chemicals within the prostate tissue or by inhibiting the action of a sex-hormone-binding protein. Without that protein binding with the cells, there's less likely to be freewheeling growth of the prostate gland, says Dr. Sahelian.

Because nettle and pygeum relieve BPH symptoms differently, they're often used in combination with each other or with saw palmetto for the best results, says Dr. Kruzel. One combination product that he uses has 160 milligrams of saw palmetto, 320 milligrams of pumpkin seed oil, and 20 milligrams of pygeum. Take two capsules twice a day until your symptoms improve, he suggests, then take one capsule twice a day to maintain prostate health. For men with mild BPH, he also suggests taking two 300-milligram doses of nettle twice a day until symptoms improve, then taking one capsule once or twice a day to maintain prostate health.

Zinc: A Highly Influential Mineral

Some alternative practitioners believe that zinc is probably the most important mineral for preventing and treating BPH. "The prostate has one of the highest concentrations of zinc of any tissue in the body. It's abundant in semen and in the thin, milky fluid that the prostate gland secretes in the urethra just before ejaculation to prevent infections," says Dr. Kruzel.

In one study, zinc was shown to reduce the size of the prostate, and it alleviated symptoms in the majority of men who were taking it. A laboratory study found that zinc could inhibit the activity of a critical enzyme that converts the male hormone testosterone to DHT. What's more, other laboratory studies have shown that zinc influences a hormone that helps control the production of DHT. By helping to lower the production of that growth factor, even indirectly, zinc does the prostate a favor.

If you have BPH, consult your doctor for the appropriate zinc dosage. Doses higher than 20 milligrams daily should be taken only with medical supervision. Depending on the severity of your condition, your doctor may prescribe up to 60 milligrams a day. At that level, take your zinc in divided doses, says Ian Bier, N.D., a naturopathic doctor and licensed acupuncturist at the Institute for the Advancement of Natural Medicine in Portsmouth, New Hampshire.

Fatty Acids for Prostate Maintenance

Some naturopaths believe that men who supplement their diets with fatty acids can reverse BPH and kiss irritating symptoms goodbye.

The human body can make all but two fatty acids. Those two must come from plant food and are known as essential fatty acids. In our bodies, they act as components of substances called prostaglandins, the regulators of inflammation, pain, and swelling. One, linoleic acid, is an omega-6 fatty acid, while the other, alpha-linolenic acid, belongs to the omega-3 group. "Essential fatty acids can inhibit cell growth in the prostate, therefore stopping its growth. They rebalance the appropriate fatty acid ratios in the gland," says Dr. Bier.

These fatty acids, especially omega-3's, are essential in helping to promote healthy cell growth and function. They also help prevent up to 60 illnesses, including prostate disease, says Dr. Kruzel.

The richest source of omega-3's is flaxseed oil, and some naturopaths recommend one tablespoon a day if you're trying to control or prevent a prostate problem. Dr. Kruzel has some concern, however, that flaxseed oil may increase testosterone levels in the body and that not everyone can metabolize the oil properly to reap the benefits. He suggests taking 1,000 to 2,000 milligrams of fish oil daily for one to two weeks if you are being treated for BPH.

For maintaining prostate health rather than treating BPH, the recommended dose is 500 to 1,000 milligrams, he says. The role of essential fatty acids in cancer prevention is the focus of ongoing studies. Check with your doctor before taking fish oil capsules.

Amino Acids for Symptom Relief

The combination of the amino acids alanine, glutamic acid, and glycine has been shown in some studies to relieve many symptoms of BPH. "There are many amino acids that are present in the prostate gland, but these three, in particular, are key in developing and maintaining prostate health," says Dr. Kruzel.

In one study, 45 men were given this combination of supplement. At the end of the study, researchers saw a reduction in nighttime bathroom visits in 95 percent of the participants. Eighty-one percent said they didn't have the urge to urinate as often, and 73 percent made fewer daily trips to the bathroom.

For symptom relief, Dr. Kruzel suggests taking combination products that contain herbs and vitamins as well as 50 milligrams of alanine and glycine and between 50 and 100 milligrams of glutamic acid. He suggests taking two capsules twice a day for 10 to 14 days and then reducing the dose to one capsule once or twice a day as a maintenance dose.

You may need to get this specific formula from a holistic practitioner, but similar products are available commercially. Dr. Kruzel recommends talking to your doctor before you begin taking these amino acids.

Raynaud's disease

If you have Raynaud's disease, your hands overreact to cold, and your feet may, too. Stepping outdoors on a wintry day, you feel as if all your fingers or toes go numb instantly. Odder still, the numbness can assault your fingers even if you're just rummaging around in the freezer for a package of frozen carrots. When you look at your numb toes or fingers, they appear dead white, as if all the blood had left them. Even after you've rescued your hands or feet from the arctic temperatures and tried to warm them up, the numbness can linger.

It's thought that people who have Raynaud's disease have something slightly awry in the way their nervous systems function. The nerves that are connected with the muscles that control blood flow somehow screw up their messages.

The sympathetic nervous system is responsible for expanding or shrinking blood vessels in response to temperature. Normally, if your body gets cold, the blood vessels that lead to your arms and legs will open up, allowing warm blood to flow to fingers and toes. In Raynaud's disease, blood vessels get the wrong message and constrict instead, sending already cold fingers to the deep freeze.

Women seem to have Raynaud's more then men do. Often, someone with Raynaud's has other problems as well that seem to be associated with the disease, such as migraines, carpal tunnel syndrome, or mitral valve prolapse, a condition that occurs when one part of a heart valve malfunctions.

Raynaud's can also be associated with lupus, a disease related to a defective immune system, or scleroderma, a problem of abnormally thickening skin. All of this suggests to scientists that there may be a genetic link between some of these other conditions and Raynaud's.

While Raynaud's is usually not much more than an annoying problem, some of the related conditions mentioned above are serious. If you think that you may have Raynaud's, you should see your doctor to get a proper diagnosis.

Doctors subscribe to a number of procedures. If you learn relaxation techniques and biofeedback, you might teach your body to send more blood to your fingers and toes even when your jumpy nervous system is telling the blood vessels to slam shut.

Some doctors recommend warm-water exercises. If you periodically submerge your hands in a tub of warm water while standing in a cold room, you can retrain your body to warm up rather than cool down when it's exposed to a cool environment. Your doctor can give you more information about the conditioning procedures that sometimes prove effective.

Whether or not you try a conditioning regimen, there are some supplements that may help. The ones that are most likely to be beneficial are those that relax and open blood vessels. Here are some natural ways to support proper circulation.

Try Magnesium for Relaxed Blood Flow

The mineral magnesium is known for relaxing smooth muscle, the kind that lines the insides of blood vessels. "Magnesium can counter the inappropriate activation of the sympathetic nervous system," says Jay Lombard, M.D., assistant clinical professor of neurology at Weill Medical College of Cornell University in New York City and co-author of *The Brain Wellness Plan*. Instead of shutting down, the blood vessels may be encouraged to open up when they're under the influence of magnesium.

Take 1,000 milligrams of magnesium a day, Dr. Lombard recommends. One form that he suggests is magnesium gluconate, which won't give you the diarrhea that may be caused by other forms. Avoid magnesium oxide or magnesium chloride, he advises.

Turn Up the Heat with Niacin

Niacin is a supplement with side effects. The most noticeable one is what's referred to as flushing, a sensation of heat and tingling that comes from high doses of the pure form of the nutrient. It's just this side effect that can be helpful in Raynaud's disease, says Ross Hauser, M.D., director of Caring Medical and Rehabilitation Services at Beulahland Natural Medicine Clinic in Thebes, Illinois.

Doses many times higher than the Daily Value of niacin make the capillaries dilate. That's what causes the famous side effect, says Dr. Hauser.

While the feeling can be uncomfortable or even frightening if it happens un-expectedly, a controlled niacin flush can help bring warmth to frigid digits, he notes.

Niacin has two chemical structures, but only one, nicotinic acid, causes flushing. Nicotinamide or niacinamide, the form of niacin usually found in multivitamins, won't cause the desired effect, says Dr. Hauser. To see if niacin helps, you'll need to find pure niacin or nicotinic acid. Check labels to be sure.

Before taking supplements, you should check with your doctor. With your doctor's consent, you can start with 100 milligrams of nicotinic acid a day, suggests Dr. Hauser, although he sometimes recommends higher and more frequent doses to some patients. He recommends that you see your doctor for re-evaluation after two months of this treatment.

restless legs syndrome

If you have restless legs syndrome, you may not know it, but your bed partner probably does. When you—and your legs—are ready to rest, restless legs are ready to run. Sensations of jumpiness, itchiness, burning, aching, or twitching are all common in people with restless legs.

"It's often an unrecognized cause of insomnia," explains Jay Lombard, M.D., assistant clinical professor of neurology at Weill Medical College of Cornell University in New York City and co-author of *The Brain Wellness Plan*. You may think that you "just can't sleep," but in fact, it's the annoyance of your overactive limbs that is robbing you of your rest.

Calming restless legs can require some patience. If you're a pregnant woman, your legs will probably feel better after you've had your baby. Smokers with restless legs should quit smoking to give their leg circulation a chance to flow full force. For some people with severe restless legs, a trial of medication may be in order. Then, there are also some leg-soothing supplements that are definitely worth trying.

A Mineral Trio to Calm Cranky Muscles

A combined deficiency of three minerals could be responsible for the annoying jumpiness of restless legs syndrome, according to Ross Hauser, M.D., director of Caring Medical and Rehabilitation Services at Beulahland Natural Medicine Clinic in Thebes Park, Illinois. "A lack of calcium, potassium, and magnesium can make the large muscles in the legs hyperirritable," he says.

Calcium, magnesium, and potassium all have an effect on muscle contraction and relaxation. In addition, they help nerve transmission.

Experts say that you can help calm your legs and get some rest by making sure that you're getting enough of all three minerals. Dr. Hauser recommends taking a daily dose of between 800 and 1,000 milligrams of calcium, 300 milligrams of potassium, and 500 milligrams of magnesium at bedtime.

Try 5-HTP for a Good Night's Sleep

Have you ever noticed the little jerking movements that you (or your partner) make just as you're shifting into sleep? Those are outward signs that your brain is closing the gate on muscle movement for the night. If those muscles didn't voluntarily shut down, they'd go on obeying your brain impulses even in the midst of deep sleep. Without that safety switch, if you dreamed of running a marathon, you might end up about 26 miles from where you went to sleep.

For people with restless legs syndrome, that gating mechanism may not be functioning at 100 percent efficiency, says Dr. Lombard. Some movement impulses are getting through, keeping your legs active all night long and leaving you exhausted come morning.

"An interesting supplement called 5-hydroxytryptophan (5-HTP) seems to work well," says Dr. Lombard. Experts believe that 5-HTP is used to make serotonin, a chemical messenger in the brain that can affect sleep quality.

"The rationale behind using 5-HTP for restless legs is that raising serotonin levels will raise the gating effect," says Dr. Lombard. Essentially, it helps to separate mind from body, thus making it easier for your legs to lie still through the night.

Some people with restless legs who try 5-HTP notice a change for the better right away, but you might have to take the supplements for two weeks to a month before you'll know whether it will work for you, according to Dr. Lombard.

Start by taking 100 milligrams about 20 minutes before you go to bed, he suggests. You can increase the dose to 200 milligrams if you don't see results after the first few weeks, but don't take any more than that, he advises. Larger doses can cause disturbing dreams and nightmares.

You shouldn't take 5-HTP for longer than three months without consulting a doctor. You should also avoid it if you are currently taking antidepressants or have taken them recently. The combined effects could cause a possibly fatal condition called serotonin syndrome. Do not take supplements of 5-HTP if you are pregnant or trying to conceive.

Stabilize Membranes with Horse Chestnut

Preparations of horse chestnut leaves, bark, and seeds are used in Europe for their good effect on vein health. There's reason to consider standardized extracts of this herb for the treatment of restless legs as well, according to Dr. Hauser.

"Horse chestnut is unique in its ability to stabilize vascular membranes," he says. This may give restless legs extra blood flow that can prevent sensations of itchiness or burning.

Give this herbal remedy a try by taking 400 milligrams of standardized extract twice a day, says Dr. Hauser. Generally, people respond within a month, he adds. If your symptoms don't improve in that amount of time, stop taking it and see your doctor for an evaluation.

Horse chestnut is not for everyone. It may interfere with the action of other drugs, especially blood thinners such as warfarin (Coumadin). It may also irritate the gastrointestinal tract. As with other herbs, you should not take it if you are pregnant or breastfeeding.

"You must obtain a standardized extract and follow package directions if you're going to use horse chestnut as a healing herb," says James A. Duke, Ph.D., botanical consultant, former ethnobotanist with the U.S. Department of Agriculture who specializes in medicinal plants, and author of *The Green Pharmacy*. "It's simply not safe to use otherwise."

rheumatoid arthritis

If you have rheumatoid arthritis, your body's infection-fighting immune cells decide that *you're* the enemy. They attack your joints and cause inflammation, with pain, redness, heat, swelling, and tissue damage. The inflammation doesn't always confine itself to joints, either, says Andrew Rubman, N.D., director of the Southbury Clinic for Traditional Medicine in Connecticut and consultant to the Office of Complementary and Alternative Medicine at the National Institutes of Health. "Other organs, such as the skin, heart, and lungs, can be affected," he says.

Rheumatoid arthritis is usually treated with aspirin, ibuprofen, naproxen sodium, or various other, more powerful versions of anti-inflammatory drugs. If necessary, your doctor may call on steroid drugs to knock out inflammation.

Alternative practitioners attack rheumatoid arthritis on several additional fronts, says Jody Noé, N.D., a naturopathic doctor at the Brattleboro Naturopathic Clinic in Vermont. They use anti-inflammatory nutrients and herbs. Often, these supplements are prescribed in large doses, so you'll need the advice of a practitioner or doctor before you start taking them.

Some of the recommended supplements also work to restore proper immunity and to get the adrenal glands functioning better. These glands, located above the kidneys, are powerful little organs that secrete hormones such as epinephrine and steroids that affect many organ functions and influence the use of energy throughout your body.

Alternative practitioners also try to address what they believe are potential triggers of autoimmune diseases such as rheumatoid arthritis. Naturopathic doctors believe that one of the triggers is increased intestinal permeability, or "leaky gut," a condition that occurs when molecules of incompletely digested food or bacterial fragments appear to be seeping through the walls of the intestine, setting off an immune response.

People also have allergic reactions to foods, and if you see an alternative practitioner about rheumatoid arthritis, you're likely to be questioned closely about what foods you eat and when. Realizing that adrenal gland problems can arise from too much physical or emotional stress, alternative practitioners may try to treat the stress as a way of avoiding an autoimmune reaction. If you've been diagnosed with rheumatoid arthritis and want to try these options, get your doctor's approval first.

Antioxidants That Ax Inflammation

Any time you have inflammation, there's production of free radicals, unstable molecules that can harm surrounding cells, causing what's called oxidative damage. Some nutrients that may help stop free radicals and prevent that damage include vitamins E and C, beta-carotene, selenium, and zinc.

Several studies have shown that the risk of rheumatoid arthritis is highest among people with the lowest blood levels of these nutrients. Other studies suggest that whether or not people are deficient, these nutrients may help reduce the arthritis symptoms.

In a Belgian study, 15 women with rheumatoid arthritis who took 160 micrograms of selenium or 200 micrograms of selenium-enriched yeast every day for four months experienced significant improvement in joint movement and strength. Another study showed that people with rheumatoid arthritis who took 600 international units (IU) of vitamin E twice a day had a significant reduction in pain compared with people who took pills with no vitamin E (placebos).

Researchers at the University of Washington in Seattle found that people with rheumatoid arthritis who took 50 milligrams of zinc three times a day for three months experienced significant improvement in joint swelling and morning stiffness with the aid of the supplements. With the zinc, it also took them less time to walk certain distances than when they were not taking it.

"Zinc helps your body make an important inflammation-fighting enzyme called superoxide dismutase," says Dr. Noé. She cautions, however, that this doesn't mean that you should take the amounts of zinc that were used in the study. This amount of zinc should not be taken without medical supervision.

Dr. Noé recommends a daily mixture of antioxidant nutrients, including

1,000 to 3,000 milligrams of vitamin C in divided doses, 400 to 1,000 IU of vitamin E, 200 to 400 micrograms of selenium, and 15 to 30 milligrams of zinc picolinate or citrate.

You can also take 1 to 2 milligrams a day of copper and 5 to 15 milligrams of manganese, suggests Dr. Noé. Both of these trace minerals help the body make its own antioxidants. Be careful not to take higher doses of these two, however, as they can be toxic in large amounts.

"A good multivitamin/mineral will cover a lot of these nutritional basics," Dr. Noé says. To maximize absorption from a multi, she suggests taking capsules with meals.

Friendly Fats

You might reduce the amount of inflammation-generating chemicals that your body produces by changing the kinds of fats you eat, Dr. Noé says. "Meat and other animal foods provide your body with something called arachidonic acid, which is used to make pro-inflammatory biochemicals," she explains.

There are other oils that don't have the effect of stimulating inflammation. Oils from cold-water fish such as mackerel as well as certain plant oils follow a chemical pathway that is pretty much neutral, according to Dr. Noé. Thus, if those are your primary sources of fat, you'll be a lot less likely to aggravate arthritis symptoms.

At least six studies have shown that diets rich in fish oil, which contains omega-3 fatty acids, help reduce the pain and stiffness of rheumatoid arthritis as well as the biochemical signs of inflammation. Evidence so far suggests that taking 3,000 to 6,000 milligrams of these fatty acids a day seems to have an anti-inflammatory effect, Dr. Noé says. Good food sources are herring, salmon, tuna, sardines, mackerel, and anchovies.

Two studies also suggest that gamma-linolenic acid (GLA), a kind of fatty acid found in certain plant oils, may reduce the symptoms of rheumatoid arthritis. In one study, people took 2.8 grams a day of GLA for one year. At the end of that time, 76 percent showed improvement.

Dr. Noé recommends taking 1,000 to 1,500 milligrams a day of eicosapentaenoic acid (EPA) and 500 to 700 milligrams a day of docosahexaenoic acid (DHA), both of which are active ingredients in fish-oil supplements. She also suggests supplementing with 500 to 1,000 milligrams of GLA from evening primrose, borage, or black currant oil.

Reining In Radicals with C and E

In our bodies, inflammation is usually a protective response brought on by an infection or injury. If your immune system is in good operating order, it detects any foreign organism that's been able to invade at the site of the wound or infection, and your body begins setting up its defense. The response is designed to wall off the infection or foreign matter from the rest of the body, destroy any organisms involved, and break down any injured tissue, clearing the way for new construction.

The classic signs of inflammation are heat, redness, swelling, and pain. These symptoms are the result of increased blood flow into the affected area. The blood vessels actually change size, making room for immune cells to travel through the bloodstream to the site of injured or infected tissue. This process also produces a number of chemicals that orchestrate the process and that can cause pain and fatigue.

In this process, free radicals are normally generated, according to Maret G. Traber, Ph.D., principal investigator at the Linus Pauling Institute and associate professor of nutrition at Oregon State University in Corvallis. Free radicals are molecules that can cause damage to healthy cells by stealing electrons from other molecules in cells. "Immune cells, such as lymphocytes, macrophages, and neutrophils, generate oxygen and hydrogen peroxide as part of the clean-'em-up, move-'em-out process," notes Dr. Traber.

Macrophages are amoeba-like cells that engulf bacteria and foreign

Nutrients to Improve Digestion

Some kinds of arthritis have a clear link with inflammatory bowel disease. Two with confirmed links are arthritis of the knees, ankles, and wrists and ankylosing spondylitis (rheumatoid arthritis of the spine).

These links, as well as other clues, have suggested to doctors of alternative medicine that digestive problems can play a role in rheumatoid arthritis. Here's where the leaky gut theory comes in. If incompletely digested food and bacterial fragments are seeping through the intestinal lining into the bloodstream, so the thinking goes, maybe they're setting off an improper immune response that ends up causing rheumatoid arthritis.

"It's possible to do tests that can confirm if someone is having an im-

matter. Inside the voluminous macrophages are sacs of hydrogen peroxide, and when the invaders are trapped in these sacs, they're killed by the interaction with hydrogen peroxide.

As inflammation progresses, some free radicals end up on the wrong side of the battlefield. They may react with the membranes of cells that are essentially innocent bystanders, damaging some of the molecules in those otherwise healthy cells. If the healthy cells' membranes are damaged enough, the cells may be killed or maimed.

If there are antioxidants in the neighborhood during this reaction, less damage may occur. Some antioxidants, such as vitamin E, act as shields. They are incorporated into cell membranes and can give up one of their own electrons, thus neutralizing a free radical and making it settle down rather than hunting for other electrons.

Vitamin C can collaborate in neutralizing free radicals. If vitamin C is available to give vitamin E one of its electrons, vitamin E can put the damper on free radical activity. "It actually travels through the cell membrane, and each molecule of vitamin E can protect about 1,000 molecules in the membrane," Dr. Traber says.

Other antioxidants act in different ways, but the end result is the same: More cells are protected and emerge unscathed despite being under assault from the free radicals that have been unleashed during inflammation.

mune reaction that could cause rheumatoid arthritis," Dr. Noé says. Your rheumatologist or a naturopathic doctor can order these tests.

In addition, she recommends nutritional supplements that nourish and rebuild the intestinal lining and restore good bacteria to the bowel. Some foods that commonly aggravate leaky gut are wheat gluten, corn, and dairy products.

"I may also recommend enzymes that help break down food for proper digestion if tests suggest that someone's pancreas is not producing enough for normal digestion," Dr. Noé says.

To provide nourishment directly to intestinal cells, she suggests a large number of supplements that are specifically used to treat autoimmune diseases like rheumatoid arthritis and lupus. They include:

- 500 to 750 milligrams of the amino acid glutamine.
- 100 to 300 milligrams of gamma-oryzanol, a component of rice bran oil.
- 50 to 100 milligrams of fructooligosaccharides (FOS), taken two or three times a day between meals. (Fructooligosaccharides are naturally occurring sugars that help to promote the growth of friendly bacteria in the intestines.)
- One or two capsules two or three times a day of a supplement containing various forms of lactobacillus and other so-called friendly bacteria—*Lactobacillus acidophilus*, *L. rhamnosus*, *L. casei*, *L. plantarum*, *Bifidobacterium bifidum*, *B. longum*, and *B. breve*. The recommended dose has two to five billion active organisms per capsule.
- 500 to 1,000 milligrams of 10X U.S.P. of digestive enzymes. (10X U.S.P. is a measure of strength, listed on the bottle.)
- A mixture of other enzymes derived from plants, including 12,500 to 18,000 U.S.P. of protease, 2,675 U.S.P. of lipase, 12,000 to 27,000 U.S.P. of amylase, and 175 CU(2) of cellulase.

Dr. Noé says that these supplements are safe to take on a continuous basis as long as you get your doctor's approval and remain under supervision. Some of the supplements may only be available through a naturopathic physician or holistic doctor.

A Spicy Way to Ease Aches

Turmeric, an Indian spice, contains an anti-inflammatory and antioxidant compound called curcumin that might be helpful for people with rheumatoid arthritis, especially during flare-ups, says Dr. Rubman. "In animals, curcumin has excellent anti-inflammatory and antioxidant effects, without any toxicity," he says.

When curcumin is present, the body is much less likely to form the compounds that are instrumental in causing inflammation, according to Dr. Rubman. Research with humans is still sketchy, but some preliminary studies have suggested benefits.

The recommended dose of curcumin is 400 to 600 milligrams three times a day with or without food, Dr. Rubman says. If you don't notice some relief within 10 days, stop taking it. It is safe to take indefinitely as long as you don't have a digestive problem, but for best results, he recommends seeking the care of a naturopathic physician. Curcumin is available from naturopathic doctors and is also sold at health food stores.

Bringing in Bromelain

To enhance absorption of curcumin and add more anti-inflammatory power, supplement manufacturers sometimes mix curcumin with bromelain, an enzyme found in pineapple, Dr. Rubman says.

"Bromelain can activate compounds that break down fibrin, tissue that blocks off areas of inflammation," Dr. Rubman explains. He points out that the fibrin blocks blood vessels, which can prevent tissues from draining and cause them to swell.

Bromelain also blocks the production of compounds produced during inflammation that increase swelling and cause pain.

The usual dosage for bromelain, according to Dr. Rubman, is 400 to 600 milligrams three times a day, taken at the same time as curcumin on an empty stomach. Mixtures of bromelain and curcumin in a ratio designed to reduce inflammation are available at some health food stores or from a naturopathic doctor.

Going with Ginger

Ginger, a relative of curcumin and the same spice used in baking, has anti-inflammatory and antioxidant properties that make it helpful for rheumatoid arthritis, Dr. Rubman says. In two small studies, ginger helped to reduce muscle stiffness, pain, and swelling.

You can take ginger instead of curcumin if you prefer, he says. The doses he recommends are 100 to 200 milligrams three times a day of ginger extract standardized to contain 20 percent gingerol and shogaol, the active ingredients. You also have the option of 8 to 10 grams (about 1½ tablespoons) of fresh ginger or 2 to 4 grams (about one teaspoon) of dry powdered ginger daily. Do not use the dried root or powder if you have gallstones.

Ginger can be especially soothing if your rheumatoid arthritis includes gastrointestinal problems. If you tend to "run hot," as Dr. Rubman puts it—if you tend to sweat a lot or have hot, swollen joints—you're better off avoiding ginger, he says.

sciatica

If all your nerves were a network of roads, the sciatic nerve would be a busy interstate highway. All of the nerve impulses transmitted to and from the lower half of your body must pass through the sciatic nerve, the largest and longest in the body. From its roots in the spinal cord, the thick conduit branches through the buttocks and down the back of each leg to the foot. Pain that follows this route is called sciatica.

Pressure on the nerve in the spinal area is normally the cause of sciatica. The sensation can vary from mild tingling in your foot to searing pains that shoot down your leg.

Sciatica often begins after you've done some customary movement that never caused pain previously. Smokers, people who do a lot of heavy lifting, and people with osteoporosis or arthritis are at highest risk for developing sciatica.

To discover what's causing your pain, you'd have to look closely at an x-ray of your spinal column, particularly the circular sections of cartilage called disks that are assigned the job of cushioning the bones and sheltering the nerve that runs alongside your spine. If you're under age 40 and you get sciatica, it's likely that one of those disks has slipped and is bulging between the vertebrae in your spine. Since the nerve runs alongside the spine, the off-kilter disk puts pressure on it.

If you're hit with sciatica when you're over 40, the cause is also disk-related, but in a somewhat different way. At that age, your disks are starting to become dehydrated. The shrinking disks can cause the spine to compress, increasing pressure on the nerve.

Do you get the pain most when you cough or sneeze? That's just one sign that your sciatic nerve is probably pinched. You really can't diagnose yourself from that clue alone, however, so you should see a doctor to be sure of the origin of the pain, says Barbara Silbert, D.C., N.D., a chiropractor and naturopathic doctor in Newburyport, Massachusetts. Low back pain and intermittent claudication—pain in the legs caused by poor arterial blood flow—are often mistaken for sciatic pain, notes Dr. Silbert.

Because sciatica almost always involves a mechanical problem with your back, you may need massage or chiropractic adjustment. In severe cases, surgery may be necessary to free the nerve. More often, your doctor will simply prescribe some bed rest. You might also want to try some natural supplements that can help relieve inflammation and relax spastic muscles, says Dr. Silbert.

Helping Your Body Douse Inflammation

The key to drug-free relief is to turn on your body's natural inflammation-fighting powers, says David Perlmutter, M.D., a neurologist in Naples, Florida, and author of *Lifeguide*. While drugs like aspirin and ibuprofen work by reducing inflammation and thus reducing the sensation of pain, nutritional supplements can reprogram the chemical process that produces pain signals. Moreover, nutrients influence the complicated inflammation process.

"Obviously, the body must have its own ways of reducing inflammation," says Dr. Perlmutter. "The entire process of turning inflammation on and off is controlled by a group of hormone-like molecules called prostaglandins."

According to Dr. Perlmutter, there are basically two groups of prostaglandins. One group is the starter kit that initiates inflammation. The other is a "tone group" that reduces the flare-up.

Dr. Silbert explains that there are four key supplements in nature's arsenal of inflammation fighters that may help sciatica—bromelain, the bioflavonoid quercetin, essential fatty acids, and the herb turmeric. They inhibit the production of bad prostaglandins that start inflammation, and they promote the production of good prostaglandins that fight it. In other words, they stop the bad guys and help the good guys.

Fight the Flames

Bromelain, an enzyme found in pineapple, is the jack-of-all-trades when it comes to fighting inflammation.

In a study of 146 boxers, researchers showed that bromelain significantly speeded up the healing process when the boxers were injured. Bromelain was given to 74 of the boxers four times a day, while the remaining 72 took an inactive substance (placebo). In 58 of the boxers taking bromelain, all signs of bruising disappeared in four days. In the group taking the placebos, only 10 healed completely in four days.

Quercetin, just one of more than 800 bioflavonoids that have been identified, works best with bromelain to block the inflammation process. Naturopathic doctors believe that bromelain helps your body absorb the quercetin, so they often prescribe the two together, says Dr. Silbert. Quercetin is rich in powerful antioxidants that stop the damaging effects of free radicals, the unstable molecules that damage cells.

When the pain of sciatica strikes, take up to 1,000 milligrams of bromelain and 500 milligrams of quercetin four times a day between meals, says Dr. Silbert. The strength of a particular batch of bromelain is measured in milk clotting units (mcu) or gelatin-dissolving units (gdu). The higher the mcu number, the greater its strength. Look for a supplement with a strength between 1,800 and 2,400 mcu or 1,080 and 1,440 gdu.

Beware of bromelain supplements that merely list weight in milligrams; if the measurement isn't listed on the label, you can assume that you are getting a cheap, ineffective preparation, cautions Jacob Schor, N.D., a naturopathic doctor in Denver and president of the Colorado Association of Naturopathic Doctors.

Any type of inflammation responds well to the essential fatty acids found in fish oil, flaxseed oil, and evening primrose oil.

To reprogram your pain process, take one tablespoon of flaxseed oil and 500 milligrams of black currant oil (or three capsules of evening primrose oil) every day, says Dr. Perlmutter. These two supplements are rich in omega-3 and omega-6 essential fatty acids that your body needs but cannot make. By adding them to your diet, you can stimulate your body to produce increased levels of good prostaglandins and reduce inflammation.

If you want to use fish oil instead of flaxseed oil, take 1,000 milligrams two to four times a day, says Priscilla Evans, N.D., a naturopathic doctor at the Community Wholistic Health Center in Chapel Hill, North Carolina.

Turmeric Time?

During intense flare-ups, add some turmeric. This yellow spice contains one of nature's most powerful anti-inflammatory drugs, a chemical called curcumin. The herb has been used for thousands of years in India's traditional Ayurvedic medicine to treat pain and inflammation.

Several clinical studies show that curcumin has an anti-inflammatory action. Don't reach into your spice cupboard for relief, however. Instead, opt for capsules of standardized extract that contain 97 percent pure curcumin.

When pain is acute, Dr. Evans advises people to take 250 to 500 milligrams three times a day. But you shouldn't take turmeric as a remedy if you are pregnant or have severe stomach acid, ulcers, gallstones, or a bile duct obstruction.

If you're taking natural supplements, you should start to see some improvement in about two weeks. Stick with the dosages to get the desired effect, says Dr. Evans.

"We lose sight of the fact that many nutritional and herbal supplements are more like foods than drugs. Dosages are important because taking just one capsule a day is not going to do much for your symptoms," she says. "In many cases, you have to take a pretty large dose of fish oil or curcumin to get an effect. Our culture, though, has conditioned us to taking just a pill or two for relief."

A Recipe for Relaxation

Sometimes, pain and tingling can be due to muscle spasms in the piriformis muscle, a pear-shaped muscle in the buttocks that surrounds the sciatic nerve. Relaxing this muscle can help relieve pain, says Dr. Evans.

Naturopaths often use a mixture of soothing herbs such as valerian, passionflower, and kava kava to promote muscle relaxation. Although valerian has become a staple on drugstore shelves, where it is sold as a sleep aid, its powers of reprieve go beyond sleep.

"Valerian is also great for easing tension and for general pain relief," says Dr. Evans. It contains substances known as volatile oils that work together to make you sleepy and relax your muscles.

Sometimes, your sciatic nerve is in the grip of a spastic muscle, and that no-win tug-of-war is at the root of the pain. Your doctor will need to confirm if a spastic muscle is the source of your pain. If it is, taking 150 milligrams of valerian three times a day may help, says Dr. Evans.

scleroderma

Scleroderma means, literally, "hard skin." It occurs when cells called fibroblasts, concentrated in the skin but also found in other organs, begin to replicate overtime.

The fibroblasts crank out a connective tissue called collagen. "They literally overgrow parts of the body with collagen, the same way these cells would form new tissue to heal a wound," says Richard Silver, M.D., head of the rheumatology division at the Medical University of South Carolina in Charleston. Unfortunately, the excess collagen isn't needed for anything. It just messes things up.

No one knows exactly what triggers scleroderma, but "it is considered an autoimmune disorder, meaning that something is wrong with a person's immune system," Dr. Silver says. Certain immune cells secrete chemicals that make the fibroblasts more active than they should be. Genetics and environment both play roles. "Some cases may have been triggered by exposure to organic solvents such as trichloroethylene, a solvent that's used mainly to degrease machinery but can also be found in drinking water," Dr. Silver says. For many cases, though, no cause is ever found.

The immune system first produces inflammation that can make the joints hurt and cause the hands to become puffy. Ultimately, scar tissue forms and makes the skin thick, hard, and shiny. The muscles can become weak, and organs that depend on muscles, such as the esophagus and intestines, can begin to go haywire. Moreover, almost everyone with scleroderma also has Raynaud's disease, an extreme sensitivity to cold in their hands and feet caused by constricted blood vessels that cut off blood flow to the fingers and toes.

Scleroderma is most often treated with drugs that reduce inflammation and muscle spasms, improve blood flow, or reduce high blood pressure if the kidneys are damaged, Dr. Silver says. "Scleroderma can be controlled somewhat, but not cured."

Alternative treatments for scleroderma include nutritional supplements that help reduce inflammation and improve circulation. Some can also address possible underlying causes, including digestive problems, says Andrew Rubman, N.D., director of the Southbury Clinic for Traditional Medicines in Connecticut and a consultant to the Office of Complementary and Alternative Medicine at the National Institutes of Health. If you've been diagnosed with scleroderma, you should get your doctor's approval before you take supplements.

Antioxidants against Early Damage

At least in its earlier stages, scleroderma involves inflammation. While tissues are becoming inflamed, your body begins to form an excessive number of free radicals. These are the free-roaming, unstable molecules that cause cell damage.

Antioxidant nutrients such as vitamins E and C, beta-carotene, and selenium, as well as zinc (which acts like an antioxidant), can help stop free radical damage, according to Dr. Silver.

Dr. Rubman recommends a total of 35,000 to 50,000 international units (IU) of vitamin A equivalents, from a combination of vitamin A and beta-carotene. He prefers a supplement with 15,000 to 20,000 IU of retinal palmitate and 20,000 to 30,000 IU of beta-carotene, but other combinations can be substituted, he notes. He also recommends 600 to 800 IU of vitamin E, about 2,500 milligrams of vitamin C, and 50 milligrams of zinc for men and 35 milligrams for women. While these are the amounts he recommends to his patients, you need to get your doctor's approval before supplementing with antioxidants at these dosage levels.

"Zinc is an important part of the mix because it helps the body make its own antioxidants, such as superoxide dismutase," Dr. Rubman says. It also helps to maintain a healthy lining in the intestinal tract, which is important for anyone with an autoimmune disease, he notes.

The Right Fats

Naturopathic doctors often ask patients with scleroderma to cut back on saturated fat and add omega-6 and omega-3 fatty acids, says Dr Rubman. Both of these fatty acids act in the body to reduce inflammation.

Although there are no studies that show the impact of omega-3's and omega-6's on scleroderma, researchers do know something about how these fatty acids affect people with Raynaud's syndrome. Since Raynaud's is an early symptom of scleroderma, the link could be important.

Dr. Rubman has people take eicosapentaenoic acid (EPA), which is an omega-3, starting with 2,000 to 5,000 milligrams a day of fish oil. He also recommends omega-6 which you can get by taking 2,000 to 5,000 milligrams of evening primrose, borage, or black currant oil. "I think the best way to tell whether these oils are having a positive effect is to dose fairly liberally with them initially and see if you perceive a change," he says. "It can take as long as five or six weeks at these quantities before people notice a difference."

That difference might be a reduction in inflammation that results in less painful, more functional joints. You might also experience fewer muscle spasms, and you may find that your skin is less sensitive to touch and temperature changes, Dr. Rubman says.

An Enzyme-Spice Combination

Naturopathic doctors will sometimes recommend supplements of bromelain, an enzyme derived from pineapple. Some doctors also suggest curcumin, a component of the Indian spice turmeric. "I'll recommend these if a person needs good short-term control over acute inflammation," Dr. Rubman says.

Both bromelain and curcumin act to quiet inflammation. Bromelain has the additional talent of inhibiting the body's production of fibrin, or scar tissue, Dr. Rubman says. Much of its anti-inflammatory action is achieved by activating compounds that break down fibrin. Bromelain also blocks compounds produced by immune cells that increase swelling and cause pain.

Dr. Rubman recommends 1,000 milligrams of bromelain and 500 milligrams of curcumin powder a day during periods of acute inflammation. "If it's going to help, it will work in fairly short order, within a week or so," he says.

In research at the Medical University of South Carolina, scientists are studying curcumin's effect on fibroblasts. Test-tube observations of this spice have led them to wonder if curcumin could inhibit collagen production in these cells, Dr. Silver says.

Supplements to Aid Digestion

Some doctors believe that people with autoimmune diseases such as scleroderma have increased permeability in their intestines, or "leaky guts." If so, they surmise, there's a possibility that molecules from foods and bacterial fragments are seeping through the intestinal walls and getting into the bloodstream. "The molecules set off an improper immune response that can manifest itself in any number of ways—as rheumatoid arthritis, lupus, or, potentially, as scleroderma," Dr. Rubman says.

The treatment for leaky gut problems can be extensive, Dr. Rubman says. It includes a complete stool analysis to check for too much bacteria or yeast, among other problems.

To discourage unchecked growth of bacteria, Dr. Rubman may recommend *Lactobacillus acidophilus*. These "good bacteria," found in some foods like cultured yogurt, can crowd out bad bacteria in the intestines. If you want to take lactobacillus supplements, look for a brand that contains live cultures and lists "no animal or fish derivatives" on the label, says Dr. Rubman.

Dr. Rubman also recommends getting plenty of fiber, especially soluble fibers such as pectin, glucomannan, oat bran, and psyllium, which are associated with the growth of good bacteria in the gut. "I encourage people to get 30 grams or more of fiber a day, from foods and supplements if necessary," he says.

Depending on the results of a stool analysis, Dr. Rubman may also suggest various digestive enzymes, such as hydrochloric acid (betaine hydrochloride) and pancreatin, to help break down food for proper absorption. You can find various mixtures of enzymes at health food stores. If you're seeing a naturopathic doctor, the doctor may recommend particular enzymes, Dr. Rubman says. "These can vary widely in quality and activity, so sometimes it's good to have some educated help in making a selection."

In a 40-year study, long-term high doses of PABA (para-aminobenzoic acid) were observed to prolong life compared to untreated patients. The dose was 3 grams 4 times daily. This shold be taken for at least 4 to 6 months. High doses may cause a rash or hypoglycemia and should be used under physician supervision. Also, centella asiata (gotu kola) has been shown to decrease skin hardness, improve mobility , and decrease pain.

shingles

If you had childhood chicken pox, your parents probably told you that you'd never get it again. That's good news to any kid who has just endured the little blisters, the itching, and the fever that are all signs of chicken pox.

It's too bad that your parents were wrong.

The same virus that causes chicken pox—the varicella-zoster virus—can continue to live an undercover existence in your nerve cells, and it may emerge later. The second time around you don't get the childhood version of itchy, blotchy chicken pox. Instead, you get the adult version, shingles, which is characterized by searing pain and lesions that can leave a good-size scar.

It's hard to tell why the virus re-emerges in some people and not others and impossible to tell when it's going to crop up again. Certainly, elderly people get it more often than young people, and some individuals are more likely to develop shingles when they're under severe stress or when their immune systems have been weakened. Adults may get shingles after an illness. For cancer patients who are undergoing chemotherapy, compromised immune systems may be a factor in bringing on shingles.

What characterizes all of these situations is a weakened immune system in which your body's disease-fighting soldiers, the antibodies, are in short supply.

"The virus looks for the right opportunity when your antibody production is down," says William Warnock, N.D., a naturopathic doctor in Shelburne, Vermont. "Stress is one of the biggest causes of reduced antibody production. When people become stressed, they don't eat right, they don't sleep well, and their immune systems just don't function as well."

Typically, during a shingles outbreak, you have tingling and pain around your torso, neck, or face. Lesions, or small blisters, may break out on the skin near the site of the infected nerve. The pain often lasts from two to four weeks, but in some cases, it can last for months. If it does, you've moved from shingles to a condition known as postherpetic neuralgia.

624

Fighting the Virus

Once it gets loose, there's no cure for the varicella-zoster virus, but there may be ways to slow it down or limit damage during the outbreak. Medical doctors frequently prescribe an antiviral drug such as acyclovir (Zovirax) or famciclovir (Famvir) to shorten the course of the infection.

In order to hasten healing, treatment should be started within two to three days of the first appearance of the small blisters. In addition, you may be able to boost your immunity and help fight the virus with some herbs, says Dr. Warnock.

Herbalists believe that astragalus and echinacea are most effective. They work best if you take them as soon as you know you have an outbreak of the virus, says Dr. Warnock. Although you can take an herbal tincture, he recommends taking one 300-milligram capsule of standardized extract three times a day.

If you use capsules of dried echinacea root, he recommends 2,000 milligrams three times a day. Since echinacea is also safe at higher doses, you can take even more than the specified dose if you find it effective. "I'd do a high dose for a short period—just a few days. That's when it's most effective," he says.

Support from Astragalus

While echinacea speeds white blood cells to the infection site, you can add astragalus to help with the healing process. This herb provides what is known as deep immune support, working within the bone marrow where immune cells are manufactured, says Anne McClenon, N.D., a naturopathic doctor at the Compass Family Health Center in Plymouth, Massachusetts. You can take astragalus in capsule form, following the directions on the label.

"Astragalus provides immune support on a long-term basis. That's important because people who get shingles may have a weakened immune system that needs to be built up again," she says. "I'd recommend taking it for four to six months."

Some Licorice Aid

Licorice also has strong antiviral properties. During the course of the infection, Dr. Warnock recommends taking 500 milligrams of standardized licorice extract in capsule form three times a day. If you take powdered licorice root in capsules, however, the dose should be 2,000 milligrams three times a day. Continue the treatment for two weeks after the lesions have healed, Dr. Warnock says.

Take licorice with caution, and don't take it at all if you are pregnant or nursing or if you have diabetes, high blood pressure, liver disorders, or kidney problems. In general, you shouldn't take high doses of licorice for more than four to six weeks unless you're under the supervision of a qualified health-care practitioner.

On the High Cs

High doses of vitamin C have been shown to keep the varicella-zoster virus from replicating, according to some studies involving people who were given intravenous injections. There have not been any studies that showed similar effects from taking oral supplements. Dr. Warnock believes, however, that you can help keep the virus from taking hold with a daily dose of 10,000 milligrams of vitamin C. Dr. Warnock recommends five doses of 2,000 milligrams each, taken three hours apart. "The dosage goes beyond being a simple immune booster," he says. "The point is to interrupt the virus."

Dr. Warnock thinks vitamin C might prevent the virus from multiplying and spreading along the infected nerve. At the same time, vitamin C may ease inflammation in the nerve and lessen the outbreaks of the lesions, he says.

With a dose this high, you might experience an upset stomach and diarrhea, which is a frequent side effect of excess vitamin C. If so, just reduce the dose until you reach a level that's more tolerable, says Dr. Warnock.

"Also, you need to take this treatment early in the infection," he says. "Once there are millions of virus particles floating around, it becomes a much harder task to keep them from reproducing."

Starve the Virus

Varicella-zoster belongs to a larger family of herpesviruses, all of which share an important characteristic: They multiply with the help of the amino acid arginine and are inhibited by another amino acid called lysine. Lysine may work by blocking the virus's ability to absorb and use arginine.

To keep shingles at bay, doctors advise, you should avoid arginine-rich foods such as chocolate, legumes, and nuts, especially peanuts, and eat more foods that are rich in lysine, such as fish, tofu, eggs, lean beef, and lean pork.

You can also boost your lysine levels by taking a supplement. Dr. Warnock suggests taking 2,000 milligrams of lysine daily until the infection runs its course.

Beat the Pain with a B Vitamin

Shingles is not just painful, it's *intensely* painful. Because your nerves carry the virus and the virus causes inflammation, having shingles is like having a raw wound inside your nervous system. Even a light touch can give you a jolt, while something as innocuous as a tight shirt can give you a full day of misery.

Vitamin B_{12} seems to maintain the fatty membranes that sheathe and insulate the nerves, says Dr. McClenon. There's also evidence that it reduces the inflammation of the nerve where the virus is causing pain, and it may even shorten the length of the illness.

Some people with shingles take vitamin B_{12} injections, says Dr. Mc-Clenon. If the idea of an injection doesn't appeal to you, you can get B_{12} tablets to place under your tongue (sublingual). Although some people have difficulty absorbing B_{12}, most people can absorb at least some of the vitamin this way.

"It definitely speeds healing," says Dr. McClenon, "and it may lessen the chance of a person getting the postherpetic neuralgic pain." She suggests taking a 2,000-microgram dose of sublingual B_{12} each day during the course of the infection.

Limit the Lesions

The skin outbreaks and pain of shingles can sometimes be eased with herbal treatments that you can apply directly to the surface of the skin. Among these topical treatments are licorice root extract, capsaicin, and St. John's wort oil.

Licorice root comes in a gel or ointment form that you rub directly on painful skin areas. It seems to interfere with the spread of the virus, says Dr. Warnock. Licorice gel (Licrogel) is available from your physician or chiropractor. You can also ask your health food store to order a brand called Licroderm.

Although naturopathic doctors find that St. John's wort oil applied to the unbroken skin acts as an anti-inflammatory, it also is used to relieve pain and strengthen nerves, says Dr. McClenon. "Thus, it's a good topical treatment for any kind of nerve pain. I would continue to use it for the residual pain that may linger after the outbreak."

Fight Fire with Fire

Many over-the-counter ointments for shingles contain capsaicin, the substance that makes hot peppers hot. Like St. John's wort, capsaicin cannot be used on open lesions, so use it after they've cleared to relieve the pain of postherpetic neuralgia, says Dr. Warnock. Capsaicin cream is available in a number of different strengths, ranging from 0.025 percent to 0.075 percent.

Capsaicin works by stimulating and then exhausting Substance P, the nerve-related transmitter that sends pain messages to your brain, in the skin. After two to three days of applying capsaicin, you should begin to feel the pain subsiding. The cream itself is irritating to the skin, so start with a tiny amount, and if a high-strength concentration burns too much, just switch to a lower strength, says Dr. Warnock.

Because capsaicin can burn the skin, however, he advises people to use it carefully. "I tell them to apply it four times a day to the affected area," he says. "You should always wear gloves when you apply it, and if you get it somewhere where you don't want it, don't try to wash it off with water. That just reactivates it and makes it worse. Instead, you can lessen the burning by rubbing the area with olive oil."

stress

Daily traffic. Work deadlines. Family squabbles. Rebellious teenagers. Illness. Injury. All of these life experiences add up to big-time stress that can knock you off your feet, spin you around, and keep you dazed. Without some relief, you may feel as if each morning is the beginning of a new melodrama.

Poking fun at stress is one way to help you de-stress. But the truth is, that stress is no laughing matter. Whenever you're filled with tension and anxiety, your adrenal glands, located above your kidneys, pump out stress hormones such as adrenaline and cortisol, which give your body that burst of energy it needs to escape danger. Long-term stress causes chronically high levels of stress hormones, which can weaken your immune system, tax your heart and blood vessels, tire you out, and make you more susceptible to illness.

Fortunately, certain dietary and lifestyle changes can help relieve stress and release tension. For starters, get at least 20 minutes of aerobic exercise three to five times a week to lift your spirits and melt away feelings of pressure and anxiety. Also, don't overlook weight lifting and brisk walking, as they can have similar effects.

Another tip for stress control: Limit your intake of caffeine, alcohol, high-fat foods, and sugar. Caffeine and alcohol can raise the levels of stress hormones in the blood and alter brain chemistry. Caffeine also causes nervousness, anxiety, and irritability. Moreover, when you replace nutritious foods with refined carbohydrates like sugar, you lower the amount of vitamins and minerals in your diet, depleting your body of essential nutrients that protect you from the dangers of stress.

Once you have made these changes, you can try a variety of nutritional supplements as added stress protection. Certain vitamins can build up your immune system to prevent stress-related illnesses. Others can boost your energy and lift your mood. Even some herbs can help to calm your nerves, increase stamina, and keep you mentally and physically strong in the midst of turmoil.

Vitamin C: What Happens

Vitamin C gives your immune system the fighting power it needs to prevent many stress-related health problems such as headaches, high blood pressure, diabetes, and heart disease, says C. Norman Shealy, M.D., Ph.D., founder of the American Holistic Medical Association and director of the Shealy Institute, an alternative medicine clinic in Springfield, Missouri.

What's more, vitamin C is required to manufacture stress hormones, which can flow excessively if you're stressed for a long time. After a while, your adrenal glands become exhausted from overwork, and your body's ability to produce stress hormones declines, says Ray Sahelian, M.D., a physician in Marina del Rey, California, and author of *Kava: The Miracle Antianxiety Herb*. Once this happens, you could experience excessive fatigue, low blood pressure, and low blood sugar. Supplementing with extra vitamin C is one step that you can take to keep your adrenal glands healthy.

When the going gets tough, take 3,000 milligrams of vitamin C in divided doses daily, says Dr. Shealy.

Welcome the B Family

The B-complex vitamins are a treasure trove of stress relief. They can give you more energy, strip away fatigue, make adrenal gland hormones, and manufacture brain chemicals responsible for keeping you alert and lifting your mood, says Dr. Sahelian. "The B vitamins work in concert with each other, and they play hundreds of biochemical roles in the body," he says.

The members of this close-knit family include thiamin, riboflavin, niacin, pantothenic acid, and vitamins B_6 and B_{12}. Pantothenic acid, in particular, plays a major role in the making of adrenal gland hormones and energy production, says Dr. Sahelian.

If you want to combat stress, check with a doctor or naturopath about taking a daily high-potency B-complex vitamin formula that includes 100 to 500 milligrams of pantothenic acid, 50 to 75 milligrams of vitamin B_6, and 500 micrograms of B_{12}, says Joseph E. Pizzorno Jr. N.D., president of Bastyr University in Bothell, Washington.

Ginseng: A Stress-Busting Powerhouse

Ginseng is considered the most notable medicinal herb used to restore vitality, boost energy, reduce fatigue, improve mental and physical perfor-

Food for Your Adrenal Glands

For a nutritional supplement that claims to zap fatigue, boost energy, and help you cope with stress, some people are turning to adrenal gland extracts.

These extracts fall into a category called glandular supplements because they come from the glands of animals such as cows and pigs, on the assumption that what helps them will help you. Advocates of these products claim that adrenal gland extracts can put life back into your own adrenal glands, which have become tired out from pumping so much stress hormone during long periods of stress.

At first glance, it seems sensible to assume that an adrenal booster can do some good. Doctors know that unless we have a healthy pair of adrenal glands, we're more prone to infections and stress-related illnesses. When you're under a lot of stress, your glands need all the help they can get.

The results aren't certain, however. "It's believed that adrenal extracts can help people who are under a great deal of stress or who have chronic fatigue, but very little research has been done to prove their effectiveness, and dosages aren't standardized across the board," says C. Norman Shealy, M.D., Ph.D., founder of the American Holistic Medical Association and director of the Shealy Institute, an alternative medicine clinic in Springfield, Missouri. He notes that some people could benefit, however.

To find the right dosage, you may need to try products with various potencies and qualities, according to Joseph E. Pizzorno Jr., N.D., president of Bastyr University in Bothell, Washington. "I suggest taking one-third of the recommended dosage on the label and slowly increasing it every two days unless you notice any signs of irritability, restlessness, or insomnia," he says. "If you experience any of these symptoms, simply reduce your dosage until they go away. Over time, you should notice an increase in energy and better resistance to stress." If you don't feel better in two to three weeks, the supplements are probably not working for you.

mance, and protect the body from the negative effects of stress. With ginseng, your initial reaction to stress is likely to be less intense. It's often referred to as a tonic for the adrenal glands because it tones and maintains their overall health.

You can find different varieties of the herb, including Siberian ginseng, Asian ginseng, and American ginseng. Asian ginseng is the most widely used for medicinal purposes. They all have similar properties, although Asian ginseng is more of a stimulant than its Siberian cousin, says Dr. Pizzorno. Thus, if you're acutely stressed or recovering from a long illness, Asian ginseng would be the way to go.

In one study, nurses who had switched from day shift to night shift were given either Asian ginseng or an inactive substance (placebo). Their competence, mood, and general well-being were rated. This study showed that the nurses who took the ginseng were more competent, upbeat, and alert than those who didn't take the herb.

Because potency varies, as does the concentration of active ingredients, you'll need to adjust the amount you take depending on which product you buy. You can take 1,000 to 2,000 milligrams one to three times a day if you choose a high-quality crude Asian ginseng root, says Dr. Pizzorno. If you take an extract standardized to 5 to 7 percent ginsenosides, take 100 milligrams one to three times a day.

If you're taking Siberian ginseng root, says Dr. Pizzorno, you probably should take somewhere between 2,000 and 3,000 milligrams a day in divided doses. If you take the extract, take 100 to 200 milligrams of a product that is standardized to 0.8 percent eleutherosides three times a day. Because everyone's response to ginseng is different, start off with the lower dosage and increase it over time, he suggests.

Women taking Asian ginseng may experience breast tenderness. You can simply reduce the dose or discontinue use to make the symptoms go away, says Dr. Pizzorno.

Cool Out with Kava Kava

This time-honored herb, which has soared in popularity as the best natural stress buster, can calm your nerves and help you unwind. Not only that, it's fast-acting, so you may see the effects in as little as 30 to 60 minutes.

Kava can actually preempt stress if you take it prior to an expected stressful situation. It's also a post-stress soother: You can take it to relax tense muscles and wind yourself down after an especially stressful day. You'll feel at peace and maybe even a little euphoric, says Dr. Sahelian.

The secret behind kava is its anxiety-reducing effect on your brain, says

Dr. Sahelian. It contains a group of chemicals called kavalactones that are responsible for its anti-anxiety effects. Animal studies show that kavalactones act on the limbic system, the part of the brain that is the center of emotions.

What's more, kava isn't addictive, it won't lose its effectiveness over time, and your mind will remain alert and sharp even when you take it during the day.

Dr. Sahelian suggests taking one capsule that contains between 40 and 70 milligrams of kavalactones two or three times a day. Start with the lower dosage first to determine whether you feel any of the soothing effects, he says. If you don't feel any stress relief in two to three hours, you can take another capsule. See page 239 for important information about kava.

sunburn

Sunburn is an inflammation of the skin that results from overexposure to ultraviolet radiation. Get a mild burn, and you might be uncomfortable overnight, but the redness and stinging will dissipate pretty quickly. If you really fry yourself and end up with what's called a second-degree burn, though, your skin will actually blister and ooze.

For a second-degree roasting, see a physician, but for mild sunburn, you can do a number of things to help reduce your day-after discomfort.

When you've been out in the sun too long, the first thing you need is immediate relief from the burning. There are several effective topical treatments for sun exposure, beginning with the old folk remedy of taking an oatmeal bath, says Kathy Foulser, N.D., a naturopathic doctor at the Ridgefield Center for Integrative Medicine in Connecticut. Simply pour about 1½ ounces of ground oatmeal, which is sold under brand names like Aveeno, into comfortably warm water and soak for 15 minutes.

Another home-style treatment for sunburn is aloe gel. If you have an aloe plant, break a leaf, squeeze out the gel, and gently rub it into the damaged skin. You can also purchase the gel at drugstores. "The gel is great for cooling and soothing the skin," says Dr. Foulser.

In a study at the University of Texas in Galveston, scientists found that aloe vera inhibited the formation of a substance known as TxA2. This substance is responsible for a lot of the skin damage that results from burns, electrical injuries, and frostbite. By inhibiting TxA2, aloe relieves pain and increases blood supply to the injured area, researchers report.

Oil Your Burn

Because sunburn essentially produces skin inflammation, it's helpful to take herbs with strong anti-inflammatory properties, says Dr. Foulser.

She recommends evening primrose oil, which contains gamma-linolenic acid (GLA). The body transforms GLA into hormonelike compounds called prostaglandin, which have anti-inflammatory effects. When you put more GLA into your system, your body has increased power to reduce inflammation.

The essential fatty acids in this oil provide another benefit: They are good for overall skin health, says Dr. Foulser. She recommends taking six capsules daily of evening primrose oil for long-term use.

"If you want, you can take more, because this oil is quite safe," she adds. Be sure to check the labels of the supplement for information on recommended dosages.

Up Your Antioxidants

Whenever your skin burns, cells are damaged. This damage is caused by free radicals, which are free-roaming, unstable molecules that are seeking to stabilize themselves by stealing electrons from healthy cells. As a result of this cell damage, free radicals can cause premature wrinkling, and in the case of repeated sun exposure, even skin cancer. If you take antioxidants, substances that scavenge free radicals in the body, you can speed healing and prevent rapid cell damage.

At your drugstore or health food store, you will find plenty of antioxidant combination products on the shelf. Alternatively, you can choose to take separate supplements of vitamin C, vitamin E, and beta-carotene, all of which have strong antioxidant properties, says Dr. Foulser.

For a mild sunburn, take 50,000 international units (IU) of beta-carotene a day, Dr. Foulser advises. If your sunburn is more severe, you could take 100,000 IU of beta-carotene for a few days and then reduce it to 50,000 IU as the burn heals. Dr. Foulser also suggests taking 800 IU daily of vitamin E, which is known to aid in the repair of damaged skin.

"You should keep this up for about a couple of weeks, even after you think the burn has healed," she says. The exceptions are pregnant women and people with liver problems, who should never take high doses of beta-carotene, even for short periods. To be safe, consult a holistic physician before starting this program, Dr. Foulser suggests.

Vitamin E also can be used topically on sun-damaged skin along with other salves and skin conditioners, says Dr. Foulser.

Guarding against Sun Singe

Of course, we all know that a milligram of prevention is worth many pounds of cure when it comes to sunburn. The best way to prevent sunburn is to simply use common sense by avoiding excess exposure and using sunscreen. You can also help your skin by taking some supplements when you know you're going to be exposed to the sun.

Vitamin C has qualities that can help protect skin from sunlight, and it's also well-known for its antioxidant properties, says Leon Hecht, N.D., a naturopathic doctor at the North Coast Family Health Center in Portsmouth, New Hampshire.

For people who spend a lot of time in the sun, Dr. Hecht suggests up to 1,000 milligrams of vitamin C three or four times a day. "Vitamin C stimulates repair of sun-damaged skin," he says.

In a controlled study, 10 people took either 2,000 milligrams of vitamin C with 1,000 IU of vitamin E a day or an inactive substance (placebo). The sunburn reaction after eight days of treatment revealed that the skin of people in the treatment group showed less damage than that of those in the placebo group.

Dr. Hecht also states that vitamins C and E used in topical sunscreens prove effective as well. "Early studies show that it is prudent to add vitamins C and E to your sunscreen to protect against ultraviolet phototoxic injury to your skin," he says. Sunscreens with these vitamins already added can be found in drugstores.

You can also prepare your skin to withstand the harmful effects of ultraviolet rays by taking a beta-carotene supplement, says Dr. Hecht. He recommends taking 100,000 IU of beta-carotene for a month or two before you plan to expose yourself to intense sunlight—before the first beach day, for instance, or before a midwinter skiing vacation. This preventive works particularly well for light-skinned people, says Dr. Hecht. You should talk to your doctor, though, before taking this amount.

"It pigments the skin a little bit and just gives you a kind of base. It's no substitute for protecting yourself from the sun, but it does help prevent some burning," he says.

taste and smell loss

"Take time to stop and smell the roses," goes the saying.

That's very good advice, but it's impossible to follow if you're losing your sense of smell.

If you don't smell things as well as you once did, there could be many explanations. Advancing age can be a contributing factor, possibly because infection has taken its toll or because you've sniffed too many noxious fumes over the years. Moreover, you shouldn't be surprised if you temporarily lose your sense of smell because you've had an infection such as a bad cold.

Head injury is another possible cause if the delicate nerves leading from your nose to your brain are damaged. Also, certain prescription drugs can rob you of some ability to enjoy the fragrance of flowers, perfume, or fresh-baked apple pie.

As smell slips away, your sense of taste may suffer, too. The two senses are so closely related that people who complain of not being able to smell often say that they also have trouble tasting.

Depending on the cause, disturbances of taste and smell are sometimes permanent. Yet you might regain these senses after a while, says Charles P. Kimmelman, M.D., associate professor of otolaryngology at Weill Medical College of Cornell University in New York City and attending physician at Manhattan Eye, Ear and Throat Hospital. If smell loss is linked to a head cold, for instance, you can expect your nose to work normally after you've shaken off the cold.

When the problems last longer, talk to your doctor. "Disturbances of the taste and smell senses are best treated by a physician," says Barbara Silbert, D.C., N.D., a chiropractor and naturopathic doctor in Newburyport, Massachusetts.

She adds, however, that people who are deficient in zinc often have taste and smell problems, and in those cases, supplementing with zinc is an excellent remedy to the problem.

Taste for Heavy Metal

Not having enough zinc can make smelling and tasting things like a festive holiday meal a real challenge. Here's why: The cells in your tastebuds and nose that help you to smell depend on zinc. In fact, cells in the salivary glands make a zinc-dependent protein called gustin that is secreted into your saliva. An important contributor to your sense of taste, gustin helps develop cells that can distinguish among different flavors.

Although zinc deficiencies are pretty rare in the United States, it's worth asking your doctor to test for a deficiency if you are experiencing taste and smell loss. Many things can lead to a deficiency, including poor eating habits, alcoholism, certain drugs, kidney disease, and the stress of surgery or serious burns.

"If I discover a zinc deficiency, I typically recommend 25 milligrams of zinc picolinate twice a day to start," says Dr. Silbert. Of course, you can also eat more of the foods that contain zinc. Your best bet is seafood such as cooked oysters and crab. Meats such as lean beef and lean pork also provide zinc, but they're not really recommended because they are high in saturated fat. Other sources include eggs, whole grains, nuts, and yogurt. If you plan to take more than 20 milligrams of zinc a day, it's best to do so under your doctor's care.

tinnitus

Imagine having the whoosh of a vacuum cleaner, the roar of the breaking surf, or even the innocent chirping of a cricket inside your head. You can't turn it off, walk away, or stomp on it. Earplugs won't help. It's there when you wake up, when you're trying to fall asleep, and when you're talking or trying to watch TV.

That's tinnitus in a nutshell: It's ringing in the ears. While this condition can be caused by a buildup of ear wax or by allergies, it is often due to damage to the nerve cells in the ears.

Exposure to loud noises can cause ear damage. Some medicines can contribute to it. Alcohol abuse can also lead to tinnitus, as can an overdose of caffeine. Or it could be the result of direct damage to some portion of the ear, such as blockage in the tiny arteries that feed blood to the ears, hardening of the tiny bones in the inner ear, or viral infections that damage the inner ear. Even high blood pressure can be a contributing factor.

With so many possible causes, you and your doctor should try to figure out what's causing your tinnitus, says William H. Slattery III, M.D., director of clinical studies at the House Ear Institute in Los Angeles. Once that's established, some natural remedies may be helpful for improving blood circulation to the ear, if that's your problem, or protecting ear nerves from further damage. Here's what some experts recommend.

Magnesium Shields against Noise Damage

An essential mineral, magnesium, can help protect your ears from noise-induced damage, Dr. Slattery says. "I would recommend that everyone, especially those who already have some hearing loss, make sure they are getting adequate amounts of magnesium."

When magnesium-deficient laboratory animals were exposed to noise, their inner ears were damaged far more than the ears of animals that had adequate magnesium. When magnesium is in short supply and there's a lot of exposure to noise, the inner-ear cells can become exhausted. That in turn can lead to cell damage or destruction.

Low magnesium levels can also cause blood vessels to constrict, affecting the tiny arteries leading to your inner ear. When the arteries constrict even farther in reaction to loud noises, the result is tinnitus.

Israeli researchers found that soldiers who got an additional 167 milligrams of supplemental magnesium daily during two months of basic training had less inner ear damage than those getting inactive substances (placebos). Extra magnesium from supplements can also protect against long-term noise exposure.

If you're often in a noisy environment, make sure you're getting the Daily Value of magnesium, which is 400 milligrams from food and supplements, Dr. Slattery says. Most people get less than this amount from food, with men averaging about 329 milligrams and women 207 milligrams a day. Make sure that your multivitamin/mineral supplement has enough magnesium to make up the difference, he advises.

Go after Ginkgo

If there's a blockage in the tiny arteries that go to your ears, the herb ginkgo may help your tinnitus symptoms, says Jennifer Brett, N.D., a naturopathic doctor at the Wilton Naturopathic Center in Stratford, Connecticut.

"Ginkgo works a number of ways to improve blood flow, especially in tiny blood vessels," says Dr. Brett. It also acts as an antioxidant, which means that it helps to protect your cells from all kinds of damage, including damage from drugs like quinine (Quinamm), furosemide (Lasix), and some antibiotics, such as streptomycin and gentamicin (Garamycin). Ginkgo also stabilizes cell membranes. With more stable membranes, your nerve cells conduct signals more efficiently, so it's quite possible that the nerves in your ears will work better even if they're damaged.

Ginkgo also enhances the use of oxygen by cells. Even if blood flow is restricted so that a cell isn't getting all the oxygen it needs, the cell may function better if you're taking ginkgo. "In my experience, ginkgo improves symptoms in about half the people who try it," says Dr. Brett. Even if you've had tinnitus for more than three years, ginkgo can be effective, although it seems to be more helpful in people who haven't had tinnitus that long.

Take 40 to 80 milligrams of ginkgo extract three times a day. Dr. Brett recommends a concentration of 24 percent ginkgoflavoglycosides, a product that is available in many health food stores.

"Try it for about six weeks and see if you notice an improvement in your symptoms," she says. If you do, continue taking it.

Bet on the Bs

Your body needs vitamin B_{12} to manufacture myelin, the fatty sheath that wraps around nerve fibers, insulating them and allowing them to conduct their electrical impulses normally. That's apparently important for ears as well as the rest of your body.

The same Israeli researchers who found that magnesium helped protect ears also found that 47 percent of a group of 113 army personnel with tinnitus had a B_{12} deficiency. All of the people low in B_{12} received injections of 1,000 micrograms weekly for about four months. At the end of that time, all of them reported some improvement in their tinnitus, including a decrease in loudness.

If your tinnitus is accompanied by memory problems, depression, or difficulty walking, talk to your doctor about having your blood levels of B_{12} or zinc checked. It's possible that you may not be absorbing the vitamin or mineral properly, and you may need injections.

vaginitis

If you're a woman who's never had a bout of vaginitis, you're lucky, but the odds are good that you'll have to deal with it at some point in your life. It's all part of being a woman.

Vaginitis is an umbrella term for inflammation, irritation, and redness of the vulva and vagina. The most common form is bacterial vaginosis, an infection characterized by a yellowish, fishy-smelling discharge. Yeast infection is another form, which reveals itself with a white, cottage cheese–like discharge, intense itching, and burning.

Trichomoniasis is yet another type, an inflammation triggered by a single-celled organism that's transmitted sexually and causes itching, burning, and a frothy green or yellowish, foul-smelling discharge. Due to hormone level changes, women are more likely to be plagued by vaginitis before menstruation, during pregnancy, or after menopause, when thinning vaginal walls caused by decreasing estrogen become more susceptible to infection. This same lack of estrogen also causes vaginal dryness, which can lead to irritation, inflammation, and a higher risk of developing a bacterial infection.

Whatever the cause or the symptoms, vaginitis needs attention. If left untreated, trichomoniasis can put you at risk for other sexually transmitted diseases, and untreated bacterial vaginosis may lead to urinary tract infections and pelvic inflammatory disease, which can cause infertility. Be sure to see your doctor without delay if you have any of these symptoms. After a proper diagnosis, your doctor can help you decide if supplements are right for you.

If you're plagued by chronic yeast infections that are causing vaginitis, you can make some dietary changes that could help prevent recurrences. Try to eliminate sugar and milk and other dairy products from your diet, naturopathic doctors advise. You also should avoid foods that contain mold and yeast, including alcoholic beverages, cheeses, dried fruit, melons, mushrooms, and peanuts.

There's a clear rationale behind the ban on these foods, naturopathic doctors believe. *Candida albicans*, the fungus that causes yeast infections, thrives on sugar, and because milk is high in lactose—also a sugar—it may contribute to a yeast infection.

While you're dodging those foods, naturopathic doctors say that you can also take a number of nutritional supplements that have been known to clear up more than one stubborn case of vaginitis. Vitamins and minerals can reduce the severity of symptoms and boost your immune system at the same time. Supplementing with a type of "good bacteria" called *Lactobacillus acidophilus* can create a more stable and healthy environment in your vaginal area, thus quickly chasing out the yeast infection.

Certain herbs such as licorice and black cohosh, which contain estrogen-like compounds, can restore the vaginal moisture that some women lose when they have hormonal changes during menopause. Other herbs laced with powerful immune-stimulating properties, such as garlic, can destroy fungi and bacteria on contact.

Fight Back with Vitamin A

Whether your bout with vaginitis is caused by bacteria, yeast, or hormonal changes, supplementing with a powerful arsenal of vitamins and minerals may help shorten the duration and lessen the severity of the infection, says Pamela Jeanne, N.D., a naturopathic doctor and owner of Mount Hood Holistic Health in Gresham, Oregon.

Among these stars are vitamins A, C, and E, beta-carotene, and zinc. Taken together, they can help reduce the pain and inflammation associated with vaginitis, says Dr. Jeanne.

Vitamin A is a renowned infection fighter that will keep vaginal tissues healthy. It cranks up your immune system, stimulates growth of healthy vaginal tissues, strengthens cell membranes, and protects the vagina from further infection, she says. But it does have some drawbacks, she notes. If you take too much, it could affect your liver, and if pregnant women take high doses for long periods of time, there's a chance that their babies may have birth defects.

As an alternative, you can take beta-carotene. It helps to produce more vitamin A in your body, but unlike vitamin A, beta-carotene can be taken in large doses without the worry of side effects.

If you have a vaginitis infection, you can take 5,000 to 10,000 international units (IU) of vitamin A daily if you're not pregnant, not trying to conceive, and are using a reliable method of birth control, Dr. Jeanne advises. Alternatively, you can take 100,000 IU of beta-carotene daily, she says. But you need to talk to your doctor if you're taking this much beta-carotene.

Get C and E on Your Side

Similar to vitamin A, vitamin C kicks your immune system into high gear, strengthening your body's ability to fight off the infection. Vitamin C helps reduce the inflammation and strengthens capillary walls and mucous membranes lining your vagina so they can ward off infection, says Dr. Jeanne. "Make sure the vitamin C you take contains bioflavonoids or rose hips," she says. "Bioflavonoids prevent the infected vaginal cells from releasing immune system chemicals called histamines, which cause the inflammation."

Take 2,000 milligrams of vitamin C daily to maintain a healthy vagina, Dr. Jeanne suggests. If you suffer from chronic vaginal infections, take 3,000 to 4,000 milligrams a day over a two-week period until symptoms improve.

Vitamin E should be the number one nutrient for women during and after menopause, says Dr. Jeanne. Estrogen levels drop and remain low once menopause is under way, leading to the irritation, inflammation, and other vaginal problems related to low estrogen. Dr. Jeanne believes that vitamin E can lower this risk by strengthening the cell membranes lining your vagina. The stronger the membranes, the less likely it is that bacteria will invade them and wreak havoc.

With your doctor's consent, you can take 400 to 800 IU of vitamin E daily, says Dr. Jeanne. Sometimes, higher dosages are recommended, depending on your condition.

More Zinc?

The trace mineral zinc is another powerful healer and protector against vaginal infection. It will support your immune system so you can battle the infection. It's vital for the production of collagen, the connective tissue that helps wounds heal, and it can create new skin.

During an infection, take 30 to 60 milligrams of zinc daily in divided doses, says Dr. Jeanne. Since zinc can cause stomach upset, you might want to take a partial dose with each of your meals. You shouldn't take zinc if you have certain health conditions, however, so talk to your doctor before starting these dosages.

Strike a Balance with Lactobacillus

When vaginitis is caused by a yeast overgrowth, the best supplement to take is *Lactobacillus acidophilus*, says Liz Collins, N.D., a naturopathic doctor and co-owner of the Natural Childbirth and Family Clinic in Portland, Oregon. It's the predominant type of bacteria that keeps the vagina healthy and helps keep other vaginal bacteria in balance. Without enough acidophilus, yeast organisms can grow uncontrollably.

Naturopathic doctors believe that acidophilus keeps the yeast population under control by producing lactic acid and natural antibiotic substances. "There is almost always yeast inside the vagina, and that's okay," says Dr. Collins. "The problem starts when your vaginal immune system is weak, and you don't have enough acidophilus in there to maintain a balance in the vaginal flora."

To restore that balance, take three capsules of acidophilus or eat eight ounces of acidophilus yogurt daily, says naturopathic doctor Tori Hudson, N.D., professor at the National College of Naturopathic Medicine in Portland, Oregon, and author of *Women's Encyclopedia of Natural Medicine*. Continue to take the supplements throughout the infection and for a couple of days afterward, Dr. Hudson says. She recommends taking one capsule a half-hour before each meal with a large glass of water.

To make sure you get the live cultures, which are what you need, buy refrigerated capsules, and read the label to make sure that you're getting one to two billion live organisms daily.

Herbs to Wipe Out Yeast and Bacteria

To clear up bacterial infections and control yeast, consider taking some garlic or echinacea. Whether you take them together or separately, naturopaths believe that these herbs can muster up a tough defense against bacterial offenders. They also help to restore the natural flora to the vagina, reinforcing the efforts of good bacteria to defend you from the bad and the ugly.

Garlic strengthens the immune system so that your body can fight off the infection on its own, plus it has both antifungal and antibacterial properties, says Dr. Hudson. When garlic comes on the scene, invading bacteria and overgrowing yeast don't have a chance to survive. The number one ingredient in garlic that kills bacteria and stunts the growth of yeast is allicin, and experts believe this is one of the plant kingdom's most potent antibiotics.

Echinacea also deserves high praise. This powerful immune system stimulant has antiviral powers as well. It increases levels of a chemical in the body called properdin, which activates the part of the immune system responsible for destroying bacteria and viruses.

During an acute infection, take one or two capsules of garlic daily for 3 to 14 days, or until the infection clears up, says Dr. Hudson. Take two capsules daily for four weeks or longer if your infection is chronic. Products that contain at least 4,000 micrograms of allicin may be the most effective, she says.

Take 300 milligrams of echinacea three times a day for at least one week, says Dr. Jeanne. When symptoms subside, drop the dosage to 300 milligrams twice a day. Dr. Jeanne says that this dose can be taken for four to six weeks, but after that it's best to stop for a while.

Licorice for Vaginal Dryness

Most women in their twenties and thirties probably take their abundant supply of estrogen for granted. It's only when the supply runs low as they get older that they begin to notice the effects of a shortfall.

During and after menopause, women produce less estrogen, which is one of the "basics" that's needed to prevent vaginal problems. "Estrogen feeds the vaginal tissue and promotes circulation and natural lubrication, which protects the vagina from bacteria," says Dr. Collins.

Herbs can replenish some of the estrogen that's lost during the menopausal and postmenopausal years and give you the moisture and protection you need. Naturopathic doctors recommend herbs like licorice, dong quai, and black cohosh. But none of these should be taken by women who are pregnant.

Licorice contains natural estrogen-like compounds. Like the isoflavones in soy foods, its active ingredient glycyrrhizin seems to help adjust estrogen in both directions, reducing levels that are too high and increasing them when they're too low. "Licorice is a good herb for the menopausal and post-menopausal changes in a woman's life," says Dr. Jeanne.

Licorice helps support the function of the adrenal glands, located just above your kidneys, where your body's supply of estrogen is produced, she explains. The adrenal production of estrogen becomes increasingly important as women approach menopause. Licorice also helps with adrenal function during stress in menopause.

To relieve vaginal dryness, take 200 to 300 milligrams of licorice two or three times a day for one to two months, says Dr. Jeanne. For the best effects, she recommends taking black cohosh and dong quai along with the licorice. It's not advisable to take excessive doses, however. High daily doses of licorice for more than four to six weeks may cause your body to react by retaining too much sodium and water. Doctors warn that high doses of licorice may also lead to high blood pressure or impaired heart or kidney function.

Another Use for Cohosh

Black cohosh also contains estrogen, and studies show that this herb relieves vaginal dryness, hot flashes, and depression. "Black cohosh really helps a lot of women," says Dr. Collins. You can combine black cohosh with dong quai to get better results if taking the herbs individually doesn't eliminate symptoms. Dr. Collins suggests taking 250 to 300 milligrams of black cohosh three times a day. If you combine it with dong quai, take up to 4,000 milligrams of each per day for up to six months. Some women start with 4,000 milligrams per day and then, once their symptoms are under control, decrease the dose slowly to find the minimum dose that maintains control, says Dr. Collins.

Try a Woman's Tonic

Dong quai is a Chinese herb with a centuries-old reputation as a woman's tonic. Herbalists say that it relieves vaginal dryness associated with menopause and menstrual problems. Sometimes promoted as the "female ginseng," this herb is a general tonic for the female reproductive system.

Many women find great relief from using dong quai, which is sometimes called dang gui, tang kwei, or Chinese angelica. It also helps lower blood pressure and relieve headaches and arthritis, and it has been shown to stimulate immunity," says Dr. Jeanne.

Take 300 milligrams of dong quai two or three times a day along with licorice for one to two months, says Dr. Jeanne. Be patient: It may take several months before the herb begins to relieve symptoms. You shouldn't take it while you're menstruating, however, since it can increase blood loss. It also contains substances that can cause a rash or severe sunburn if you're exposed to sunlight.

varicose veins

Varicose veins aren't just a cosmetic problem. They can make your legs swell or make them feel heavy and tired. They can also aggravate muscle cramps.

When you have varicose veins, it means that the blood returning to your heart is extremely sluggish. Within the veins, valvelike mechanisms that help maintain upward blood flow aren't doing their job any more. It may get to the point where blood is simply pooling in the veins rather than moving along as it should.

Blood vessel damage can set the stage for thrombosis, or clotting, so be sure to see your doctor for a proper diagnosis. If your veins present a real danger to your health, your doctor may recommend sclerotherapy, a procedure that shuts them off, says Decker Weiss, N.M.D., a naturopathic doctor with the Arizona Heart Institute in Phoenix. While that may seem drastic, Dr. Weiss points out that sclerotherapy could relieve discomfort. "The veins aren't helping you in any way," he says. "They are just creating pain."

Most doctors' nutritional recommendations for varicose veins are limited to "Lose weight and eat more fiber." That's good advice, but some naturopathic doctors also recommend nutrients that help to strengthen blood vessel walls or reduce the likelihood of blood clots that could block the veins. Just be sure to talk to your own doctor before you start taking supplements for this condition.

Take Fiber for Vein Strain

Straining to have a bowel movement puts a lot of pressure on the veins of your lower body, and over time, it can promote the development of varicose veins in your legs, Dr. Weiss says. "I've had patients who, once they have their constipation problems under control, see their varicose veins improve, especially the hemorrhoid type."

The "Compression Stocking" Herb

Which would you rather do to treat your varicose veins: wear surgical compression stockings that make you feel like you're encased in elastic or take a herbal tincture of horse chestnut seed extract?

In a study, people with varicose veins were divided into two groups. One group took an extract of horse chestnut that provided 50 milligrams a day of escin, one of the active ingredients. The other group used compression stockings, which are commonly recommended by doctors as a way to relieve the discomfort of varicose veins. After 12 weeks, researchers found that both groups had an almost identical reduction of swelling in their legs.

Horse chestnut contains compounds called bioflavonoids. When you take this herb, the bioflavonoids seem to move into the bulging varicose veins, says Decker Weiss, N.M.D., a naturopathic doctor at the Arizona Heart Institute in Phoenix. "I'd recommend it as a first-line treatment along with correcting constipation," he says.

Horse chestnut seed extract—the supplement form that's used—has anti-edema properties, which means that it helps prevent the buildup of fluids. It also helps prevent inflammation, and it can decrease fluid leakage from capillaries by reducing the number and size of the small pores in the capillary walls.

Horse chestnut also improves the tone of blood vessels so veins become more elastic. With this boost in elasticity, they can contract more strongly and relax better, Dr. Weiss says.

How much you'll need to take depends on what kind of horse chestnut you buy. If you get a standardized extract of horse chestnut seed, use an amount that provides you with a daily dose of 50 milligrams of escin, Dr. Weiss says. Reduce the dosage after symptoms improve, he advises.

"I haven't had many problems with it, and I've had people on it for seven or eight months at a time," says Dr. Weiss. There have been some reports of side effects such as itching, nausea, and stomach discomfort. If you experience these side effects, simply stop taking horse chestnut for a while until the symptoms go away. If you are pregnant, don't take this herb without your doctor's okay. Since horse chestnut may also interfere with the action of other drugs, especially blood thinners such as warfarin (Coumadin), also check with your doctor.

To prevent constipation, it's best to eat foods that contain a mixture of fiber, such as beans, fruits and vegetables, and whole grains. If you also need to take a fiber supplement, find one that contains both soluble and insoluble fibers, Dr. Weiss advises. Whatever kind of fiber you're getting, also make sure you drink at least eight glasses of water and other fluids every day.

Bromelain Breaks Up Bumps

Bromelain, an enzyme that's extracted from green pineapple, can help prevent the development of the hard and lumpy skin found around varicose veins, says Joseph E. Pizzorno Jr., N.D., president of Bastyr University in Bothell, Washington.

People with varicose veins have a decreased ability to break down fibrin, one of the compounds involved in formation of blood clots and tissue scarring. In healthy veins, a substance called plasminogen activator helps break down fibrin, but veins that are varicose have decreased levels of this substance.

Bromelain acts similarly to plasminogen activator to help break down fibrin, so it's particularly helpful for varicose veins, says Dr. Pizzorno. It can also help people who have a tendency to develop phlebitis, or blood clots in leg veins.

Try taking 500 to 750 milligrams of bromelain on an empty stomach two or three times a day, Dr. Pizzorno recommends. If you take it with meals, it simply works as a digestive enzyme and is used up in your intestines rather than passed along to your bloodstream.

Bioflavonoids Keep Veins Strong

Even if you seem destined to get varicose veins, the powerful antioxidant and anti-inflammatory properties of bioflavonoids might help make the walls of your veins stronger, says Stephen T. Sinatra, M.D., a cardiologist and director of medical education for Manchester Memorial Hospital in Connecticut.

"Bioflavonoids can help protect the structural integrity of the vascular walls and help prevent free radical stress inside the vessel," he says. Two bioflavonoids that seem to promote vascular health are grapeseed and pycnogenol, commonly called oligomeric proanthocyanidins, or OPCs. In one study, OPCs demonstrated powerful antioxidant activity by being able to trap the free-roaming, unstable molecule that can do so much cell damage. In fact, the antioxidant ability of OPCs was found to be many times greater than that of vitamin C and vitamin E.

If you have varicose veins, you should take about 200 to 300 milligrams of grapeseed extract or pycnogenol a day with meals for at least six months, says Dr. Sinatra. If your discomfort improves, you can continue taking the supplement indefinitely.

C and B

Vitamin C is needed to help your body manufacture two important connective tissues, collagen and elastin. "Both of these tissues help to keep vein walls strong and flexible," says Dr. Pizzorno. Vitamin C may be especially important if you bruise easily or have broken capillaries, which may show up on your skin as tiny spider veins, he says. He recommends 500 to 3,000 milligrams of vitamin C daily.

Some doctors also recommend a combination of B vitamins, especially to people who have a history of blood clots. It's particularly important to make sure that you're getting sufficient amounts of folic acid, B_{12}, and B_6, Dr. Weiss says.

"I recommend B vitamins to all my patients with heart or circulatory problems as part of a high-potency multivitamin," says Dr. Weiss. If people have absorption problems, he will suggest B_{12} injections. Otherwise, you can take B-vitamin supplements in pill or capsule form.

Bring on the Es, Too

Vitamin E can also help, Dr. Pizzorno says. "Vitamin E helps keep platelets, blood components involved in clotting, from sticking together and from adhering to the sides of blood vessel walls," he says.

Research shows that reducing platelet stickiness with vitamin E may help people who are at particularly high risk for blood-clotting problems, such as those with type 1 (insulin-dependent) diabetes.

Taking 200 to 600 international units of vitamin E a day should be sufficient, Dr. Pizzorno says. If you've had bleeding problems, however, or are taking prescription anticoagulants to help prevent clotting, get your doctor's okay before you take vitamin E.

Get Your Gotu Kola

The herb gotu kola is particularly good for varicose veins and also has a reputation as an anti-aging herb, says Roberta Bourgon, N.D., a naturopathic doctor at the Wellness Center in Billings, Montana. This herb seems to be able to strengthen the sheath of tissue that wraps around veins, reduce formation of clogging scar tissue, and improve blood flow through affected limbs.

"It's really more of a preventive measure than a cure," says Dr. Bourgon. "If you know you're prone to varicose veins, this can help you slow down or perhaps prevent the problem."

Even if it doesn't help the varicosity itself, gotu kola often improves the symptoms of varicose veins, including pain, numbness, and leg cramps, Dr. Bourgon says. Try taking 60 to 120 milligrams a day in capsules.

water retention

Fluid retention, or edema, is an excess of water in the body's tissues. It occurs when fluid that normally circulates in blood vessels and lymph ducts is diverted into the tiny channels between cells, called interstitial spaces. This makes the tissue swell.

Fluid accumulates for two primary reasons, says David B. Young, Ph.D., professor of physiology and biophysics at the University of Mississippi in Jackson. First, increased blood pressure in your veins causes increased pressure in the tiny capillaries that form a network throughout your tissues. This causes fluid to filter out of the capillaries and into the tissues.

"Increased blood pressure in the veins is usually caused by heart failure, often to the right side of the heart," Dr. Young says. "During the later stages of pregnancy, a woman may also experience swollen ankles because the baby is pressing against veins in her abdomen, hindering blood flow back from the legs and increasing pressure."

You don't have to be carrying a baby to have edema, however. Just standing for a long period of time can also increase blood pressure in veins. That's why your feet may be swollen at the end of the day.

Anything that changes the permeability of the capillaries can also cause swelling. Allergic reactions, such as a reaction to a bee sting, is one common cause. Also, if you have an injury that causes the capillaries to leak, that will create swelling.

No doubt you've heard that an ice pack or cold pack will reduce the swelling. There's much more than wishful thinking behind that advice. "Ice is so effective at reducing swelling because it constricts blood vessels, helping to reduce the flow of fluid from capillaries to tissue," Dr. Young says.

While leakage from capillaries is one clear cause of swelling, it's less clear why women often have fluid retention premenstrually for a few days each month. No one knows exactly why that happens, Dr. Young says. "It's a huge question, and certainly hormonal changes are involved, but nobody has a clue as to exactly how to explain it."

An Herb That Gets the Bloat Out

"Many herbs act as diuretics—that is, they help your kidneys to remove water from your body," says Michael DiPalma, N.D., a naturopathic doctor and director of natural medicine at the Village at Newtown Medical Center in Pennsylvania. One of the best at getting the bloat out is dandelion, he says.

In an animal study, dandelion leaf removed fluid from the body as well as furosemide (Lasix), a powerful diuretic often used for congestive heart failure. Dandelion leaf also supplies potassium, which other diuretics tend to drain out of your body. Dr. DiPalma praises it as "a natural potassium-sparing diuretic."

For temporary bloating such as that which may occur premenstrually, you can drink two to four cups of dandelion leaf tea per day. Although teas work better as diuretics, you can also take one or two capsules of dried dandelion leaf, says Dr. DiPalma.

You'll find alcohol-based tinctures of dandelion on store shelves, but because they're not as effective as teas or capsules, you have to take an extremely high dose, and that means you're dosing up with too much alcohol, he says.

If you have fluid retention due to heart problems, you'll want to work with your doctor. You may be able to slowly increase your dosage of dandelion and decrease your dosage of pharmaceutical diuretics, Dr. DiPalma says. If you have gallbladder disease, however, do not use dandelion preparations without medical approval.

Normally, a healthy body eventually recovers from swelling on its own. If you put your feet up for an hour or get a night's rest, your feet shrink to normal size. If you put a cold pack on a sprained ankle, the swelling goes down. Once hormones shift and menstruation starts, most women find that bloating quickly disappears. Additionally, there are ways that you can help your body to recover or to not be so prone to fluid retention. Here's how.

The Potassium Connection

Your body uses a balance of dissolved minerals to help regulate fluids. Two of the most important minerals in this regard are sodium and potassium, Dr. Young says. For optimal fluid regulation, your body needs to have a proper balance of both.

Unfortunately, most people get too much sodium and barely enough potassium. This can raise your blood pressure and your potential for fluid retention, Dr. Young says.

He suggests that you double your potassium intake to about 5,000 milligrams a day by consuming potassium-rich foods such as fruits and vegetables. It is possible to get potassium from supplements, but by law, over-the-counter supplements contain only 99 milligrams per tablet, because large doses have the potential to cause stomach irritation. For tablets that contain more potassium, you'll need a doctor's prescription. As for sodium, "your body needs very little and is very good at conserving it, so the less, the better," Dr. Young says.

Try B₆ for Hormone-Related Bloating

Vitamin B_6 plays a role in the body's use of hormones associated with fluid retention in women, including estrogen and progesterone, says Marilynn Pratt, M.D., a doctor in Playa del Rey, California, who specializes in women's health. "By helping the liver to metabolize, or break down, these hormones, B_6 may help the body remove excess amounts that may be present during the premenstrual period," Dr. Pratt says.

In one study, 500 milligrams a day of vitamin B_6 relieved the breast tenderness, headaches, and weight gain associated with water retention in 215 women.

If you'd like to try B_6 for hormone-related fluid retention, take 50 milligrams four times a day for the five days before your period begins, Dr. Pratt suggests. In addition, take a supplement containing the rest of the B vitamins. "These nutrients interact and tend to work better as a team than individually," she says. Look for a supplement that contains a total of about 50 milligrams of most of the other B vitamins.

Vitamin B_6 can cause nerve damage in large doses if you take it for a number of weeks without a break, so generally, it's best not to take more than 100 milligrams on a daily basis, Dr. Pratt says.

For monthly edema related to menstruation, Dr. Pratt recommends up to 200 milligrams daily. Taking it during the five days around your period, "when you don't want to feel like a water balloon." If your hands or feet start to feel numb or clumsy, stop taking B_6 and tell your doctor, she cautions.

wrinkles

We don't like wrinkled sheets. We don't like wrinkled apples. And we sure don't like wrinkled skin.

What is it about wrinkles? They suggest two things that we'd rather not think about—age and overuse. Of course, when it comes to wrinkles caused by aging, we have to accept a certain number as an inevitable part of the process. But your skin can defy the passage of years if you take certain precautions.

If you smoke, drink alcohol, eat poorly, and spend a lot of time in the sun, you can expect your face to become as lined and craggy as any weathered mountain. If, however, you take better care of your overall health, protect your skin from the sun, and feed it the proper nutrients and vitamins, you'll still age, but you will look younger than your years.

"You can definitely take better care of your skin, and that can make a difference in the number of wrinkles you eventually get," says Hope Fay, N.D., a naturopathic doctor in Seattle. "The number one advice is: Don't stay in direct sun for long periods."

Undoing the Damage

When your skin is exposed to the sun, cells are damaged. These damaged cells give off free radicals, unstable molecules that cause cell damage.

By taking antioxidants, medicines that scavenge free radicals in the body, you can prevent further cell damage and protect your skin, says Dr. Fay. Three of the most common antioxidant vitamins are vitamin C, vitamin E, and beta-carotene.

If you've gotten a sunburn, Dr. Fay recommends taking between 25,000 and 50,000 international units (IU) of vitamin A for a few days, along with 400 to 800 IU of vitamin E per day. Be sure to talk to your doctor before taking these high doses of vitamin A and vitamin E, however.

"Vitamins A and E are really good for preventing free radical damage to the skin. They are very protective, and vitamin A is especially important for healing damaged skin," says Dr. Fay.

Vitamin C may be even more powerful because not only is it an antioxidant, it's an essential developer of connective tissue. It aids in the formation of collagen, a protein in all connective tissues, including skin. Collagen binds cells together somewhat like mortar binds brick. It maintains the integrity and firmness of the skin, and firmer skin means fewer wrinkles.

You can get vitamin C from citrus juices, red bell peppers, and broccoli, says Michael Gazsi, N.D., a naturopathic doctor in Ridgefield, Connecticut. "If your goal is healthy connective tissues and skin, taking 500 milligrams of vitamin C each day may help," he adds.

Selenium for Skin

Like the antioxidant vitamins, the trace mineral selenium is very effective at consuming free radicals caused by sun damage. You have to be careful when taking a selenium supplement, however, Dr. Gazsi warns. "I'd start with a multivitamin that contains some selenium—usually less than 100 micrograms," he says. "Then you can work your way up to a higher dosage." The maximum he recommends is 200 micrograms.

The dose that's right for you may depend on how much selenium you have in your diet, he adds. Selenium is found in the soil and makes its way into our bodies through plants and animals. Regions in the Great Lakes and Atlantic Seaboard have little selenium in the soil, while vast swatches of the Great Plains and Midwest have rather high amounts. If you live in one of the high-selenium areas and eat lots of local produce, you probably get enough selenium from your diet.

Hormone Helpers

Although we all get wrinkles as we age, sometimes they seem to come on more suddenly after pregnancy, menopause, or emotional stress. These triggering events may upset the balance of hormones in the body. Proper regulation and production of these chemical messengers are essential to maintaining soft, elastic skin.

To prevent hormone imbalances, you can begin by eating more legumes and soy products such as tofu, says Dr. Gazsi. These foods contain phytoestrogens, plant compounds that mimic the biological activities of female hormones.

Other important building blocks for hormone production are essential fatty acids, which are also generally good for the health of the skin, says Dr. Gazsi.

Upping Your Fatty Acids

Fatty acids aren't manufactured by the body but must be obtained from food sources like eggs, nuts, vegetables, butter, and whole milk. Some people who have poor, unbalanced diets don't get enough fatty acids for healthy skin, says Dr. Gazsi, and "unhealthy skin can lead to permanent wrinkles."

Whether your diet is deficient or not, you can help your skin fight off the effects of aging and sun exposure by taking a supplement of either flaxseed oil or evening primrose oil, which are sources of essential fatty acids, says Dr. Gazsi. He recommends four capsules per day of evening primrose oil or two tablespoons of flaxseed oil. "I'd probably start with the flaxseed oil and see how it works." he says. "It may take several months, however. Skin responds pretty slowly."

yeast infections

Few people would sign up to do battle with microscopic plant life, especially if they knew that the plant life would use guerrilla tactics at every opportunity.

Unfortunately, most women are destined to fight this battle. An estimated 75 percent of women get at least one yeast infection during their lives. To deal with yeast infection, many women head for the local drugstore and buy an over-the-counter treatment such as miconazole nitrate (Monistat). But if treatments address only vaginal symptoms, you're getting at only half of the problem, says Lorilee Schoenbeck, N.D., a naturopathic doctor with the Champlain Centers for Natural Medicine in Shelburne and Middlebury, Vermont.

When it comes to chronic or recurring infections, the heart of the problem is often the intestines rather than the vaginal area, according to many naturopaths. *Candida albicans*, the organism that most frequently causes yeast infections, can sometimes become overgrown in your intestines. Yeast that exits the gastrointestinal tract can migrate into the vagina. That area can become infected repeatedly, says Dr. Schoenbeck.

Yeast infections can also mimic urinary tract infections or sexually transmitted diseases, so it's important to get an accurate diagnosis from a medical practitioner before beginning treatment. Also, you should definitely consult your doctor if this is your first experience with symptoms of a yeast infection or if you are pregnant and have an underlying condition such as diabetes. Your doctor can determine whether you have a yeast infection.

Fortunately, there are many things that you can do to ward off yeast infections in the first place. Limit the amount of sweets you eat, suggests Dr. Schoenbeck. Candida breeds even more profusely when you ingest a lot of sugar.

Another preventive measure is spelled d-r-y. Candida loves a warm, moist environment. Panty hose, tight jeans, wet bathing suits, and sweaty exercise clothes all provide the yeast with an ideal set of moist conditions.

If you get damp clothes off as fast as you can and change into something dry and airy, you just might discourage the little diehards. Also, wear only pure cotton underwear and change it daily, says Dr. Schoenbeck.

Apart from these precautions, fighting off a chronic yeast infection usually requires a combined approach. With the correct diet, herbs, and a good topical treatment regimen, most women can expect to begin winning the battle in about a month, says Dr. Schoenbeck. As for supplements, consider them potent allies in this battle. Some can help clear up a minor infection, and others can actually help ward off a yeast invasion.

Acidophilus—The Right Stuff

Because the vaginal itching, redness, and pain can drive you absolutely nuts, you have to take care of the immediate outbreak first, says Dr. Schoenbeck. *Lactobacillus acidophilus* is your ally because it's a type of good bacteria that helps keep candida in check.

When the level of acidophilus is down, candida starts growing like wild. This is frequently the case if you have recently taken antibiotics for an infection or are continuously taking them for acne. In the process of killing off infectious bacteria, antibiotics inadvertently kill off acidophilus as well, giving candida an extra chance to flourish. One way to get more acidophilus is to eat live-culture yogurt. Acidophilus also comes in supplement form.

Acidophilus capsules can help re-establish normal intestinal health, says Dr. Schoenbeck. Take the capsules only when you have an active yeast infection or are having a problem with recurring infections.

Taking oral doses of acidophilus for just two to four weeks can help decrease candida in both your vagina and your intestines, she says. That makes you less prone to repeat infections.

Look for acidophilus capsules that are refrigerated and contain at least one billion organisms per capsule. Dr. Schoenbeck recommends two capsules before breakfast and two before dinner, one hour before each meal, for one month. At the end of the month, see your medical practitioner to be certain that the infection is gone.

Acidophilus capsules can also help with prevention. If your doctor prescribes antibiotics, you can help prevent a yeast outbreak by starting the acidophilus capsules at the same time as your prescription. Continue taking the capsules for just two weeks, says Dr. Schoenbeck.

Turning to Herbs

"Garlic is one of the best things to take for yeast infections," says naturopathic doctor Tori Hudson, N.D., professor at the National College of Naturopathic Medicine in Portland, Oregon, and author of *Women's Encyclopedia of Natural Medicine*. It is both antifungal and immunity-boosting, she says.

In a laboratory study, researchers gave some animals with yeast infections a solution of aged garlic extract and others a plain saltwater solution with no active ingredients. After two days, the animals that received the garlic extract showed no signs of yeast infection. The other group still had infection.

In humans, two garlic capsules a day are enough to protect against yeast, according to Dr. Hudson. It's best to take enteric-coated capsules because the coating prevents the active ingredients in garlic from breaking down in the stomach. Look for garlic capsules with 4,000 milligrams of allicin-alliin, which is the antifungal agent found in garlic, she says.

Herbs such as Oregon grape root extract, teatree oil extract, and lavender extract all help reduce the amount of candida growing in the intestines. "There are supplements that contain all of these extracts, but they are hard to find. I'd ask an alternative practitioner to prescribe one," Dr. Schoenbeck says. She recommends taking two tablets three times a day. After a month, see your practitioner to be sure the infection is gone.

Echinacea is beneficial, too. A German study found that women taking antifungal medicine plus echinacea extract had only a 10 percent recurrence of yeast infections. In the study, this group was compared to women who took only antifungal medicine. Nearly 60 percent of that group had recurrent infections.

Another great anti-yeast herb is goldenseal, says Dr. Schoenbeck. Like Oregon grape, goldenseal contains berberine, a chemical that has antibiotic properties and works particularly well against yeast. You can buy echinacea and goldenseal separately or in combination capsules. Whichever you choose, take them daily as directed on the product you buy. If the capsules are 450 milligrams of an echinacea and goldenseal combination, a typical dose would be two or three capsules daily with water. Do not use goldenseal if you are pregnant, however.

Drinking a tea made with pau d'arco bark or taking a supplement may also bring relief, says Kathleen Head, N.D., a naturopathic doctor in Sandpoint, Idaho, and senior editor of *Alternative Medicine Review*.

Index

Underscored page references indicate boxed text.